Medical Neurosciences

Medical Neurosciences

An Approach to Anatomy, Pathology, and Physiology by Systems and Levels

Second Edition

Jasper R. Daube, M.D.
Professor of Neurology

Thomas J. Reagan, M.D.
Formerly Associate Professor of Neurology; now
Neurologist, Newport News, Virginia

Burton A. Sandok, M.D.
Professor of Neurology

Barbara F. Westmoreland, M.D.
Professor of Neurology

Mayo Medical School
Rochester, Minnesota

Little, Brown and Company
Boston/Toronto

To the students of the Mayo Medical School and the residents in the Department of Neurology who have provided the stimulus for this venture by teaching us as we have taught them, who have helped us to refine our objectives and methods of presentation, and who through their enthusiasm have encouraged us to write this book.

Contents

Preface

The first edition of *Medical Neurosciences* was published in 1978. Its primary objective was to present integrated introductory background knowledge that medical students could readily apply in their study and understanding of clinical neurologic problems. The text also contained an organizational framework for more advanced students and residents in neurology that could be utilized as a starting point on which to build new knowledge. The first edition provided a clinically relevant survey of the nervous system rather than an in-depth study of basic neuroscience. Our hope was that, once stimulated by a basic understanding of the structure and function of the nervous system, the student would seek further information about the mechanisms underlying the clinical phenomena being described.

The past decade has seen a dramatic increase in interest and knowledge in the neurosciences, and this created a difficult decision about the direction to be taken in this second edition. Although the temptation to alter our basic goals and expand the scope of the text was great, our experience has supported the choice of our original objective, and we have again elected to provide an integrated, clinically oriented overview rather than a comprehensive collage of new information. In reaching this decision, we recognize that we have taken on an added responsibility to our own medical students who utilize this text as the basis for their introductory neuroscience course. We must, by our presence and actions, instill the feeling of excitement that now permeates the ever-widening field of neuroscience and provide the resources that will allow the student to learn more about the nervous system. We hope that others who decide to use this introductory text also will share in this responsibility.

The second edition retains the same basic organization as the first. Each chapter has been reviewed and updated. Major sections have been rewritten and new information and illustrations added. A list of selected additional readings has been included with each chapter. Although any such list is personal and somewhat arbitrary and many other references could have been selected, the readings provide sources for the student to study the subject in greater depth.

This edition is the product of the authors; however, many others have contributed significantly to its development and evolution. We are grateful to the many students and faculty, both at Mayo Clinic and elsewhere, who have taken the time to share their suggestions with us. This is an exciting time in the world of neuroscience; we hope our readers will be stimulated to further explore that world.

J. R. D.
T. J. R.
B. A. S.
B. F. W.

Integrated Neuroscience for the Clinician

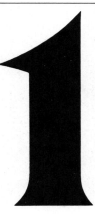

Neurologic disorders are common, and clinicians must be capable of dealing confidently with them. Many steps are required in accomplishing this task. Patients seldom present to their physician with a well-defined diagnosis for which appropriate therapy can be readily dispensed. Instead they arrive with a vast array of symptoms and signs that constitute a clinical problem which the physician must attempt to resolve. The solution of a clinical problem in neurology, as in any area of medicine, requires a knowledge of anatomy, physiology, and pathophysiology. This book is an attempt to organize the body of information contained in the basic neurologic sciences into the format used by clinicians in dealing with diseases of the nervous system.

The process used by a clinician who examines a patient with a neurologic disorder (that is, one involving the brain, spinal cord, nerves, or muscles) is that of inductive reasoning. It is a familiar process in which a number of distinct pieces of information are put together to reach a general conclusion. For example, if a woman has a 1-year history of slowly progressive numbness and weakness of the left side of her face, left arm, and left leg, the physician concludes that the patient may have a neoplastic lesion at the supratentorial level on the right side. The physician utilizes the data obtained by interviewing and examining the patient to produce a history that is a chronologic account of the patient's symptoms and their evolution with time (the temporal profile). The specific symptoms in the history can be categorized into broad groups and related to particular anatomic structures and certain disease categories. In a patient with neurologic disease, these symptoms often are identified with changes in sensation, activity, movement, thinking, or consciousness. And often the physical examination of a patient with neurologic disease allows an even more precise definition of abnormal function, which, based on the clinician's knowledge of anatomic structure and function, can be related to specific areas of the nervous system.

Throughout the interview and the examination, the clinician is constantly organizing and reorganizing the collected data in order to arrive at hypotheses about the nature of the disorder. In the previous example, the hypothesis of a right cerebral tumor was reached because the temporal profile of slow progression is common with neoplastic disorders, and weakness and numbness on the left side of the body often are due to disease of structures that are controlled at the supratentorial level on the right.

The physician must answer three questions. Is there disease involving the nervous system? If so, where is the disease located? And what kind of disease is it (that is, what is the pathologic nature of the disease)? The first question is often one of the most difficult to answer, since an answer depends not only on the knowledge to be presented in this book but also on experience with disease involving all other body systems. This book will focus primarily on answering the two simpler questions: "Where is the lesion located?" and "What is its pathologic nature?"

Objectives

Neurologic diseases include all the major pathologic categories seen in other organ systems and can involve one or several areas within the complex human nervous system. However, adequate management of neurologic problems can be based on answering the questions: "Where is the problem?" and "What is the problem?" The elaboration and analysis of these specific questions form the major objectives in the study of the neurosciences. The answers to these questions are based on a knowledge of the gross anatomic structures of the nervous system (Fig. 1-1), their function, the usual patterns of disease, and the forms of treatment available. This simplified approach to neurologic disease is the one customarily used by many neurologists, and it includes four questions:

1. Is the responsible lesion located at
   a. The supratentorial level
   b. The posterior fossa level
   c. The spinal level
   d. The peripheral level
   e. More than one level
2. Is the responsible lesion
   a. Focal, and located on the right side of the nervous system
   b. Focal, and located on the left side of the nervous system
   c. Focal, but involving midline and contiguous structures on both sides of the nervous system
   d. Diffuse, and involving homologous, symmetric, noncontiguous areas on both sides of the nervous system
3. Is the responsible lesion

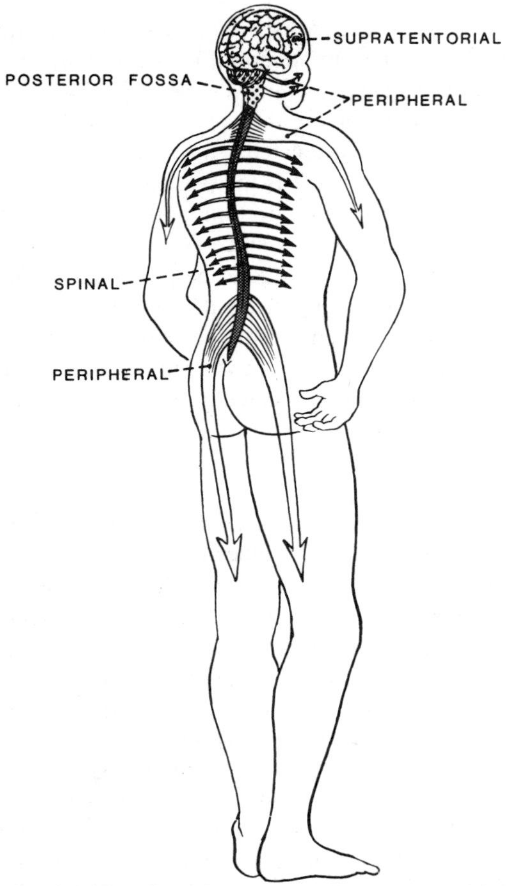

Fig. 1-1. Levels of the neuraxis. Supratentorial level includes cerebral hemispheres and portions of cranial nerves I and II within the skull. Posterior fossa level includes brain stem, cerebellum, and portions of cranial nerves III through XII within the skull. Spinal level includes spinal cord and portions of nerve roots contained within the vertebral column. Peripheral level includes portions of both cranial and peripheral nerves that lie outside the skull and spinal column, and structures innervated by these nerves.

    a. Some form of mass lesion
    b. Some form of nonmass lesion
4. Is the lesion most likely
    a. Vascular
    b. Degenerative
    c. Inflammatory
    d. Neoplastic
    e. Toxic-metabolic
    f. Traumatic
    g. Congenital-developmental

The major objective of this text therefore is to provide the information necessary to answer these questions for any clinical problem involving the nervous system and to provide a description of the mechanism by which the patient's symptoms and findings are produced by the underlying disorder.

Organization

The solution of a neurologic problem requires three levels of knowledge, and this text is therefore organized into three sections. Section I provides general information necessary to understand how neurologic disorders are diagnosed. The remainder of the text is organized to enable a precise topographic and etiologic diagnosis. Topographic localization initially requires relating the patient's functional impairment to one of six major longitudinal systems (Section II) and then localizing the lesion at a well-defined level of the nervous system (Section III).

Each chapter begins with an introduction and overview and ends with a listing of objectives and clinical problems for self-assessment. Additional suggested readings are provided.

Survey of the Neurosciences
The clinician must first have an understanding of the methods utilized in diagnosing a neurologic disorder. How is a lesion localized, and to what do the general anatomic terms used to describe localization refer? How is a pathologic or etiologic diagnosis determined, and what do the terms used to describe them mean? These questions require a general knowledge of the diagnostic principles of neurologic disorders as these principles relate to the anatomy, physiology, and pathology of the nervous system. Chapters 2 through 5 provide a common basic vocabulary and the background knowledge necessary to begin solving clinical problems. These chapters cover the following subjects:

Chapter 2: Organization of the Nervous System: Neuroembryology
Chapter 3: Diagnosis of Neurologic Disorders: Anatomic Localization
Chapter 4: Diagnosis of Neurologic Disorders: Neurocytology and the Pathologic Reactions of the Nervous System
Chapter 5: Diagnosis of Neurologic Disorders: Transient Disorders and Neurophysiology

Longitudinal Systems

Increasingly detailed knowledge öf the anatomy and physiology of the nervous system is required for a precise diagnosis of a neurologic disorder. The clinician usually first identifies the patient's symptoms and signs as indicative of disease involving one or more of six major longitudinal subdivisions of the nervous system. These longitudinally organized groups of structures are called *systems* within the nervous system, each subserving a specific function. In this section the anatomy, physiology, and clinical expression of disease as it affects the following six major longitudinal systems are described:

Chapter 6:   The Cerebrospinal Fluid System
Chapter 7:   The Sensory System
Chapter 8:   The Consciousness System
Chapter 9:   The Motor System
Chapter 10:   The Visceral System
Chapter 11:   The Vascular System

The name of each system characterizes its function. Correlation of the symptoms and signs with the appropriate system permits localization of the disease process in one dimension.

Levels of the Neuraxis

The final step in localizing a lesion requires identification of an additional dimension—determining its location along the length of the systems involved. Although a precise localization can be made in many cases, most clinicians classify the disorder according to one of four major regions defined by the bony structures surrounding much of the nervous system. The final part of the text explores the ways in which functions in each major system are integrated and modified at each of the following levels:

Chapter 12:   The Peripheral Level
Chapter 13:   The Spinal Level
Chapter 14:   The Posterior Fossa Level
Chapter 15:   The Supratentorial Level

In all these sections, there is repetition of material, with each subsequent section building on the basic information presented earlier to provide amplification and reemphasis. This approach to clinical neurologic problems can be used with any of the problems that may be encountered and is particularly useful in problems that are new, unfamiliar, or unusual to the clinician. While the identification of diseases by recognition of a particular syndrome sometimes can be very efficient, the method of inductive reasoning presented herein is consistently more accurate and more reliable.

Survey of the Neurosciences

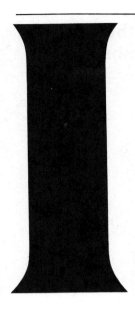

Organization of the Nervous System: Neuroembryology

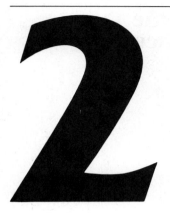

The study of neurosciences begins with a survey of neuroembryology because it provides a framework and background for understanding the anatomy of the nervous system in the adult. The eventual location of the structures in the brain is not a random occurrence, but is a reflection of the orderly development of the primitive nervous system. Neuroembryology also serves as an aid in understanding the pathogenesis of developmental neurologic abnormalities that are encountered not only in the newborn and pediatric periods but also in later life.

Overview

By the eighteenth day of embryonic development, the early stage of gastrulation has been completed. The embryo consists of two layers, ectoderm and endoderm, with mesoderm growing outward between them from the midline primitive streak. The notochord, a specialized column of mesodermal cells, grows forward from the anterior end of the primitive streak (Hensen's node). The ectoderm overlying the notochord is induced to form the neural plate, which thickens and folds into the neural tube, from which the entire central nervous system develops. Cell columns derived from the junction of skin ectoderm and neuroectoderm, the neural crests, separate from the neural tube and later form major portions of the peripheral nervous system.

The neural tube undergoes longitudinal differentiation into six regions: telencephalon (cerebral hemispheres), diencephalon (thalamus and hypothalamus), mesencephalon (midbrain), metencephalon (pons and cerebellum), myelencephalon (medulla), and the spinal cord. These subdivisions of the neural tube are the precursors of the four major anatomic levels in the adult: supratentorial (telencephalon and diencephalon), posterior fossa (mesencephalon, metencephalon, and myelencephalon), spinal (spinal cord), and peripheral.

The neural tube also undergoes transverse differentiation with the formation of a dorsal region, the alar plate, which will subserve sensory functions, and a ventral region, the basal plate, which will subserve motor functions. At each level, the cavities of the tube are modified to form the fluid-filled spaces, the ventricular system. Mesodermal tissues grow into the neural tube and form blood vessels. These transverse subdivisions are the basis of the major functional systems: sensory, consciousness, motor, visceral, cerebrospinal fluid, and vascular.

Throughout the length of the neural tube, cells differentiate into neurons and supportive cells (ependyma, astrocytes, and oligodendroglia). The cells of the neural crest differentiate into the dorsal root ganglia, the autonomic ganglia, and Schwann cells.

Disorders of development of the nervous system may occur in any of these steps. These disorders can be classified as failures of fusion of the neural tube (for example, spina bifida and myelomeningocele) or failure of proliferation and migration (for example, lissencephaly and polymicrogyria).

Formation of the Neural Tube

The nervous system is commonly divided into central and peripheral components. The central nervous system is that part located within the spinal column and skull. It is formed from the neural tube between the eighteenth and the twenty-fifth day of gestation. Before these structures are formed, at the end of the second week of gestation, gastrulation has been completed. The longitudinal axis of the two-layered embryonic disk is established by the formation of an area of rapidly proliferating cells, the *primitive streak*. The midline of the embryo is defined by the growth of the *notochord*, a group of mesodermal cells that grow forward from one end of the primitive streak (Hensen's node) in a plane between the ectoderm and the endoderm. The mesoderm of the remainder of the embryonic disk is formed by the outgrowth of mesodermal cells from the lateral margins of the primitive streak. As the notochord and mesodermal tissues grow forward, the primitive streak becomes incorporated into the tailbud, and a three-layered embryo with a clearly delineated longitudinal axis is formed. These early changes set the stage for the subsequent events that establish the *neural tube*, the morphologic substrate of the adult nervous system.

The neural tube is formed in approximately 1 week, beginning on the eighteenth day. The initial step in its formation is a thickening of the ectoderm in the dorsal midline overlying the notochord to form the *neural plate* (Fig. 2-1A, B). The lateral edges of the neural plate thicken more rapidly than the center and begin to roll toward the midline, creating the *neural groove*, which has lateral margins, the *neural folds*. With continued growth, the neural folds meet in the midline to form a hollow tube, the neural tube, which closes first in the middle of the embryo (Fig. 2-1C, D) (the future cervical region)

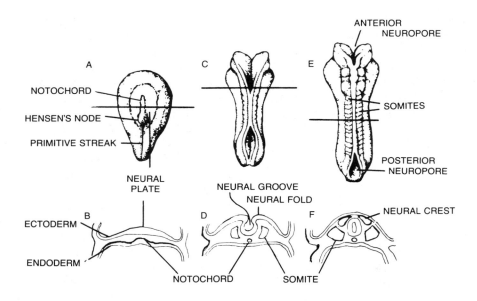

Fig. 2-1. Formation of neural tube (eighteenth to twenty-fifth day). A. Dorsal view of neural plate forming over notochord, which has grown forward from Hensen's node between ectoderm and endoderm. B. Cross section through neural plate shown in A. C. Dorsal view of early closure of neural tube. D. Cross section through neural tube shown in C. E. Dorsal view of almost complete closure of neural tube, and formation of well-defined somites. F. Cross section through E.

and then proceeds toward the head (cephalad) and toward the tail (caudad), until the entire tube is closed. The unfused areas at the two ends of the tube before complete closure are *neuropores* (Fig. 2-1E). As the neural tube is being formed by the fusion of the margins of the neural folds, the skin ectoderm also fuses and covers its dorsal surface. Ultimately, the two ectodermal derivatives, neural tube and skin, become further separated by the growth of intervening mesodermal derivatives, bone and muscle. Cell columns derived from the original junction of skin and neuroectoderm form the neural crests, which later differentiate into important components of the peripheral nervous system.

Even before the neural tube is entirely closed, longitudinal differentiation begins. Parallel to the neural tube, the mesodermal cells segment longitudinally into aggregates, the *somites*, from which bones and muscle will arise (Fig. 2-1E, F). At the same time the cephalic or head end of the neural tube becomes larger than the caudal end, resulting in an irregularly shaped tubal structure. Continued

differential growth along the length of the neural tube results in the formation of three cavities at the cephalic end of the tube. These are the primary brain vesicles: the *prosencephalon*, the *mesencephalon*, and the *rhombencephalon* (Fig. 2-2A, B). These three vesicles will further differentiate into five subdivisions, which will persist in the brain of the mature nervous system (Fig. 2-2 C, D). The remaining caudal end of the neural tube undergoes much less modification as it forms the spinal cord. A central remnant of the internal cavity of the tube remains in each of these derivatives.

The subdivisions of the primitive neural tube evolve, through the processes of cellular proliferation, migration, and differentiation (described in the next section), into the major elements in the adult nervous system listed in Table 2-1.

Differentiation of the Central Nervous System

The primitive neural tube consists of multipotential *neuroepithelial cells*, derived from ectoderm. These cells undergo a process of multiplication, differentiation, and migration to establish three concentric layers in the neural tube. Cell division occurs in the inner layer, from which cells migrate outward, undergoing further differentiation, growth, and maturation.

The *ependymal layer*, which arises by local cell proliferation, lines the primitive neural cavities. This layer persists in the mature nervous system, lining the ventricular system as a single layer of cil-

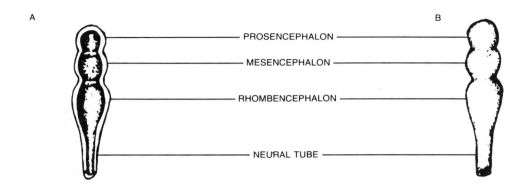

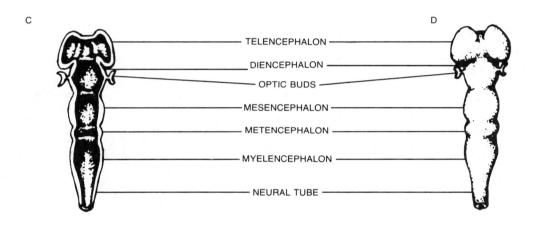

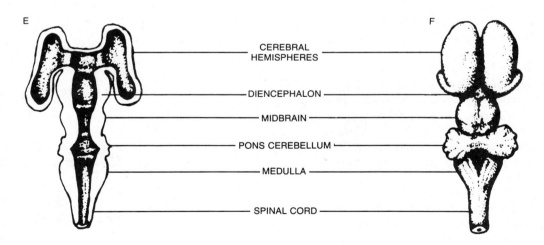

Fig. 2-2. Formation of major brain vesicles of neural tube (twenty-fifth to thirtieth day) in horizontal section (left) and dorsal view (right). A, B. Stage of three primary vesicles. C, D. Stage of five major vesicles. E, F. Differentiation of specific structures by cell migration and overgrowth.

Table 2-1. Major Elements in Adult Nervous System Derived from the Neural Tube

Level	Primary divisions	Subdivisions	Major derivatives	Cavities
Supratentorial	Prosencephalon	Telencephalon	Rhinencephalon Basal ganglia Cerebral cortex	Lateral ventricles
		Diencephalon	Thalamus Hypothalamus Optic nerves Neurohypophysis Pineal	Third ventricle
Posterior fossa	Mesencephalon	Mesencephalon	Midbrain	Aqueduct of Sylvius
	Rhombencephalon	Metencephalon	Cerebellum Pons	Fourth ventricle
		Myelencephalon	Medulla	Fourth ventricle
Spinal	Primitive neural tube	Neural tube	Spinal cord	Central canal
Peripheral		Neural crest	Peripheral nerve Ganglia	None

iated, columnar cells known as the *ependyma*. The *mantle layer* is formed by the outward migration of the cells proliferating in the ependymal layer (Fig. 2-3). Further proliferation and maturation of cells will occur in this layer. Some of the cells in the mantle layer send out processes toward the periphery of the neural tube. The *marginal layer* is a relatively acellular outer layer made up of the processes of cells in the mantle (Fig. 2-3E, F).

Cell Differentiation
The original neural plate is a single layer of cells. As these primitive neuroepithelial cells proliferate in the ependymal layer and migrate into the mantle layer, they differentiate into neuroblasts and spongioblasts and finally mature into the two major types of cells found in the adult nervous system, neurons and supporting cells.

The neurons, derived from neuroblasts, perform the primary function of the nervous system, that is, processing information. They have long extensions called *axons*, which pass via the marginal layer as nerve fibers, forming connections with other areas of the central or peripheral nervous system. The supporting cells derived from spongioblasts are the ependyma, astrocytes, and oligodendroglia. They are referred to as *glial cells. Ependymal cells* line the cavities of the brain. *Astrocytes* maintain the proper environment and provide nutritional support for the neurons. *Oligodendroglia* form the insulation (myelin) on the axons of the neurons by wrapping layers of cytoplasm around the axons along

Fig. 2-3. Differentiation of cell layers in primitive neural tube, with high-power view on the right and cross section of tube shown on the left. A, B. Early neural plate is a single layer of cells. C, D. Formation of layers of cells by outward migration of cells proliferating in inner ependymal layer. E, F. Formation of outer acellular marginal layer by growth of processes (axons) peripherally from cells.

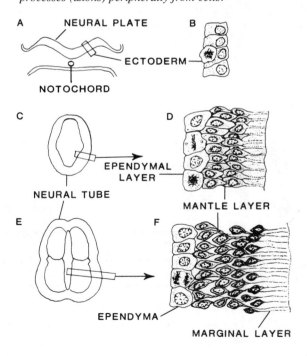

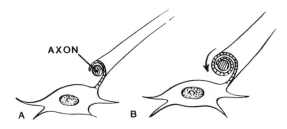

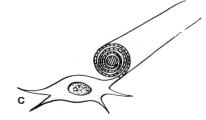

Fig. 2-4. Process of myelination of nerve fibers in central and peripheral nervous system. Layer of cytoplasm wraps around an axon (A) and then encircles it repeatedly (B). Condensation of layers of cytoplasm forms myelin (C).

their length (Fig. 2-4). Cells of mesodermal origin also grow into and surround the neural tube. Blood vessels extend throughout the nervous system. Other mesodermal cells form covering layers, the *meninges*, which surround and protect the brain. *Microglial cells*, also of mesodermal origin, migrate into the neural tube and act as scavenger cells.

Transverse Differentiation

As the neural tube enlarges, it undergoes differentiation in the transverse plane. In a transverse section, the region of the neural tube nearest the thoracic and abdominal cavities is called *ventral*; that farthest from them is *dorsal*. (These are also sometimes referred to as anterior and posterior, respectively.) As the neurons proliferate, more of them accumulate laterally in the neural tube, leaving relatively thin areas middorsally and midventrally. These thin areas are the *roof plate* and *floor plate* (Fig. 2-5). Differential proliferation of cells in the dorsal and ventral regions results in the formation of a longitudinal groove, the *sulcus limitans*, on each lateral wall of the central canal. The sulcus limitans divides the neural tube into dorsal and ventral halves.

The cells that are separated into groups by this differential growth will have different functions in the mature brain. These differences in function are the basis for the separation of the brain and spinal cord into longitudinal systems. The portion of the mantle layer that lies dorsal to the sulcus limitans is the *alar plate* (Fig. 2-6). The neurons in this area will differentiate primarily into sensory relay neurons, which transmit information coming into the central nervous system. They are *afferent*, that is,

conducting inward. They receive information coming from somite derivatives (skin, bones, joints, and muscles) and endoderm derivatives (all the internal organs). The neurons that carry afferent information from somatic structures will form the *sensory system*.

The part of the mantle layer ventral to the sulcus limitans is the *basal plate*. The neurons in this area will differentiate into motor neurons, which initiate the activities of the body such as limb movement and organ secretion. They are *efferent*, that is, conducting outward. Neurons concerned with the control of muscle and body movement will form the *motor system*.

Afferent and efferent neurons involved in the function and control of internal organs are derived from the alar and basal plates close to the sulcus limitans. They are considered functionally distinct from the somatic sensory and motor systems al-

Fig. 2-5. Transverse section of neural tube at 30 days, with early regional differentiation.

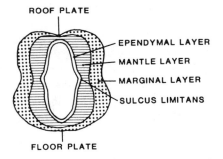

ROOF PLATE

EPENDYMAL LAYER

MANTLE LAYER

MARGINAL LAYER

SULCUS LIMITANS

FLOOR PLATE

Fig. 2-6. Transverse section of spinal cord at fourth (left) and fifteenth (right) weeks.

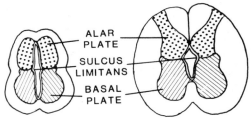

ALAR PLATE

SULCUS LIMITANS

BASAL PLATE

ready mentioned and together constitute the *visceral system*.

Functionally related to the sensory system at cephalic levels and comprised of structures largely elaborated from the alar plate is the *consciousness system*.

In addition to these four longitudinal systems (sensory, consciousness, motor, and visceral), two other systems are formed from the cavities in the neural tube and the addition of mesodermal tissues. The mesodermal cells joining the neural tube form either connective tissue layers surrounding it (the meninges) or blood vessels ramifying within it. These blood vessels will form the *vascular system*. The meninges surrounding the brain form fluid-filled spaces that are continuous with the fluid-filled cavities of the brain; together, these spaces will form the *cerebrospinal fluid system*. This basic plan of organization of the longitudinal systems is modified somewhat at each level of the neuraxis with further development. These modifications will be considered at each level of the central nervous system.

Longitudinal Differentiation

Between the third and the fifth week of gestation, development differs significantly along the length of the neural tube. The most complex changes occur at the cephalic end, where the brain is forming. These changes are the result of three processes: flexure formation, development of special structures in the head, and regional overgrowth.

Three bends, or flexures, occur in the neural tube (Fig. 2-7). The *cervical flexure* occurs between the spinal cord and the myelencephalon in a ventral direction, the *pontine flexure* occurs in the metencephalon in a dorsal direction, and the *midbrain flexure* occurs in the mesencephalon in a ventral di-

rection. These flexures produce a widening in the transverse configuration of the neural tube in the rhombencephalon, with lateral displacement of the alar plates (Fig. 2-8C, D). The sum of the three flexures leaves only slight bends in the mature brain at the diencephalon-mesencephalon junction and at the medulla–spinal cord junction.

Two types of specializations occur in the cephalic region of the embryo. The first of these is the development of *branchial arches*, phylogenetic remnants of the gill system in lower animals. These arches contribute to the formation of structures in the head and neck, such as the facial muscles. The motor and sensory cells that provide axonal innervation of structures derived from the branchial arches are located in the rhombencephalon but are aggregated in groups distinct from the somatic and visceral, sensory, and motor neurons. The second specialization is the appearance of complex sensory structures such as the eyes, the ears, balance receptors (vestibular), and smell and taste receptors. Separate groups of sensory neurons develop for each of these structures. Neurons concerned with vision and smell are located in the prosencephalon, while those concerned with balance, hearing, and taste are located in the rhombencephalon.

Finally, certain areas of the cephalic portions of the neural tube undergo marked proliferation of cells, with overgrowth of surrounding structures. This overgrowth and accompanying migration of cells produce complex rearrangements of the basic plan of the neural tube. For example, overgrowth of the alar plates of the prosencephalon results in large cerebral hemispheres, which almost completely surround the derivatives of the diencephalon. The cerebellum also arises by overgrowth of cells of the alar plate in the metencephalon and eventually covers the dorsal surface of the entire rhombencepha-

Fig. 2-7. *Flexures of neural tube as primary brain vesicles are forming* (arrows).

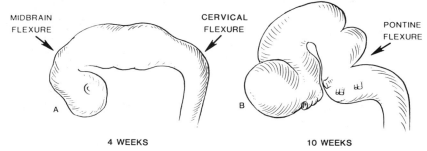

MIDBRAIN FLEXURE   CERVICAL FLEXURE   PONTINE FLEXURE

A

B

4 WEEKS   10 WEEKS

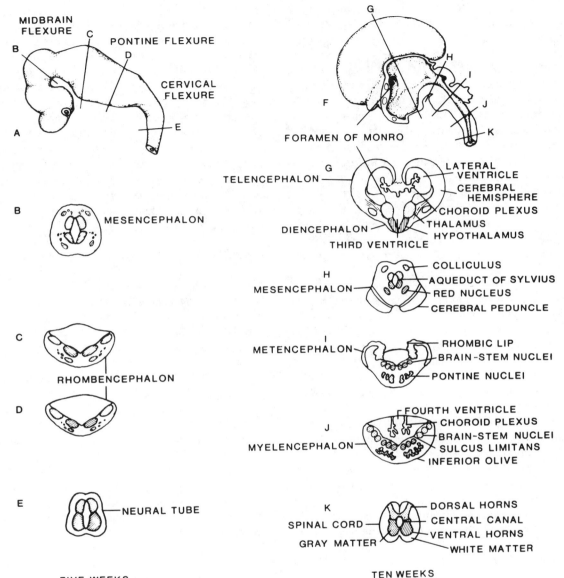

FIVE WEEKS

TEN WEEKS

Fig. 2-8. Longitudinal differentiation along neural tube at fifth (A through E) and tenth (F through K) weeks seen in whole embryo and transverse section. (Redrawn from K. L. Moore. The Developing Human: Clinically Oriented Embryology *[2nd ed.]. Philadelphia: Saunders, 1977.)*

lon. The unique changes occurring at each major level during the fourth to sixth weeks of development will be considered separately for each level.

SPINAL LEVEL.   The caudal end of the neural tube, as it develops into the spinal cord, remains basically the same as that seen in the primitive nervous system (Fig. 2-8E, K). The central canal becomes obliterated, and the shape of the cellular areas of the mantle layer, now called *gray matter*, is modified. The marginal layer becomes the *white matter*, a dense layer of nerve fibers or tracts carrying axons longitudinally. The meninges surround the spinal cord and form a subarachnoid space. Bone surrounding the cord forms the spinal column. At the spinal level, therefore, the sensory, motor, visceral, cerebrospinal fluid, and vascular systems are all present.

POSTERIOR FOSSA LEVEL.   The mesoderm that surrounds the cephalic end of the embryonic nervous system forms the skull and meninges that enclose and protect the brain within the cranial cavity. In concert with the formation of the primary brain vesicles and flexures, folds of meninges that ultimately become tough dural septae are formed. A major horizontal fold of dura forms at the level of the mesencephalon. This fold will ultimately cover the dorsal surface of the cerebellum and is called the *tentorium cerebelli*. The region of the cranial cavity below the plane of the tentorium is the posterior cranial fossa and contains the rhombencephalon and mesencephalon and their derivatives.

In the rhombencephalon, as the flexures occur, the alar plates of the myelencephalon and metencephalon rotate laterally; the roof plate becomes greatly thinned; and the central cavity opens out into a rhombic-shaped space, the fourth ventricle. This rotation results in a change in the relationship of the alar and basal plates, so that the alar plate lies lateral to the basal plate, with the sulcus limitans running in the floor of the fourth ventricle in the adult derivatives—the medulla and pons (Fig. 2-8C, D, I, J). The junction between the thinned roof plate and the alar plate is the *rhombic lip*. Proliferation, migration, and overgrowth of cells from the rhombic lip result in the formation of *inferior olives*, nuclei at the base of the pons, and portions of cerebellum that come to overlie the entire fourth ventricle and rhombencephalon. The neurons innervating branchial arch derivatives and the special

sensory structures for hearing, balance, and taste also are located at this level.

In the mesencephalon, which becomes the midbrain, the basic relationships seen in the spinal cord persist (Fig. 2-8B, H). The central cavity here is a small canal, the *aqueduct of Sylvius*. As the alar and basal plates differentiate into specialized sensory and motor structures, they become known as the *tectum* and *tegmentum*, respectively. Dense bundles of longitudinal axons beneath the tegmentum become the cerebral peduncles, a part of the motor system. In addition to the motor system other longitudinal systems in the posterior fossa are the sensory, cerebrospinal fluid, visceral, consciousness, and vascular systems.

SUPRATENTORIAL LEVEL.   The portion of the cranial cavity located above the tentorium contains the two derivatives of the prosencephalon, the *diencephalon* and *telencephalon*. The general rule, that the sensory structures are dorsal and arise from the alar plate whereas the motor structures are ventral and arise from the basal plate, does not hold true in the diencephalon and telencephalon because most of the structures that arise from these regions are derived from the alar plate. Only some of the ventral diencephalon (hypothalamus and subthalamus) is derived from the basal plate.

The central canal in the diencephalon becomes a slitlike cavity, the third ventricle. Only a small portion of the telencephalon remains as a midline structure, its central canal becoming the anterior third ventricle. Most of the telencephalon develops from paired lateral evaginations that undergo tremendous growth to become the largest portions of the mature brain, the cerebral hemispheres (Fig. 2-8F, G). The orifice of each lateral evagination is the *foramen of Monro*, which leads into the lateral ventricles, the cavities within the cerebral hemispheres (Fig. 2-8G).

The cerebral hemispheres are seen initially as two lateral evaginations of the prosencephalon. However, the rapid rate of proliferation of the cells in the dorsal parts of these outpouchings results in a sweeping of tissue posteriorly, laterally, and ventrally. This broad sweep and cellular migration give the hemispheres and ventricles a C-shaped configuration (see Fig. 2-2F). As these cellular areas are forming the major lobes of the cerebral hemispheres, they pull along with them deep midline groups of cells and fiber pathways connected to the

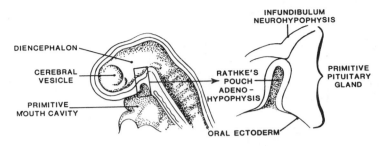

Fig. 2-9. Embryogenesis of pituitary gland at junction of invaginated oral ectoderm and evagination of diencephalon.

hypothalamus in the diencephalon. These cells and pathways will become the limbic system, which is also C-shaped. Continued proliferation of cells in the enclosed space of the skull leads to the complex folds in the surface of the hemispheres known as *gyri* (ridges) and *sulci* (grooves).

Two specialized cranial structures are derived from the diencephalon, and each depends on an interaction of neural tissue with other tissue. The eye develops from tissue that is derived from paired lateral outgrowths of the diencephalon and from the overlying ectoderm in contact with these outgrowths. The pituitary gland, an endocrine gland, is derived from a midline ventral outgrowth of the diencephalon, the *infundibulum*, a ventral neural ridge, and oral ectoderm, *Rathke's pouch* (Fig. 2-9). The mature pituitary gland has three divisions, the *adenohypophysis* (anterior pituitary gland), the *neurohypophysis* (posterior pituitary gland), and the *intermediate lobe*.

There is one group of specialized sensory structures derived from the telencephalon, the group concerned with olfaction. As at the posterior fossa level, all the major longitudinal systems are represented at the supratentorial level.

Differentiation of Peripheral Structures

The derivatives of the neural tube outlined in the previous sections become the central nervous system contained within the bony skull and spinal column. While the peripheral nervous system is largely a derivative of the neural crest, the peripheral neuromuscular structures of interest to us are derived from three sources: neural crest cells, somites, and outgrowths of the central nervous system. All these structures outside the spinal column and skull are at the *peripheral level*.

Neural Crest

As the neural tube closes, cells split away from the neural tube and ectoderm, forming two columns of cells along the junction between the surface ectoderm and the neural tube (Figs. 2-10, 2-11). These are the *neural crests*. As the neural tube separates from the overlying ectoderm, the cells of the neural crests proliferate and migrate laterally. As they differentiate, they form three of the four major components of the peripheral nervous system: dorsal root ganglia, visceral (autonomic) ganglia, and Schwann cells. The fourth component is an outgrowth of the neural tube, the motor axons. The somatic structures innervated by both components, the muscles and the dermis of the skin, are derivatives of somites.

Dorsal root ganglia are collections of cell bodies of sensory neurons. These neurons send axons peripherally to all areas of the body to gather sensory information, and they send other axons centrally into the alar plate to carry this information to the central nervous system. These neurons are therefore the initial transmitters of sensory information and are *primary sensory neurons*.

The *autonomic ganglia* are collections of cell bodies of visceral neurons in the trunk and head that send out axons to innervate all the internal organs. They receive connections from axons of visceral neurons in the central nervous system and from sensory neurons in the internal organs. These ganglia mediate motor and sensory activities of the visceral organs.

Schwann cells form the myelin, or insulation, surrounding the axons in the peripheral nervous system, just as the oligodendroglia do in the central nervous system (see Fig. 2-4). Schwann cells are located serially along the length of all peripheral axons and envelop them. Neural crest cells also give rise to an endocrine organ, the adrenal medulla.

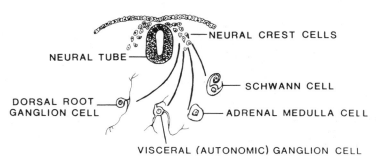

Fig. 2-10. Derivatives of neural crest cells formed at junction of neural tube and covering ectoderm.

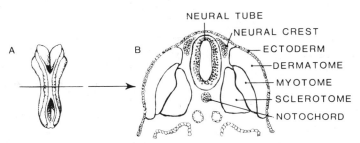

Fig. 2-11. Formation of myotome, sclerotome, and dermatome from somites in embryo of 4 weeks, in whole embryo (A) and transverse section (B).

Somites

As the neural tube closes, the embryonic mesoderm lateral to the tube becomes segmented into cell masses known as *somites* (Fig. 2-11). These masses differentiate into three components: the sclerotome, myotome, and dermatome. The ventromedial portion of the somite forms the *sclerotome*, which will differentiate into the cartilage and bone, forming the vertebrae of the spinal column and base of the skull surrounding the central nervous system. The notochord becomes incorporated into the ventromedial extensions of the sclerotome and thus remains ventral to the tube. The notochordal remnant within the vertebral column is the nucleus pulposis in the intervertebral disk. The dorsomedial portion of the somite forms the *myotome*, which gives rise to the striated skeletal muscle of the body, with the exception of that muscle formed from the branchial arches in the head and neck. The primordial muscle cells of the myotome migrate peripherally, reaching their eventual location in the trunk and limbs. The lateral portion of the somite forms the *dermatome*. Cells from the dermatome migrate peripherally to form the dermis, the connective tissue layer of the skin.

Peripheral Nerves

Connections between the central nervous system and the peripheral structures derived from the somites and the neural crest are established by growth of axons from the dorsal root ganglia into the alar plate of the neural tube and by outgrowth of axons from neurons in the basal plate. These distally growing motor axons join the peripherally growing sensory axons of the dorsal root ganglia to form a nerve that innervates the somite at the same level (Fig. 2-12). The nerves formed in this fashion at the

Fig. 2-12. Formation of spinal nerves by combination of axons from basal plate and dorsal root ganglia.

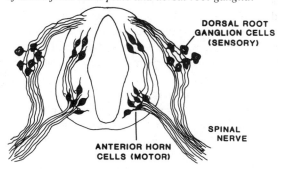

Table 2-2. Classification of the Functional Components
of Nerves on Basis of Embryologic Origin and Destination

Type	Category	Tissue innervated	Tissue origin	Abbreviation*
Afferent (sensory)	General	Skin, muscle, bone, joints	Somites	GSA
		Visceral organs	Endoderm	GVA
	Special	Ear, eye, balance	External receptors (ectoderm)	SSA
		Taste, smell	Visceral receptors (endoderm)	SVA
Efferent (motor)	General	Somatic striated muscle	Somites	GSE
		Glands, smooth muscle, visceral organs	Nonsomite (mesoderm and endoderm)	GVE
	Special	Head and neck muscle	Branchial arches	SVE

*GSA = general somatic afferent; GVA = general visceral afferent; SSA = special somatic afferent; SVA = special visceral afferent; GSE = general somatic efferent; GVE = general visceral efferent; and SVE = special visceral efferent.

spinal level are the *spinal nerves*; those formed at the posterior fossa and supratentorial levels are the *cranial nerves*. Both types are composed of mixtures of sensory and motor axons. In these nerves, the motor axons from cells in the central nervous system innervate the myotomal derivatives and autonomic ganglia, while the sensory axons innervate the dermatomes and endoderm derivatives. As the embryo develops and the cells forming the muscles, skin, and internal organs migrate to their adult locations, these neural processes will be pulled along with them to establish the pattern of innervation of peripheral nerves.

The functions of the axons in peripheral nerves are classified into systems just as are those in the central nervous system. *Afferent* fibers are those that conduct information toward the central nervous system (sensory), and *efferent* fibers are those that carry information away from the central nervous system. Axons are also subdivided on the basis of the type of structure they innervate. Fibers that innervate tissues derived from somites (muscles and skin) are designated *somatic*; fibers that innervate endodermal or other mesodermal derivatives (internal organs) are called *visceral*. Thus, afferent axons that carry sensations such as pain, temperature, touch, and joint movement from the body surface and supporting structures are *general somatic afferent* (GSA). Afferent axons that carry sensations such as pain, fullness, and blood chemical levels from the internal organs are *general visceral afferent* (GVA). Motor axons to skeletal muscle of somite origin are *general somatic efferent* (GSE). Motor axons that innervate smooth muscle of viscera, glands, and blood vessels are *general visceral efferent* (GVE).

Each of these types of fibers is found in the pe-

ripheral and cranial nerves. The cranial nerves also have fibers that mediate special sensations and fibers that innervate branchial arch derivatives. Those to the branchial arch derivatives, especially facial muscles, are *special visceral efferent* (SVE); those mediating sensations of taste and smell are *special visceral afferent* (SVA). The fibers that carry the other special sensory information of vision, hearing, and balance are *special somatic afferent* (SSA). The somatic afferent fibers will be considered in detail in the discussion of the sensory system; the somatic efferent fibers will be considered in the discussion of the motor system; and the visceral afferent and efferent fibers will be considered in the discussion of the visceral system. Other special functions will be presented in the discussion of the posterior fossa and supratentorial levels. Table 2-2 summarizes the classification of the functional components of nerves on the basis of embryologic origin and destination.

Clinical Correlations

In a number of ways, knowledge of the embryology of the nervous system is relevant to the study of neurologic diseases and clinical practice. Understanding the anatomy of the nervous system, an essential part of clinical diagnosis, is greatly aided by knowing the manner in which the nervous system is formed and how various relationships in the adult nervous system develop in the embryo. For example, knowledge of the myotomal and dermatomal distribution of nerves is needed for precise localization of damage in the nervous system. In addition, many neurologic disorders can be understood only in terms of the developmental anatomy of the nervous system and related tissue.

The most common disorders in this category are

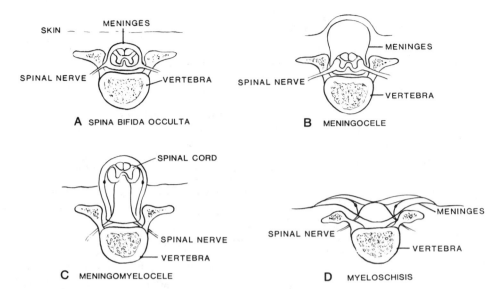

Fig. 2-13. Examples of failure of fusion at spinal level. A. Spina bifida occulta with incomplete vertebral arch. B. Meningocele with outpouching of fluid-filled sac of meninges and skin. C. Meningomyelocele with sac containing abnormal neural tissue. D. Myeloschisis with no closure and a deformed neural plate open to the surface. (Redrawn from B. Pansky and E. L. House. Review of Gross Anatomy *[3rd ed.]. New York: Macmillan, 1975.)*

the congenital malformations. Although this disease category includes many seemingly complex conditions, they may be grouped into a few categories on the basis of the stages of development during which they are thought to arise. The two most conspicuous aspects of neuroembryology are neural tube formation with fusion of the neural folds in the dorsal midline, and proliferation and migration of neuroepithelial cells. Most congenital anomalies can be viewed as abnormalities in one of these two processes, that is, failure of fusion or failure of proliferation and migration of cells.

The first group leads to disorders in dorsal midline structures, often obvious on the surface. Varied degrees of severity of the defect are seen, especially in the caudal (lumbosacral) regions (Fig. 2-13). Thus, *spina bifida occulta*, failure of fusion of the vertebral arch (Fig. 2-13A), *meningocele*, protrusion of a meningeal sac through the skin and bone defect (Fig. 2-13B), *meningomyelocele*, inclusion of herniated spinal cord in the sac (Fig. 2-13C), and *myeloschisis* (rachischisis), a completely open spinal cord (Fig. 2-13D), are viewed as increasingly

severe manifestations of the same disorder. They are associated with increasingly severe neurologic deficits that vary from no deficit to paralysis of the lower extremities, with impaired bladder or bowel function. Similar defects occur in the rostral end of the neural tube, and the resulting defects are termed *cranium bifidum*, *cranial meningocele*, *meningoencephalocele*, and *cranioschisis* or *anencephaly*. The most severe form of this type of defect is a completely open neural tube and dorsal midline—*craniorachischisis*.

Failures in the proliferation and migration of cells result primarily in abnormalities of the form and architecture of the cerebral hemispheres. These abnormalities range from failure of gyri to form (lissencephaly) through the formation of abnormally large gyri (pachygyria) to the formation of numerous abnormally small gyri (polymicrogyria). Clinically, these defects are often associated with severe mental retardation. There are many other forms of congenital malformation of the brain, some of which cannot be grouped easily into either of these major categories and which require further research to determine the mechanism of formation.

Because skin and nervous system both evolve from the ectoderm, a genetically determined disorder that affects one of these systems may affect the other. A group of diseases, the neuroectodermal dysplasias or the neurocutaneous syndromes, is characterized by specific changes in both the skin and the nervous system. Common manifestations of three of the most frequently seen disorders of this type are outlined in Table 2-3.

Table 2-3. Examples of Some Neuroectodermal Dysplasias
and Some of Their Common Skin and Nervous System Manifestations

Disease	Skin	Nervous system
Von Recklinghausen disease	Neurofibromas Café-au-lait spots	Schwannomas Gliomas Meningeal angioma
Sturge-Weber syndrome	Port-wine nevus of face	Cortical calcification
Tuberous sclerosis	Adenoma sebaceum Subungual fibromas Depigmented patches	Periventricular tumors Cortical giant cell tumors Gliomas

The retina of the eye is also a derivative of the central nervous system. As with the skin, the retina may be affected by disorders that involve the nervous system, and observation of the retina with an ophthalmoscope may provide information as to the nature of the disorder. An example of this association is *Tay-Sachs disease*, the lipid-storage disease in which neurons of the central nervous system accumulate large amounts of gangliosides. This accumulation is reflected in the retina by a "cherry red spot" in the macula, due to the storage of lipids and the relative opacification of retinal ganglion cells surrounding the macula. Retinal tumors also may be seen in the neuroectodermal dysplasias, and malformations of the eye sometimes accompany anomalies of the nervous system.

As the central nervous system develops, it is surrounded by the vertebral column; but there is a notable difference in the growth rate of the spinal cord and the vertebral column, with the latter growing faster. As a result, while in the third fetal month the spinal cord completely fills the vertebral canal, at birth it terminates at the lower border of the third

Fig. 2-14. Location of caudal end of spinal cord in vertebral column at 12 weeks (A), birth (B), and adulthood (C). (Redrawn form K. L. Moore. The Developing Human: Clinically Oriented Embryology *[2nd ed.]. Philadelphia: Saunders, 1977.)*

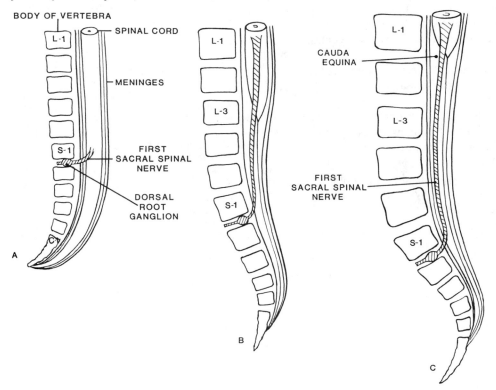

lumbar vertebra, and in adults it terminates near the upper border of the second lumbar vertebra (Fig. 2-14). Therefore a lumbar puncture in newborn infants must be done at a very low level in order to avoid puncturing the spinal cord.

The differential rate of growth of the cord and the spinal column also places the spinal cord segments, particularly in the lower half of the body, above the vertebral segments of the corresponding number. Because the spinal nerves emerge between the embryologically established vertebral bodies, there is a progressive elongation of the lower nerve roots that is known in the adult as the *cauda equina* (Fig. 2-14).

Objectives

1. Describe the primitive streak, notochord, neural plate, neural folds, neural tube, and neural crest in the early development of the nervous system.
2. List the five major subdivisions of the cephalic portion of the neural tube, their associated central cavities, and major adult structures derived from them.
3. On a cross section of the neural tube, identify the alar plate, the basal plate, the ependymal, marginal, and mantle layers, and the neural crest, and name the derivatives of each of them.
4. Describe the formation of the peripheral nervous system and its connections with the central nervous system.
5. Name the structures in the embryo found at the supratentorial, posterior fossa, spinal, and peripheral levels.
6. Describe the embryologic distinctions between the major longitudinal systems (sensory, consciousness, motor, visceral, cerebrospinal fluid, and vascular).
7. List the two major types of developmental abnormality of the nervous system, and name examples of each of them.

Clinical Problems

1. A newborn child has a large bulging mass over the lower portion of the spinal column. There is no skin overlying this mass, and through the glistening membranes of the fluid-filled mass, ill-defined neural structures can be seen. The infant does not move his legs.
   a. What embryologic process was not completed in this child?
   b. What primitive structure was involved and at what stage in the development?
   c. Which types of functions are probably absent in this child?
   d. What is the origin of the structures involved in this defect?
   e. What primitive layers of the spinal cord might be involved?
   f. Name the disorder.
2. A 4-year-old boy has white spots (phakomas) in the retina of his eyes, as seen with an ophthalmoscope, and red lesions over his face. He also has convulsions and mental retardation.
   a. How could these findings all be on a congenital basis?
   b. From what primitive structures does the eye develop?
   c. What are the two primitive neural cell types from which tumors might arise?
   d. What is the functional embryologic classification of the nerve fibers from the eye?
   e. Name the disorder.

Suggested Reading

Cowan, W.M. The development of the brain. *Sci. Am.* 241: 112, 1979.

Crelin, E. S., Netter, F. H., and Shapter, R. K. Development of the nervous system: A logical approach to neuroanatomy. *Clin. Symp.* 26 (2):1, 1974.

Langman, J. *Medical Embryology* (4th ed.). Baltimore: Williams & Wilkins, 1981.

Moore, K. L. *The Developing Human: Clinically Oriented Embryology* (3rd ed.). Philadelphia: Saunders, 1982.

Tuchmann-Duplessis, H., Auroux, M., and Haegel, P. *Illustrated Human Embryology*. Vol. III: *Nervous System and Endocrine Glands*. New York: Springer-Verlag, 1974.

Diagnosis of Neurologic Disorders: Anatomic Localization

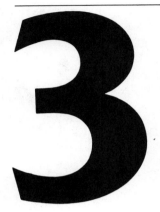

The diagnosis of neurologic disorders is a skill that requires the application of basic scientific information to a clinical problem. As knowledge of the nervous system grows, more complicated neurologic problems can be solved in more sophisticated ways; however, the basic approach to the solution of all neurologic problems remains unchanged. In arriving at a solution, three questions must be answered: (1) Is there a lesion involving the nervous system? (2) Where is the lesion located? (3) What is the (histopathologic) nature of the lesion?

Answering the first question is undeniably the most difficult since it requires a familiarity not only with clinical neurology but also with other disciplines of medicine. In time, as the manifestations of neurologic disorders become better known, the neurologic origin of certain symptoms will be identified with increasing confidence.

To answer the question "Where is the lesion located that has caused the signs and symptoms?" requires an understanding of the organization of the nervous system and an ability to relate the patient's description and the physician's observations of dysfunction to a particular area or areas within the nervous system.

In addition to localizing a lesion in an area in the nervous system, the physician must determine the nature of the lesion. An infarct (stroke), tumor, or abscess may lead to similar signs and symptoms. The manner in which these symptoms evolve, the temporal profile, provides the clues to distinguish these disorders and predict the histopathologic changes responsible for the observed abnormality.

A physician highly skilled in neurologic-anatomic diagnosis is capable of localizing a lesion in the nervous system to within millimeters of its actual site. Although this type of skill is laudable, it is often more than is required of even the practicing neurologist. In most clinical situations, for proper patient management it is sufficient to decide whether the responsible lesion is producing dysfunction in one or more longitudinal systems, to relate those abnormalities to one (or more) of several gross anatomic levels, and to determine whether the presumed lesion is on the right side, on the left side, or in the midline or is diffuse and involves homologous areas bilaterally. Neurologic disorders may affect one or more of the following systems:

1. Cerebrospinal fluid system
2. Sensory system
3. Consciousness system
4. Motor system
5. Visceral system
6. Vascular system

and may occur at one or more of the following levels:

1. Supratentorial level
2. Posterior fossa level
3. Spinal level
4. Peripheral level

Familiarity with these major systems and levels will aid in the diagnosis of neurologic disorders. Each system and level will be discussed in further detail in subsequent chapters; this chapter will emphasize the anatomy of the levels.

Overview

The major structures of the central nervous system—the brain and the spinal cord—are surrounded by three fibrous connective tissue linings called *meninges* and are encased within a protective bony skeleton. The brain, consisting of derivatives of the primitive telencephalon, diencephalon, mesencephalon, metencephalon, and myelencephalon (Fig. 3-1), is enclosed within the *skull;* the spinal cord is situated in the spinal column. Cranial and peripheral nerves must pass through these surrounding investments to reach the more peripheral structures of the nervous system.

The major anatomic levels to be discussed are defined by the meninges and bony structures to which they are related. The divisions between the anatomic levels used in this book are not exact, and there will be some divergence from strict anatomic definitions found in other textbooks. The levels as they will be defined, however, have boundaries that are clinically useful in understanding neurologic disorders.

Supratentorial Level

The floor of the human skull (Fig. 3-2) is divided into three distinct compartments (*fossae*) on each side: anterior, middle, and posterior. A rigid membrane, the *tentorium cerebelli,* separates the ante-

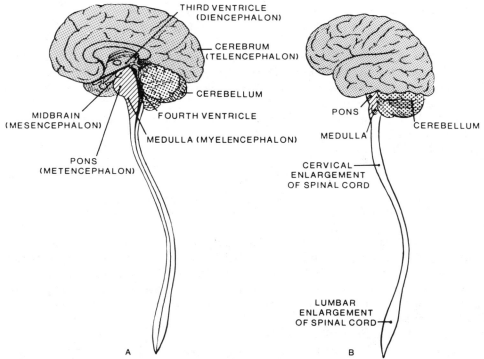

Fig. 3-1. *Medial (A) and lateral (B) views of sections through brain and spinal cord illustrating major levels: supratentorial (dark shading), posterior fossa with brain stem (lines) and cerebellum (dots), and spinal (clear area). Peripheral level is not shown.*

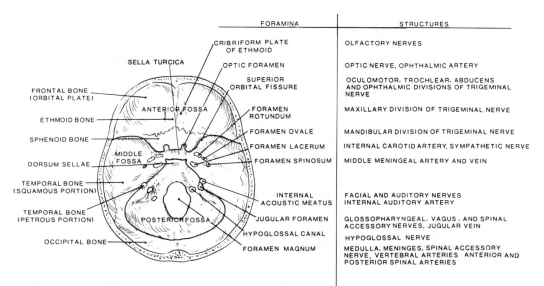

Fig. 3-2. *Base of cranial cavity, viewed from above, illustrating major cranial fossae, bones of base of skull, foramina, and their associated structures.*

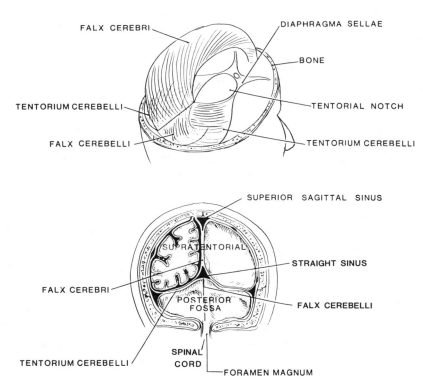

FALX CEREBRI — DIAPHRAGMA SELLAE
— BONE
TENTORIUM CEREBELLI —
— TENTORIAL NOTCH
FALX CEREBELLI —
— TENTORIUM CEREBELLI

SUPERIOR SAGITTAL SINUS
SUPRATENTORIAL
— STRAIGHT SINUS
FALX CEREBRI —
POSTERIOR FOSSA
— FALX CEREBELLI
TENTORIUM CEREBELLI —
SPINAL CORD
— FORAMEN MAGNUM

Fig. 3-3. Reflections of dura mater forming falx cerebri and tentorium cerebelli (top). Structures located above tentorium are part of supratentorial level; those below tentorium but above foramen magnum are part of posterior fossa level (bottom). (Redrawn from B. Pansky and E.L. House. Review of Gross Anatomy [3rd ed.]. New York: Macmillan, 1975.)

rior and middle fossae from the posterior fossa (Fig. 3-3). The tentorium lies in a nearly horizontal plane and attaches laterally to the petrous ridges and posteriorly to the occipital bone. The portion of the nervous system located above the tentorium cerebelli constitutes the *supratentorial level*. The major anatomic structures of this level are derivatives of the telencephalon and diencephalon and consist primarily of the cerebral hemispheres, basal ganglia, thalamus, hypothalamus, and cranial nerves I (olfactory) and II (optic).

Posterior Fossa Level

Structures located within the skull, below the tentorium cerebelli but above the *foramen magnum* (the opening of the skull to the spinal canal), constitute the *posterior fossa level*. These structures—the midbrain, pons, medulla, and cerebellum—are the derivatives of the mesencephalon, metencephalon,

and myelencephalon. Cranial nerves III through XII are located in the posterior fossa. Anatomically and physiologically, these nerves are analogous to other peripheral nerves; however, functionally they are intimately related to the mesencephalon, metencephalon, and myelencephalon and are therefore studied along with the structures of the posterior fossa. Those segments of cranial nerves contained within the bony skull are considered part of the posterior fossa level. After these nerves emerge from the skull, they are part of the peripheral level.

Spinal Level

The portion of the central nervous system located below the foramen magnum of the skull but contained within the vertebral column constitutes the *spinal level* (Fig. 3-4). This level has a considerable longitudinal extent, reaching from the skull to the sacrum. However, the spinal cord itself (the major structure at the spinal level) does not extend that entire length. A series of spinal nerves arises in the spinal canal and exits through the intervertebral foramina. Nerves contained within the bony vertebral column and within the intervertebral foramina are part of the spinal level. After these nerves leave the vertebral column, they become part of the pe-

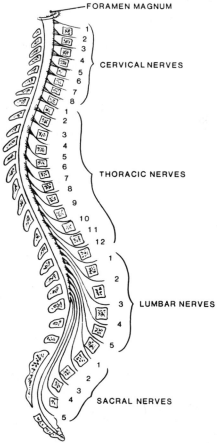

FORAMEN MAGNUM

CERVICAL NERVES

1
2
3
4
5
6
7
8

THORACIC NERVES

1
2
3
4
5
6
7
8
9
10
11
12

LUMBAR NERVES

1
2
3
4
5

SACRAL NERVES

1
2
3
4
5

Fig. 3-4. Structures at spinal level include spinal cord, nerve roots contained within vertebral column, and vertebral column itself.

ripheral level. The vertebral column itself is part of the spinal level.

Peripheral Level

The *peripheral level* includes all neuromuscular structures located outside the skull and vertebral column, including the cranial and peripheral nerves, their peripheral branches, and the structures (including muscle) that are innervated by these nerves. The autonomic ganglia and nerves are also part of the peripheral level.

Gross Neuroanatomy—Introduction to Anatomic Levels

The major anatomic features of each of the major levels of the nervous system will be reviewed. Prior to doing so, however, it is useful to discuss individually certain structures that may be related to more than one of the major levels previously defined.

The Skull

The skull (Fig. 3-5) is formed by the union of a number of bones and can be grossly subdivided into (1) the facial bones and orbits, (2) the sinus cavities within the bones that form the anterior aspect of the skull, and (3) the cranial bones. The cranial bones surround the brain in the cranial cavity and provide a nonyielding protective covering for the brain. In contrast to other protective structures in the body, the cranial bones severely limit the expansion of the brain, even when expansion becomes necessary in response to specific pathologic processes. The cranial cavity is formed by the *frontal, parietal, sphenoid, temporal,* and *occipital* bones. The bones forming the base of the cavity are shown in Figure 3-2. A roentgenogram of the skull shows the bones as lighter areas, and structures on the opposite sides of the skull are overlapped (Fig. 3-6).

When the base of the cranial cavity is viewed from above, three distinct areas are noted: the *anterior, middle,* and *posterior* fossae. In addition there are symmetrically placed holes (foramina) located in the base of the skull, through which the cranial nerves emerge to innervate peripheral structures.

Meningeal Coverings

The meninges are an important supporting element of the central nervous system and include the dura mater, arachnoid, and pia mater (Fig. 3-7). The outermost fibrous membrane, the *dura mater,* consists of two layers of connective tissue that are fused, except in certain regions where they separate to form the *intracranial venous sinuses.* The dura mater is folded into the cranial cavity in two areas to form distinct fibrous barriers: the *falx cerebri,* which is located between the two cerebral hemispheres, and the *tentorium cerebelli,* which demarcates the superior limit of the posterior fossa. The delicate, filamentous *arachnoid* lies beneath the dura mater and appears to be loosely applied to the surface of the brain. *Pacchionian granulations* (arachnoid villi) are small tufts of arachnoid, invaginated into dural venous sinuses, especially along the dorsal convexity of the cerebral hemispheres, superior to the longitudinal (interhemispheric) fissure. Many of the major arterial channels can be seen on the surface of the brain beneath the arachnoid. The innermost layer, the *pia mater,* is composed of a very thin layer of mesoderm that is so closely attached to the brain surface that it cannot be seen in gross specimens.

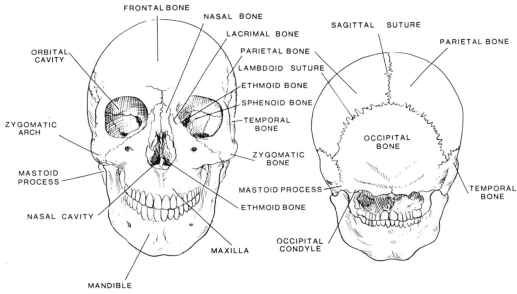

Fig. 3-5. Anterior (left) *and posterior* (right) *views illustrating major bones of skull. Hollow sinus cavities are located within frontal, ethmoid, sphenoid, and maxillary bones.*

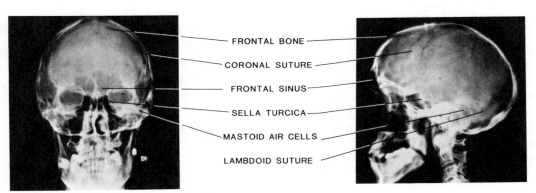

Fig. 3-6. Anterior (left) *and lateral* (right) *views illustrating major bones of skull. Air-filled sinuses and nasal cavities appear darker. Compare with Figure 3-5.*

Several important potential and actual spaces are found in association with these meningeal coverings (Fig. 3-7). Between the bone and the dura mater is the *epidural space*, and beneath the dura mater is the *subdural space*. The bone, dura, and arachnoid are normally closely applied to one another so that the epidural and subdural spaces are potential spaces in which blood or pus may accumulate. Beneath the arachnoid is the *subarachnoid space*, which surrounds the entire brain and spinal cord and which is filled with cerebrospinal fluid. The subarachnoid space communicates with the in-

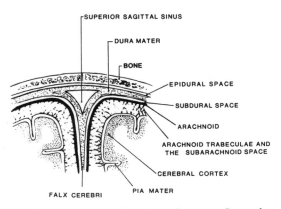

Fig. 3-7. Meninges and meningeal spaces. Coronal section through parasagittal region of cerebral hemispheres.

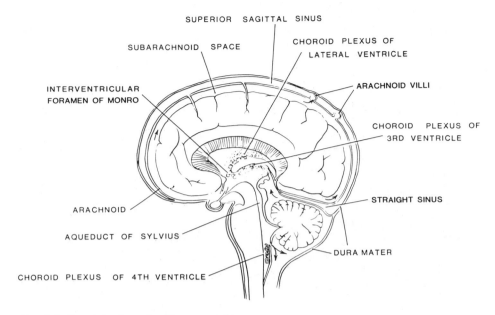

Fig. 3-8. Cranial subarachnoid space and its communication with both spinal subarachnoid space and ventricular system.

terior of the brain via the ventricular system (Fig. 3-8).

The Ventricular System

Located within the depth of the brain is the ventricular system (Fig. 3-9), a derivative of the primitive embryonic central canal. *Cerebrospinal fluid* is formed within the ventricles by the *choroid plexus* (located in each ventricle) and is circulated throughout the ventricles and subarachnoid space.

The cavity contained within each cerebral hemi-

sphere is the *lateral ventricle,* which communicates with the cavity of the diencephalon, the *third ventricle,* via the *foramen of Monro.* The caudal end of the third ventricle narrows into the cavity of the mesencephalon, the *aqueduct of Sylvius,* which leads into the *fourth ventricle.* Communication with the subarachnoid spaces is via the two lateral *foramina of Luschka* and the central *foramen of Magendie* (all contained within the fourth ventricle). The portion of the primitive central canal of the spinal cord becomes obliterated in the mature human nervous system and is usually identified only as a cluster of ependymal and glial cells in the central regions of the spinal cord.

Fig. 3-9. Ventricular system. Cerebrospinal fluid is formed by choroid plexus within ventricles. This fluid circulates and communicates with subarachnoid space via foramina of Luschka and Magendie.

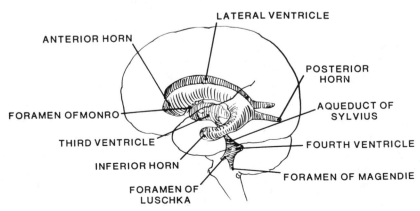

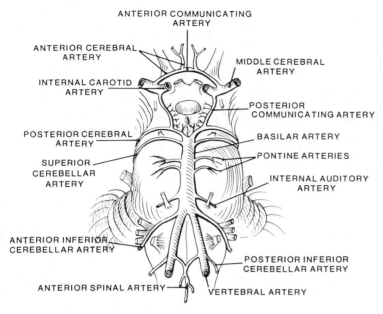

ANTERIOR COMMUNICATING ARTERY

ANTERIOR CEREBRAL ARTERY

MIDDLE CEREBRAL ARTERY

INTERNAL CAROTID ARTERY

POSTERIOR COMMUNICATING ARTERY

POSTERIOR CEREBRAL ARTERY

BASILAR ARTERY

SUPERIOR CEREBELLAR ARTERY

PONTINE ARTERIES

INTERNAL AUDITORY ARTERY

ANTERIOR INFERIOR CEREBELLAR ARTERY

POSTERIOR INFERIOR CEREBELLAR ARTERY

ANTERIOR SPINAL ARTERY

VERTEBRAL ARTERY

Fig. 3-10. Arterial supply to brain as viewed from base. Major arterial supply is via internal carotid and vertebrobasilar systems, which communicate with each other via series of anastomotic channels known as the circle of Willis.

Blood Vessels

Blood enters the skull via two arterial systems (Fig. 3-10). The brain is supplied by the posteriorly located *vertebrobasilar system* and the anteriorly located *carotid system*. A series of anastomotic channels lying at the base of the brain, known as the *circle of Willis*, permits communication between these two systems.

The *internal carotid artery* and its major branches, the *anterior cerebral* and *middle cerebral* arteries, can be seen at the base of the brain (Fig. 3-10). The anterior cerebral arteries are connected to each other by the small *anterior communicating artery* and continue in the midline between the two hemispheres to supply blood to their medial surfaces. The middle cerebral artery courses laterally between the temporal and the frontal lobes and emerges from the *insula* between the frontal and temporal lobes, where its branches spread over and supply blood to the lateral surface of the hemisphere (Fig. 3-11).

Additional blood is carried to the brain by the two *vertebral arteries,* which enter the skull via the foramen magnum and join at the caudal border of the pons to form the *basilar artery* (see Fig. 3-10). Branches from these arteries normally provide the

sole arterial supply to the occipital lobe, undersurface of the temporal lobe, thalamus, midbrain, pons, cerebellum, medulla, and portions of the cervical spinal cord. The *posterior inferior cerebellar arteries* are branches of the vertebral arteries, whereas the *anterior inferior cerebellar arteries* and *superior cerebellar arteries* are branches of the basilar artery.

The basilar artery continues cephalad until it divides into the *posterior cerebral arteries*. The *posterior communicating arteries* usually arise as branches of the posterior cerebral arteries and join those vessels with the internal carotid arteries to complete the circle of Willis.

Blood leaves the head by way of veins (Fig. 3-12) that course over the cerebral hemispheres to converge into large channels, the *venous sinuses,* contained within the layers of the dura mater. The most prominent of these sinuses are the *superior sagittal sinus* and *inferior sagittal sinus,* which run longitudinally from front to back in the falx cerebri between the hemispheres. The major venous channels merge in the occipital region and form the *transverse* and *sigmoid sinuses*, which exit through the skull via the jugular foramen as the *internal jugular veins.*

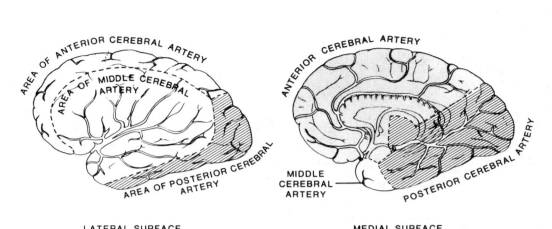

LATERAL SURFACE   MEDIAL SURFACE

Fig. 3-11. Lateral and medial surfaces of cerebral hemispheres illustrating distribution of blood supply of major arteries. Anterior and middle cerebral arteries are branches of internal carotid arteries; posterior cerebral arteries are branches of basilar artery. (Redrawn from B. Pansky and E.L. House. Review of Gross Anatomy *[3rd ed.]. New York: Macmillan, 1975.)*

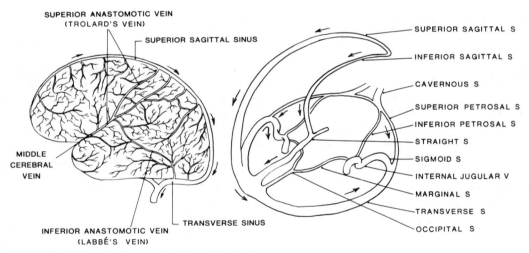

Fig. 3-12. Venous drainage of cerebral hemispheres. Blood circulating over cortex collects in superior sagittal sinus (left); blood from deeper structures enters other venous sinuses (right). Direction of flow is toward confluence of sinuses in occipital region and then toward internal jugular veins by way of transverse and sigmoid sinuses. (S = sinus; V = vein.) (Redrawn from B. Pansky and E.L. House. Review of Gross Anatomy *[3rd ed.]. New York: Macmillan, 1975.)*

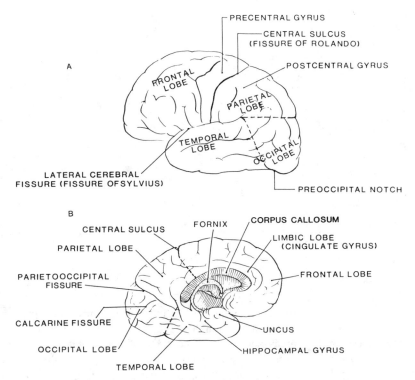

Fig. 3-13. Lateral (A) and medial (B) surfaces of cerebral hemispheres illustrating major gyri and sulci and division of hemispheres into five major lobes: frontal, parietal, temporal, occipital, and limbic.

The Supratentorial Level

The major structures at the supratentorial level are the telencephalic derivatives (the cerebral hemispheres), the diencephalon, and cranial nerves I and II.

CEREBRAL HEMISPHERES.   Through a process of growth and proliferation, the telencephalic structures differentiate into the cerebral hemispheres. The *longitudinal (interhemispheric) fissure* separates the cerebrum into two cerebral hemispheres. The surface of each hemisphere is convoluted: the folds are known as *gyri* and are separated from one another by grooves or *sulci*. Certain grooves are more prominent, deeper, and more constant and are known as *fissures*. The fissures must be identified in order to locate the four major lobes into which each hemisphere is divided: *frontal, parietal, temporal*, and *occipital*. As shown in Figure 3-13, the following serve as important landmarks in defining the limits of each lobe: *lateral fissure (fissure of Sylvius), central sulcus (fissure of Rolando), parietooccipital fissure*, and *preoccipital notch*. The

calcarine fissure divides the occipital lobe. Within the fissure of Sylvius is buried a portion of the cortex known as the *insula*. The central sulcus separates the *precentral gyrus* of the frontal lobe from the *postcentral gyrus* of the parietal lobe. A line drawn from the end of the fissure of Sylvius to the preoccipital notch serves to demarcate the limits of the temporal lobe, whereas a similar line from the preoccipital notch to the parietooccipital fissure delineates the occipital lobe.

Certain structures, best seen on the mesial surface of the hemispheres, are not included within the traditional division of the brain into four lobes. The *corpus callosum* represents a prominent fiber tract for transfer of information from one hemisphere to another. A number of the remaining prominent structures seen on the mesial surface have been found to be functionally and anatomically related to the processing of memory and emotion. These structures have been grouped into a fifth lobe of the brain, the *limbic lobe* (Fig. 3-13). Some of the major structures within this lobe are the *uncus* (located on the medial aspect of the temporal lobe), the *hip-*

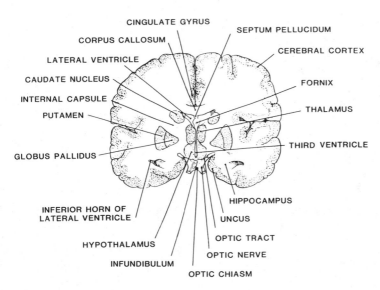

Fig. 3-14. Coronal section through cerebral hemispheres. The gray matter is shown as stippled area.

pocampal gyrus (also on the medial temporal lobe), the *fornix* (a fiber bundle connecting the hypothalamus with the hippocampus), and the *cingulate gyrus* (located above the corpus callosum).

A coronal (Fig. 3-14) and a horizontal (Fig. 3-15) section through the cerebrum reveal several important structures within the substance of the brain. Computed tomographic (CT) scans usually show the brain in horizontal sections (see Fig. 6-17). The

two lateral ventricles and the third ventricle occupy a central position. The *gray matter* (mainly nuclear areas and cerebral cortex) and *white matter* (regions where fiber tracts are traveling) can be differentiated. Several distinct, large gray nuclear masses can be seen. The *thalamus* (an important relay nucleus for the motor and sensory systems) is located lateral to the third ventricle. The *basal ganglia*, composed of the *caudate nucleus*, *putamen*, and *globus pallidus*, are all part of the motor system. A large and important area of white matter, the

Fig. 3-15. Horizontal section through cerebral hemispheres at the level of the thalamus (right); areas of gray matter are stippled. The cerebellum beneath the occipital lobes can be seen in the midline. Computed tomographic scan (left) is through the hemispheres at a slightly different angle. Bone, falx, and choroid calcification are white on CT.

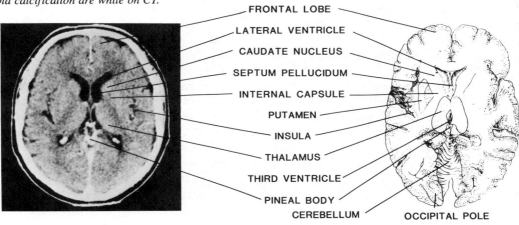

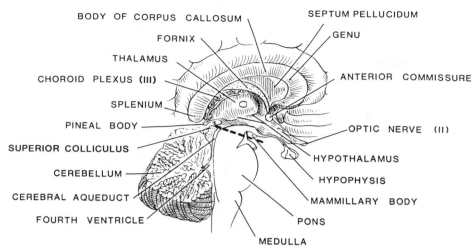

Fig. 3-16. Median sagittal section through diencephalon, brain stem, and cerebellum. Dotted line above level of superior colliculus separates supratentorial and posterior fossa levels.

internal capsule, passes between these central nuclear masses and transfers information between the *cerebral cortex* and the lower structures.

DIENCEPHALON. The diencephalon represents a zone of transition between the cerebrum at the supratentorial level and those structures in the posterior fossa. The diencephalon consists of the *third ventricle* and those structures related to it, including the *thalamus, hypothalamus, optic pathways,* and *pineal body* (Fig. 3-16). At the base of the hypothalamus is an important neuroendocrine structure, the *hypophysis* or *pituitary gland*. It is located in the middle of the skull in the bony sella turcica. All these structures are at the supratentorial level.

CRANIAL NERVES I AND II. The *olfactory bulb* and *tract* (I) are located at the base of each frontal lobe. The olfactory nerves are filaments passing from the nasal cavity through the cribriform plate to connect to the olfactory bulb. The *optic nerves* (II) develop as an outgrowth from the primitive diencephalon. The optic pathway from the orbit consists of the *optic nerve, optic chiasm*, and *optic tract*. The intracranial portions of these nerves are at the supratentorial level.

The Posterior Fossa Level
The major structures contained within this level are the *brain stem*, the cerebellum, and the origins of cranial nerves III through XII.

BRAIN STEM. The term *brain stem* is not a precise anatomic term and therefore has been defined in different ways. However, the term is so commonly used in neurologic discussions that one must be familiar with it. As defined herein, the *brain stem* consists of the portion of the brain that remains after removal of the cerebral and cerebellar hemispheres (see Fig. 3-1). Cephalad from the spinal cord, the brain stem includes the *medulla oblongata* (myelencephalon), *pons* (metencephalon), and *midbrain* (mesencephalon). Only the pontine portion of the metencephalon is part of the brain stem; the cerebellum is excluded. The upper portion of the brain stem is continuous with the diencephalon, where overlapping structures make precise definition difficult. In this text, the diencephalon is not included as a part of the brain stem; the *superior colliculus* is used to demarcate the upper border of the brain stem. The *red nucleus* and the substantia nigra are both present in the upper mesencephalon and extend into the posterior diencephalon, thereby overlapping the supratentorial and posterior fossa levels.

The longitudinal separation of the brain stem into midbrain, pons, and medulla is made primarily by a large bundle of prominent crossing fibers on the ventral and lateral surfaces of the brain stem that connect the brain stem to the cerebellum (Fig. 3-17). These fibers demarcate the extent of the pons. The medulla is immediately caudal, and the midbrain is cephalad to these fibers. The brain stem at

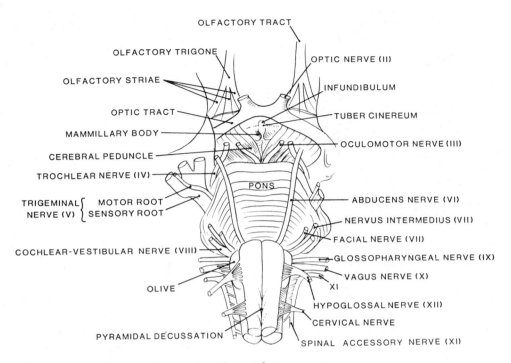

OLFACTORY TRACT

OLFACTORY TRIGONE

OLFACTORY STRIAE

OPTIC TRACT

MAMMILLARY BODY

CEREBRAL PEDUNCLE

TROCHLEAR NERVE (IV)

TRIGEMINAL { MOTOR ROOT
NERVE (V) { SENSORY ROOT

COCHLEAR-VESTIBULAR NERVE (VIII)

OLIVE

PYRAMIDAL DECUSSATION

OPTIC NERVE (II)

INFUNDIBULUM

TUBER CINEREUM

OCULOMOTOR NERVE (III)

PONS

ABDUCENS NERVE (VI)

NERVUS INTERMEDIUS (VII)

FACIAL NERVE (VII)

GLOSSOPHARYNGEAL NERVE (IX)

VAGUS NERVE (X)

XI

HYPOGLOSSAL NERVE (XII)

CERVICAL NERVE

SPINAL ACCESSORY NERVE (XI)

Fig. 3-17. Ventral aspect of brain stem and cranial nerves. Cranial nerve I is not shown. It ends at the olfactory bulb, from which the olfactory tract arises. Cranial nerves I and II arise at the supratentorial level; cranial nerves III through XII arise in the posterior fossa. (Redrawn from B. Pansky and E.L. House. Review of Gross Anatomy *[3rd ed.]. New York: Macmillan, 1975.)*

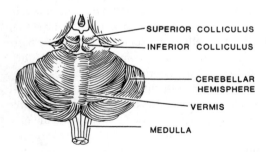

SUPERIOR COLLICULUS

INFERIOR COLLICULUS

CEREBELLAR HEMISPHERE

VERMIS

MEDULLA

Fig. 3-18. Cerebellum as viewed from its dorsal surface.

the midbrain and pons is divided dorsoventrally into three regions. The area dorsal to the aqueduct of Sylvius is the *tectum*, whose major structures are the superior and inferior colliculi (corpora quadrigemina). The area of multiple nuclei and intermingled pathways ventral to the aqueduct and fourth ventricle is the *tegmentum*. The large distinct cerebral and cerebellar white matter pathways in the most ventral regions below the tegmentum make up the *base* or *basal region* of the midbrain and pons.

CEREBELLUM. The cerebellum consists of two *hemispheres* and a midline *vermis* (Fig. 3-18). The cerebellar surface is much more highly convoluted than is the surface of the cerebrum, with folds known as *folia*. The cerebellum is metencephalic in derivation and therefore is associated structurally with the pons. The cerebellum lies dorsal to the fourth ventricle, the pons, and the medulla.

CRANIAL NERVES III THROUGH XII. Emerging from the brain stem are 10 pairs of nerves, which can be identified in Figure 3-17. (Cranial nerves I and II are *not* contained within the posterior fossa.) The names, location, and general function of all the cranial nerves are summarized in Table 3-1.

The Spinal Level

The major structures contained within this level are the spinal cord, the origins of the spinal nerves within the vertebral column, and the vertebral column itself.

The *spinal cord* is surrounded by meninges similar to those that surround the brain (Fig. 3-19). Outside the dura mater is the *epidural space*, an actual space that contains fat and venous plexuses. The *arachnoid* adjacent to the inner surface of the dura

Table 3-1. Location and General Function of the Cranial Nerves

Nerve	Anatomic relationship	Function
I Olfactory	Cerebral hemispheres	Smell
II Optic	Diencephalon, cerebral hemispheres	Vision
III Oculomotor	Midbrain	Eye movement
IV Trochlear	Midbrain	Eye movement
V Trigeminal	Pons	Facial sensation, jaw movement
VI Abducens	Pons	Eye movement
VII Facial	Pons	Facial movement
VIII Cochlear-vestibular	Pons, medulla	Hearing and balance
IX Glossopharyngeal	Medulla	Throat movement
X Vagus	Medulla	Throat and larynx movement, and control of visceral organs
XI Spinal accessory	Medulla, spinal cord	Shoulder and neck movement
XII Hypoglossal	Medulla	Tongue movement

mater forms the subarachnoid space, which contains the cerebrospinal fluid. The spinal *pia mater* is closely applied to the surface of the spinal cord but is visible as the *dentate ligaments* extending on either side between the origins of the spinal nerve roots. These ligaments join the arachnoid at intervals and are inserted into the dura mater. The dural sac and *subarachnoid space* end at the level of the second sacral vertebra (Fig. 3-20). The pia mater continues caudally as a filamentous membrane (the *filum terminale*) from the end of the spinal cord (the *conus medullaris*). It fuses with the dural sac at the second sacral vertebral level and is attached to the dorsal surface of the coccyx as the *sacrococcygeal ligament*.

The adult spinal cord begins rostrally from the caudal margin of the medulla at the level of the foramen magnum and terminates opposite the cau-

Fig. 3-19. Cross sections of vertebral column at cervical and lumbar vertebral levels. (Redrawn from B. Pansky and E.L. House. Review of Gross Anatomy *[3rd ed.]. New York: Macmillan, 1975.)*

dal margin of the first lumbar vertebra. The spinal cord, therefore, does *not* extend the entire length of the spinal canal. Throughout much of the length of the cord a spinal segment is *not* adjacent to its corresponding vertebral segment.

The spinal cord exhibits *cervical* and *lumbosacral enlargements*. Cross section shows a relative increase in gray matter in these two regions, to account for the relative enlargement in these areas. Thirty-one pairs of *spinal nerves* are attached to the spinal cord via *dorsal* (posterior) and *ventral* (anterior) *nerve roots*. Segmentally there are 8 cervical, 12 thoracic, 5 lumbar, 5 sacral, and 1 coccygeal spinal nerve on each side. At their origins, the nerve roots consist of multiple filaments, which, on the posterior (dorsal) surface of the cord, exit from a relatively constant groove, the *posterior lateral sulcus*. The dorsal and ventral roots of each spinal nerve join as they enter the intervertebral foramen of the spine. After leaving the spinal cord, the roots of the lumbar and sacral spinal nerves run caudally a number of segments toward their exit. The collec-

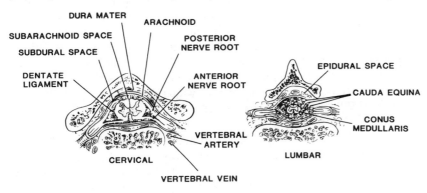

DURA MATER
ARACHNOID
SUBARACHNOID SPACE
SUBDURAL SPACE
POSTERIOR NERVE ROOT
DENTATE LIGAMENT
ANTERIOR NERVE ROOT
EPIDURAL SPACE
CAUDA EQUINA
CONUS MEDULLARIS
VERTEBRAL ARTERY
CERVICAL
VERTEBRAL VEIN
LUMBAR

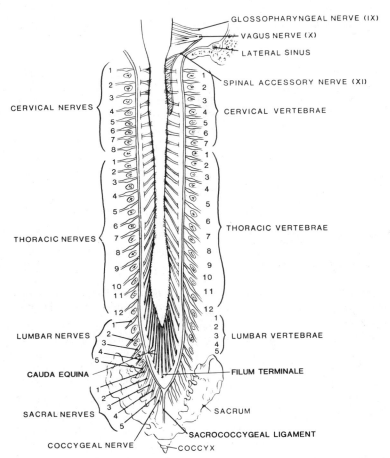

GLOSSOPHARYNGEAL NERVE (IX)

VAGUS NERVE (X)

LATERAL SINUS

SPINAL ACCESSORY NERVE (XI)

CERVICAL NERVES

CERVICAL VERTEBRAE

THORACIC NERVES

THORACIC VERTEBRAE

LUMBAR NERVES

LUMBAR VERTEBRAE

CAUDA EQUINA

FILUM TERMINALE

SACRAL NERVES

SACRUM

COCCYGEAL NERVE

SACROCOCCYGEAL LIGAMENT

COCCYX

Fig. 3-20. Dorsal view of spinal level. Note spinal cord itself terminates between the L-1 and L-2 vertebrae. Caudal end of spinal cord is conus medullaris, and collection of nerve roots in lumbar region is cauda equina. (Redrawn from B. Pansky and E.L. House. Review of Gross Anatomy [3rd ed.]. New York: Macmillan, 1975.)

tion of spinal nerve roots contained within the lumbosacral spinal canal is known as the *cauda equina* (see Fig. 3-19). Although most of the spinal nerves have both a ventral (motor) and a dorsal (sensory) root, often the first cervical nerve has only a motor root, while the first coccygeal nerve and the fifth sacral nerve have only a sensory root. Surrounding the spinal cord is the *vertebral column*, consisting of 7 cervical, 12 thoracic, and 5 lumbar vertebrae, the fused sacrum, and the coccyx (Fig. 3-20).

The Peripheral Level
The major structures of the peripheral level are the somatic nerves, the autonomic nerves and ganglia, the neuromuscular junction, the muscles of the

skeleton, and the peripheral sensory receptors. The spinal nerves, as they emerge from the vertebral column, enter the peripheral level. These spinal nerves, which were formed by the joining of dorsal and ventral roots, contain somatic and autonomic motor and sensory nerve fibers and branch into posterior and anterior divisions as they enter the peripheral level. Fibers of the anterior divisions en route to the limbs gather together and are rearranged in plexuses. The *brachial plexus,* located in the axillary region, redistributes the fibers to the major nerves of the upper extremities: median, ulnar, radial, axillary, and musculocutaneous. The *lumbosacral plexus,* located in the lower abdominal cavity and pelvis, redistributes the fibers to the major nerves in the lower extremities: femoral, obturator, and sciatic, which divides into the tibial and peroneal nerves.

Gross Neuroanatomy—Introduction to the Longitudinal Systems
The gross anatomic features of each of the major levels have been reviewed. At this point, some of

these same structures should be related to the major longitudinal systems, which will be studied in further detail in subsequent chapters.

The Cerebrospinal Fluid System

Structures included in the cerebrospinal fluid system are the meninges (dura, pia, and arachnoid), meningeal spaces (epidural, subdural, and subarachnoid), the ventricular system, and the cerebrospinal fluid. This system, present at the supratentorial, posterior fossa, and spinal levels, provides both cushioning and buffering for the central nervous system and helps maintain a stable environment for neural function.

The Sensory System

This system receives somatosensory information from the external environment and transmits it to the central nervous system (afferent), where it can be processed and utilized for adaptive behavior. Elements of the somatosensory system are found at all major levels and include the peripheral receptor organs; afferent fibers traveling in cranial, peripheral, and spinal nerves; dorsal root ganglia; ascending pathways in the spinal cord and brain stem; portions of the thalamus; and the thalamocortical radiations that terminate primarily in the sensory cortex of the parietal lobe. In addition, structures related to the special sensory systems (vision, taste, smell, hearing, and balance) are located at the supratentorial, posterior fossa, and peripheral levels.

The Consciousness System

Functioning as an additional afferent system, the consciousness system allows a person to selectively attend to and perceive isolated stimuli and maintains various levels of wakefulness, awareness, and consciousness. Structures contained within this system are found only at the posterior fossa and supratentorial levels and include portions of the central core of the brain stem and diencephalon (reticular formation and ascending projectional pathways), portions of the thalamus, and pathways that project diffusely to widespread areas of cerebral cortex. All lobes of the brain are part of this system.

The Motor System

The motor system initiates and controls activity in the somatic muscles via efferent connections of the motor cortex and other areas of the frontal lobes; descending pathways that traverse the internal capsule, cerebral peduncles, medullary pyramids, and other areas of the brain stem; portions of the spinal cord, including the ventral horns; ventral roots; efferent fibers traveling in both peripheral and cranial nerves; and muscle, the major effector organ of the motor system. Also included in this system are the cerebellum and basal ganglia and related pathways. The motor system is thus present at all major levels and is directly involved in the performance of all motor activity mediated by striated musculature.

The Visceral System

The visceral system is composed of the structures in the nervous system that regulate the function of visceral glands and organs. It contains both afferent and efferent components which interact to maintain the internal environment (homeostasis). The system has major representation at all levels of the nervous system. Important structures include areas of the limbic lobe and hypothalamus (supratentorial); the reticular formation and fibers traveling in cranial nerves (posterior fossa); longitudinal pathways in the spinal cord and brain stem; and numerous ganglia, receptors, and effectors found at the peripheral level.

The Vascular System

Each organ in the body must have blood vessels to provide a relatively constant supply of oxygen and other nutrients as well as a means for removal of metabolic wastes. The vascular system is therefore found at all major levels of the nervous system and includes the arteries, arterioles, capillaries, veins, and dural sinuses. These supply supratentorial, posterior fossa, spinal, and peripheral nervous system structures.

Clinical Correlations

Neurologic diagnosis includes identification of the anatomic location and pathology of the disorder. Through the utilization of problem-solving skills that are already familiar, and the assignment of some functional significance to the anatomic structures discussed in this chapter, the reader can begin to solve clinical neurologic problems by identifying the anatomic location.

In certain respects, an analogy may be drawn between the nervous system and an electrical circuit. The nervous system may be considered to be a series of electrical cables laid out in a specific plan (Fig. 3-21). Leading to and from the cerebral hemispheres are two parallel cables (representing a lon-

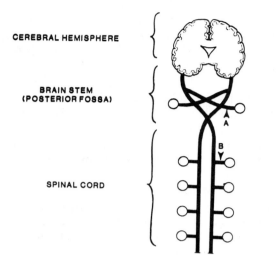

Fig. 3-21. Major nervous system connections. (A = cranial nerves; B = *peripheral nerves.) Note long intersegmental pathways leading to and from higher centers and multiple, short segmental pathways (cranial and peripheral nerves) to the peripheral level.*

gitudinal system) that conduct impulses from one segment to another. Scattered along these *intersegmental* cables are several smaller branching *segmental* wires. As in basic electricity, damage (a lesion) anywhere along the course of the main inter-

segmental cables will cause malfunction in all areas beyond that point, whereas damage to the segmental wires will cause malfunction only within that specific segment. In applying this analogy to humans, we note that the higher centers exert control or receive information from the body segments through long *intersegmental pathways* and that one side of the brain is associated with function on the *opposite* side of the body.

Anatomic diagnosis first requires the ability to relate the patient's signs and symptoms to specific longitudinal systems within the nervous system. Neurologic diagnosis relies mainly on the symptoms of dysfunction in the sensory, motor, and consciousness systems, whose organization is similar to the schematic pathways seen in Figure 3-21. Symptoms of dysfunction in the sensory system consist of altered sensation, described by the patient as pain, numbness, tingling, or loss of sensation. Symptoms of dysfunction in the motor system consist primarily of weakness, paralysis, incoordination, shaking, or jerking. Lesions of the consciousness system, which is located only at the supratentorial and posterior fossa levels, are expressed as altered states of consciousness and coma. The presence of any of these or related symptoms identifies the longitudinal system involved in a disease.

Localization is determined by the level of the

Fig. 3-22. Summary of functions associated with the major anatomic levels.

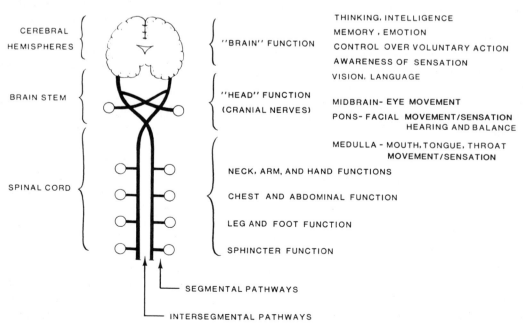

nervous system in which the pathway function is interrupted. To aid in localization, the functions of each of the major anatomic levels are described in the following sections and are schematically represented in Figure 3-22.

Peripheral Level

The spinal and cranial nerves, after they emerge from the vertebral column and skull, and the structures they innervate, constitute the major components of the peripheral level. Each emerging nerve defines a specific *segment*. A lesion in one of these pathways alters all function within that segment but has no effect on functions carried to and from other segments. Thus, in the presence of a peripheral lesion, *loss of sensation and muscle weakness* in a focal area are common. Often, peripheral nerve damage is not complete and the sensation of *pain* is produced. Therefore, in addition to sensory loss and weakness, pain in a segmental distribution is an important clue to a lesion at the peripheral level.

Spinal Level

The spinal cord has two functions. It is the structure from which individual segments of the limbs and trunk originate, and it transmits information to and from higher centers. Therefore, lesions at the spinal level may alter *segmental* functions in the region of the abnormality and alter *intersegmental* function below the lesion. Except in complete transections of the spinal cord, all functions are not altered equally; however, even under those circumstances, the characteristic combination of segmental loss of function at the site of the lesion and intersegmental loss below it usually can be identified.

The spinal cord is a narrow structure that contains the major intersegmental pathways for both sides of the neuraxis (nervous system). Therefore, in spinal lesions, bilateral involvement from a single focal lesion is not uncommon. Furthermore, because of the length of the spinal column, specific segmental functions can be assigned to certain areas of it. The upper portion (cervical) is related primarily to arm function, the midportion (thoracic) to the trunk, the lower portion (lumbar) to the legs, and the lowermost area (sacral) to anal-genital-urinary functions.

Posterior Fossa Level

The cranial nerves mediate segmental function for the head and arise in the posterior fossa. Lesions at the posterior fossa level therefore will produce segmental and intersegmental disturbances, just as occur at the spinal level. The *segmental* nerves of the brain stem are the cranial nerves, which control movement and sensation in the head (see Table 3-1). Brain-stem lesions often will alter these segmental functions. In addition, since the brain stem is also an area where intersegmental pathways cross, or have crossed, to the opposite side of the brain, a characteristic pattern is often seen with focal lesions. Lesions of the posterior fossa will cause loss of segmental head function *ipsilateral* (same side) to the lesion; if the lesion also involves intersegmental pathways, it will cause loss of intersegmental function on the side of the body *contralateral* (opposite) to the lesion (Fig. 3-22). Extensive lesions in the brain stem may affect the consciousness system and produce coma.

Supratentorial Level

Each cerebral hemisphere exerts its control over the opposite side of the body. Therefore, supratentorial lesions are associated with loss of intersegmental sensory or motor function on the opposite side of the body. In addition, some functions are associated almost exclusively with the supratentorial level and may be considered segmental functions of this level. These functions are language (almost always localized to the left side of the brain), memory, intelligence, cognition, olfaction, and vision. When abnormal, they serve to further localize the disorder to the supratentorial level (Fig. 3-22). Extensive lesions involving the structures of the supratentorial level may alter consciousness and produce coma.

Precise localization is possible when an area can be identified where both segmental and intersegmental functions are altered in one or more systems.

The major features to be determined in the anatomic diagnosis of neurologic disorders are whether:

1. The responsible lesion is *focal*, strictly confined to a single well-circumscribed area. If the lesion is focal, the *anatomic level* and whether the abnormality is located on the right or left or in the midline of the nervous system must be defined.
2. The responsible lesion is *diffuse* and nonfocal. A diffuse lesion may involve only a single level or may involve multiple levels. In general, a le-

sion is considered to be diffuse if it involves bilateral regions in the nervous system without extending across the midline as a single, circumscribed lesion.

Objectives

1. Define the boundaries of the major anatomic levels (supratentorial, posterior fossa, spinal, and peripheral), and identify on gross specimen, photograph, or other reproduction the major anatomic structures contained in each level.
2. Given a cross-section specimen, drawing, or reproduction, identify the approximate area of the neuraxis to which the specimen belongs (that is, cerebral hemisphere; mesencephalon; pons; medulla; cerebellum; cervical, thoracic, lumbar, or sacral spinal cord).
3. Given a clinical problem, answer the following two questions:
   a. The signs and symptoms contained in the protocol are most likely the manifestation of disease at which of the following *levels* of the nervous system?
      (1) Supratentorial level
      (2) Posterior fossa level
      (3) Spinal level
      (4) Peripheral level
      (5) More than one level
   b. Within the level you have selected, the responsible lesion is most likely:
      (1) Focal, on the *right* side of the nervous system
      (2) Focal, on the *left* side of the nervous system
      (3) Focal, but involving the *midline* and *contiguous* structures on both sides of the nervous system
      (4) Nonfocal and diffusely located

Clinical Problems

The following is a series of case histories of neurologic disorders. The problems were selected to illustrate examples of involvement in different regions of the nervous system. Read each history carefully. On the basis of the information presented, try to localize the lesion in accordance with the objectives above. When you have arrived at a conclusion for each case, review the pertinent anatomic structures in that area.

1. A 19-year-old man was involved in an automobile accident 4 months earlier. He sustained only minor bruises about the head and face. When he returned to school in the fall, he seemed to be uninterested in his schoolwork and began to complain of headaches. He dragged his right foot when he walked and used his right hand clumsily. He had a slight droop to the right side of his face. (Answers refer to items under a and b of objective 3.)
2. A 68-year-old man awakened one morning and noted that he was unable to speak clearly. He wanted to ask for help but could utter only the words "go now." His wife noted some weakness of the right side of his face and right arm and leg. He seemed unable to answer the questions that his wife posed to him.
3. A 26-year-old man awoke and noted that all the muscles on the left side of his face seemed to be paralyzed. Sensation was normal, although he was aware of an inability to taste on the left side of his tongue. He had no other difficulties. Six weeks later, he noted gradual and continued improvement.
4. A 42-year-old man noted, over a period of several years, the onset of ringing in his right ear and loss of hearing in that ear. In addition, he experienced right facial weakness and decreased sensation. In the weeks before his examination, he noted stiffness and weakness of his left arm and leg.
5. A 24-year-old woman was involved in an automobile accident. When examined, she had complete loss of sensation from the arms downward. She could not move her hands or legs and had no sensation below the armpits. She was incontinent.
6. For no apparent reason, a 64-year-old woman began to experience pain beginning in her back and encircling the right side of her chest about the level of her breast. A rash later appeared in the same distribution. She continued to have pain in that region, and sensation in that region was greatly diminished.
7. The patient, a 46-year-old woman, described a pain that was similar to the one noted in problem 6. The pain involved the left side of her chest. (No rash was present.) Her symptoms increased over several months but remained localized in a rather circumscribed region of her chest. She

was concerned about "heart trouble." In addition, she complained of difficulty in walking. Her left leg seemed to be weak and stiff, and at times the left leg felt "numb."

Suggested Reading

Brodal, A. *Neurological Anatomy in Relation to Clinical Medicine* (3rd ed.). New York: Oxford University Press, 1981.

DeArmond, S. J., Fusco, M. M., and Dewey, M. M. *Structure of the Human Brain: A Photographic Atlas* (2nd ed.). New York: Oxford University Press, 1976.

Heimer, L. *The Human Brain and Spinal Cord: Functional Neuroanatomy and Dissection Guide*. New York: Springer-Verlag, 1983.

Moyer, K. E. *Neuroanatomy*. New York: Harper & Row, 1980.

Netter, F. *Ciba Collection of Medical Illustrations*. Vol. 1: *The Nervous System*. Part I: Anatomy and Physiology, 1962.

Villiger, E. *Atlas of Cross Section Anatomy of the Brain*. New York: Blakiston, 1951.

Watson, C. *Basic Human Neuroanatomy. An Introductory Atlas* (2nd ed.). Boston: Little, Brown, 1977.

Diagnosis of Neurologic Disorders: Neurocytology and the Pathologic Reactions of the Nervous System

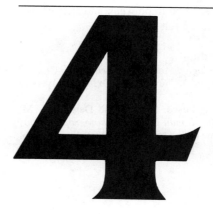

The principles of anatomic localization have been introduced in Chapter 3. Anatomic localization, however, is but one part of the diagnosis of neurologic disorders; it is also necessary to determine the pathologic features of the lesion involved. Identification of the pathology requires knowledge of the cellular elements of the nervous system (neurocytology) and the ways in which these cells react to noxious stimuli (pathologic reactions).

Two major parameters must be considered in describing lesions of the nervous system:

1. The topography of the lesion. The anatomic location of the pathologic process and a judgment as to whether the abnormality is
   a. *Focal.* Strictly confined to a single circumscribed anatomic area.
   b. *Diffuse.* Distributed over wide areas of the nervous system. A diffuse lesion may involve only a single level (for example, supratentorial or spinal level), or it may be distributed over multiple levels. A diffuse lesion involves bilaterally symmetric areas in the nervous system, without extending across the midline as a single, circumscribed lesion.
2. The morphology of the lesion. The gross and histologic appearance of the abnormal area and a judgment as to whether the pathologic process is
   a. *Nonmass.* One that is altering cellular function in the area of the lesion but is not significantly interfering with neighboring cell performance. In this type of lesion, the pathologic process is not, by virtue of its size or volume, compressing, destroying, or damaging nearby structures.
   b. *Mass.* One that not only alters cellular function in the area of the lesion but also is of sufficient size and volume to interfere with neighboring cell functions by compressing, destroying, or altering nearby cells.

Integration of the *topographic* and *morphologic* descriptions provides a precise pathologic diagnosis. When patients are examined clinically, tissue is not available for study, yet on the basis of the signs and symptoms and their evolution, the nature of the responsible pathologic lesion can be deduced. This chapter will provide the information necessary to accomplish that task.

Overview

The nervous system is composed of neurons, supporting cells of neuroectodermal origin, and supporting cells of mesodermal origin. *Neurons* are derived solely from ectoderm and are the functional units of the nervous system, capable of generating and conducting the electrical activity that underlies nervous system performance. Mature neurons do not undergo proliferation; therefore most disease processes that affect neurons produce only neuronal degeneration and loss.

The *supporting cells of neuroectodermal origin* are the oligodendroglia, Schwann cells, astrocytes, and ependymal cells. *Oligodendroglial cells* are responsible for the formation of the myelin sheaths that invest and surround axons in the central nervous system, while *Schwann cells* serve a similar function in the peripheral nervous system. Disease processes affecting these cells are associated with myelin breakdown and loss (demyelination). *Astrocytes* are widely distributed throughout the central nervous system, lie near both the neurons and the blood vessels, and thus help to provide much of the metabolic support of neural elements. Disease processes are often associated with astrocytic proliferation, which results in gliosis, the scar tissue of the central nervous system. Astrocytes also may react to metabolic disturbances in more specific ways. *Ependymal cells* line the entire ventricular system and provide a selective barrier between the ventricular fluid and the brain substance. Noxious stimuli may produce a loss of ependymal cells. Epithelium of the choroid plexus is a derivative of the ependyma and has an important role in the formation of cerebrospinal fluid.

The *supporting cells of mesodermal origin* are microglia and connective tissue cells. *Microglia* migrate into the central nervous system, and although normally present in small numbers, they can proliferate rapidly to become scavenger cells, or *macrophages*, which remove damaged tissue. With the exception of vascular structures, the parenchyma of the brain is almost devoid of elements of *connective tissue;* however, the nervous system is surrounded by the meninges, which are of mesodermal, connective tissue origin.

Disease processes may affect one or more of

these cytologic elements, and differences in their histologic features form the morphologic basis for the various clinical features of neurologic diseases. The signs and symptoms produced by these disorders reflect the anatomic location and histologic evolution (temporal profile) of the underlying pathologic lesion.

Degenerative disorders are characterized by a gradual neuronal damage in widespread areas of the nervous system, and therefore are seen clinically as chronic, progressive, and diffuse diseases. *Neoplastic disorders* present clinically as chronic, focal, progressive disorders. Any cell type in the nervous system can undergo neoplastic change to form a gradually enlarging, localized mass of proliferating cells (a neoplasm).

Vascular diseases may be of several pathologic types, but they all are associated with sudden alteration in structure and function. Therefore, disorders of this etiologic category are always acute in onset, but they may be either focal (infarct, intracerebral hemorrhage) or diffuse (subarachnoid hemorrhage, anoxic encephalopathy) in distribution. Because foreign pathogens invading the nervous system generally produce a rapid but not immediate cellular response, *inflammatory disease*, which may be either focal (abscess) or diffuse (meningitis, encephalitis), commonly presents as a progressive, subacute disorder.

Toxic or metabolic diseases alter neural function over widespread areas and therefore present with diffuse signs and symptoms. However, depending on the responsible agent, the resultant symptoms may make their appearance as acute, subacute, or chronic disorders. *Traumatic lesions* of the nervous system usually are focal and of acute onset, reflecting the effects of the immediate damage of tissue produced by the offending agent. At times, however, delayed effects of a traumatic lesion may produce clinical symptoms and present a pattern of a chronic, progressive lesion.

Structural Elements of the Nervous System

The nervous system is composed of three basic categories of cells: (1) nerve cells, called *neurons*, which are the major functional units of the nervous system; (2) supporting cells of neuroectodermal origin (oligodendroglia, Schwann cells, astrocytes, and ependymal cells); and (3) supporting cells of mesodermal origin (microglia and connective tissue elements).

The first two categories of cells, the neurons and the supporting cells of neuroectodermal origin, are derived from the primitive neuroepithelium that lines the neural tube and from the cells of the neural crest. The processes of differentiation and migration followed by these cells are outlined in Chapter 2. The third category, mesodermal supporting tissue, is derived from the mesoderm that surrounds the neural tube during development.

The structure of these cells and their interrelationships have been studied extensively at the light microscopic and electron microscopic levels. Any description of their microscopic appearance, therefore, must include a statement of the method on which the description is based. Nerve tissue is routinely studied at the light microscopic level by using thin sections of tissue to which stains are applied. Stains have been developed that will emphasize certain features of cells while obscuring others. Some of these stains are dyes that react with and bind to certain chemical groups in the tissue, rendering them colored. Other stains are salts of heavy metals, especially silver salts, which undergo a physicochemical reaction with and "impregnate" certain structural elements in the tissue. Table 4-1 outlines the uses of some of the stains commonly employed in the study of nerve tissue.

Neurons

The neuron is the most important structural element of the nervous system because it generates and conducts the electrical activity that is associated with the function of the nervous system.

Unlike most other cells of the body, normal nerve cells in the fully developed human do not undergo division and replication. Neurons vary greatly in their size and shape from one region of the nervous system to another (Fig. 4-1).

However, they possess certain common features that are most readily demonstrated in the largest neurons; for example, the large motor neurons of the anterior horns of the spinal cord (Figs. 4-2, 4-3). In routine preparations, the cell bodies of these neurons, which may be 100 μm in diameter, are irregular in outline because of the numerous processes that extend outward from the cell body at irregular intervals. Neurons possess a large nucleus within which a conspicuous nucleolus can be found. Otherwise the nucleus appears to be relatively clear, or vesicular, because of the dispersion of the nuclear chromatin. The cytoplasm surround-

Table 4-1. Stains in Neuropathology

Use	Stain	Comment
Routine	Hematoxylin and eosin (H & E)	General tissue stain; nuclei stains blue, cytoplasm stains red
Nissl bodies	Nissl (for example, cresyl violet)	Stains nuclei and Nissl bodies blue; faint or no staining of cytoplasm
Neurofibrils (axons)	Silver impregnations (for example, Bodian or Bielschowsky)	Stains intracellular neurofibrils and axis cylinders black
Myelin sheaths	Luxol-fast blue; Weigert	Stains normal but not degenerating myelin
Myelin (degenerating)	Marchi (osmium tetroxide)	Intense staining of degenerating myelin; faint staining of normal myelin
Astrocytes	Cajal (gold sublimate)	Astrocytes stain black
Glial fibers	Mallory's phosphotungstic acid-hematoxylin; Holzer (crystal violet)	Stains astrocytic fibers and is useful for demarcating reactive astrocytes
Microglia and oligodendroglia	Variations of Hortega's silver-impregnation methods	Stains microglia or oligodendroglia black depending on method

Fig. 4-1. Neurons of different sizes and configurations from various areas of nervous system.

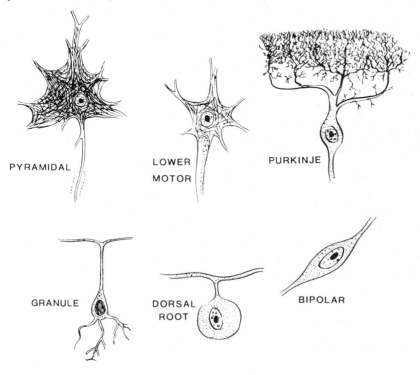

PYRAMIDAL

LOWER MOTOR

PURKINJE

GRANULE

DORSAL ROOT

BIPOLAR

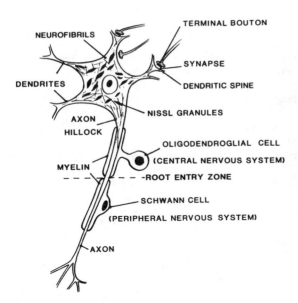

Fig. 4-2. *Spinal motor neuron.*

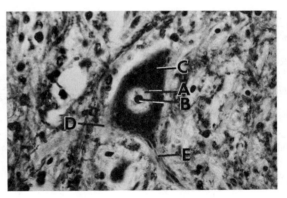

Fig. 4-3. *Spinal motor neuron showing* (A) *nucleus,* (B) *nucleolus,* (C) *cytoplasm filled with Nissl granules,* (D) *axon hillock,* (E) *dendrite. (Nissl stain; ×400.)*

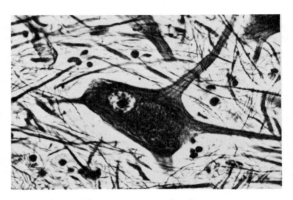

Fig. 4-4. *Spinal motor neuron showing numerous fibrils streaming through cytoplasm of cell body and processes. Background contains processes of other neurons. (Bodian stain; ×400.)*

ing the nucleus constitutes the main cell body, or *perikaryon,* and contains the same types of organelles for metabolism as do other cells in the body, for example, mitochondria, Golgi apparatus, lysosomes, and endoplasmic reticulum. However, two types of organelles are unusually conspicuous in neurons and distinguish them from other cells in the body.

The endoplasmic reticulum is heavily laden with ribonucleoprotein granules (rough endoplasmic reticulum). Concentrations of these rough endoplasmic reticulum membranes produce the appearance, at the light microscopic level, of dense basophilic bodies (Fig. 4-3). These structures are called *Nissl granules* (named after the German pathologist, Franz Nissl, who first described them). Various basic blue dyes, which stain Nissl granules as the most conspicuous element in brain tissue, are called Nissl stains; the Nissl granules also are well seen in routine preparations with hematoxylin and eosin.

The second type of organelle that is conspicuous in neurons is the fibrillar component of the cytoplasm. With the light microscope, neurofibrils can be seen only with silver-impregnation stains (Fig. 4-4). The fibrils demonstrated in this manner correspond to two ultrastructural components of the cell: (1) neurofilaments, which are 100 Å in diameter and are distributed through the cell body and all its processes, and (2) neurotubules, which are 200 to 300 Å in diameter and are similarly distributed,

except that they are relatively more numerous in dendrites than in axons. The function of the former is uncertain, although a skeletal-supporting function for the cell has been proposed. The latter seem to function as a cytoplasmic transport mechanism.

Processes of nerve cells extend outward from the cell body into the surrounding tissue. These processes are called either *dendrites* or *axons,* and the number, length, and branching of these processes vary markedly from one type of neuron to another. Neurons possess only one axon; the remaining processes are dendrites. The region of the cell body that forms the root of the axon, the *axon hillock,* does not have Nissl granules and appears to be relatively pale on Nissl and hematoxylin and eosin staining (see Fig. 4-3). From this region, the axon extends outward for distances that vary from a few millimeters to several feet. In general, the diameter of an axon varies with its length. Functionally, the axon is the portion of the neuron that conducts electrical activity away from the cell body, toward an effector organ (muscle, glands) or toward the next neuron in a chain or circuit.

Neurons of the central nervous system have one or, usually, many dendrites. Nissl granules in at least the proximal portions of the dendrites make them visible in routine preparations. The dendrites extend a relatively short distance from the cell body and usually branch repeatedly. Dendrites are, in a sense, the antennae of the nerve cell, and they transmit incoming signals toward the cell body.

Communication between neurons is accomplished at specialized regions of these cells called *synapses* (see Fig. 4-2). Synapses are the anatomic basis for the transfer of a signal from one neuron to another. The axon of a nerve cell usually terminates on and forms a synapse with the dendrites or cell body of another. At the region of the synapse, the axon terminal may be enlarged (*terminal bouton*) and the dendrite may present a small projection (*dendritic spine*) for the axon to terminate upon. Electron micrographs show that the axonal (presynaptic) and dendritic (postsynaptic) membranes are thickened. They do not actually touch but are separated by a space, the *synaptic cleft*, which is 200 to 300 Å wide. Rare synapses in the human brain have bridges across the synaptic cleft, providing the opportunity for direct electrical contact. In the axon terminal are tiny vesicles (synaptic vesicles) that contain the chemical neurotransmitters responsible for the transfer of the signal from the presynaptic to the postsynaptic cell. The dendritic tree and cell body of the neuron may be covered by hundreds of synapses from multiple sources. Its axon may branch repeatedly and form synapses on many other neurons. This is partly the basis for the complexity and the flexibility of the function of the nervous system. In the periphery, axons may terminate not only on other nerve cells but also on gland or muscle cells where synapse-like structures are also found.

Certain neurons have characteristic appearances that bear the names of the neuroanatomists who originally described them. Examples include the Betz cells of the inner pyramidal layer of the cerebral cortex and the Purkinje cells in the middle layer of the cerebellar cortex. In addition, Golgi recognized two distinct types of neurons. Axons of type I neurons project well outside the dendritic field of the cells and travel some distance away from the cell body of origin. These cells can conduct information for long distances within the central nervous system. Type II neurons have very short axons that terminate on cells near (and often within) the dendritic field of the cell body of origin. These cells are probably more involved in data processing than in data conduction.

Supporting Cells of Neuroectodermal Origin

OLIGODENDROGLIA AND SCHWANN CELLS.   These two cell types are discussed together because they share a very important function: They form the insulating sheaths (called myelin) that surround the axons in the central and peripheral nervous systems (see Fig. 4-2).

Myelin formation around peripheral axons is performed by the Schwann cells. In routine histologic sections of the axons in peripheral nerves, nuclei of Schwann cells are recognized as elongated structures oriented in the direction of the axis cylinders (Fig. 4-5). In transverse sections of peripheral nerves, most of the axons are surrounded by a myelin sheath (Fig. 4-6), but the relationship among the myelin sheath, Schwann cell, and axon is not obvious with the light microscope. In transverse sections of a peripheral myelinated axon viewed in the electron microscope, the relationship becomes more apparent. The plasma membrane of the Schwann cell invests the axon and is wound around it (Fig. 4-7). The cytoplasm is squeezed out, and the internal surfaces of the membranes are fused. In each successive turn, the outer surfaces of adjacent turns also fuse. Thus, a spiral of fused-Schwann-

Fig. 4-5. Longitudinal section of peripheral nerve showing Schwann cell nuclei oriented in long axis of nerve fibers. (H&E; ×250.)

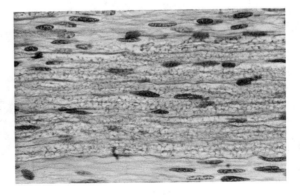

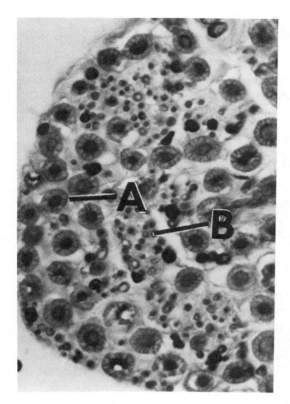

Fig. 4-6. Transverse section of spinal nerve showing (A) large myelinated fibers and (B) small myelinated and unmyelinated fibers. (Luxol-fast blue–Bodian stain; ×250.)

Fig. 4-7. Progressive steps in myelination of axon by Schwann cell.

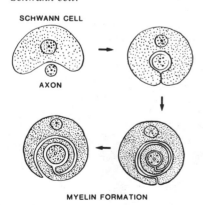

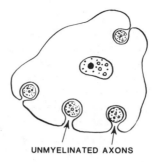

UNMYELINATED AXONS

Fig. 4-8. Relationship between Schwann cell and unmyelinated axons. Many unmyelinated axons may be invested by single Schwann cell.

cell cytoplasmic membrane is formed. The resulting multilayered protein-lipid substance is called myelin. The number of spirals that the Schwann cell process makes around the axon determines the thickness of the myelin sheath. In very small axons, the Schwann cell membrane may simply invest them once and make no turns at all. These axons are considered unmyelinated fibers. A single Schwann cell may invest a segment of several unmyelinated fibers in this way (Fig. 4-8). However, in myelinated fibers, a Schwann cell is related to a segment of only one axon. The physiologic significance of the thickness of the myelin sheath and of unmyelinated fibers is discussed in later chapters.

If myelinated axons of a peripheral nerve are "teased" apart so that a single fiber may be studied, there are numerous Schwann cells along its length, each forming the myelin sheath over a short segment of the axon (Fig. 4-9). Each segment of myelin belongs to a single Schwann cell along a given axon. There is a minute gap between each myelin segment, where the fiber appears to be constricted. These gaps are the *nodes of Ranvier*. The myelin segment is therefore often referred to as an internode, and the distance between the nodes of Ran-

Fig. 4-9. Schwann cell-myelin-axon relationship in longitudinal section. Portions of three myelin segments (internodes) separated by two nodes of Ranvier are represented.

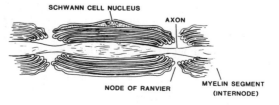

SCHWANN CELL NUCLEUS   AXON

NODE OF RANVIER   MYELIN SEGMENT (INTERNODE)

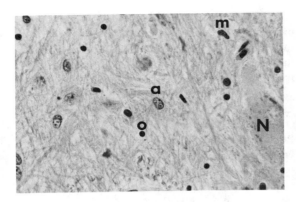

Fig. 4-10. Section of brain tissue in which nuclei belonging to various types of glial cells are seen, including oligodendroglia (o), astrocytes (a), and microglia (m). A portion of neuron (N) is seen at right of picture. (H&E; ×250.)

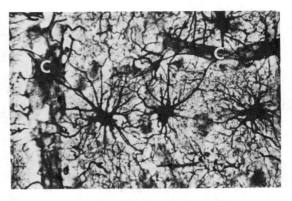

Fig. 4-11. Astrocytes as seen with gold sublimate stain (Cajal). Note many processes ending on walls of capillaries (C). (Cajal stain; ×400.)

vier as the internodal length. The internodal length varies directly with the thickness of the myelin sheath along any given fiber, approaching 1 mm in length in the largest fibers.

In routine preparations of the central nervous system, oligodendroglial cells are recognized as small, round nuclei with a dense chromatin network (Fig. 4-10). With no cytoplasm being stained, the nuclei seem to be surrounded by a clear halo. Oligodendroglial cells lie in both gray and white matter. In gray matter, they lie near neurons (perineuronal satellites) and their function is unknown. In white matter, the oligodendroglia lie among the myelinated fibers, but their precise relationship to myelin is not apparent at the light microscopic level. With the electron microscope, the same relationship of oligodendroglia cell to myelin that is present between Schwann cell and peripheral myelin can be demonstrated. The oligodendroglial cell sends out cytoplasmic extensions that wrap themselves around an axon and fuse (see Figs. 4-2, 4-7). A major difference between the central and the peripheral nervous system is that a single oligodendroglial cell may myelinate a segment of several axons in its vicinity, whereas a Schwann cell myelinates a segment of only one axon.

ASTROCYTES. Easily recognized in sections of central nervous system tissue stained with hematoxylin and eosin, astrocytes show oval nuclei, slightly larger and less densely stained than oligodendroglial nuclei (Fig. 4-10). Cytoplasm and processes of normal astrocytes are not seen with these methods. With metallic impregnation stains, however, notably the gold sublimate stain of Cajal, astrocytes show an elaborate radiating system of processes from which their name is derived (Fig. 4-11). There are minor anatomic variations by which astrocytes may be separated into different types, for example, protoplasmic astrocytes, which predominate in gray matter, and fibrous astrocytes, which predominate in white matter. These minor morphologic differences have no known functional significance.

The most important function assigned to astrocytes is deduced from their relation to blood vessels. At least one process of an astrocyte abuts on the wall of a capillary. Cerebral capillaries, in turn, have an almost continuous covering of astrocytic processes called *end feet* (Fig. 4-11). The capillary wall and astrocytic processes are separated by a basement membrane. The remaining processes terminate in relation to nonsynaptic zones of neurons and to other parenchymal cells in the central nervous system. This anatomic arrangement immediately suggests that astrocytes serve to transport substances between the blood and the parenchyma of the central nervous system. There is physiologic and biochemical support for this hypothesis, and this selective transport process is at least part of the phenomenon called the blood-brain barrier. The only other major known function of astrocytes is their reaction in certain stereotyped ways to disease processes.

EPENDYMAL CELLS. When the epithelium of the neural tube has proliferated in the ependymal zone, and the major portion of its cells have differentiated and migrated, a single layer of ciliated columnar epithelial cells (the *ependyma*) is left lining the cavity of the neural tube (Fig. 4-12).

In the cerebrum and brain stem of the mature brain, the ependyma lines the entire ventricular system. The central canal of the spinal cord is usually obliterated as an open cavity when development is complete, and the central region of the adult cord is represented by a nest of ependymal cells with a disorganized appearance. The ependymal lining of the ventricular system forms a selective barrier between the ventricular fluid and the brain substance, since tight junctions between the plasma membranes of adjacent ependymal cells serve to inhibit the passage of certain substances.

The choroid plexus is formed when the thinned roof plate, consisting of a layer of ependymal cells, invaginates the ventricular cavity ahead of a vascular-connective-tissue component derived

Fig. 4-12. Ependyma lining the third ventricle of an infant. Note continuous layer of columnar cells with cilia on their free (ventricular) border. (H&E; ×100.)

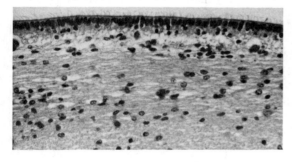

Fig. 4-13. Choroid plexus. Each tuft consists of core containing dilated capillary surrounded by small amount of connective tissue and covered by choroidal epithelial cells. (H&E; ×100.)

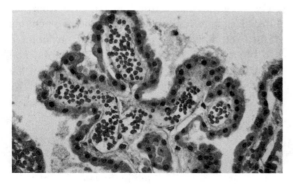

from the pia mater. Enormous elaboration of these evaginations leads to the formation of many small tufts, each of which has essentially the same structure (Fig. 4-13). The ventricular surface of a choroidal tuft is lined by cuboidal epithelial cells, which are modified ependymal cells. The free surface of a choroidal cell displays numerous microvilli on electron microscopic examination. Beneath the surface epithelium is a core of richly vascular connective tissue.

The function of the choroid plexus is to form the ventricular and the cerebrospinal fluid. It does this by filtering water and selected molecules out of the blood that passes through its capillaries and by passing this solution through its epithelial cells into the ventricular system.

Supporting Cells of Mesodermal Origin

MICROGLIA.   These cells are not derived from the neuroepithelium; they are mesodermal cells that migrate into the central nervous system, along with blood vessels from the mesoderm that surround the neural tube. They are seen as small, elongated, darkly staining nuclei in hematoxylin and eosin-stained sections (see Fig. 4-10). Normally they are present only in small numbers and are widely scattered in the nervous system. Their major function becomes manifest only when a destructive process affects the central nervous system, at which time the cells proliferate rapidly and become scavenger cells, or macrophages, ingesting and removing damaged tissue.

CONNECTIVE TISSUE.   Fibroblasts derived from the mesoderm have an important role in the normal structure and function of the nervous system. The brain and spinal cord are permeated by a rich network of blood vessels which, except at the capillary level, have a thin collagenous investment making up the adventitia. Other than the vascular structures, the parenchyma of the central nervous system is almost devoid of fibrous connective tissue elements, which accounts for its extremely soft consistency. Thus, fibroblasts rarely participate in reactive or reparative processes (scar formation) in diseases of the central nervous system.

The central nervous system is surrounded by three connective tissue membranes called *meninges*. The two inner membranes, the pia mater and arachnoid, are the *leptomeninges* and are very thin and delicate. The outer membrane, the *dura mater* or the pachymeninx, is thick and tough.

The peripheral nerves are rich in fibrous connective tissue. Each myelinated nerve fiber in a peripheral nerve is invested by a thin layer of collagen, the *endoneurium*. Groups of nerve fibers are bound together in fascicles by a *perineurium*. Finally, the fascicles that comprise a nerve trunk are surrounded by a thick sheath, the *epineurium*. The three connective tissue sheaths of a peripheral nerve are analogous to the three layers of the meninges (pia mater, arachnoid, and dura mater) and are continuous with them at the spinal nerve level.

Pathologic Reactions of the Structural Elements

Each of the cellular elements of the nervous system may undergo physical change in response to disease states. In some disorders, the pathologic alteration may be primarily functional (physiologic)—there may be little change in the physical appearance of the cell, yet the cell cannot function normally. In many diseases of the nervous system, however, the physical appearance of the cell is altered. When the nervous system is affected by disease, the cells undergo changes that reflect either the damage done to them by the pathologic process or their reaction to it. Some of these morphologic changes are "nonspecific" and may be seen in many entirely different types of diseases. Other changes may be "specific" and indicate a particular type of disease or even a specific disease entity. In this section, we will review some of the more common and important pathologic changes seen in the individual cell types studied previously. In most pathologic conditions, the various cell types react in concert, and the pathologic diagnosis is derived from analysis of the total tissue reaction.

Pathologic Reactions of Neurons

NONSPECIFIC REACTIONS. Almost any disease leading to the death of a patient is associated with changes in body chemistry and physiology that may affect the appearance of neurons. In addition, catabolic processes that proceed after death (autolysis) and the mechanical procedures involved in obtaining and processing tissue can distort the appearance of neurons. It is not surprising, then, that almost any histologic section of brain tissue will contain some neurons that deviate from "normal" in size,

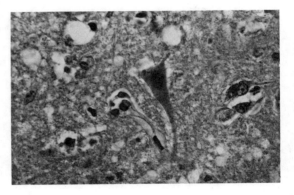

Fig. 4-14. Ischemic cell change. Neuron is shrunken, nucleus is pyknotic, and cytoplasm is diffusely eosinophilic. (H&E; ×400.)

shape, and affinity for stains. Shrunken, dark-staining neurons, as well as swollen, pale-staining cells, are often encountered. Although these neurons are not normal in the strict sense, the factors responsible for their nonspecific change are usually not identifiable. Neuronal loss is another nonspecific change that may result from any form of severe damage to a neuron. Under pathologic circumstances, neuronal loss is usually accompanied by a reaction of other tissue elements (astrocytes, microglia) which marks the site of damage. Neuronal changes of a more specific type can accompany certain pathologic processes and, when present, can help to define the pathophysiologic basis for those disorders.

Ischemic cell change (Fig. 4-14) takes place in response to deprivation of oxygen and cessation of oxidative metabolism; the neurons undergo a readily recognized morphologic change. Eight to twelve hours after the insult, the neuron becomes smaller and its outline becomes more sharply angular. The cytoplasm becomes distinctly eosinophilic. The nucleus shrinks and becomes homogeneously darkly stained. This is an irreversible change, and the end result is complete dissolution of the cell. Ischemic cell change may be brought about by any condition that deprives the neuron of oxygen, including loss of blood flow, lack of oxygen in the blood, lack of substrates necessary for oxidative metabolism, or the presence of a poison such as cyanide, which blocks oxidative metabolism. The typical morphologic change of ischemic damage may be preceded briefly by certain nonspecific changes, such as acute swelling of the neuron.

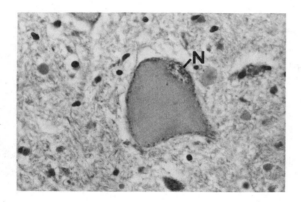

Fig. 4-15. Central chromatolysis. Cell is swollen, nucleus (N) is eccentric, and Nissl granules have disappeared except at periphery. (H&E; ×400.)

Central chromatolysis (Fig. 4-15) is a change in neuron cell bodies after severe injury to their axons. Thus, it is sometimes called the *axonal reaction*. In human pathology, this change is usually recognized only in large motor cells, such as the spinal anterior horn cells and motor nuclei of cranial nerves when their axons are injured close to the central nervous system. The reaction consists of swelling of the cell body and dissolution of the Nissl granules, beginning close to the nucleus and spreading to the periphery of the cell, where a rim of Nissl granules may be found intact. The nucleus migrates to the periphery of the cell body. These changes usually begin 2 to 3 days after injury and reach a maximum in 2 to 3 weeks. Unlike ischemic cell change, central chromatolysis is reversible, and the neuron may revert to a normal appearance in a few months.

Wallerian degeneration occurs in the distal part of an axon, when its parent cell body is destroyed or separated from the axon by disease or injury along its course. In both the central and peripheral nervous systems, an axon cannot survive when it is separated from its cell body. The process of degeneration of the axon and its myelin sheath is called *wallerian degeneration* (after Waller, who in 1850 first described it in peripheral nerves).

The changes seen in the degenerating axon are the rapid disappearance of the neurofibrils, followed by the breaking up of the axon into short fragments that eventually disappear completely (Fig. 4-16). As axonal fragmentation proceeds, the myelin sheath begins to fragment in a similar manner into oval segments (ovoids). Each oval segment of myelin, containing a fragment of axon, is called a *digestive chamber* because the axon seems to be digested within it. At the same time, the myelin fragment is undergoing biochemical changes including breakdown into its component lipids. These lipids are eventually removed by phagocytosis.

Some notable differences exist between this process in the central and peripheral nervous systems. Wallerian degeneration proceeds more rapidly in peripheral nerves, where degenerative changes are completed in a few weeks, whereas in the central nervous system the degeneration proceeds over several months. More importantly, in the peripheral nervous system, regeneration of the nerve is possible if the parent cell body survives; this regeneration does not occur in the central nervous system. Each axon and myelin sheath in a peripheral nerve is surrounded by a basement membrane, which belongs to the Schwann cell, and

Fig. 4-16. Sequence of events in wallerian degeneration and early peripheral nerve regeneration. After degeneration and removal of myelin and axonal debris, sprouts from severed end of axon may find their way into tube of regenerated Schwann cell.

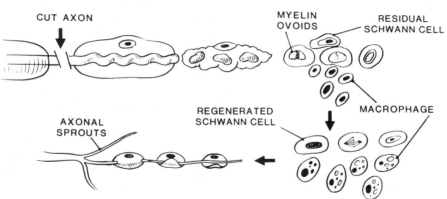

CUT AXON

MYELIN OVOIDS

RESIDUAL SCHWANN CELL

AXONAL SPROUTS

REGENERATED SCHWANN CELL

MACROPHAGE

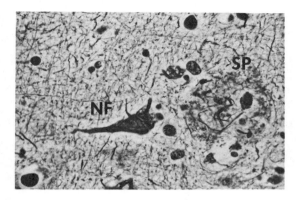

Fig. 4-17. Neuron showing neurofibrillary degeneration (NF). Note tangle of thickened neurofibrils in cell body and axon. Senile plaque (SP) is seen on right. (Bodian stain; ×400.)

by a delicate connective tissue sheath, the *endoneurium*. These structures maintain their integrity even as the axon and myelin degenerate. In addition, the Schwann cells, with the potential of forming new myelin, proliferate along the length of the degenerating fiber. Thus, the distal portion of a damaged nerve provides a superstructure that is ready to receive and myelinate new axonal sprouts growing from the proximal portion. If these axonal sprouts can find their way into one of these "tubes," they will continue to grow at a rate of about 3 mm per day, and function may be restored eventually. In the central nervous system, there are no basement membranes or collagen sheaths surrounding nerve fibers, and oligodendroglia are incapable of proliferation. Thus, new axonal growth, even if it should begin, has no path to follow, and functionally significant regeneration of tracts does not occur after damage to the central nervous system.

Injury of an axon generally results in no change in the postsynaptic cell. There are exceptions: for example, when the motor innervation of a muscle is destroyed, the muscle becomes atrophic. A similar phenomenon, *transneuronal degeneration*, has been observed in certain pathways in the central nervous system. The process apparently depends on the removal of some "trophic" influence by which the axon maintains the condition of the postsynaptic element. The nature of such trophic influences is unknown.

The processes of chromatolysis and wallerian degeneration are often utilized in experimental studies for the purpose of tracing neuroanatomic pathways. When the axons of a functional group of neurons are sectioned or otherwise damaged, the cell bodies of the neurons from which the axons originate can be located by finding which neurons undergo chromatolysis. Conversely, the neuroanatomist may destroy a group of neuronal cell bodies within a particular nucleus of the central nervous system and may then trace the route taken by the axons by staining the degenerating fibers with techniques designed to demonstrate either degenerating myelin or degenerating axons.

Neurofibrillary degeneration is the formation of clumped masses of neurofibrils within the cytoplasm (Fig. 4-17) and is a common, readily recognized change in neurons of the central nervous system. This change, *Alzheimer's neurofibrillary degeneration*, is best seen with silver-impregnation stains. It is a neuronal degeneration that is most closely associated with clinical dementia. The change is seen to some extent in hippocampal neurons of many "normal" aged people and is found throughout the cerebral cortex and in other parts of the brain in a severe dementing process known as Alzheimer's disease. Alzheimer's degeneration is also a prominent change found in a few other conditions classed as "degenerative" diseases. The senile plaque is a closely associated pathologic change noted primarily in senile dementia and Alzheimer's disease. Typical senile plaques consist of a central deposit of amyloid (the core) surrounded by a halo of degenerated nerve processes and reactive elements, such as astrocytic fibers and microglia.

Inclusion body formation refers to abnormal, discrete deposits in nerve cells (Fig. 4-18) and, when present, often identifies the type of disease and sometimes the specific disease. Inclusion bodies can be divided into intranuclear and intracytoplasmic types. The appearance and significance of the most important types of neuronal inclusions are outlined in Table 4-2.

Storage cells refer to the accumulation of metabolic products within nerve cells. A number of metabolic diseases of the nervous system are associated with this accumulation. Most of these disorders involve the storage of lipids. As these lipid products accumulate, the cell body swells so much that it is referred to as a "balloon" cell (Fig. 4-19). Identification of the specific disease requires biochemical identification of the stored material.

Pathologic Reactions of Oligodendroglia
The oligodendroglial cells, as identified in routine

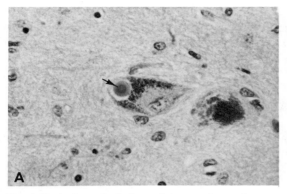

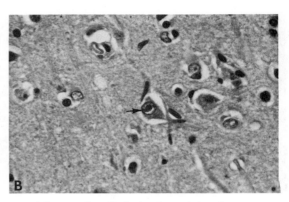

Fig. 4-18. A. Lewy body (arrow) in cytoplasm of pigmented neuron in Parkinson's disease. B. Cowdry type A intranuclear inclusion (arrow) in subacute sclerosing panencephalitis. (H&E; ×400.)

Table 4-2. Inclusion Bodies

Location	Name	Staining characteristics	Disease association
Cytoplasm	Lewy body	Eosinophilic with concentric lamination	Parkinson's disease
Cytoplasm	Pick body	Metallophilic (silver, gold)	Pick's disease
Cytoplasm	Lafora body	Basophilic	Myoclonus epilepsy
Cytoplasm	Negri body	Eosinophilic	Rabies
Nucleus	Cowdry type A inclusion	Eosinophilic	Viral infections: herpes simplex, subacute sclerosing panencephalitis, cytomegalic inclusion disease

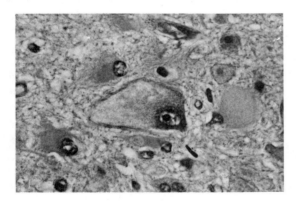

Fig. 4-19. Neuron in Tay-Sachs disease (lipid-storage disease). Note ballooning of cytoplasm with stored material, forcing nucleus and Nissl granules to one corner of cell. (H&E; ×400.)

preparations, undergo few reactions of pathognomonic importance. They seem to be extremely sensitive to injury and, when affected by a pathologic process, oligodendroglial nuclei simply shrink or break up and vanish. The myelin that they form, however, is an extremely important indicator of disease of the central nervous system. Just as the oligodendroglial cell is readily damaged by most pathologic processes, the myelin sheaths are also extremely sensitive to injury. Partial or complete loss of myelin in an area of injury is easily seen in myelin stains such as the Luxol-fast blue stain (see Fig. 4-21A). Sections stained in this way provide the most reliable method of studying the topography of most disease processes.

In addition to the nonspecific injury to myelin associated with most kinds of disease, there are two groups of diseases that specifically affect myelin sheaths. The first group is called the *demyelinating* or *myelinoclastic* diseases. In these disorders, normal myelin is attacked by some exogenous agent, usually unknown, and broken down into its component lipids (as in wallerian degeneration) and absorbed. The axons that the myelin surrounds are left relatively intact. The most common and important disease in this group is multiple sclerosis.

The process of demyelination in multiple sclerosis and some other diseases of the central and peripheral nervous system, such as postvaccinal encephalomyelitis and the Guillain-Barré syndrome, involves immunologic mechanisms. While details of the pathogenesis of these disorders remain to be clarified, humoral- and cell-mediated immunologic reactions involving myelin components set in motion the cytotoxic and inflammatory processes that lead to demyelination.

The second group of diseases are the *leukodystrophies*, or *dysmyelinating* diseases. In these disorders, myelin is abnormally formed owing to a genetically determined error in metabolism. Because the myelin is abnormally constituted, it is un-

Fig. 4-20. Reactive astrocytes at border of infarct. Note expansion of cytoplasm, producing plump appearance and dense tangle of fibers in background. (H&E; ×250.)

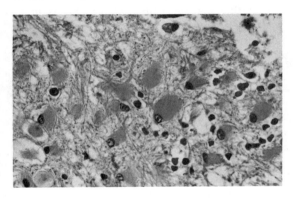

Fig. 4-21. Transverse section of pons of patient with multiple sclerosis. A. Myelin stain (Luxol-fast blue) showing plaques of demyelination (light areas). (Luxol-fast blue; ×4.) B. Glial fiber stain showing gliosis of demyelinated areas (dark areas). (Holzer stain; ×4.)

stable and breaks down. The type of metabolic defect often can be determined by histochemical staining reactions and biochemical analysis of the tissue.

Pathologic Reactions of Schwann Cells

Disease processes affecting the Schwann cells that surround peripheral axons produce segmental loss of myelin (segmental demyelination). If the disease is severe, there also may be associated secondary axonal destruction and wallerian degeneration. In certain genetic disorders affecting peripheral nerve (hypertrophic neuropathies), there is repeated demyelination and remyelination of nerve fibers. Each episode leaves a layer of connective tissue, forming concentric layers around the axon. Such nerves become large and firm; the axons may finally be lost, leaving only the stroma of the connective tissue.

Pathologic Reactions of Astrocytes

Almost any injury to central nervous system tissue can produce a reaction of astrocytes. The terms *astrocytosis*, *astrogliosis*, or *gliosis* refer to this nonspecific response whereby astrocytes form "scars" in injured neural tissue. Strictly speaking, astrocytosis refers to the early stages of the reaction in which astrocytes proliferate and increase greatly in number. As this occurs, their cytoplasm becomes visible with hematoxylin and eosin stains as an eosinophilic apron of cytoplasm with somewhat irregular margins. At this stage, they are known as "plump" or *gemistocytic* (from the German *gemaste* = stuffed) astrocytes (Fig. 4-20). These plump astrocytes then form progressively longer and thicker processes which form a dense network in the damaged tissue. This network of tissue is the

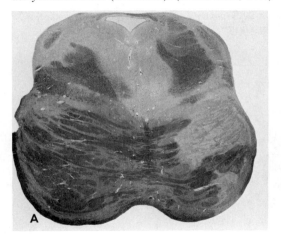

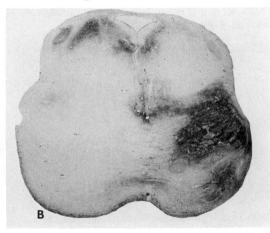

equivalent of a scar formed by fibroblasts in other body tissues. The fibers of reactive astrocytes, while readily visible in hematoxylin and eosin stains, are seen even more clearly with special stains like Mallory's phosphotungstic acid-hematoxylin or Holzer stain. With the latter techniques, an area of gliosis can be seen in a section even without the aid of a microscope, which is of advantage in mapping the topography of a large lesion (Fig. 4-21).

Astrocytes also may react in more specific ways to certain injuries, especially metabolic disturbances. The most notable example is the presence of acutely swollen astrocytic nuclei, called Alzheimer's type 2 astrocytes, in hepatic failure. Astrocytes may also form intranuclear inclusion bodies in certain viral infections.

Pathologic Reactions of Microglia

Microglial cells react in a stereotyped way to most diseases that affect the central nervous system. Injury to other cellular constituents of the central nervous system usually leads to multiplication of nearby microglial cells (Fig. 4-22). The nuclei of these microglial cells become elongated and form *rod* cells. If actual tissue necrosis does not occur, the reaction may progress no further. The presence of many rod cells then usually indicates the presence of low-grade chronic irritation of the tissue. An example of such a condition is the chronic encephalitis associated with syphilis (general paresis).

If tissue necrosis occurs, the microglial cells continue to proliferate and their nuclei become rounded. Their cytoplasm becomes evident as it begins to engulf the debris of the necrotic tissue. Be-

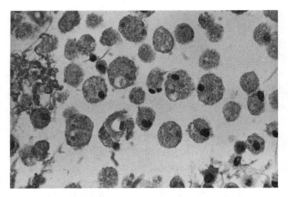

Fig. 4-23. Lipid-laden macrophages (gitter cells) in area of necrosis. Note small eccentric nuclei and foamy cytoplasm. (H&E; ×250.)

cause of the high fat content of central nervous system tissue, most of the engulfed material is lipid, and the cytoplasm assumes a foamy appearance. At this stage, the cells are referred to as *lipid-laden macrophages*, or gitter cells (Fig. 4-23). In large lesions, many, perhaps even most, of the gitter cells probably are not microglial cells originally but rather were blood-borne macrophages that migrated into the lesion. Eventually, most of the macrophages in a destructive lesion of the central nervous system are reabsorbed back into the bloodstream. At times, microglia attack isolated, damaged neurons. This process is called *neuronophagia* (Fig. 4-24). When the neuron has been engulfed, the cluster of microglia remaining in its place is a *microglial nodule*.

Other Pathologic Reactions

Ependymal cells react in a very limited way to noxious stimuli (which most often are infectious).

Fig. 4-22. Margin of recent infarct showing proliferating microglial cells. (H&E; ×100.)

Fig. 4-24. Damaged neuron undergoing neuronophagia by cluster of microglial cells. (H&E; ×250.)

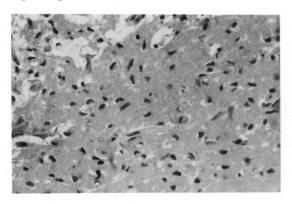

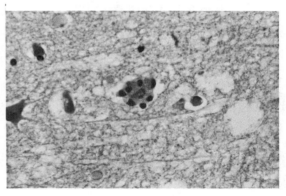

There is often loss of ependymal cells; however, proliferation of the subependymal astrocytes is frequently associated with this loss to form *ependymal granulations* that may be seen along certain areas of the ventricular system.

In response to injury, blood vessels may respond by capillary proliferation, and when inflammation is present, infiltration of leukocytes occurs, as it does in other tissues.

Cerebral edema is the result of accumulation of fluid, primarily in white matter, and may be caused by a wide variety of factors. The edema may occur diffusely or be localized in and surround an area of focal abnormality. The precise mechanism of fluid accumulation is not known, but microscopic study has shown that the fluid is present within swollen astrocytes, in the perivascular and extracellular spaces, and in the myelin lamellae. These varied locations of the edematous fluid may reflect different types of cerebral edema due to different pathophysiologic mechanisms. The net result of this accumulation of fluid is to increase the size and volume of the responsible lesion.

Uncontrolled cellular proliferation of any of the cellular elements results in a *neoplasm* (a localized accumulation of abnormal tissue, a mass lesion). The type of neoplasm is named after the predominant cell type (such as astrocytoma, oligodendroglioma, or schwannoma).

Clinicopathologic Correlations

Clinical diagnosis in neurology requires the analysis of two types of data. The first type is obtained from both the history and the neurologic examination and enables localization of the disease process within the nervous system. On this basis, neurologic disease may be classified as *focal*, involving a single circumscribed area or group of contiguous structures in the nervous system; *multifocal*, involving more than one circumscribed area or several noncontiguous structures; and *diffuse*, involving portions of the nervous system in a bilateral, symmetric fashion.

The localization of the pathologic process depends partly on a knowledge of the functional anatomy of the nervous system, outlined in Chapter 3. Vastly different types of pathologic processes located in the same anatomic structure may produce similar symptoms and signs. Since the manifestations of disease are dependent on where a lesion is located and not on its pathologic nature, the pathologic diagnosis must utilize a second type of data—information obtained from the patient's history that relates to the onset and evolution (temporal profile) of the disease. The development of symptoms can be classified in the following terms: *acute*, within minutes; *subacute*, within days; and *chronic*, within weeks or months. The evolution (course of symptoms after the onset) may be categorized as *transient*, when symptoms have resolved completely after onset; *improving*, when symptoms have decreased from their maximum, but have not completely resolved; *progressive*, when symptoms continue to increase in severity or when new symptoms make their appearance; and *stationary*, when symptoms remain unchanged after reaching maximum severity and show no significant change during a period of observation.

Combining the above terms allows clinical differentiation between mass and nonmass lesions. Although other clues for differentiation will be discussed in later chapters, the presence of a *mass lesion* should be considered when the signs and symptoms, whether acute, subacute, or chronic in onset, suggest progression of a focal lesion. A *nonmass* lesion should be considered when the lesion is diffuse in location or when the symptoms and signs suggest a nonprogressive focal abnormality.

As the text proceeds, qualification of these definitions will be required; an attempt to explain exceptions to these general statements will be made at appropriate times.

Interpretation of the temporal profile of disease depends on an understanding of the way in which pathologic processes affect nerve tissue and the rates at which various destructive and reparative processes proceed. Knowledge of the basic types of cellular and tissue reactions is a prerequisite to making this type of analysis. For the purposes of recognizing and understanding clinical neurologic disease, it is sufficient to become familiar with six types of pathologic changes that occur within the nervous system: (1) degenerative disease, (2) neoplastic disease, (3) vascular disease, (4) inflammatory disease, (5) toxic-metabolic disease, and (6) traumatic disease. In the following paragraphs, the temporal and spatial characteristics of these major disease categories will be outlined.

Degenerative Disease

The term *degenerative* is applied to a large group of neurologic diseases for which no cause is apparent.

As causes of these diseases are found (viral infection, metabolic error), they will be moved to the appropriate disease category; many conditions in this group are familial biochemical disorders. These disorders are characterized by a gradual decrease in neuronal function. Sometimes the pathologically altered neurons show specific changes, such as neurofibrillary tangles or inclusion body formations; more often, the neurons simply atrophy and disappear. The neuronal degeneration is accompanied by astrocytic proliferation in the central nervous system. Topographically, degenerative diseases affect the nervous system in a diffuse manner in that they are usually bilateral, symmetric, and may affect multiple levels of the nervous system. The clinical correlation of degenerative diseases, therefore, can be summarized by the terms *chronic*, *progressive*, and *diffuse*.

Neoplastic Disease

Any cell type in the nervous system can undergo neoplastic change and proliferate in an unrestrained manner. Generally, the causes of neoplasia are obscure although certain genetic, infectious, and chemical factors have been implicated in some neoplasms. Tumors are named by adding the suffix *-oma* to the name of the constituent cell type. Cells of the nervous system vary greatly in their apparent potential to undergo neoplasia.

There is a general correlation between the normal capacity of a cell to undergo cell division and its tendency to undergo neoplasia. Nerve cells are normally incapable of cell division after differentiation is complete, and neoplasms of nerve cells (neurocytomas) are extremely rare. Astrocytes are the most reactive cells of the central nervous system, and astrocytomas are the most common primary tumors of the central nervous system. Oligodendrogliomas, ependymomas, and microgliomas occur less frequently. The cells of the leptomeninges and the Schwann cells of nerve roots and peripheral nerves give rise to meningiomas and schwannomas, respectively.

All these tumor types are believed to arise from relatively mature cell types that are normally present in the nervous system. In each cell type, however, tumors vary in the rapidity of growth, the likelihood of recurrence after surgery, and the length of patient survival. These factors correspond fairly well to the histologic malignancy of the tumor. Tumors of the central nervous system, except in extremely rare instances, do not metastasize outside the central nervous system; thus, one of the major criteria of malignancy in other forms of neoplasia does not apply to tumors of the central nervous system. The degree of malignancy of these tumors may be graded by considering the degree of pleomorphism (lack of uniformity of appearance and nuclear-cytoplasmic ratio) of tumor cells, frequency of mitotic figures, proliferation of tumor vessels, and necrosis of tumor tissue. Especially in infants and children, tumors of immature cellular elements or tumors of cells not normally present in the nervous system (teratomas) are often seen. In children, the medulloblastoma of the cerebellum is especially common and is probably derived from immature cerebellar stem cells, with both neuroblastic and spongioblastic potential. In addition, systemic cancer can spread as secondary growth (metastasize) to the central nervous system.

A neoplastic mass progressively increases in size and alters the function of the region in which it lies. It may also alter the function of adjacent structures by compression or by the formation of edema around the primary mass. The cardinal topographic feature of a neoplasm, therefore, is its *focal* character. The clinical correlate of neoplastic disease may be summarized by the terms *chronic*, *progressive*, and *focal*. It must be mentioned at this point that not all progressively expanding (mass) lesions in the nervous system are composed of neoplastic cells. Blood clots (hematomas) and edema may be produced by different basic disease processes, and they represent common examples of nonneoplastic mass lesions.

Vascular Disease

Neurons deprived of metabolic support from the blood in the form of oxygen and glucose cease functioning in seconds and undergo pathologic change in minutes. Therefore the hallmark of a vascular disease process is its *sudden onset*. Neurologic function will be altered abruptly and usually maximally at the time of the initial insult. Vascular disease, however, is of several types, and although this will be dealt with more fully in the section on the vascular system, certain general distinctions must be drawn at this time. The most common type of vascular disease is the *infarct*. The chronologic, microscopic events that occur in a region of an infarct may be listed as follows:

6 to 12 hours	Nerve cells may show acute swelling with staining pallor; as the process progresses, the neurons show the typical ischemic change described earlier in this chapter.
24 to 48 hours	Leukocytes appear from the blood vessels and begin migrating into the brain substance.
48 to 72 hours	Microglia proliferate and macrophages begin to appear and steadily increase in number up to the third week, after which they gradually diminish in number; the early stage corresponds only to the gross softening of the lesion (encephalomalacia) and then later to cyst formation.
4 to 5 days	In the region of astrocyte survival, the astrocytes begin to proliferate and show the changes described on page 57; this process goes on, reaching a peak at about 6 weeks, and a glial scar is formed.
2 weeks	During the second week, surviving capillaries also proliferate and take part in the attempted repair process.

The characteristic ischemic cell change is the hallmark of infarction. Although diffuse anoxic insults may occur, infarcts usually result from the cessation of the blood supply to a specific area of the nervous system and are generally *well localized*. The histologic events are primarily attempts at repair and, therefore, the course of a patient's symptoms is generally one of stabilization or improvement. Clinical progression of symptoms, when it occurs, usually indicates cerebral edema or, more rarely, continuing infarction of adjacent tissue after the initial event (progressing stroke).

The second type of vascular disorder is the *cerebral hemorrhage*. Instead of an interruption of vascular supply to an area, a blood vessel may rupture within the brain tissue, with localized accumulation of a blood clot within the neural tissues (an intraparenchymal hemorrhage). In this situation, both the symptoms and pathologic changes would be expected to appear abruptly and be focal, but because of the continuing pathologic changes that occur in response to a localized hemorrhage compressing neighboring tissue, progression might be seen.

A third type of vascular change occurs when a blood vessel, usually on the surface of the brain, suddenly ruptures and blood is spread over the surface of the brain and throughout the subarachnoid space (a subarachnoid hemorrhage). In this situation, the symptoms and pathologic changes are of abrupt onset, but diffusely distributed in the nervous system.

Although seemingly complex, the clinical correlates of vascular disease can be summarized as follows: (1) vascular disease is always acute in onset; (2) vascular disease may be focal or diffuse in distribution; (3) if diffuse in distribution, a condition like a subarachnoid hemorrhage or a diffuse anoxic process is considered; and (4) if distribution is focal, the lesion is likely to be an infarct or a hemorrhage, and if it shows features of progression, it is likely to be a hemorrhage.

Inflammatory Disease

In response to microorganisms, immunologic reactions, and toxic chemicals, a complex series of events called the *inflammatory response* occurs in any system or organ of the body, including the nervous system. This response usually occurs rapidly but not suddenly and may therefore be termed *subacute* in its temporal profile. The pathologic hallmark of the inflammatory response is the outpouring of white blood cells. In certain types of infections, especially bacterial, the major component of the exudate is polymorphonuclear leukocytes. In immunologic reactions and indolent infections, the predominant cells are mononuclear cells, especially lymphocytes.

Most inflammatory diseases of the central nervous system, particularly infections, are diffusely distributed either in the leptomeninges and cerebrospinal fluid (meningitis) or in the parenchyma of the brain (encephalitis). Other inflammatory diseases in the central nervous system are more likely to be focal, such as inflammation in the spinal cord, which occurs in multiple sclerosis. Inflammation also may occur in the peripheral nervous system, either in single nerves (mononeuritis) or in multiple nerves (polyneuritis). Infections sometimes localize in a specific area of the brain. In response to this localized area of inflammation, astrocytes proliferate in the surrounding tissue, and a wall of glial fibers is formed in an attempt to limit the spread of the infection. The inflamed brain becomes softened and liquefied, and eventually there may be a cavity. This process is called *abscess formation*. A brain abscess can exert a mass effect and progressively expand and compress neighboring structures.

The clinical correlates of inflammatory disease may be summarized as follows: (1) the course is usually subacute and progressive and (2) it may be diffuse in distribution, as in meningitis or encephalitis, or focal, as in an abscess, myelitis, or mononeuritis.

Toxic-Metabolic Disease

Various chemical agents, both endogenous and exogenous, may alter neuronal function. Vitamin deficiencies, genetic biochemical disorders, and the encephalopathies of kidney and liver disease are examples. When function is altered, the manifestations are almost always diffusely distributed throughout the nervous system. Depending on the nature of the specific toxin or metabolic abnormality, the effect may be exerted on the nervous system *acutely*, *subacutely*, or *chronically*. Pathologic changes vary with the noxious agent, but may include such reactions as ischemia, edema, demyelination, and cell death.

Traumatic Disease

Trauma to the nervous system is almost always acute in onset, with a clearly identifiable precipitating event (automobile accident, fall, missile wound). Injuries to the peripheral nervous system are focal. Injuries to the central nervous system are frequently diffuse in their initial manifestations, presenting as the syndrome of concussion, which reflects widespread physiologic damage to the central nervous system. Traumatic damage is usually maximum at onset, and the natural course is one of resolution or improvement. This type of disturbance usually improves, until only the areas of severe anatomic damage (contusions, lacerations, hematomas) become clinically manifest, and the symptoms therefore become focal.

An important exception to the rule of trauma being maximal at onset and improving thereafter is that of delayed intracranial hemorrhage. The two most common forms are the epidural and the subdural hemorrhage. The epidural hematoma usually

Table 4-3. Summary of the Most Important Temporal and Spatial Features of the Major Disease Categories[a, b, c]

	Acute	Subacute	Chronic
Focal	Vascular (infarct or intraparenchymal hemorrhage)	Inflammatory (abscess, myelitis)	Neoplasm
Diffuse	Vascular (subarachnoid hemorrhage, anoxia)	Inflammatory (meningitis, encephalitis)	Degenerative

[a]Metabolic and toxic disorders are usually diffuse and may follow any temporal profile, depending on the toxin or metabolite involved.
[b]Traumatic disorders are usually acute in onset, but their localization and course depend on the site of trauma, severity of trauma, and delayed complications.
[c]Almost all focal, progressive disorders are *mass lesions*; in general, the type of mass determines the course. For example, hemorrhages are acute, abscesses subacute, and neoplasms chronic. The basic distinction between *mass* and *nonmass* lesions carries extremely important therapeutic as well as diagnostic implications.

results from fracture of the temporal bone and a tear in the middle meningeal artery, which runs in a groove in the inner table of the skull. Bleeding then occurs between the temporal bone and the dura mater. The bleeding is arterial and therefore brisk, and a significant hematoma accumulates within minutes to hours after the injury. Symptoms progress rapidly. Subdural hematomas result from tears in the veins that cross the subdural space in passing from the brain surface to the dural sinuses. The bleeding is venous and therefore under low pressure. The slow accumulation of blood with progression of symptoms may not manifest itself for days, weeks, or even months after the trauma.

The clinical correlates of traumatic disease may be summarized as follows: (l) in the peripheral nervous system, the symptoms are focal; in the central nervous system, they may be focal, but are often diffuse at onset and later become focal; (2) the onset is usually acute; and (3) the usual course is one of improvement or stabilization, but the symptoms may be subacutely or chronically progressive.

The most important temporal and spatial features of the major disease categories are summarized in Table 4-3.

Objectives

1. Define the general functional role and embryonic origin of neuron, astrocyte, oligodendrocyte, microglial cell, ependymal cell, and Schwann cell.
2. Describe ischemic cell change, neurofibrillary degeneration, inclusion body formation, central chromatolysis, wallerian degeneration, astrocytosis, demyelination, and cerebral edema.
3. Describe the clinical and pathologic features of degenerative disease, neoplastic disease, vascular disease, inflammatory disease, toxic-metabolic disease, and traumatic disease.
4. On a photograph, be able to recognize neuron, astrocyte, oligodendrocyte, microglial cell, ependymal cell, ischemia and infarction, neoplasia, diffuse inflammation, abscess formation, and degenerative disease.
5. In a clinical situation, be able to answer the following four questions:
   a. The signs and symptoms contained in the protocol are most likely the manifestation of disease at which of the following *levels* of the nervous system?
      (1) Supratentorial level
      (2) Posterior fossa level
      (3) Spinal level
      (4) Peripheral level
      (5) More than one level
   b. Within the level you have selected, the responsible lesion is most likely:
      (1) Focal, on the *right* side of the nervous system
      (2) Focal, on the *left* side of the nervous system
      (3) Focal, but involving *midline* and *contiguous structures* on both sides of the nervous system
      (4) Nonfocal and diffusely located
   c. The principal pathologic lesion responsible for the symptoms is most likely:
      (1) Some form of *mass* lesion
      (2) Some form of *nonmass* lesion
   d. The cause of the responsible lesion is most likely:
      (1) Vascular
      (2) Degenerative
      (3) Inflammatory
      (4) Neoplastic
      (5) Toxic-metabolic
      (6) Traumatic

Clinical Problems

For each of the following problems, identify the level, lateralization, presence of mass, and cause as outlined in objective 5.

1. A 68-year-old, right-handed man noted heaviness in his left arm while reading a newspaper. He tried to stand up but could not support his weight on his left leg. He was able to call for help. When his wife came to the room, she noted that the left side of his face was sagging.
2. A 6-year-old, right-handed girl with known congenital heart disease began to complain of headaches. Several days later, the severity of the headaches increased, and she was noted to have a left hemiparesis and a left homonymous hemianopia.
3. A 54-year-old, right-handed woman noted some difficulty in expressing her thoughts. This difficulty was mild, and she paid little attention to it. Weeks later, she complained of clumsiness and weakness in her right arm and leg, but the results of an examination by her physician were considered to be normal. Headaches appeared several months later, along with increasing right-sided weakness. She was also aware of an inability to see the right half of the visual field with either eye.
4. A 46-year-old, left-handed woman suddenly noted the onset of a severe bitemporal-occipital headache. On lying down, she became violently ill, with nausea and vomiting. She complained of a stiff neck. She was taken immediately to the hospital, where she was noted to be somnolent but to respond appropriately when stimulated. She could move all four extremities with equal facility. Her level of consciousness deteriorated, and she became deeply comatose.
5. A 4-year-old, right-handed boy complained of a sore throat, chills, and fever. He was put to bed and given aspirin and fluids. The next morning, he noted headache and an increasingly stiff neck. His temperature was 105°F (40.5°C). When seen at a physician's office later that afternoon, he was difficult to arouse. He was confused and delirious when stimulated. He held his neck rigid, but moved his extremities on command.
6. A 50-year-old, right-handed woman, formerly an executive secretary for a local banker, un-

derwent neurologic evaluation because she had had a marked personality change during the past several months. Her memory was poor. She could no longer do even simple calculations, and she had difficulty in following commands. She seemed ill informed about current events and no longer seemed interested in her personal appearance. Results of the remainder of the examination were unremarkable.

7. A 54-year-old, right-handed woman suddenly became dizzy, with nausea and vomiting. Examination revealed dysarthria, difficulty in swallowing (with weakness of the left palate), loss of pinprick sensation over the left side of the face and the right side of the body, and marked ataxia on using the left extremities.

8. A 62-year-old, right-handed man began to note generalized muscle cramps, which he attributed to a charley horse. In the ensuing months, he became aware of weakness in his arms and legs as well as some difficulty in speaking and in swallowing. Examination revealed weakness and atrophy and fasciculations of nearly all muscle groups, with no sensory changes. Bilataral Babinski's signs were present.

9. A 68-year-old, right-handed man noted the sudden onset of severe pain in the chest and abdomen. Almost immediately after the pain he became weak and was unable to support any weight on his right leg. Examination revealed marked weakness of the right lower extremity, with a decrease in the perception of pinprick in the left leg to about the level of the umbilicus.

10. A 46-year-old, right-handed woman noted (in the absence of back pain) gradually increasing pain and numbness extending down her right leg. After these symptoms had been present for 12 months, she consulted her physician, who found slight weakness of the plantar-flexor muscles, absent ankle reflex, and decreased sensation in the posterior aspect of the calf—all on the right side.

Suggested Reading

Blackwood, W., and Corsellis, J. A. N. *Greenfield's Neuropathology* (3rd ed.). London: Arnold, 1976.

Escourolle, R., and Poirier, J. *Manual of Basic Neuropathology*. Philadelphia: Saunders, 1973.

Haymaker, W., and Adams, R. D. *Histology and Histopathology of the Nervous System*. Springfield, Ill.: Thomas, 1982.

Hirano, A. *Color Atlas of Pathology of the Nervous System*. New York: Igaku-Shoin, 1980.

Hirano, A. *A Guide to Neuropathology*. New York: Igaku-Shoin, 1981.

Okazaki, H. *Fundamentals of Neuropathology*. New York: Igaku-Shoin, 1983.

Diagnosis of Neurologic Disorders: Transient Disorders and Neurophysiology

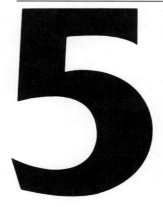

Knowing the location and function of the structural components of the nervous system presented in Chapter 3 permits localization of the site of a lesion. The temporal profile of the major types of disease, as presented in Chapter 4, assists in identifying the cause of the disorder. However, one temporal profile has not yet been considered, that of the *transient* or rapidly reversible abnormality. Many diseases that produce signs or symptoms of brief duration may not produce destructive changes in cells and may occur without demonstrable histologic abnormality of the involved structures. To understand transient manifestations of disease, it is necessary to understand the mechanism by which the many cells of the nervous system process information and, specifically, to understand their physiology. Transient alterations in the physiology of the cells cause transient symptoms and signs. This chapter will provide an introduction to the physiology of neurons, axons, and muscle fibers, which is the basis for information transmission in the central and peripheral neural structures and for the transient symptoms and signs that accompany disease states.

Nerve and muscle cells, like those of other body tissues, carry on many metabolic activities. They generate energy from glucose and oxygen, using aerobic metabolic pathways, and they synthesize proteins and lipids making up the structural components of the cells. Such activities, important for maintaining the integrity of the cells, are disrupted in some diseases. But these metabolic processes are only indirectly involved in accomplishing the major function of the nervous system, which is the transmission and processing of information. This function is accomplished by the generation, conduction, and integration of electrical activity and by the synthesis and release of chemical agents.

Information is conducted from one region to another as electrical activity, commonly known as nerve impulses, which are *generated* by neuronal cell bodies or axons and *conducted* by axons. Information is *transmitted* between cells by neurotransmitters, the chemical agents that convey the signals from one cell to the next. Information is *integrated* by the interaction of electrical impulses in single cells and in groups of cells. Although this chapter will discuss only the physiology of single cells, it must be remembered

that the activity of the central and peripheral nervous systems never depends on the activity of a single neuron or axon but is always mediated by a group of cells or nerve fibers. Information is represented in the nervous system by a change in activity in a group of cells or fibers, as they respond to some change in their input. The interactions of neurons in large groups will be considered in later sections.

Overview

Normal function in a single neuron as it participates in the processing of information is manifested as electrical potentials. These potentials are called membrane potentials and are present in the cell bodies and axons of all neurons and in muscle fibers. They include the following types of membrane potentials: resting potentials; action potentials; and such local potentials as synaptic potentials, generator potentials, and electrotonic potentials.

The *membrane potential* is the difference in electrical potential between the inside and the outside of a cell. All neurons, axons, and muscle fibers have a membrane potential. The *resting potential* is the baseline level of the membrane potential when the cell is at rest and not processing information. This potential depends primarily on potassium ions. When a cell is active in the processing of information, the membrane potential varies. These variations are either local or action potentials.

Action potentials are the electrical signals or nerve impulses by which information is conducted from one area to another within a single cell. The action potential is an all-or-none change in membrane potential in the body or axon of a neuron, or within a muscle fiber. It either occurs fully or not at all and depends on sodium ions. When this potential occurs, it spreads to all other parts of the cell in which it arises. The function of action potentials is thereby to conduct bits of information from one place to another. The action potential is initiated by one form of local potential, the electrotonic potential.

Local potentials are localized changes in the membrane potential that occur in response to stimuli. They are graded signals whose size varies in proportion to the size of the stimulus. They remain localized in the area of the cell in which they are generated; that is, they do not spread to

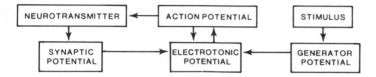

Fig. 5-1. Initiation of electrical potentials in nervous system. Arrows indicate potentials that may be initiated by each element.

involve the entire cell. Local potentials can be summated and integrated by single cells and are thereby an integral part of the processing of information by the nervous system. They are generated in one of two ways: (1) by a change in the characteristics of the membrane—synaptic potentials and generator potentials—or (2) by the flow of electrical current, the electrotonic potentials.

Synaptic potentials are variations in the membrane potential that occur at *synapses,* the specialized areas of cells where adjacent cells are in intimate contact. Synaptic potentials are local potentials arising in postsynaptic cell membranes in response to the action of a neurotransmitter released by presynaptic cells. Neurotransmitters, released when an action potential reaches the synaptic region, serve to transmit information from one cell to another by converting the electrical signal (action potential) into a chemical signal (neurotransmitter release) and then back into an electrical signal (synaptic potential). In turn, synaptic potentials produce electrotonic potentials, which can then initiate another action potential.

Generator potentials are the variations in membrane potentials that occur in receptors—those neural structures in the body, such as the touch receptors in the skin or the light receptors in the eye, that respond to specific stimuli. Generator potentials are also local potentials and are localized and graded. They can generate electrotonic potentials and thereby initiate action potentials (Fig. 5-1).

A localized change in membrane potential will result in current flow to surrounding areas of membrane. This current flow will produce a small change in the membrane potential of adjacent areas. This change is called an *electrotonic potential*. The main features of these potentials are summarized in Table 5-1.

Transient alterations in function in the neuromuscular system may be due to a disruption of the mechanisms underlying the normal generation of the resting potential, the synaptic potential, the generator potential, or the action potential.

Resting Potential

The resting potential is the *absolute difference* in electrical potential between the inside and outside of an inactive neuron, axon, or muscle fiber. If an electrical connection is made between the inside and the outside of a neuron, the cell acts as a battery, and an electrical current will flow. The potential is generally near 80 mV, with the inside of the cell being *negative* with respect to the outside. The resting potential can be measured directly by using a microelectrode. The tip of such an electrode must be less than 1 μm in diameter to be inserted into a nerve or muscle

Table 5-1. Characteristics of Different Membrane Potential Variations

| Characteristic | Action potential | Local potentials | | |
		Electrotonic	Synaptic	Generator
Graded and localized	−	+	+	+
All-or-none spread	+	−	−	−
Active membrane channel	Na^+, K^+	None	Na^+, K^+, or Cl^-	Na^+, K^+
Initiated by	Electrotonic potential	Action, synaptic, or generator potentials	Chemical neurotransmitter	Stimulus

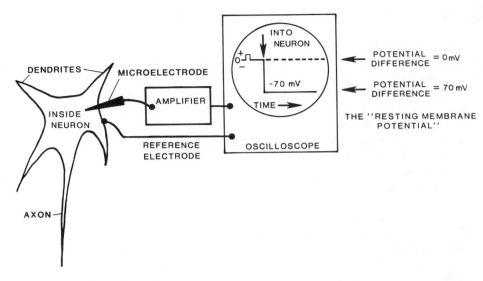

Fig. 5-2. Oscilloscopic recording of membrane potential from neuron.

cell. By connecting the microelectrode to an appropriate amplifier, the membrane potential can be recorded and displayed on an oscilloscope (Fig. 5-2).

The oscilloscope registers the potential difference between the two electrical inputs and is displayed as a vertical deflection of a spot of light that moves continuously from left to right across the cathode ray tube of the oscilloscope. A negative membrane potential is registered as a downward deflection, and thus when a microelectrode enters a neuron or muscle fiber, the oscilloscope beam moves down to a new position.

Because the resting potential is the absolute difference in potential between the inside and the outside of the cell, a negative sign need not be included in describing the value of a resting potential. In addition, a "fall" or "reduction" in resting potential will mean *less negativity* inside, and the oscilloscope beam will move up toward the baseline.

The resting potential in nerve and muscle cells depends on two factors: (1) the cell membrane is a *semipermeable membrane* with different permeabilities for different ions and (2) the cell membrane contains an *energy-dependent mechanism that moves ions* from one side of the membrane to the other, producing different concentrations of ions on the inside and outside of the cell. An understanding of the manner in which these two characteristics of cell membranes result in the

generation of the resting potential requires some knowledge of semipermeable membranes and the biophysics of ionic solutions.

Biophysical Considerations

When a material is dissolved in water, its molecular motion will result in the material spreading from a region of higher concentration to a region of lower concentration, until it is equally distributed throughout the solution. The molecular motion is thus a source of energy that does work on the molecules and is referred to as the *diffusion pressure*. The diffusion pressure is a function of the molecular motion and the relative concentration of the material in different areas. (The molecular motion increases with temperature.)

Body fluids contain charged ions in solution. Sodium (Na^+), potassium (K^+), chloride (Cl^-), and calcium (Ca^{++}) are of particular importance in nerve and muscle cells. Ions with a positive charge such as Na^+ and K^+ are *cations;* those with a negative charge are *anions*. In addition to these simple ions, there are many large intracellular ions, primarily proteins, that are negatively charged and referred to as anions (A^-). Since ions have an electrical charge, they are acted on by differences in electrical potential. Anions move toward the positive pole (the anode), and cations move toward the negative pole (the cathode) of an applied voltage. Thus, a voltage produces an *electrical pressure,* which also can act as a source of energy that does work on ions in solution.

A *semipermeable membrane* permits the passage of some substances but not others. The ease with which a molecule can move through a membrane is called the *membrane permeability*. The ease with which a charged molecule (ion) can move through a membrane is its *conductance*. The conductance of an ion is the reciprocal of the electrical resistance to movement of that ion through the membrane. The permeability and conductance are generally similar for any given ion.

If a salt is dissolved into two ions of opposite charge on one side of a semipermeable membrane, the membrane may be permeable to neither of the ions, to one of the ions, or to both of the ions. If it is permeable to neither, water will move across the membrane and reduce the concentration (osmotic pressure). If the membrane is permeable to both of the ions, they will both move across the membrane by diffusion pressure until they are both equally distributed on the two sides of the membrane. If the salt dissolves into two ions of different sizes, one with a high conductance and the other with a low conductance, an interesting phenomenon occurs. The diffusion pressure moves the diffusible ion across the membrane into the area of lower concentration. As this occurs, a separation of charges develops because the nondiffusible ions all remain on one side of the membrane and have a charge opposite that of the diffusible ions, which move through the membrane.

Two regions that accumulate different charges have an electrical potential difference. Therefore, as the diffusible ions move across the membrane, an electrical potential develops that resists the movement of the diffusible ions across the membrane. The net ionic movement will continue until *the diffusion pressure equals the electrical pressure*. At this time, the system will be in equilibrium. At equilibrium, there will continue to be random ionic movements, but no net movement of ions will occur. The electrical potential developed across the membrane at equilibrium is called the *equilibrium potential*. An algebraic representation of the equilibrium potential can be derived because the physical determinants of the diffusion pressure and electrical pressure are known. The final equation is the Nernst equation.

Electrical pressure is defined by:

$$W_e = E_m \cdot Z_i \cdot F$$

in which W_e = electrical pressure (work required to move an ion against a voltage)
E_m = absolute membrane potential
Z_i = valence (number of charges on the ion)
F = faraday (number of coulombs per mol of ion)

Diffusion pressure is defined by:

$$W_d = R \cdot T \cdot (\ln[C]_{hi} - \ln[C]_{lo})$$

in which W_d = diffusion pressure (work required to move an ion against a concentration gradient)
R = universal gas constant
T = absolute temperature
$\ln$ = natural logarithm
$[C]_{hi}$ = ion concentration on the more concentrated side of the membrane
$[C]_{lo}$ = ion concentration on the less concentrated side

At equilibrium:

$$W_e = W_d \text{ and therefore}$$

$$E_m \cdot Z_i \cdot F = R \cdot T \cdot (\ln[C]_{hi} - \ln[C]_{lo})$$

By rearrangement, the equilibrium potential is:

$$E_m = \frac{R \cdot T}{F \cdot Z} \cdot \ln\left(\frac{[C]_{hi}}{[C]_{lo}}\right)$$

The *Nernst equation* is an important relationship that defines the equilibrium potential, E_m, inside the cell for any ion in terms of its concentration on the two sides of a membrane. From the Nernst equation the polarity of the potential will depend on whether the ion is an anion or a cation: E_m for a cation will be $(+)$ on the low concentration side, and E_m for an anion will be $(-)$ on the low concentration side. By substituting for the constants at room temperature, converting to a base 10 logarithm, and converting to millivolts, we get a useful form of the equation:

$$E_m = 58 \log_{10} \frac{[C]_{lo}}{[C]_{hi}} \text{ for cations}$$

$$E_m = 58 \, \log_{10} \frac{[C]_{hi}}{[C]_{lo}} \text{ for anions}$$

We may use these equations to calculate the equilibrium potential for any ion if we know the concentrations of that ion on the two sides of the membrane. This potential will only develop if the membrane is permeable to the ion. A more precise representation of the actual voltage developed across a membrane with unequal concentrations of an ion on the two sides of the membrane also must include the permeability (P) since the membrane potential (E_K) depends on the ease with which the ion can diffuse across the membrane. Algebraically, for potassium in which P_K = potassium conductance:

$$E_K = \frac{R \cdot T}{F \cdot Z} \cdot \ln \frac{P_K \cdot [K^+]_o}{P_K \cdot [K^+]_i}$$

If a membrane is permeable to multiple ions that are present in differing concentrations on either side of the membrane, the resultant membrane potential will be a function of the concentrations of each of the ions and of their relative permeabilities. The *Goldman equation* combines these factors for the major ions that influence the membrane potential in nerve and muscle cells:

$$E_m = \frac{R \cdot T}{F \cdot Z} \cdot \ln \frac{P_K \cdot [K^+]_o + P_{Na} \cdot [Na^+]_o + P_{Cl} \cdot [Cl^-]_i}{P_K \cdot [K^+]_i + P_{Na} \cdot [Na^+]_i + P_{Cl} \cdot [Cl^-]_o}$$

The Goldman equation permits the calculation of the membrane potential for various neurons or muscle fibers. Such calculations, on the basis of the actual ionic concentrations and ionic permeabilities, agree with measurements of these values in living cells. Since the potassium permeability in most living cells is much greater than the sodium permeability, the resting potential is near the equilibrium potential of potassium.

These equations also show that a change in either ionic permeability or ionic concentrations can alter membrane potential. If the *concentration gradient* of an ion is reduced, there will be a lower equilibrium potential for that ion. If the resting membrane potential is determined by the equilibrium potential of that ion, the resting potential will decrease. In contrast, if the *permeability* for an ion is increased, the membrane potential will approach the equilibrium potential of that ion, and it may increase or decrease, depending on whether the membrane potential is above or below the equilibrium potential. The movements of ions that occur with normal cellular activity are not sufficient to produce significant concentration changes, and therefore membrane potential fluctuations are normally due to permeability changes.

The Cell Membrane

The membranes of excitable cells contain separate channels for individual ions that differ in permeability to different ions. The ion channels are protein structures embedded in the lipid membrane (Fig. 5-3) and are of various sizes and shapes. They are lined with electrical charges that repel or attract the ions. Voltage-sensitive gates or gating potentials at the entrance of the channels regulate the movement of the ions into them. When there is a strong gating potential, the ions are repelled; when the gating potential is weak, ions can pass into the channels. In the resting state, the gates of the sodium channels are almost completely closed, whereas those of the potassium channels are partially open, making the membrane approximately 50 to 100 times more permeable to potassium than to sodium ions. The gating potential can be altered by a neurotransmitter, a physical stimulus, or a change in the membrane potential that can cause the gates to open or close and thereby allow or prevent more ions from entering the channels. For example, a decrease in the membrane potential can cause an opening of the sodium gates, with an increase in the permeability of the membrane to sodium ions.

Fig. 5-3. Diagram of cell membrane with ion channels formed by protein structures embedded in the lipid membrane.

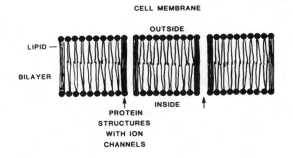

CELL MEMBRANE

OUTSIDE

LIPID —

BILAYER

INSIDE

PROTEIN
STRUCTURES
WITH ION
CHANNELS

In addition to the sodium and potassium channels, there are calcium channels that allow the movement of calcium ions into the nerve membrane. These are most abundant at the nerve terminals, where the influx of calcium ions is necessary for the release of neurotransmitter substances. Calcium ions also help regulate the sodium gates by producing an electrical field or gating potential that blocks the entry of sodium ions into the membrane. When calcium ions are decreased in the extracellular fluid, the sodium gates fail to close and sodium ions continue to leak in.

The movement of ions through the membrane is also dependent on the hydration charge. Most ions are bound to water molecules, which must be removed before the ions can pass through the channel. The amount of energy necessary to remove the water molecules is referred to as the *hydration energy.* This energy is less for potassium ions than for other ions, thus allowing for an easier transfer of potassium ions through the membrane.

The density of ion channels differs along a cell membrane in some cells, which adds differences in permeability. Other factors affecting the movement of ions across the membrane are the potential difference and the concentration gradients across the membrane.

Active Transport

Nerve and muscle cells obtain energy from glucose and oxygen via the glycolytic pathways, the Krebs cycle, and the electron transport system. These pathways provide the energy for normal cell function in the form of adenosine triphosphate (ATP). ATP is partly consumed in generating the resting potential by a mechanism in the membrane, which moves potassium in and sodium out of the cell, with slightly more sodium being moved than potassium. This movement is referred to as *active transport,* and the system through which it occurs is the *sodium pump.* The sodium pump moves sodium out of the cell and potassium into the cell against their concentration gradients. Chloride moves out of the cell passively with sodium. The large internal anions are nondiffusible and remain intracellular. A defect in the energy-producing system due to anoxia or to an enzyme block results in cessation of active

transport and in an inability to generate and maintain a resting potential.

The Resting Potential

Active transport across the cell membrane results in unequal concentrations of the ions on opposite sides of the membrane and in a diffusion pressure to move the ions back down their concentration gradients. *Potassium* diffuses through the membrane most readily because its conductance is much higher than that of the other ions. Therefore, potassium is the largest source of separation of positive and negative charges (voltage) as it diffuses out and leaves the large anions behind. This is illustrated schematically in Figure 5-4. In Figure 5-4, the ionic concentrations have been established with a high external and a low internal concentration of sodium, and a high internal and a low external concentration of potassium initially (A), with large, nondiffusible anions shown inside. The conductance of potassium is much greater than that of sodium, and potassium diffuses out of the cell to produce the separation of positive and negative charges which establishes a membrane potential (B). However, the potential difference resists this redistribution of ions, and a balance between A and B occurs (C), with a resultant resting potential at equilibrium.

In the living cell, there is a continuous small influx of sodium and an efflux (outward flow) of potassium ions, which are transferred back across the membrane by the sodium pump. Because the net diffusion of ions is continuous across the membrane, and the ions are returned by the sodium pump, a true equilibrium does not occur. However, as long as the pump keeps up with the inward leak of sodium and an outward leak of potassium, a steady membrane potential is established, which is referred to as the *steady state.* The resting potential in living cells therefore is a steady state and not an equilibrium potential. The normal ionic concentrations in mammalian neurons are shown in Table 5-2.

Similar mechanisms are at work in all nerve and muscle cells, although the actual concentrations of the ions vary widely in different cells. Some examples of the determination of the resting potential from ionic concentrations by the Nernst equation are shown in Table 5-3, which also illustrates that, despite different ionic con-

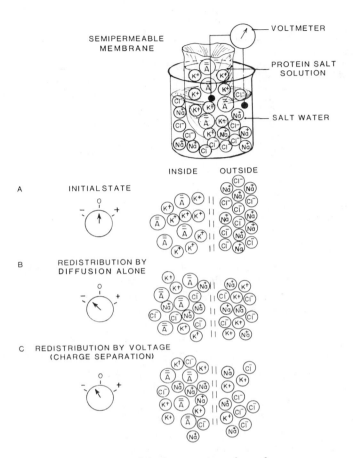

Fig. 5-4. Theoretic model of generation of membrane potential by diffusion across semipermeable membrane. A. Equal amounts of anions and cations dissolved on each side of membrane—no voltage gradient. Membrane is permeable to all ions except large anions (A^-). B. K^+, Na^+, and Cl^- redistribute themselves solely by diffusion; this results in a charge separation, with greater negativity inside. C. Electrical pressure due to charge separation and diffusion pressure due to concentration differences are balanced at resting membrane potential.

Table 5-2. Relative Ionic Conditions in Mammalian Neurons

Condition	Sodium	Potassium	Chloride
Internal concentration	Low	High	Low
External concentration	High	Low	High
Resting permeability	Low	High	Moderate

centrations, the similar extracellular-intracellular ratios result in similar resting potentials. Some glial cells that are potassium-dependent have also been found to have resting potentials of 70 to 90 mV.

The concentration gradient of calcium is similar to that of sodium, with an even higher positive (inside) equilibrium potential. However, calcium has such a low conductance that it does not contribute directly to the resting potential. It is, however, adsorbed on the external surface of the membrane, where it is involved in membrane changes occurring during the activity of cells. In general, calcium tends to reduce or limit changes in the sodium or potassium conductances. It acts, thereby, as a membrane "stabilizer." A calcium current mediates the conduction of some spikes in dendrites and in cardiac muscle and participates in the release of neurotransmitter.

Table 5-3. Ionic Concentration in Neurons of Various Species

Cell	Ion	Extracellular concentration (mm/L)	Intracellular concentration (mm/L)	Extracellular-intracellular ratio	Equilibrium potential inside
Squid axon (RP 70 mV)*	Na$^+$	450.0	50	9:1	+55
	K$^+$	20.0	400	1:20	−76
	Cl$^-$	560.0	40	14:1	−104
Cat motor neuron (RP 65 mV)	Na$^+$	150.0	15	10:1	+58
	K$^+$	5.5	150	1:27	−83
	Cl$^-$	125.0	9	14:1	−107
Human skeletal muscle (RP 80 mV)	Na$^+$	150.0	26	6:1	+53
	K$^+$	4.0	150	1:38	−95
	Cl$^-$	105.0	4	26:1	−85

*RP = resting potential.

Local Potentials

In the normal nerve or muscle cell with adequate sources of oxygen and glucose, the resting potential is maintained at a stable, relatively unchanging level. The resting potential, however, will readily change in response to a wide variety of stimuli. The membrane potential can change from the resting state in only two ways. It can either become more negative inside, *hyperpolarization,* or less negative inside, *depolarization.* Even if the membrane potential reverses, so that the inside becomes positive with respect to the outside, it is still referred to as depolarization, because the potential is less negative than the resting potential.

The changes in the membrane potential that occur with anoxia or a change in the concentration of the ions on either side of the membrane are relatively long lasting (minutes to hours). In contrast, rapid changes (seconds or less) can occur in response to electrical, mechanical, or chemical stimuli. These changes occur as a result of current flow through the membrane. Current in living tissues is due to the movement of charged ions, and it can flow through the membrane as a result of an applied voltage or of a change in membrane conductance.

A *local potential* is a transient shift of the membrane potential in a localized area of the cell. This may occur in response to various stimuli and may have either a hyperpolarizing or a depolarizing effect. Local potentials may result from a local change in the permeability of the membrane to one or more ions (synaptic potentials and generator potentials), or from a change in a voltage or current applied to the membrane

from some other source (electrotonic potential). The latter is the mechanism by which an action potential is initiated and is spread throughout a single cell; the former occurs in response to neurotransmitters or external stimuli and is the manner in which information is transmitted into or out of a cell. While both of these types of local potentials have characteristics in common, the ionic basis of generation is different.

Ionic Basis of Local Potentials

Local potentials result from a flow of current through the membrane that is due either to an applied voltage (electrotonic potential) or to a change in membrane permeability (synaptic or generator potential).

The synaptic potential occurs with change in membrane permeability induced by *neurotransmitters* by one of four mechanisms acting on ion channels:

1. An increase in conductance of potassium, which results in a hyperpolarization.
2. An increase in conductance of sodium, which results in a depolarization.
3. An increase in conductance of both sodium and potassium, which results in a depolarization but to a lesser degree than in 2.
4. An increase in conductance of chloride, which results in a hyperpolarization.

The generator potential occurs by mechanical or chemical activation that involves the third mechanism.

The electrotonic potential may occur in one of two ways that do not alter ion channels:

1. The application of a negative voltage to the outside of the membrane produces an outward current flow that depolarizes the membrane. (Positive ions are drawn away from the outside of the membrane in the area of the negative cathode, reducing the potential difference across the membrane.)
2. Application of a positive potential to the outside of the membrane will hyperpolarize the membrane.

When a voltage is applied to the outside of the nerve membrane, the negative pole is commonly referred to as the *cathode;* the positive pole is the *anode.* The current flow at the cathode depolarizes, whereas that at the anode hyperpolarizes a cell.

Characteristics of Local Potentials

All local potentials have certain common characteristics. Most importantly, the local potential is a *graded* potential, that is, its amplitude is proportional to the size of the stimulus (Fig. 5-5). Measurement of a local potential uses the resting potential as its baseline so that, if the membrane's resting potential is depolarized from 80 to 70 mV during the local potential, the local potential has an amplitude of 10 mV. This potential change is one of decreasing negativity or of depolarization, but it could also be one of an increase in negativity or of hyperpolarization.

Because the local potential is a graded response, proportional to the size of the stimulus, the occurrence of a second stimulus, before the first subsides, results in a larger local potential. Local potentials therefore can be *summated.* They are summated algebraically, so that similar potentials are additive, while hyperpolarizing and depolarizing potentials tend to cancel out each other. Summated potentials may reach threshold and produce an action potential when single potentials individually are subthreshold.

When a stimulus is applied in a localized area of the membrane, the change in membrane potential has both a temporal and a spatial distribution. A study of the temporal course of the local potential (Fig. 5-5) shows that the increase in the potential is not instantaneous but that it develops over a few milliseconds. After the stimulus ends, the potential subsides over a few milliseconds as well. Local potentials therefore have a temporal

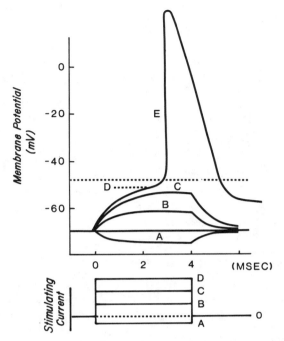

Fig. 5-5. Local potentials. These potentials are shown as upward deflection if they are a depolarization and as downward deflection if they are a hyperpolarization. Resting potential is 70 mV. At time zero, electrical currents of varied polarities and voltage are applied to the membrane (lower diagram). A is an anodal current; B, C, and D are cathodal currents. A produces a transient hyperpolarization; B, C, and D produce a transient depolarization that is graded and proportional to size of stimulus. All of these are local potentials; D has produced an action potential, E.

course that outlasts the stimulus. The occurrence of a second stimulus at the same site shortly after the first will produce another local potential, which summates with any residual of the earlier one that has not yet subsided. This summation of local potentials occurring near each other in time is called *temporal summation* (Fig. 5-6B).

Different synaptic potentials have different time courses. Most synaptic potentials range from 10 to 15 msec in duration; however, some are very brief, lasting less than 1 msec, while others may last several seconds or several minutes. The longer the duration of the synaptic potential, the more chance there is for temporal summation to occur. By means of temporal summation, the cell can integrate signals that are arriving at different times.

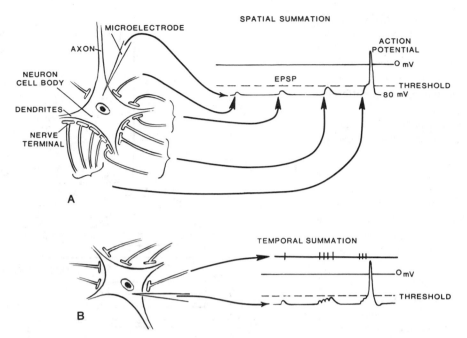

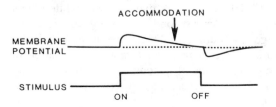

Fig. 5-6. Summation of local potentials in neuron. A. Spatial summation occurs when increasing numbers of nerve terminals release more neurotransmitter to produce larger EPSPs.   B. Temporal summation occurs when a single terminal discharges repetitively more rapidly to produce larger EPSPs.

A study of the spatial distribution of local potentials reveals another of their characteristics. As their name implies, they remain *localized* in the region where the stimulus is applied; they do not spread throughout the entire cell. However, the locally applied stimulus, because of local current flow, has an effect on the nearby surrounding membrane. The potential change is not sharply confined to the area of the stimulus but falls off over a finite distance on the membrane, usually a few millimeters. The application of a simultane-

Fig. 5-7. Accommodation of membrane potential to applied stimulus of constant strength. Note response to a sudden cessation of stimulus.

ous second stimulus near the first (but not at the same site) results in summation of the potentials in the border zones, *spatial summation* (Fig. 5-6). The membrane of the cell thereby can act as an integrator of stimuli that are arriving from different sources and are impinging on areas of membrane near one another. Spatial and temporal summation are important mechanisms in the processing of information by single neurons; when summated local potentials reach threshold, they will initiate an action potential.

If a current or voltage is applied to a membrane for more than a few milliseconds, the ionic conductances of the membrane will change in a direction to restore the resting potential to the baseline value. This phenomenon is known as *accommodation* (Fig. 5-7). Therefore, if an electrical stimulus is increased slowly, accommodation can occur and no change in the membrane potential will be seen. The changes in conductance during accommodation require a number of milliseconds, both to develop and to subside. As a result, if an electrical stimulus is gradually applied so that accommodation prevents a change in resting potential, then when the stimulus is suddenly turned off, the residual change in conductance will produce a transient change in resting potential. Accommodation thus can result in a cell responding to the cessation of a stimulus.

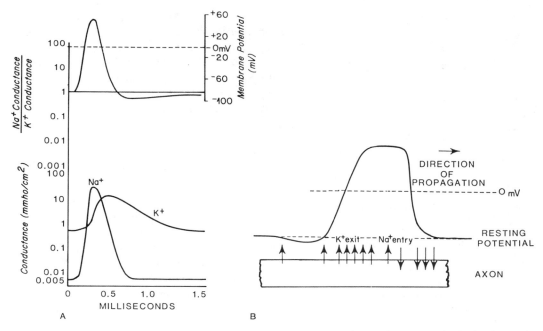

Fig. 5-8. Conductance changes during action potential. A. Temporal sequence at single site along axon is shown. Changes in conductances (permeabilities) of sodium and potassium are plotted against time as they change with associated changes in membrane potential. Note that sodium conductance changes several thousandfold early in the process, whereas potassium conductance changes only about thirtyfold during later stages and persists longer than sodium conductance changes. B. Spatial distribution of action potential over a length of axon at a single instant.

Action Potentials

Threshold

The membranes of neurons, axons, and muscle cells have another characteristic that is basic to their ability to transmit information from one area to another, their *excitability*. If a membrane is depolarized by a stimulus, there is a point at which a sudden change in the electrical characteristics of the membrane occurs. This point is known as the *threshold* for excitation (see Fig. 5-5). If the depolarization does not reach threshold, the evoked activity is a local potential, as described on page 74.

Threshold may be reached by a single local potential or by summated local potentials. When threshold is reached, there is a sudden increase in the membrane's permeability to sodium. This

change in conductance results in the action potential.

Ionic Basis of Action Potential

In the resting state, the conductance of sodium is much less than that of potassium, and the resting potential is near the equilibrium potential of potassium. At threshold, the conductance of sodium suddenly becomes greater than that of potassium, and the membrane potential shifts toward the equilibrium potential of sodium, which is approximately +60 mV. This depolarization reverses the polarity of the membrane, the inside becoming positive with respect to the outside. With the change in the sodium channel and sodium conductance, there is a flow of current with the inward movement of sodium ions. The change in sodium conductance is transient, lasting only a few milliseconds, and is followed by a change in the potassium channel and an increase in the potassium conductance and an outward movement of potassium ions. These two changes overlap, and the potential of the membrane during these changes is a function of the ratios of the conductances (Fig. 5-8). The sodium conductance increases several thousandfold early in the process, whereas the potassium conductance increases less, does so later, and persists longer. The conductance changes for these two ions result in

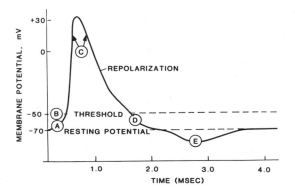

Fig. 5-9. Components of action potential with resting potential of 70 mV. A. Local, electronic potential. B. Threshold level. C. Spike. D. Negative (depolarizing) afterpotential. E. Positive (hyperpolarizing) afterpotential.

ionic shifts and current flows that are associated with a membrane potential change, the *action potential* (Fig. 5-8).

The action potential is a sudden, short-duration, all-or-none change in the membrane potential that occurs if the membrane potential reaches threshold. Its component parts are shown in Figure 5-9. The initial portion of the membrane potential change is the local potential. At threshold, the rising phase of the action potential suddenly changes because of the influx of positive ions. In most nerve and skeletal muscle tissue, the inward current during the rising phase of the action potential is carried by sodium ions because sodium conductance is markedly increased. The action potential also could be carried by calcium ions if the calcium conductance increased sufficiently. Repolarization begins as the sodium conductance decreases and the potassium conductance increases. The decreased flow of sodium ions is followed by an efflux of potassium ions. The rate of return of the membrane potential to the baseline slows after the sodium conductance has returned to baseline, producing a small residual on the negative component of the action potential, which is called the *negative afterpotential.*

The afterpotential is positive when the membrane potential is recorded with a microelectrode within the cell, but it is called negative because it is negative when recorded with an extracellular electrode. The increase in potassium conductance persists and results in a hyperpolarization after the spike component of the action potential, the *afterhyperpolarization.* The afterhyperpolarization is due to continued efflux of potassium ions, with a greater than resting difference in potential between the inside and outside of the cell. The afterhyperpolarization is positive when measured with extracellular electrodes and therefore is called a *positive afterpotential.* During the positive afterpotential, the membrane potential is near the potassium equilibrium potential, and oxygen consumption is increased with increased activity of the sodium pump.

The amounts of sodium and potassium that move across the membrane during the action potential are extremely small and do not change the concentration enough to result in a change in the resting potential. In addition, the sodium that moves in during the action potential is continually removed by the sodium pump during the relatively long intervals between action potentials.

Excitability

The excitability of a membrane is the ease with which an action potential can be generated and is usually measured in terms of the voltage required to initiate an action potential. During increased sodium conductance, the membrane cannot be stimulated to discharge again. A second stimulus at this time will be without effect, and therefore action potentials, unlike local potentials, cannot summate. This period of unresponsiveness is the *absolute refractory period* (Fig. 5-10). As sodium conductance returns to normal, the membrane again becomes excitable, but for a short period, the *relative refractory period,* it requires a larger stimulus to produce a smaller action potential. After the relative refractory period, while the negative afterpotential is subsiding, the membrane is partially depolarized, is closer to threshold, and has an increased excitability. This period is the *supernormal period.* Finally, during the positive afterpotential, the membrane is hyperpolarized away from threshold, and larger stimuli are required. This period is the *subnormal period.*

Up to now, the term *threshold* has been used to refer to the membrane potential at which changes occur that result in the generation of an action potential. The threshold of a membrane remains relatively constant. If the membrane potential be-

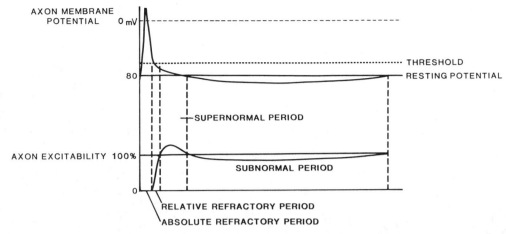

Fig. 5-10. Excitability changes during action potential. Lower portion of illustration shows ease with which another action potential can be elicited (change in threshold). During absolute and relative refractory periods, amplitude of action potential evoked is low. Subsequently, it is normal.

comes hyperpolarized, the membrane potential moves away from threshold, and the membrane is less excitable. If the membrane potential moves closer to threshold, the membrane becomes more excitable and will generate an action potential with a smaller stimulus. If the membrane potential is very near threshold, the cell may fire spontaneously. If the membrane potential remains more *depolarized* than threshold, however, the membrane cannot be stimulated to fire another action potential (Fig. 5-11).

Fig. 5-11. Effect of stimulation of neuron at different resting potentials as recorded with microelectrode. A. Membrane is hyperpolarized, and stimulus produces subthreshold local potential. B. Membrane is normally polarized at −65 mV, and stimulus produces local potential that reaches threshold and results in action potential. C. Membrane is depolarized beyond threshold, and stimulus again produces only small local potential.

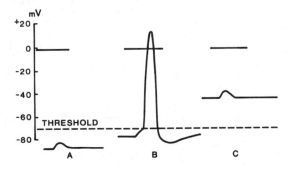

The term threshold is also used to describe the voltage required to excite an action potential. When threshold is used in this sense, an axon with an increased excitability due to partial depolarization may be said to have a lower "threshold" for stimulation, even though the actual threshold is unchanged. The first meaning of threshold is used when intracellular recordings are considered, and the second is used in reference to extracellular stimulation and recording.

The threshold of the nerve membrane differs in different parts of the neuron: it is high in the dendrite and soma and lowest at the axon hillock. Thus, an action potential is usually generated in the area of the axon hillock.

Propagation

Another important characteristic of action potentials is their propagation. An action potential initiated in any part of a neuron or muscle cell will spread to all other regions of that cell. For instance, if an action potential is initiated in an axon in the tip of the finger, the potential will spread up the entire length of that axon to its cell body in the dorsal root ganglion, and then up the central axon, ascending in the spinal cord to the brain stem. This characteristic permits the nervous system to transmit information from one area to another.

When an area of membrane is depolarized during an action potential, ionic currents will flow (Fig. 5-12). In the area of depolarization, sodium ions carry positive charges inward. There is also a longitudinal flow of current both inside and outside the membrane. This flow of positive charges (current) toward nondepolarized regions

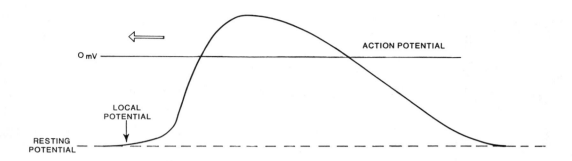

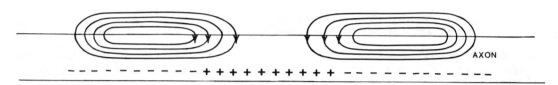

Fig. 5-12. Current flow and voltage changes in axon in region of action potential. The voltage changes along the membrane are shown in the upper part of the figure and the spatial distribution of current flow is shown in the lower part as arrows through the axon membrane.

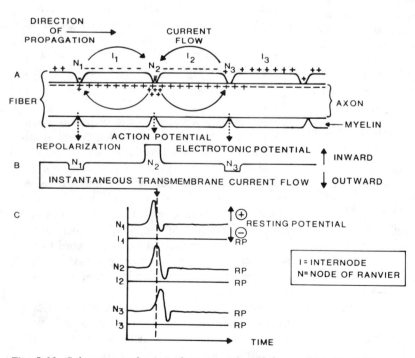

Fig. 5-13. Saltatory conduction along axon from left to right. A. Charge distribution along axon is shown with action potential (depolarization) at second node of Ranvier (N_2). Current flow spreads to next node (N_3). B. Membrane current flow along axon is shown. C. Portion of action potential found at each node is indicated by dotted lines.

internally and toward depolarized regions externally tends to depolarize the membrane in the areas that surround the region of the action potential. This depolarization is an electrotonic potential. In normal tissue, this depolarization is sufficient to shift the membrane potential to threshold and thereby to generate an action potential in the immediately adjacent membrane. The action potential thus will spread away from its site of initiation along an axon or muscle fiber. Because of the refractory period, the potential cannot reverse and spread back into an area just depolarized.

The rate of conduction of the action potential along the membrane depends on the amount of longitudinal current flow and on the amount of current needed to produce depolarization in the adjacent membrane. The longitudinal current flow can be increased by increasing the diameter of an axon or muscle fiber, since this increase reduces the internal resistance, just as a larger electrical wire has a lower electrical resistance. However, many axons in the central and peripheral nervous systems obtain an increased conduction velocity because they are insulated with a myelin sheath. A myelinated axon has its membrane bared only at the nodes of Ranvier, so that transmembrane current flow occurs almost exclusively at the nodal area. When current flow reaches threshold in the nodal area, it results in an influx of sodium ions with a generation of an action potential. The nodal area in the mammalian nervous system is unique in that it consists almost exclusively of sodium channels, with an almost complete absence of potassium channels. The potassium channels are located at the paranodal regions (adjacent to the node), which are covered by myelin. The action potential generated at the node consists predominantly of inward sodium currents with little outward potassium currents, and repolarization is achieved by means of sodium inactivation and leakage currents. An action potential at one node of Ranvier produces sufficient longitudinal current flow to depolarize adjacent nodes to threshold, thereby propagating the action potential along the nerve in a skipping manner called *saltatory conduction* (Fig. 5-13).

Synaptic Transmission

Synaptic transmission may be chemically or electrically mediated. Most of the synapses in the human nervous system use chemical transmitters. The terminations of the axons of most neurons are specialized to synthesize chemical agents which, when released, act on other cells. These are known as *neurotransmitters*. They are synthesized by enzymes that are manufactured in the cell body and transferred down the axon by an active, oxygen-dependent, axoplasmic transport system. The neurotransmitters are stored in the nerve terminals in small membranous structures (vesicles). They are released from the vesicles in discrete quantities when the nerve terminal is depolarized. The amount of neurotransmitter released is directly proportional to the change in membrane potential, that is, the amplitude of the action potential in the nerve terminal. The release of neurotransmitter from a nerve terminal is stimulated when the depolarization alters the conductance of calcium, with an inward flow of calcium ions. The calcium ions result in a fusion of the vesicle with the nerve terminal membrane and in release of neurotransmitter (Fig. 5-14).

The neurotransmitter diffuses across the synaptic cleft, the narrow space between the axon terminal and the membrane of the postsynaptic cell. The subsynaptic portion of the postsynaptic membrane is a specialized portion of the cell that responds to neurotransmitter by an alteration in the permeability of one or more ions. This change in permeability results in current flow, and the resulting local potential change in the postsynaptic membrane is the *synaptic potential*. The synaptic potential is associated with local current flow in the region around the synapse, producing an electrotonic local potential. The synaptic potential, like other local potentials, is a graded response that is proportional to the amount of transmitter released. The potential change remains localized in the area of the synapse, unless the electrotonic potential depolarizes the surrounding membrane to threshold and initiates an action potential. The postsynaptic effects of a neurotransmitter vary with the transmitter released and with the character of the postsynaptic membrane. There may be a brief, direct effect on the membrane, resulting in a transient conformational and conductance change for a few milliseconds, or a more prolonged change, lasting seconds.

In some synapses, the neurotransmitter interacts with the postsynaptic receptor to activate a

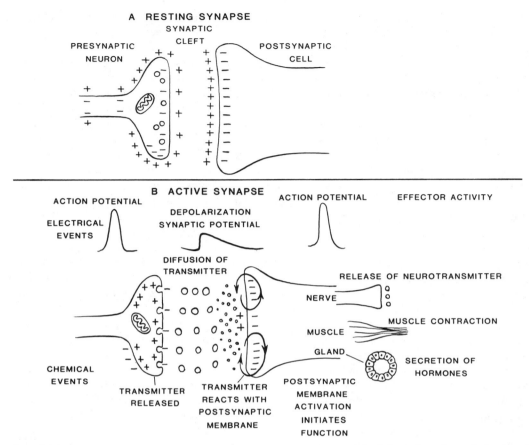

Fig. 5-14. Synaptic transmission. A. In resting synapse, both nerve terminal and muscle fiber are normally polarized. B. In active synapse, action potential invades nerve terminal from left and depolarizes it. Depolarization of nerve terminal of presynaptic neuron results in release of neurotransmitter from nerve terminal. Neurotransmitter diffuses across synaptic cleft and produces local current flow and synaptic potential in the postsynaptic membrane, which initiates the effector activity (neuronal transmission, neurotransmitter release, hormonal secretion, or muscle contraction).

second chemical substance called the *second messenger*, which in turn triggers reactions within the cell. The second messengers are cyclic nucleotides, cyclic 3′, 5′-adenosine and possibly guanosine monophosphate (cyclic AMP or cyclic GMP), which regulate membrane permeability and ion fluxes, protein synthesis, and neurotransmitter release. The second messengers act as intracellular mediators for extracellular neurotransmitters.

Since the release of neurotransmitter from the nerve terminal is a function of the amplitude of the action potential in the nerve terminal, synaptic transmission can be modified by changes in the membrane potential of the nerve terminal. Some nerve terminals synapse directly on other nerve terminals that they can partially depolarize. The partially depolarized nerve terminal will release less neurotransmitter when it is depolarized by the invading action potential. The resultant synaptic potential therefore will be smaller. This form of grading the size of the synaptic potential by reducing the amount of neurotransmitter released is called *presynaptic inhibition* (Fig. 5-15).

The synaptic potentials arising at different synapses have different names. Three of the most important are the end-plate potential, the excitatory postsynaptic potential, and the inhibitory postsynaptic potential. At the neuromuscular junction, where a motor axon innervates the muscle fiber, the release of acetylcholine acts on sodium and potassium channels to increase the conductances of sodium and potassium. The resulting current flow is seen as a depolarizing syn-

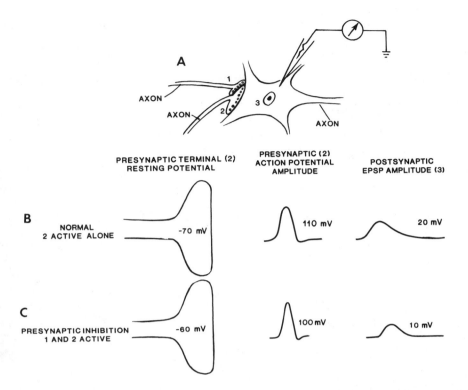

Fig. 5-15. A. Presynaptic inhibition of neuron 3 when axon 1 partially depolarizes axon 2. B. Response to axon 2 acting alone. C. Response to axon 2 after depolarization of axon 1. In the latter case, there is less neurotransmitter and a smaller EPSP.

aptic potential called the *end-plate potential* (EPP). Depolarizing synaptic potentials in the nervous system result from various neurotransmitters that act to increase conductance in sodium channels and are called *excitatory postsynaptic potentials* (EPSP). An EPSP tends to discharge a cell because it moves the membrane potential toward threshold. Other neurotransmitters produce selective increase in potassium or chloride channel conductance. The resulting synaptic potential, a hyperpolarization, is called an *inhibitory postsynaptic potential* (IPSP). It moves the potential away from threshold and makes the membrane less excitable (Fig. 5-16). EPSPs and IPSPs of longer duration are produced by the decreased conductance that occurs when the leakage channels of sodium and potassium are closed.

Many chemical agents can alter the membrane potential or other cellular functions, both in the nervous system and elsewhere. Naturally occur-

ring compounds secreted by one cell and acting on other cells are subdivided into neurotransmitters and hormones. Neurotransmitters, which have already been described, are simple compounds that are usually synthesized in the cell body, released into the synaptic cleft to act rapidly on a single adjacent cell, and then inactivated. In contrast, hormones are usually larger peptide molecules, synthesized in the cell bodies of groups of neurons or endocrine glands, and secreted into the circulation. Thus, hormones can act widely on large numbers of cells throughout the body, though they have slower actions than neurotransmitters.

A number of neurotransmitters act at synapses in the central and peripheral nervous systems. These include acetylcholine, the biogenic amines —norepinephrine, histamine, dopamine, and serotonin, and the amino acids—γ-aminobutyric acid (GABA), glutamic acid, and glycine. Some peptides also may act either as hormones when released from some cells or as neurotransmitters when released from others. Twenty-five small neuroactive peptides have been identified, including such substances as substance P, the enkephalins, the endorphins, somatostatin, vasopressin, bradykinin, angiotensin, insulin, glucagon, corti-

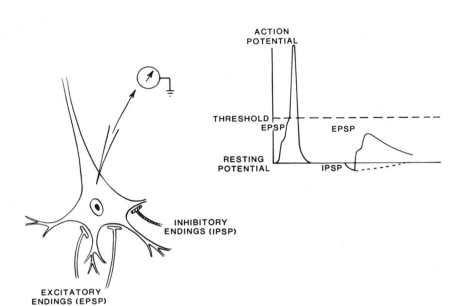

Fig. 5-16. Postsynaptic inhibition in the neuron on the left occurs when the inhibitory and excitatory endings are active simultaneously. On the right a microelectrode recording shows two EPSPs summating to initiate action potential. Where there is a simultaneous occurrence of an IPSP, depolarization is too low to reach threshold, and no action potential occurs.

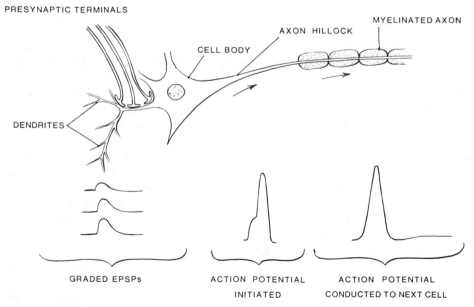

Fig. 5-17. Neuronal electrical activity from its initiation by EPSPs to its transmission as action potential to another area.

cotropin (adrenocorticotropic hormone [ACTH]), oxytocin, and thyroid-releasing hormone.

It was formerly believed that a neuron and its axon synthesized and released only one type of neurotransmitter. It is now known that some neurons release two or more neurotransmitters, by *cosecretion*, which may produce different effects on other neurons. Neurons are also now known to have more than one receptor, and these can respond to different neurotransmitters.

While the neurotransmitters at most synapses are unknown, some are well defined. Acetylcholine, for instance, is released at the neuromuscular junction, in visceral autonomic pathways, and in the basal ganglion; norepinephrine is released at other visceral autonomic nerve terminals and in the locus ceruleus, a brain-stem nucleus. Dopamine is released in the basal ganglia and hypothalamus and GABA in the cerebellum and spinal cord inhibitory neurons. Substance P may be the neurotransmitter for dorsal root ganglion cells. Since the synapses are specialized to respond to neurotransmitters, they are also very susceptible to the action of other chemical agents or drugs. Many of the drugs used in clinical medicine have their pharmacologic site of action at the synapse.

The mechanism underlying chemical synaptic transmission should make it apparent that synaptic transmission has three characteristics unique to it. First, conduction at a synapse is delayed because of the brief interval of time required for the chemical events to occur. Second, because the two sides of the synapse are specialized to perform only one function, transmission can occur in only one direction across the synapse. The cells of the nervous system are thereby polarized in their direction of impulse transmission. Third, because nerve impulses from many sources impinge on single cells in the central and the peripheral nervous system, synaptic potentials will summate both temporally and spatially. The membrane of a cell is continually being bombarded with various neurotransmitters, which will produce either EPSPs or IPSPs of varying duration. When the membrane potential reaches threshold, an action potential is generated. A single neuron thereby can integrate activity from many sources. A summary of the electrical events in a single cell underlying the transmission, integration, and conduction of information is shown in Figure 5-17.

Electrical Synapses

Although most synapses in the nervous system utilize chemical transmitters, neurons that have bridged junctions with channels from the cytoplasm of the presynaptic neuron to that of the postsynaptic neuron interact electrically. In these electrical synapses, the bridging channels mediate ionic current flow from one cell to the other. The transmission across the electrical synapse is very rapid, without synaptic delay of the chemical synapse. Electrical synapses are also bidirectional, in contrast to chemical synapses, which transmit signals in only one direction.

Clinical Correlations

The mechanisms of information transfer and processing in the neuromuscular system may be altered transiently and produce a clinical deficit of relatively short duration (seconds to hours). Such an alteration of function may be due either to a loss of activity or to an overactivity of neurons. A few examples of such changes will be described. In each of these examples, there need be no permanent or histologic damage to the cells.

The resting potential depends primarily on potassium concentration. An alteration in extracellular potassium, therefore, will have its effects mainly on the resting potential. A *reduction in extracellular potassium* will increase the concentration gradient and equilibrium potential of potassium, and thereby will increase the resting potential (hyperpolarize). Such hyperpolarized cells are less excitable because the membrane potential is farther from threshold, and fewer or no action potentials can be elicited. The function in those cells will be lost, as may occur in the case of those patients who have lost potassium because of disease or medication.

An *increase in extracellular potassium* will reduce the concentration gradient and result in a lower resting potential. Small increases in extracellular potassium will produce a resting potential closer to threshold (partially depolarized), and the cell will be more excitable and will fire action potentials in response to smaller stimuli. If the resting potential is very near threshold, the cell may fire spontaneously. However, a greater increase in extracellular potassium with a very low concentration gradient will give a persistently low resting potential at a level above threshold, resulting in a depolarization block. The cell will be unable to fire, and function will be lost. Increased extracellular potassium therefore may produce either excessive activity or a loss of activity in neurons, axons, or muscle fibers. Excessive cell discharge due to mild depolarization may present as a convulsion.

A change in potassium conductance also can occur in disease states, though the change is not associated with any specific disorders. The increase in potassium conductance during normal action potentials is associated with movement of potassium across the membrane, but the amount is not sufficient to change the potassium concentration or to alter the equilibrium potential. After prolonged excessive activity, there may be sufficient loss of potassium from the cell to partially depolarize the cell, but this is usually not sufficient to be associated with clinically recognizable abnormalities.

Extracellular potassium concentration may be elevated in a number of disorders. In particular, this elevation is considered to be one of the major mechanisms by which *anoxia* or *hypoxia* produces transient symptoms and signs, as in fainting. Without oxygen, the normal concentration gradients cannot be maintained, and the resting potential will decrease as potassium accumulates in the extracellular space. This may be associated with spontaneous firing of the cell, if mild, or with loss of function, if severe. Loss of function is seen first as the inability to generate action potentials, and when very severe, as the loss of local potentials. Anoxia also blocks the metabolic processes that maintain other cellular activity (such as movement of materials down axons) and protein synthesis. Therefore, anoxia may produce abnormalities in axons, neurons, synapses, and muscle fibers. However, the effects on the mechanisms underlying the electrical activity at the synapse (transmission of signals between cells) and the cell body (integration of signals) are altered earliest and most severely. All these changes also may be seen in severe kidney disease and in hyperkalemic periodic paralysis.

The sodium ions are of primary importance in the generation of an action potential, and anything that interferes with the flow of sodium ions can block the generation of action potentials. Interference can occur either by an alteration in sodium conductance or by a change in sodium ion concentration. If sodium conductance cannot be increased, or if the conductance is increased continuously, the membrane cannot generate action potentials and conduction of the action potential will be blocked. Tetrodotoxin, a fish toxin that blocks the sodium channel, inhibits conduction in axons and has been used to study axon physiology.

Structural changes in the membrane may result in an *increased sodium conductance* (leaky membrane), and the membrane potential will be closer to the sodium equilibrium potential (partially depolarized). The cell then will have an increased excitability if the "leak" is mild, or a block of conduction if the leak is severe.

An elevation of extracellular sodium will increase the sodium equilibrium potential, the size of the action potential, and the rate of rise of the action potential. Such increases do not have significant clinical effects. A reduction in the extracellular sodium will have the reverse effect; that is, it may lower the spike potential amplitude and slow its rate of increase. If the spike potential is low enough, it may not generate sufficient local current to discharge adjacent membrane, and action potential conduction may be blocked.

Calcium acts primarily as a membrane stabilizer, and its absence results in a reduced concentration gradient for sodium and potassium. Hypocalcemia thereby will reduce the resting potential, increase excitability, and may produce spontaneous activity. In addition, because the entry of calcium into the membrane is necessary for the release of neurotransmitter, a low calcium level may block synaptic transmission. Hypocalcemia therefore may have opposite effects; that is, it may impair synaptic transmission but produce spontaneous firing of a neuron or axon. An excess of calcium tends to block action potentials and enhance synaptic transmission. Hypercalcemia does not produce demonstrable changes, except at very high calcium concentrations, whereas even moderate hypocalcemia may produce muscle twitching or tingling.

The electrical activity of neuronal membranes is altered not only by ionic changes but also by the action of drugs. Synaptic transmission is particularly susceptible to a number of drugs that may act on the presynaptic or postsynaptic membranes. Examples of types of transmission block are illustrated in Figure 5-18. There may be a

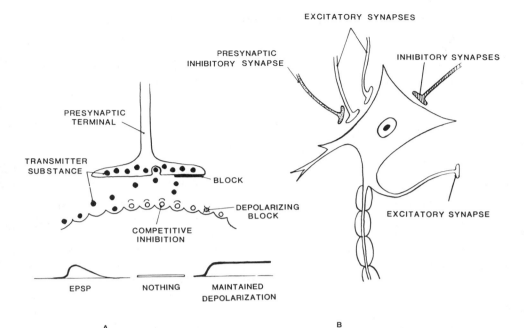

Fig. 5-18. Abnormalities of synaptic transmission may occur as shown in A. Types of transmission block include block of transmitter release (block), block of transmitter binding to postsynaptic membrane (competitive inhibition), or binding of another depolarizing agent to membrane (depolarizing block). B. These types of abnormalities may occur at each neuronal synapse shown.

presynaptic block of transmitter release or a postsynaptic block by competitive inhibition of the postsynaptic receptors, by inactivating agents, or by depolarizing substances. Drugs also may act on the axonal membrane. Local anesthetics, for example, prevent changes in sodium conductance and thereby block the conduction of action potentials.

The membrane of a cell also is altered when it loses its synaptic input. Normal function of many neurons and muscle fibers seems to depend on the release of a trophic factor from the presynaptic nerve terminal. Loss of all or most of the input to a cell may result in cell atrophy and in other structural changes in the appearance of the cell. A cell that has also lost its innervation becomes much more sensitive to neurotransmitters, a phenomenon called *denervation hypersensitivity,* in which the cellular response to a constant stimulus increases after a cell has lost some of its normal input. This phenomenon will be considered further in subsequent chapters.

Each of these types of alteration in neuronal or muscle cell physiology can produce symptoms or signs of short duration—transient disorders. The particular findings in a patient will depend on which cells are altered. If the changes are in neurons that subserve sensation, there may be a loss of sensation or an abnormal sensation such as tingling, loss of vision, or "seeing stars." In other systems, there might be loss of strength, twitching in muscles, loss of intellect, or abnormal behavior.

In all these cases, the physiologic alterations are not specific and may be the concomitant of any one of a number of diseases. Transient disorders do not permit a pathologic or etiologic diagnosis. Any of the various types of disease (vascular, neoplastic, inflammatory) may be associated with a physiologic alteration of the type described. Therefore, the pathology of a disorder cannot be deduced when its temporal profile is solely that of transient episodes.

Summary

The transmission of information in the neuromuscular system depends on the generation of a resting potential that acts as a reserve of energy poised for release when the valve is turned on. The *"valve"* is the configuration of the membrane, and the *"energy"* is the ionic concentration gradient. The release of energy is seen either as local, graded potentials or as propagated, action potentials that arise when the local potentials reach threshold. Information is moved from one area to another as action potentials conducted by single cells. The information is integrated by the interaction of local potentials generated in response to the neurotransmitters released from depolarized nerve terminals.

In this system, information can be coded either as the rate of discharge in individual cells or axons, or as the number and combination of active cells. Both of these are important mechanisms, for although the activity of the nervous system can be conveniently described in terms of the electrical activity of single cells, the combined activity of large numbers of cells and axons determines the behavior of the organism.

Objectives

1. Describe the mechanism by which the resting potential is generated and maintained.
2. List the characteristics of a local potential, and name three examples.
3. Describe the features of an action potential and the associated ionic changes.
4. Describe the events in synaptic transmission.
5. Define the following terms: depolarization, steady state, equilibrium potential, sodium pump, threshold, afterpotential, accommodation, refractory period, saltatory conduction, EPSP, EPP, conductance, active transport, spatial summation, presynaptic inhibition, and denervation hypersensitivity.
6. Describe the effect of anoxia and of an alteration in extracellular sodium, potassium, or calcium on the resting and action potentials. List which of these conditions could result in excessive electrical discharges.

Clinical Problems

1. A 64-year-old man had a sudden occlusion of a blood vessel in an area of the brain that controls speech and was unable to speak for 10 minutes. His speech then gradually returned to normal over a 15-minute period. By what mechanism could this recovery occur?
2. A 55-year-old teacher had a brain tumor, with severe right-sided paralysis and signs of brain swelling. When he was given a drug that reduced cerebral edema, his paralysis improved. (a) If the edema resulted in extracellular sodium dilution, what would be the effect on the action potential amplitude and electrotonic potential amplitudes? (b) If the osmotic pressure changes produced efflux of potassium from the cell and influx of water into the cell, what would be the effect of the edema on the resting potential?
3. A 36-year-old woman with multiple sclerosis with focal areas of loss of myelin in the central nervous system had a 2-week loss of vision in one eye. How could loss of myelin in the optic nerve have affected her vision?
4. After sitting in a biochemistry lecture for $1\frac{1}{2}$ hours and sleeping with your arm over a chair for 10 minutes, you awaken with a numb hand. As you rub it, it tingles. Which of the following could account for the tingling? (a) The resting membrane potential moves closer to threshold, (b) Hyperpolarization of the nerve membrane, (c) Increased extracellular potassium concentration, (d) Prolonged positive afterpotential.
5. Some poisons block the action of neurotransmitter at the postsynaptic membrane. What effect could this have on: (a) EPP, (b) generator potential, (c) EPSP, (d) accommodation?
6. A man named Nernst has a wooden boat with a hole in the bottom that he uses on Lake Sodium. When he wants to sit and fish, he lets the boat fill with water until no more comes in, and he keeps his feet up. This condition is one of (a) _____ . If he wants to go elsewhere, he must lower the water level in the boat, so he turns on his Lake Sodium pump, which pumps water out. He then achieves a condition in which inflow equals outflow, with little water in the boat. This he calls (b) _____ . It requires energy, so the pumping process is called (c) _____ .

Suggested Reading

Brazier, M. A. B. *Electrical Activity of the Nervous System* (4th ed.). Baltimore: Williams & Wilkins, 1977.

Brookhart, J. M., Mountcastle, V. B., and Kandel, E. R. (eds.). *Handbook of Physiology.* Section 1: The Nervous System. Vol. I: *Cellular Biology of Neurons*, Part 1. Bethesda, Md.: American Physiological Society, 1977.

Grundfest, H. Physiology of Electrogenic Excitable Membranes. In D. B. Tower (ed.), *The Nervous System*, Vol. 1. New York: Raven, 1975. Pp. 153–195.

Hille, B. Ionic channels in excitable membranes: Current problems and biophysical approaches. *Biophys. J.* 22:283, 1978.

Hodgkin, A. L. *The Conduction of the Nervous Impulse*. Springfield, Ill.: Thomas, 1964.

Jasper, H. H., and van Gelder, N. M. (eds.). *Basic Mechanisms of Neuronal Hyperexcitabil-ity*. New York: Liss, 1983.

Keynes, R. D. Ion channels in the nerve-cell membrane. *Sci. Am.* 240(3):126, 1979.

Ochs, S. *Axoplasmic Transport and Its Relation to Other Nerve Functions*. New York: Wiley, 1982.

Stevens, C. F. The neuron. *Sci. Am.* 241(3):55, 1979.

Tasaki, I. *Physiology and Electrochemistry of Nerve Fibers*. New York: Academic, 1982.

Longitudinal
Systems

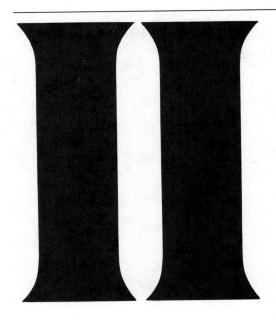

The Cerebrospinal Fluid System

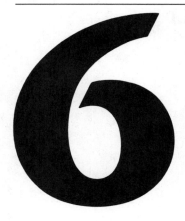

The meninges, ventricular system, subarachnoid spaces, and cerebrospinal fluid (CSF) constitute a functionally unique system that has an important role in maintaining a stable environment within which the nervous system can function. The series of membranes that constitute the meninges serve as supportive and protective structures for nerve tissue. The CSF itself provides a cushioning effect during rapid movements of the head and a mechanical buoyancy to the brain. The density of brain tissue is only slightly greater than that of CSF, and the average weight of the brain is 1,500 g. However, the CSF exerts a considerable buoyant effect on the brain. In addition, it provides a pathway for the removal of brain metabolites and functions as a chemical reservoir, protecting the local environment of the brain from some of the changes that may occur in the blood and thus ensuring the brain's continued undisturbed performance. The CSF system is found at the supratentorial, posterior fossa, and spinal levels. Because of the extensive anatomic distribution and function of the CSF system, pathologic alterations to it can occur in a wide variety of neurologic disorders.

Overview

Structures included in the CSF system are the meninges and meningeal spaces formed between the meningeal linings and the brain, the ventricular system, and the CSF itself.

The *meninges* consist of three mesodermally derived membranes: the outermost dura mater, the arachnoid, and the thin pia mater, which adheres closely to the structures of the central nervous system. The epidural space lies external to the dura mater, between it and bone. The subdural space lies between the dura mater and the arachnoid, and the subarachnoid space lies between the arachnoid and the pia mater and contains CSF. Cerebrospinal fluid is also contained in the cavities within the brain: the two lateral ventricles, the aqueduct of Sylvius, and the third and fourth ventricles.

The composition of CSF is similar but not identical to that of plasma. Cerebrospinal fluid is formed by a combination of processes, including passive diffusion, facilitated diffusion, and active transport, and is produced primarily but not exclusively by the choroid plexus of the ventricular system. There is a slow circulation of the CSF

through the ventricular system into the subarachnoid space and over the surface of the brain and spinal cord. Most of the CSF drains through the arachnoid villi into the venous sinuses.

Because of the close relationship between the CSF system and the neural tissue, pathologic processes that primarily alter the function of the CSF system may secondarily alter nervous system function. Furthermore, because the central nervous system is bathed and surrounded by CSF, disease processes that primarily affect the nervous system may be secondarily reflected by changes in the anatomy and physiology of this system. Examination of the composition of the CSF and of the structure of this system therefore becomes an important and useful neurodiagnostic tool.

Anatomy of the CSF System

Dura Mater and Its Major Folds

The *dura mater* is a tough, fibrous membrane. In the cranial cavity, it consists of two almost inseparable layers. The outer (periosteal) dura is firmly attached to the periosteum of the cranial bones. The *epidural space* between the dura mater and bone, therefore, is normally not present. It is a potential space that becomes of pathologic importance if the dura mater is separated from bone by blood (epidural hematoma) or by pus (epidural abscess). The inner (meningeal) layer of the dura mater remains attached to the outer layer except where they are separated to form venous channels, the *dural venous sinuses.*

The *falx cerebri* is a sickle-shaped reflection of meningeal dura that extends into the interhemispheric fissure to separate the two cerebral hemispheres. It extends from the base of the anterior fossa to the internal occipital protuberance. Its upper margin contains the *superior sagittal sinus,* and its lower free edge, which arches over the corpus callosum, contains the *inferior sagittal sinus* (Fig. 6-1).

At the level of the internal occipital protuberance, the dura forming the falx cerebri extends laterally to form a winglike structure, the *tentorium cerebelli.* The outer border of the tentorium is attached to the occipital bone and along the upper edges of the petrous bones. Thus, it separates the ventral surface of the cerebral hemispheres from the dorsal surface of the cerebellum and divides the cranial cavity into the supratentorial compartment (anterior and middle cranial fos-

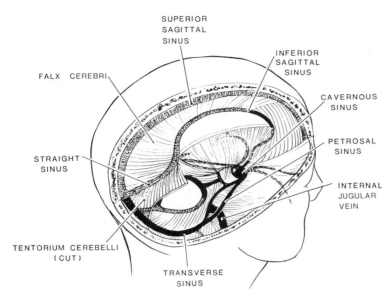

SUPERIOR
SAGITTAL
SINUS

INFERIOR
SAGITTAL
SINUS

CAVERNOUS
SINUS

FALX CEREBRI

PETROSAL
SINUS

STRAIGHT
SINUS

INTERNAL
JUGULAR
VEIN

TENTORIUM CEREBELLI
(CUT)

TRANSVERSE
SINUS

Fig. 6-1. Dura mater and its major sinuses. Dorsolateral view illustrating falx cerebri, tentorium cerebelli, and dura lining base of skull. The dural venous sinuses are stippled or black.

sae and their contents) and the infratentorial or posterior fossa compartment (see Fig. 3-3). The cerebellar hemispheres contained within the posterior fossa are partially separated by a downward extension of dura, the *falx cerebelli*. The wings of the tentorium converge and attach to the posterior clinoid process of the sella turcica. The free border of the tentorium thus forms an opening, the *tentorial notch,* which surrounds the midbrain at the transition between the posterior fossa and the middle fossa.

The two layers of the dura mater remain tightly attached as they pass through the foramen magnum into the spinal canal. At the level of the second or third cervical vertebra, the meningeal dura separates widely from the inner periosteum of bone and forms a narrow sac extending to the level of the second sacral vertebra. The spinal epidural space thus formed between the dura and the periosteum contains fat and vascular structures (principally veins). The conus medullaris, the lower end of the spinal cord (Fig. 6-2), terminates at the level of the second lumbar vertebra. A thin remnant of central nervous system tissue, the *filum terminale*, extends caudally from the conus medullaris to the termination of the dural sac at the second sacral level. The filum termi-

nale is composed of glial cells, ependyma, and astrocytes, covered by pia mater. The dura is pierced by the roots of the spinal and cranial nerves along the length of the brain stem and spinal cord.

Leptomeninges (Arachnoid and Pia Mater)

Embryologically, the leptomeninges, the arachnoid and pia mater, begin as a single membrane, which later becomes separated by numerous confluent subarachnoid spaces containing CSF. The arachnoid, however, remains attached to the pia mater by numerous weblike trabeculae (Fig. 6-3). Although the pia mater adheres tightly to the surfaces of the brain and spinal cord, the arachnoid is closely applied to the inner surface of the meningeal dura mater throughout the neuraxis. The potential space between the dura mater and the arachnoid is termed the *subdural space* and normally contains a thin layer of fluid. In pathologic states, blood may accumulate in this location and produce a *subdural hematoma*.

As a result of the relationship of the arachnoid to the dura mater, and the pia mater to neural tissue, the *subarachnoid space* varies greatly in size and shape, particularly over the surfaces of the brain and in the lumbar region of the spinal canal (see Fig. 6-2). In the cranial cavity, these enlargements of the subarachnoid space are called *cisterns,* and they are usually named for their anatomic location (for example, the interpeduncular cistern is located between the cerebral peduncles; the cisterna magna is a large space below

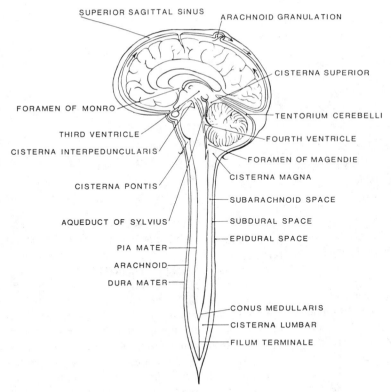

Fig. 6-2. The CSF system illustrating meningeal
layers, ventricles, and subarachnoid cisterns.
(Redrawn from C. R. Noback and R. J. Demarest.
The Nervous System: Introduction and Review. *New
York: McGraw-Hill, 1977.)*

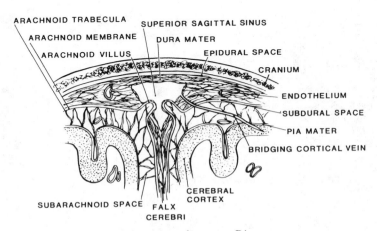

Fig. 6-3. Meninges and meningeal spaces. Diagram-
matic coronal section through parasagittal region of
cerebral hemispheres. Note bridging vein extending
from cortex to superior sagittal sinus. Tear of this
type of vein is common cause of subarachnoid and
subdural bleeding.

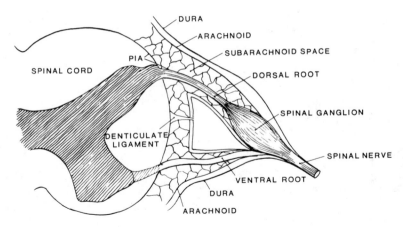

Fig. 6-4. Meningeal relationships at spinal segment. Note investments of spinal nerve root by dura mater as it leaves spinal canal. The denticulate ligaments attach spinal cord to dura laterally.

the cerebellum). In the spinal canal, where the spinal cord ends at the level of the second lumbar vertebra and the arachnoid remains closely applied to the dura mater to the level of the second sacral vertebra, a large lumbar subarachnoid space is formed that contains a reservoir of CSF, the filum terminale, and the nerve roots of the cauda equina as they pass to their intervertebral foramina. The major arterial channels of the brain are located in the subarachnoid space. Bleeding from these vessels results in a subarachnoid hemorrhage.

On gross inspection, the pia mater cannot be seen except at intervals in the spinal canal, where it extends laterally to attach to the dura mater as the *denticulate ligaments* (Fig. 6-4). Throughout the rest of its distribution, the pia mater closely invests the central nervous system, its few cell layers being separated from the outermost neural tissue, the *astrocytic glia limitans,* by a thin layer of collagen. In the trabeculae, the cells of the pia and arachnoid are contiguous and are called *leptomeninges* (see Fig. 6-2). Arterioles, as they dip into the parenchyma of the brain, are invested with a sheath of leptomeninges that disappears at the capillary level to leave only the endothelium of the blood vessel and its basement membrane in

Fig. 6-5. Detailed relationships of meninges and structures in subarachnoid space. An arteriole carries pia mater into the cortex as it penetrates.

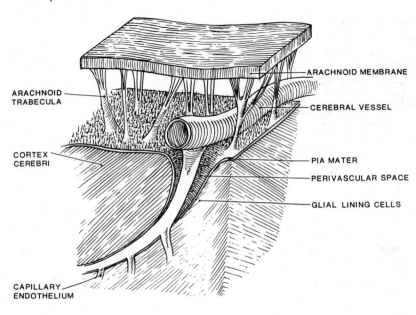

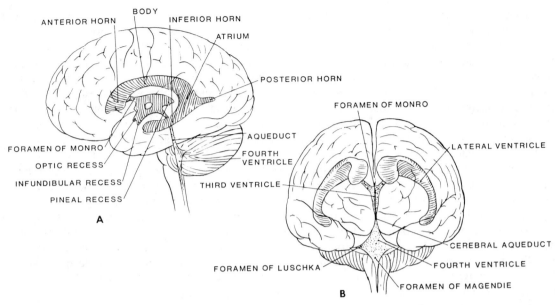

Fig. 6-6. Ventricular system. A. Lateral view. B. Anterior view. (Redrawn from C. R. Noback and R. J. Demarest. The Nervous System: Introduction and Review. *New York: McGraw-Hill, 1977.*)

direct contact with the astrocytic glia limitans (Fig. 6-5). This forms the so-called blood-brain barrier.

Blood-brain barrier is a descriptive term first used many years ago when it was observed that certain dyes injected intravenously would stain all body organs except the brain; yet the same dyes injected into the CSF would produce staining of brain tissue. It was therefore postulated that a "barrier" for the passage of the dye was located between the blood and the brain. The capillary

endothelium and astroglial membranes constitute the anatomic substrate for that barrier. They are not, however, the only blood-brain barrier, but merely part of a system of barriers (some anatomic, others physiologic) that serve to produce differences in the chemical composition of the brain, CSF, and blood.

Arachnoid villi (or granulations) (see Fig. 6-2) are invaginations of the arachnoid into the dural venous sinuses. Fluid circulating through these villi is drained into the venous blood and systemic circulation.

Ventricular System of the Brain

The ventricular system (Fig. 6-6) is lined with ciliated cuboidal epithelium (derived from ectoderm) called *ependyma*. The *choroid plexuses* are found in the lateral, third, and fourth ventricles and are multitufted vascular organs that arise embryologically when ependyma, leptomeninges,

Fig. 6-7. Detailed anatomy of ventricular system. (Redrawn from M. W. Woerdeman. Atlas of Human Anatomy: Descriptive and Regional. *Baltimore: Williams & Wilkins, 1948.*)

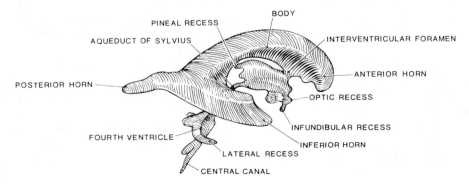

and blood vessels fold into the ventricles. These structures, rich in enzymes that are found in other secretory organs, are the main (but not the only) source for the production of the CSF.

A *lateral ventricle* (Fig. 6-7) is located in each of the cerebral hemispheres and is divided into an anterior horn located in the frontal lobe, body and atrium (or trigone) in the parietal lobe, posterior horn in the occipital lobe, and inferior horn in the temporal lobe. The lateral ventricles communicate with each other and the *third ventricle* of the diencephalon via the *interventricular foramina of Monro.* The *aqueduct of Sylvius* traverses the mesencephalon and leads from the third ventricle to the *fourth ventricle,* located dorsal to the pons and medulla. Communication of the ventricular system with the subarachnoid space is in the fourth ventricle via two *foramina of Luschka* and the *foramen of Magendie.* A small and discontinuous *central canal* extends for a short distance from the caudal aspect of the fourth ventricle. At the spinal level, this canal is usually obliterated, and therefore, in the normal adult, only a few ependymal cells remain as remnants of the once prominent central canal of the embryo.

The Cerebrospinal Fluid

Formation and Circulation of CSF

The rate of CSF formation remains relatively constant at approximately 0.35 ml per minute (500 ml/day). Because the total volume of CSF in the adult is 90 to 150 ml, the processes of CSF formation and resorption must remain in delicate balance in order to prevent alteration in structure and function of the brain.

Most of the CSF is actively secreted into the ventricular system by the choroid plexuses; however, these are not the only source of CSF. Some is derived directly from the interstitial fluid of the brain and crosses the ependyma to enter the ventricles. Additional exchange may take place between the neural tissue and the subarachnoid space across the pia mater.

Circulation of the CSF is promoted by the beating of the cilia of the ependymal cells and the pulsatile changes in the volume of intracranial blood that occurs with cardiac systole and with respiratory movements. The direction of CSF flow is from the lateral, third, and fourth ventricles to the subarachnoid space, where it then circulates in two major directions. The most important pathway is rostrally through the tentorial notch and then dorsally toward the intracranial venous system, where CSF exits through arachnoid villi that project into the dural venous sinuses, particularly the superior sagittal sinus. While the exact mechanism of transfer of CSF to venous blood through the arachnoid villi is incompletely understood, transcellular transport via giant vacuoles seems most likely. The villi act as one-way valves, preventing entrance of blood into the CSF. A hydrostatic pressure of 70 mm of water or greater forces the CSF into the sinuses. The second pathway, a quantitatively less important and slower route taken by the CSF after its exit from the ventricular system, is downward through the foramen magnum into the spinal subarachnoid space, where it is partially resorbed through the leptomeninges.

CSF Pressure

The craniovertebral cavity and its dural lining are a closed space. Any increase in the size or volume of one of the three "compartments" (blood, CSF, brain) in the cavity can occur only in conjunction with an equal reduction in the size or volume of the others, or with a consequent increase in pressure. Normally, however, the contents of the three compartments are relatively constant, producing a CSF pressure of 50 to 200 mm of water when recorded in the lumbar subarachnoid sac with the patient lying in a lateral recumbent position.

Minor oscillations occur in CSF pressure recorded in this manner in response to respiration and arterial pulsation, as varied amounts of blood enter and leave the craniovertebral cavity. Certain additional maneuvers will cause wider oscillations in CSF pressure. Compression of the jugular veins, for example, will impede the outflow of blood from the brain, expand the venous vascular bed, and cause a rapid increase in intracranial pressure. Because the lumbar subarachnoid sac is directly continuous with the intracranial subarachnoid space, this increase in pressure will be transmitted throughout the ventriculosubarachnoid system (as long as there is no obstruction to the flow of CSF). The spinal epidural venous plexuses normally contribute to the CSF pressure by continuous tamponade of the spinal dural sac.

Increased intrathoracic or intraabdominal pressure (coughing, sneezing, straining at the stool, or abdominal compression) can thereby also increase CSF pressure.

In certain pathologic conditions, the increase in the volume of some of the components of the cranial cavity cannot be compensated for by readjustments in the volume of the other constituents. In this situation, intracranial pressure increases to abnormal levels. The symptoms and consequences of increased intracranial pressure will be discussed later.

The Blood-Brain–CSF Barrier System

The central nervous system contains two basic fluid compartments: extracellular (CSF and interstitial fluid) and intracellular (primarily fluid within the cytoplasm of neurons and glial cells). The chemical compositions of these two fluid compartments are dissimilar, and the composition of each fluid differs significantly from that of blood. The chemical composition of the central nervous system fluid compartments is maintained within relatively narrow limits despite large fluctuations in the composition of extracellular fluid elsewhere in the body. Factors other than simple diffusion therefore must be responsible for the passage of chemicals from one compartment to another.

Historically, reference has been made to a blood-brain barrier, implying an anatomic structure that would explain the variable distribution of substances in each compartment. Although not the sole explanation for the blood-brain barrier, anatomic considerations do have an important role. Brain capillaries are unique in that they possess *tight junctions* that obliterate the normal intercellular clefts between capillary endothelial cells. This anatomic feature impedes the diffusion of larger molecules. Some areas of the brain, however, are excluded from this blood-brain barrier system (perhaps as a means of allowing neuronal receptors to "sample" plasma directly). In these regions, the capillary endothelium contains fenestrations that allow proteins and small molecules to pass from the blood to adjacent tissue. Three areas that lack tight junctions in the capillary endothelium and have some homeostatic function are (1) the area postrema (in the brain stem, near the "vomiting center"), (2) a region of the hypothalamus, and (3) the pineal gland.

There are also other physicochemical factors, such as lipid solubility, protein binding, and state of ionization, that alter the passage of substances from one fluid compartment to another. In addition, certain substances are transported across membranes by carrier-mediated, facilitated diffusion systems while others are transported by energy-requiring, active transport systems. Therefore, although one commonly refers to a blood-brain barrier, one is in effect referring to a wide variety of barrier systems, some anatomic, others physicochemical, which act together to maintain a homeostatic internal environment.

Composition of CSF

One additional function of the CSF is to provide a pathway for the removal of the products of cerebral metabolism. In this regard, the CSF has been referred to as a large metabolic "sink," a reservoir that allows metabolites of the brain to "drain" into it and then to enter the systemic circulation. The composition of the CSF thus is a reflection of the processes previously described as well as of the metabolic activity of the central nervous system.

APPEARANCE. The CSF is normally clear and colorless; turbidity or discoloration is always abnormal. Turbidity is most commonly due to increased numbers of red or white blood cells. The most important cause of discoloration of the CSF is bleeding in the subarachnoid space. With subarachnoid hemorrhage (usually due to trauma or rupture of an intracranial vessel), the fluid is initially pink to red, depending on the severity of the bleeding. During the 2 to 10 hours after such an event, the red cells undergo lysis, and the liberated hemoglobin is broken down to form bilirubin, which imparts a yellow color (xanthochromia) to the CSF. A yellow discoloration also may be due to a markedly elevated level of CSF protein or be secondary to an elevation in the level of plasma bilirubin.

CELLULAR ELEMENTS. Normal CSF contains no more than 5 lymphocytes per microliter. A cell count of 5 to 10 cells is very suspicious, and a count greater than 10 is definitely abnormal and suggests the presence of disease in the central nervous system or in the meninges. The presence of polymorphonuclear leukocytes is always indicative of disease.

MICROBIOLOGIC FEATURES.   Cerebrospinal fluid is normally sterile. Therefore, results of microbiologic studies (Gram's stains, cultures) should be negative.

PROTEIN.   The normal total CSF protein concentration is no greater than 45 mg per deciliter. The capillary endothelial membrane is highly effective in limiting the concentration of protein in the CSF, and elevation in the CSF protein concentration is a frequent (but nonspecific) pathologic finding, suggestive of disease involving the central nervous system or meninges.

The amount of protein normally present in CSF is much less than that in plasma, although the relative proportions of the protein fractions are similar. Most of the CSF protein is probably derived from the plasma. One protein of clinical significance is the gamma globulin fraction. Normally, gamma globulin is synthesized outside the central nervous system. The normal concentration of gamma globulin in lumbar fluid is less than 13 percent of the total CSF protein concentration. In conditions such as multiple sclerosis, neurosyphilis, and some other subacute or chronic infections of the central nervous system, the gamma globulin level increases in association with a normal or slightly elevated total protein level. (For this observation to be valid, there must be no change in the level of serum gamma globulin.) Such an increase in the gamma globulin in the CSF suggests an abnormal formation of gamma globulin by chronic inflammatory cells within the nervous system, with diffusion of the protein from brain to CSF.

Measurement of immunoglobulin G (IgG), which accounts for almost all of the gamma globulin in normal CSF and in most disease states, is a more sensitive indicator of central nervous system inflammation and immunoglobulin production than is total gamma globulin in disorders such as multiple sclerosis. Agar gel electrophoresis of concentrated CSF allows identification of qualitative changes in the IgG fraction. In normal CSF and in most noninflammatory neurologic diseases, the IgG fraction forms a diffuse, homogeneous zone of migration. In multiple sclerosis and some other subacute and chronic inflammatory diseases, two or more discrete subfractions, which represent specific antibody populations called *oligoclonal bands*, are identified within the IgG migration zone. Another protein fraction derived from the central nervous system, myelin basic protein, can be identified by radioimmunoassay. It is not present in normal CSF and is an indicator of active demyelination.

GLUCOSE.   The glucose in CSF is normally about 60 to 70 percent of that in plasma. The normal range in patients with blood levels of 80 to 120 mg per deciliter, therefore, is between 45 and 80 mg per deciliter. Values less than 35 to 40 mg per deciliter are abnormal.

Glucose enters the CSF from plasma by both simple and facilitated diffusion, and similar mechanisms are responsible for its removal. In addition, glucose is metabolized by arachnoidal, ependymal, neuronal, and glial cells, or it may leave the CSF with water (bulk flow).

Changes in levels of CSF glucose reflect similar changes in the blood, but a variable time is required before the CSF glucose equilibrates with the blood glucose. Thus, the CSF concentration does not reach a maximum for about 2 hours after the rapid intravenous injections of hypertonic glucose, and there is a similar delay in the lowering of the CSF glucose level after insulin-induced hypoglycemia. Therefore, when the CSF glucose determination is of diagnostic importance, CSF and blood levels should be obtained simultaneously, with the patient in a fasting state.

An increased CSF glucose level is of little diagnostic importance. A low CSF glucose level (in the presence of a normal blood concentration) is, however, very important. The CSF glucose level is characteristically low in acute bacterial and chronic fungal infections of the central nervous system. (It is frequently normal in viral infections.) Low CSF glucose values in the presence of bacterial infection are believed to be due to increased glycolysis by polymorphonuclear leukocytes, glucose utilization by bacteria, increased glycolysis by neural elements, or a breakdown of facilitated diffusion of glucose, which effectively slows the rate of entry of glucose into the central nervous system.

Clinical Correlations I: Disorders of the CSF System

The Syndrome of Increased Intracranial Pressure

An uncompensated increase in the volume of any of the constituents of the cranial vault results in an increase in intracranial pressure. Such an increase can occur from an increase in the total volume of brain tissue (as with diffuse cerebral edema), a focal increase in brain volume (as with an intracerebral hemorrhage, neoplasm, or other mass lesion), an increase in CSF volume without an associated loss of brain tissue (as in hydrocephalus), or diffuse vasodilatation or venous obstruction (from any of several causes). While many clinical symptoms may be associated with increased intracranial pressure, none is individually diagnostic of this condition; yet together they form a characteristic clinical pattern consisting of the following:

1. *Headache* is believed to be due to traction on the pain-sensitive structures within the cranium. Factors that tend to increase this traction, such as coughing, straining, or position change, tend to precipitate or aggravate the headache.
2. *Nausea* and *vomiting* are associated with the vagal-motor centers, which are located in the floor of the fourth ventricle and which mediate the motility of the gastrointestinal tract. Increased ventricular pressure transmitted to these centers may account for these symptoms.
3. *Bradycardia* is presumed to be due to pressure on a vagal control mechanism similar to that proposed for nausea and vomiting.
4. *Elevated blood pressure* is related to intracranial pressure; as intracranial pressure increases, the arterial blood pressure also must increase if brain blood flow is to continue. This reflex is also mediated by structures located in the floor of the fourth ventricle.
5. *Papilledema* is characterized by elevation and blurring of the optic disk margin, as viewed with an ophthalmoscope (Fig. 6-8). The subdural and subarachnoid spaces of the brain extend along the course of the optic nerve (Fig. 6-9). Increased pressure within the skull and subarachnoid space thus can be transmitted to the nerve, causing impairment of the venous drainage and edema of the nerve head.
6. *Alterations in consciousness* occur if the pressure increase is large, and as further pathologic change develops, consciousness may be lost because of brain-stem compression (see Chap. 8).
7. *Changes in the skull* occur in children and adults. In children, in whom the bones of the cranial vault have not yet permanently fused, chronic increases in pressure may be partially compensated for by a modest separation of the bones at the suture lines. In infants, in whom a "soft spot" (fontanelle) is not yet ossified, this membranous structure located at the ver-

Fig. 6-8. Optic fundus and optic nerve head. A. Normal optic disk. B. Papilledema. Disk margins are elevated and blurred; venous congestion and hemorrhages are seen surrounding disk.

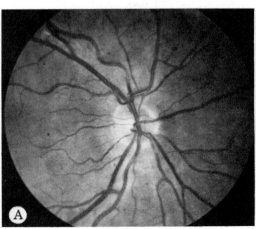
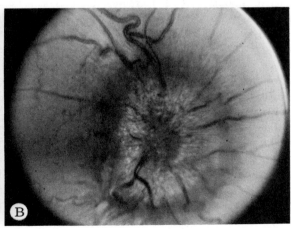

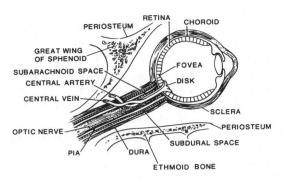

Fig. 6-9. Relationships of meninges and meningeal spaces to optic nerve. Increased intracranial pressure may result in edema of optic nerve head.

tex of the head may become tense and bulge outward. In adults, in whom bony fusion is complete and the skull is incapable of further expansion, some demineralization of bone, especially around the sella turcica, is occasionally seen.

This clinical syndrome may occur in isolation or, more commonly, it is superimposed on the signs and symptoms of the underlying pathologic lesion. If the syndrome of increased intracranial pressure occurs with signs of a focal lesion, whether acute, subacute, or chronic in their evolution, the diagnosis of a mass lesion becomes highly likely.

Hydrocephalus

In certain pathologic conditions, the pathway for CSF circulation is blocked and absorption is impaired. The rate of CSF formation by the choroid plexus remains relatively constant, and because the relative amount of CSF increases, there is a corresponding increase in ventricular pressure, and progressive dilatation of the ventricles (hydrocephalus) occurs in regions proximal to the blockage (Fig. 6-10). Signs and symptoms of increased intracranial pressure also may develop.

Before adequate techniques for visualization of the ventricular system were available, clinicians devised a method for determining the site of blockage in hydrocephalus. Histologic studies of the pathology had shown that the obstruction was most commonly either (1) within the ventricular system itself, that is, proximal to the outlets of the fourth ventricle as in, for example, aqueductal stenosis; or (2) outside the ventricular system where inadequate circulation over the convexi-

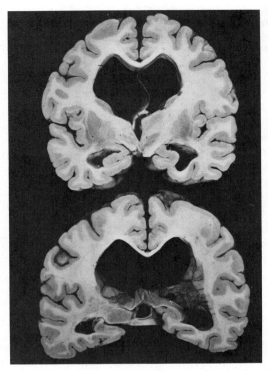

Fig. 6-10. Coronal sections of cerebral hemispheres showing hydrocephalus. Note marked dilatation of lateral ventricles, with thinning of cerebral walls at expense of white matter. In lower (more posterior) *section, the thin septum has been artificially torn.*

ties of the brain prevents adequate resorption, for example, after meningitis or subarachnoid hemorrhage. In order to differentiate these two conditions, a cannula was inserted through the skull into the ventricular system and a second cannula was inserted into the lumbar subarachnoid space. If dye that was injected into the ventricles could later be recovered in the lumbar sac, then a *communicating hydrocephalus* indicating an extraventricular blockage was present; if no dye was recovered, then a *noncommunicating hydrocephalus* indicating a blockage within the ventricular system was present. Although clinicians no longer use this method of diagnosis, the responsible lesions are still often referred to as producing either a communicating or a noncommunicating hydrocephalus.

The term *hydrocephalus* also describes the situation that occurs in brain atrophy. Coincident with the reduction in volume of brain tissue, there is enlargement of the ventricles and subarachnoid spaces, with an increase in the amount of CSF.

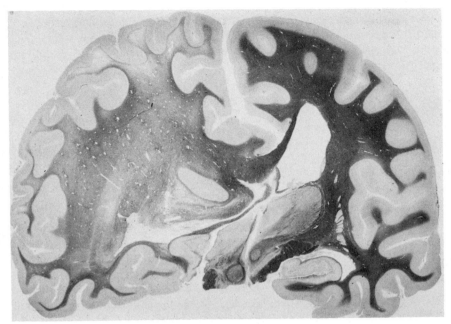

Fig. 6-11. Cerebral edema (associated with neighboring meningioma—not shown). Note pallor and swelling of white matter of left hemisphere, with marked shift of midline structures from left to right. (Luxol-fast blue stain; ×1.)

The total volume of the intracranial contents remains unchanged, however, and there is no increase in intracranial pressure. This type of process is referred to as *hydrocephalus ex vacuo.*

Cerebral Edema

Brain swelling or *edema* is an increase in brain volume due to an increase in the water content of the brain. It is a nonspecific condition that can be associated with a wide variety of cerebral disorders, including hypoxia, meningitis, neoplasm, abscess, and infarction. Two major types of brain edema have been described: (1) *vasogenic edema*, which results from an increase in permeability of brain capillary endothelial cells and produces an increase in extracellular fluid volume, and (2) *cytotoxic edema*, which is an increase in the intracellular fluid volume of the brain. This form of edema is presumably caused by a failure of the ATP-dependent sodium pump mechanism, with the result that sodium efflux is altered and water enters the cell in order to maintain osmotic equilibrium.

Although the first type of edema is most often seen surrounding focal brain lesions and the latter is seen in association with hypoxia, either type may be relatively well localized or diffuse and widespread. Both types result in an increase in intracranial volume and pressure, causing symptoms of increased intracranial pressure that may be superimposed on the underlying pathologic process (Fig. 6-11).

The Syndrome of Acute Meningeal Irritation

A number of noxious agents produce meningeal irritation, but, regardless of the cause, the clinical manifestations are similar and consist of the following:

1. *Headache* is usually prominent and severe and is due to vasodilatation or to chemical irritation or inflammation (or both) of the major pain-sensitive structures.
2. *Stiff neck* is caused by irritation of the meninges in the posterior fossa and upper cervical spinal canal, which stimulates spinal nerve roots and results in reflex spasm and contraction of the posterior neck muscles. This increased resistance to neck flexion is termed *nuchal rigidity.*
3. *Alteration in consciousness* results from a pathologic process that is widespread and severe, causing diffuse depression of cortical function and change in the level of consciousness.

The most common causes of this syndrome are

bacterial meningitis, viral encephalitis, and sub-arachnoid hemorrhage. Each of these will super-impose its own characteristic signature on the general pattern of meningeal irritation.

BACTERIAL MENINGITIS.   An inflammation of the CSF system can be caused by bacterial invasion and can be accompanied by a characteristic leukocytic exudate in the pia mater and arach-noid, as well as in structures adjacent to the lep-tomeninges (Fig. 6-12). Bacteria may be found in the CSF and within neutrophilic white blood cells. The type of leukocytic exudate reflects the nature of the invading organism. Most commonly, infections caused by meningococcus, *Haemophilus influenzae,* staphylococcus, and streptococcus organisms will be accompanied by a polymorpho-nuclear exudate, while more indolent infections, such as those caused by the tubercle bacillus, are associated with a predominance of lymphocytes. The pathologic reaction is widely distributed throughout the leptomeninges, but it may be most extensive in the basal subarachnoid cisterns. The clinical-anatomic-temporal profile of this disorder is that of diffuse, subacute, and progressive in-volvement of the nervous system, with the super-imposed features of fever and systemic reaction and the syndrome of meningeal irritation, and with or without evidence of increased intracranial

Fig. 6-12. Acute purulent bacterial meningitis. A. Brain in situ viewed from left side showing marked clouding of subarachnoid space. B. Cortex of brain showing adjacent subarachnoid space filled with acute inflammatory cells. (H & E; ×250.)

pressure. After treatment, or subsiding of the in-fection, reactive changes may occur within the CSF system, which can impair CSF absorption and result in hydrocephalus.

VIRAL ENCEPHALITIS.   Viral infections usually induce remarkably few gross pathologic changes in the brain. Vascular dilatation, congestion, and edema are not uncommon, and occasional pete-chial hemorrhages may be seen in the cortex. Histopathologically, there is necrosis of nerve cells and neuronophagia, perivascular cuffing by lymphocytes and mononuclear leukocytes, and meningeal infiltration by similar cells. The clinical-anatomic-temporal profile of this disorder is virtually identical to that noted for bacterial meningitis (diffuse, subacute, and progressive); however, because of the difference in inflamma-tory response, the findings on examination of the CSF may differ (Table 6-1).

SUBARACHNOID HEMORRHAGE.   The acute rup-ture of an intracranial vessel may produce little pathologic change in the brain itself. As red blood cells intermix with CSF, the signs and symptoms of meningeal irritation are to be ex-pected. Most commonly, subarachnoid hemor-rhage occurs as a result of trauma, rupture of an intracranial aneurysm, or leakage from an arterio-venous malformation. Although the source of bleeding is often from a single well-localized source, blood rapidly mixes with CSF and is dis-tributed throughout the neuraxis (Fig. 6-13). A diffuse, acute, and sometimes progressive disor-

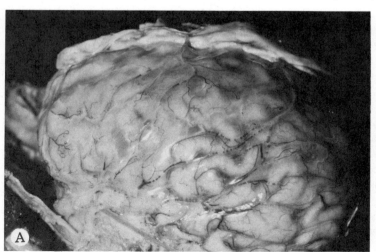
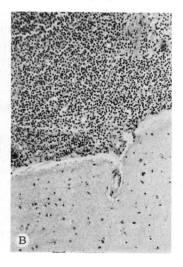

Table 6-1. CSF Findings in Syndromes Involving Meningeal Irritation

CSF	Normal	Subarachnoid hemorrhage	Bacterial meningitis	Viral encephalitis
Appearance	Clear	Bloody	Cloudy	Clear to slightly cloudy
Cell count	<5 lympho-cytes	Red blood cells present; white blood cells in proportion to red blood cells in the peripheral blood count	Usually >1,000 white blood cells; mostly polymorphonuclear leukocytes	Usually 25–500 white blood cells, mostly lymphocytes
Protein	<45 mg/dl	Normal to slightly elevated	Usually elevated >100 mg/dl	Minimally elevated, usually <100 mg/dl
Glucose	>45 mg/dl	Normal (rarely reduced)	Reduced	Normal
Microbiologic findings	Negative	Negative	Positive Gram's stain; positive cultures	Negative Gram's stain; negative viral cultures usually

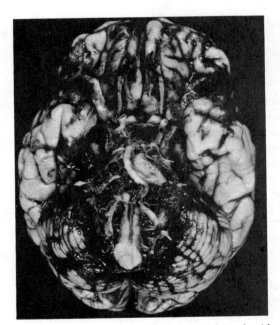

Fig. 6-13. Base of brain after acute subarachnoid hemorrhage due to ruptured aneurysm. Note blood throughout subarachnoid space concentrated in major cisterns.

der results. Only rarely does the aneurysm produce focal signs.

Examination of the CSF by lumbar puncture is the usual means of initially differentiating the disorders that produce the syndrome of meningeal irritation (Table 6-1).

Intracranial Epidural Hematoma

The epidural hemorrhage lies between the dura mater and the inner table of the skull and most commonly occurs from a skull fracture or traumatic laceration of the *middle meningeal artery*. Blood then dissects the dura mater from bone, forming a localized, rapidly expanding intracranial mass. Typically, the patient receives an injury to the head of sufficient degree to produce a period of unconsciousness. Thereafter, depending on the rate of bleeding, the patient becomes increasingly drowsy and then lapses into stupor and finally into deep coma. The cerebral hemisphere is pushed medially by the enlarging mass, thereby compressing the upper brain stem against the unyielding tentorium cerebelli. The patient will die unless emergency measures are taken to evacuate the blood clot.

The clinical-anatomic-temporal profile of this lesion is that of an acute, focal, and progressive lesion, with evidence of increased intracranial pressure. A history of trauma is often present.

Intracranial Subdural Hematoma

Subdural hematomas are most commonly seen in infants and in adults of middle age and beyond, particularly adults who are likely to suffer head injury (for example, alcoholics). The injury that produces the hematoma may be severe or so mild that it is forgotten.

At the time of injury, a tear usually occurs in a cortical vein at the point where it attaches to the superior longitudinal sinus. As a result, a small amount of bleeding occurs in the subdural space. This initial blood is often not enough to cause noticeable symptoms. Fibroblasts and capillaries proliferate and surround this blood with a fibrous membrane derived from the dura mater. Enlarge-

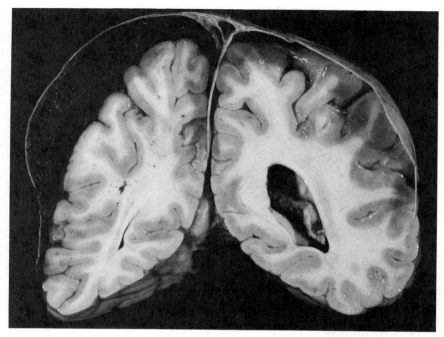

Fig. 6-14. Left subdural hematoma. Note accumulation of blood between dura mater and arachnoid, with compression of left cerebral hemisphere.

ment of the hematoma results from recurrent bleeding of the neomembrane or from increased osmotic activity of disintegrating red blood cells. With further increase in size, the intracranial volume increases, compressing the underlying brain (Fig. 6-14). The typical anatomic-clinical-temporal profile of this not uncommon and potentially treatable disorder is that of a chronic, focal, progressive lesion with symptoms of increased intracranial pressure.

Clinical Correlations II: Diagnostic Studies Utilizing the CSF System

The anatomy, physiology, and the known pathologic changes that may occur within the CSF system serve as the basis for many neurodiagnostic tests.

Lumbar Puncture

Although it is a procedure with little risk or discomfort to the patient, examination of the CSF via puncture of the lumbar subarachnoid sac is not a routine diagnostic test. Lumbar puncture is indicated only when it is necessary to obtain specific information about the cellular or chemical constituents of the CSF. The procedure is usually

contraindicated if there is known or suspected increased intracranial pressure, because in certain instances (especially those of localized mass lesions), sudden alteration in CSF pressure dynamics can lead to herniation of the brain contents through the foramen magnum and clinical decompensation or death.

The examination is usually performed in one of the three lower lumbar interspaces (Fig. 6-15). Puncture above the L-2–L-3 interspace (the region of the conus medullaris) is inadvisable. In infants or children in whom the spinal cord may be situated at a lower level, the puncture should be performed in the L-4–L-5 or L-5–S-1 interspace.

With the patient in a lateral recumbent position, the use of a simple manometer will allow measurement of CSF pressure (normally less than 200 mm of water). In order to ensure that the needle is properly placed in the subarachnoid sac, the pressure response to gentle coughing, straining, or abdominal compression should be observed. Normally, a prompt increase in pressure of at least 40 mm of water results from the elevation of central venous pressure that accompanies these maneuvers.

In patients with suspected spinal cord disease, the jugular compression test (Queckenstedt's test) may be performed. Prior to the removal of any fluid, the jugular veins are compressed manually by an assistant. There should normally be an

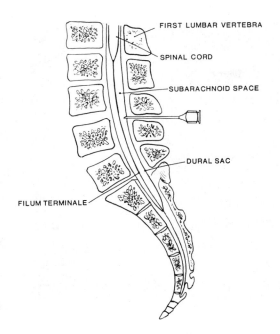

FIRST LUMBAR VERTEBRA

SPINAL CORD

SUBARACHNOID SPACE

DURAL SAC

FILUM TERMINALE

Fig. 6-15. Site of lumbar puncture. Note that, in the normal adult, caudal border of spinal cord lies at the L-1–L-2 vertebral level.

abrupt increase in spinal fluid pressure of between 100 and 300 mm of water within 10 seconds after the compression and a prompt decrease upon release. The compression procedure retards venous drainage from the skull and increases intracranial pressure. In the absence of a blockage in the spinal subarachnoid pathways, this increase in pressure will be transmitted to the lumbar subarachnoid sac. An absent or sluggish increase in pressure, with a delayed or absent decrease upon release, is suggestive of obstruction in the subarachnoid pathways, usually by a spinal mass lesion located cephalad to the needle site. Since this test is a means of determining the presence or absence of a spinal subarachnoid blockage, it is never done routinely and is *contraindicated* for all conditions other than suspected spinal cord disease. Patients with suspected intracranial disease may already have an increase in intracranial pressure, and compression of the jugular veins will further increase this pressure.

After determination of the initial pressure, the appearance of the fluid is noted, and 5 to 15 ml of CSF is removed for cell count, protein analysis, glucose determination, and microbiologic and other studies. A serologic test for syphilis is generally performed on all spinal fluid specimens because that disease, characterized partly by a chronic inflammatory reaction in the central nervous system, may mimic many other disorders.

Even with the most experienced examiners, occasionally one of the veins lying in the spinal epidural space is nicked by the lumbar puncture needle; a "traumatic tap" results, bloody fluid is obtained, and one must then differentiate this from a true subarachnoid hemorrhage. In a traumatic tap, fluid collected in successive test tubes usually shows decreasing amounts of red blood cells, while in cases of hemorrhagic disease the blood staining of fluid remains uniform. Furthermore, in a hemorrhagic disorder several hours often have elapsed between the onset of symptoms and the performance of a lumbar puncture, and xanthochromic staining of the supernatant fluid is seen in a centrifuged specimen; this staining is not noted in the case of a traumatic puncture.

Myelography

Myelography consists of the introduction of a radiopaque substance, usually via a lumbar puncture, into the subarachnoid space. Myelography can be utilized to study the spinal canal (Fig. 6-16A) and posterior fossa (Fig. 6-16B). The contrast material most commonly used is iophendylate (Pantopaque), a substance that absorbs x-rays to a much greater extent than do soft tissues or bones because of its high iodine content. Pantopaque is a nonabsorbable oil-based substance that will remain in the subarachnoid space unless removed. Most authorities recommend its removal after myelography is performed. This disadvantage is avoided by the use of more recently introduced water-soluble contrast media, such as metrizamide (Amipaque), which is absorbed into the blood. However, other factors must be weighed in the selection of an appropriate contrast agent.

Computed Tomography

Computer-assisted tomography (CT) has almost completely replaced other methods of studying the anatomy of the intracranial space in patients. This technique, which is rapid, painless, and free of risk, permits visualization of the ventriculosubarachnoid system and parenchymal structures at the posterior fossa and supratentorial levels (Fig. 6-17).

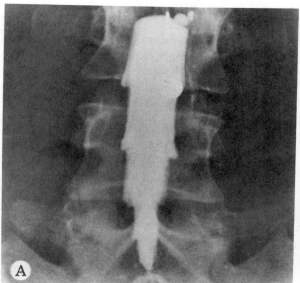
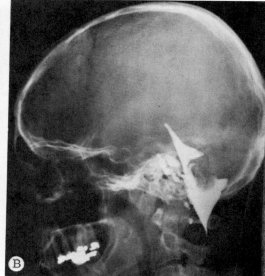

Fig. 6-16. Myelograms. A. Anteroposterior view showing filling of lumbar subarachnoid space. B. By tilting patient downward, contrast medium can be used to visualize entire spinal canal and structures contained in posterior fossa (lateral view).

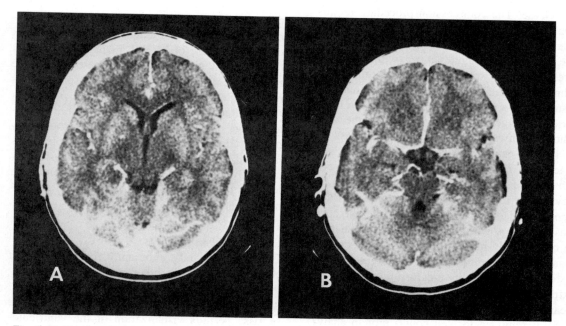

Fig. 6-17. Computed tomograms (horizontal sections). A. Level of caudate and thalamus. B. Base of brain at level of midbrain.

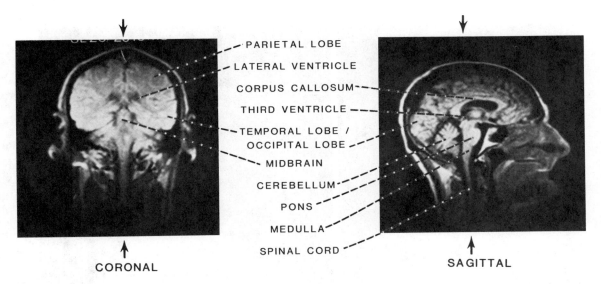

PARIETAL LOBE
LATERAL VENTRICLE
CORPUS CALLOSUM
THIRD VENTRICLE
TEMPORAL LOBE /
OCCIPITAL LOBE
MIDBRAIN
CEREBELLUM
PONS
MEDULLA
SPINAL CORD

CORONAL   SAGITTAL

Fig. 6-18. Magnetic resonance imaging of head in computer-reconstructed coronal and sagittal planes. Arrows indicate level of images of the other plane.

Computed tomographic techniques using x-rays to generate the scan were the first to be developed for clinical use. Thin beams of x-ray are passed through the patient's head, and the amount of energy transmitted (not absorbed by structures in its path) is measured by an x-ray detector on the opposite side of the head. This is repeated thousands of times (within a few seconds) from every point around the circumference of the head. The absorption data are processed by a computer, which reconstructs a horizontal section of the head about 1 cm thick. The entire cranial contents can be demonstrated by generating a series of adjacent sections. The ventricular system and any distortions and displacements can be identified. Most hemorrhages, infarcts, and tumors in the substance of the brain can be detected because their density (x-ray absorption) differs from that of normal brain. Intravenously administered contrast media (iodine-containing compounds) aid in visualizing lesions that are vascular or in which the blood-brain barrier is disturbed.

Computed tomographic techniques using physical principles and agents other than x-ray are also available. These include magnetic resonance (MR) imaging (Fig. 6-18) and positron-emission tomography (PET) scans using isotope-labeled metabolites. Magnetic resonance imaging is more sensitive than CT scanning at depicting some lesions and produces better images of structures surrounded by bone such as the spinal cord. The PET scans depict differences in metabolic activity in different brain regions.

Pneumoencephalography

In pneumoencephalography, air or another gas is introduced into the subarachnoid space, usually via a lumbar puncture. The patient is held in an upright position for a brief time, and air, being lighter than CSF, rises in the subarachnoid space through the foramen magnum and is distributed into the ventricular system and parts of the intracranial subarachnoid space (Fig. 6-19). Superior demonstration of the ventriculo-subarachnoid system by CT scanning has almost eliminated the use of pneumoencephalography.

Ventriculography

In the presence of increased intracranial pressure, it is often safer to introduce the contrast medium into the cerebral subarachnoid space and ventricular system instead of the lumbar subarachnoid space. In these situations, a small hole (burr hole) is made in the parietal bone under sterile conditions, and a needle is introduced through the brain into the lateral ventricle. Air or another contrast medium (iophendylate) may be injected, and roentgenograms taken.

Radioisotope Brain Scan

Normally, large molecules are prevented from entering into brain tissue by the blood-brain barrier system. Many focal injuries to the brain are accompanied by a local breakdown in this barrier

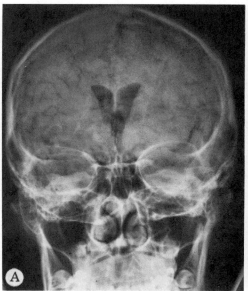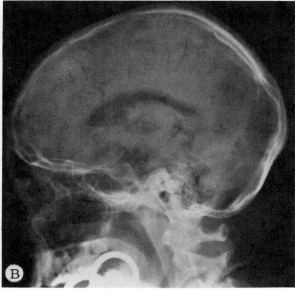

Fig. 6-19. Pneumoencephalograms. A. Anteroposterior view outlining lateral ventricles and third ventricle. Some extraventricular air is seen outlining cortex. B. Lateral view of ventricular system.

Fig. 6-20. Radioisotope brain scan (right lateral scan; face is to the right). Lesion is indicated by area of abnormal accumulation of indicator noted in right parietal lobe.

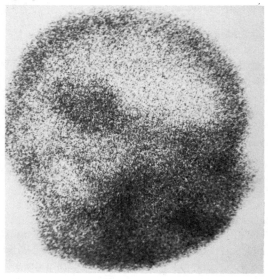

system, with subsequent diffusion of larger molecules into brain tissue. If a normally nondiffusible molecule is labeled with a radioisotope and is injected intravenously into a normal person and the brain is scanned for evidence of radioactive accumulation, the activity will be concentrated primarily in the regions of normal blood flow (that is, the venous sinuses). If, however, the patient has an area of focal disease, with normal blood flow but breakdown of the barrier system, some of the indicator will leak out from the normal vascular compartment and accumulate in the region of injury. This accumulation results in an abnormal area of increased radioactivity in the brain scan that corresponds to the area of disease. The brain scan is a sensitive indicator of neoplastic disease but is a less sensitive indicator of cerebral infarction (Fig. 6-20).

Radioisotope Cisternography

By injecting a radioisotope into the lumbar subarachnoid space, physiologic observations can be made of the circulation of CSF. Normally, the injected material will rise and accumulate both within the ventricular system and over the convexity of the brain. Localization of the indicator within the ventricles and failure to circulate over the brain surface after 48 hours are suggestive of a blockage in the extraventricular CSF pathways. Both signs are frequently seen in cases of a communicating hydrocephalus.

Neurologic Examination of the CSF System

As part of the neurologic examination of patients with suspected disease of the CSF system, it is necessary to search specifically for signs of increased intracranial pressure and meningeal irritation. In addition, assessment of this system will at times require the performance of a lumbar puncture.

An increase in intracranial pressure is suspected on the basis of the anatomic-clinical-temporal profile of the illness and the constellation of signs and symptoms outlined previously. Not all patients with increased intracranial pressure will have papilledema; however, ophthalmoscopic visualization of the optic nerve head in search of papilledema should be carefully performed on all such patients. One must be cautious; although the presence of edema of the nerve head should always raise the possibility of an elevation in intracranial pressure, it may be associated with other conditions.

The presence of meningeal irritation is best determined by examining for *nuchal rigidity.* When there is meningeal irritation, the side-to-side movement of the neck causes little discomfort, and frequently the first 10 to 15 degrees of neck flexion meet with little resistance; but with additional flexion, resistance and discomfort increase rapidly. In order to reduce the effects of traction on the lumbosacral roots when the neck is flexed, a patient with meningeal irritation may automatically flex the hips and knees. (This type of abnormal response seen with meningeal irritation is referred to as *Brudzinski's sign.*) An additional and related test can be performed with the patient recumbent and the legs flexed at the hips and knees. In this position, the lumbosacral nerve roots are relatively slack, and maneuvers designed to stretch these nerve roots (such as extension of the knee) normally produce no discomfort. In the presence of meningeal irritation, there is pain and increased resistance (Kernig's sign). When Kernig's sign is encountered in the absence of nuchal rigidity (and especially if it is unilateral), it is indicative of an irritative process involving the lumbosacral nerve roots rather than of a diffuse meningeal irritation.

Objectives

1. Define or identify the following: dura mater, arachnoid, pia mater, epidural space, subdural space, subarachnoid space, dural sinuses, falx cerebri, tentorium cerebelli, blood-brain barrier, choroid plexuses, lateral ventricles, foramen of Monro, third ventricle, aqueduct of Sylvius, fourth ventricle, and foramina of Luschka and Magendie.

2. Describe and trace the formation, circulation, and absorption of cerebrospinal fluid.

3. Define communicating hydrocephalus and noncommunicating hydrocephalus, and give an example of each type, describe its location, and state the pathologic-anatomic consequences of a lesion in that location.

4. Discuss the relationship between the contents of the cranial cavity and intracranial pressure, and give examples of general pathologic states that may result in increased pressure.

5. Interpret the significance of abnormalities in the CSF color, cellular composition, serologic findings, total protein level, gamma globulin concentration, sugar level, and culture, and list the CSF findings in meningitis, encephalitis, subarachnoid hemorrhage, and traumatic puncture.

6. Describe or list the features of the syndrome of meningeal irritation.

7. Describe or list the features that indicate increased intracranial pressure.

8. Describe the neuroanatomic basis for the following neurodiagnostic studies: myelography, pneumoencephalography, ventriculography, computed tomography, magnetic resonance imaging, radioisotope brain scan, and radioisotope cisternography.

Clinical Problems

1. A 10-month-old infant presents with an enlarging head and a delay in reaching developmental milestones. The neurologic examination confirms the developmental delay and also reveals a tense, bulging, enlarged anterior fontanelle, normal ophthalmoscopic examination of the fundi, and a head circumference of 50 cm. An opening pressure of 200 mm H_2O is found on lumbar puncture. Based on these findings, answer the following questions:

a. How do we know the head is abnormally large?
b. What are the possible causes of a large head?
c. What tests might be useful in obtaining information about the infant's ventricular system?
d. Does the lesion found in this patient (see answer to previous question) produce a communicating or noncommunicating type of hydrocephalus?
e. What changes would you expect to find in the configuration of the ventricular system in a ventriculogram performed on
(1) This patient
(2) A patient with chronic obstruction of the foramina of Luschka and Magendie
(3) A patient with inflammatory obliteration of the intracranial arachnoid villi
(4) A patient with an acute subarachnoid hemorrhage
2. A 38-year-old man with the same pathologic condition as the infant in problem 1 has a normal head size, papilledema, and an opening pressure of 500 mm H$_2$O on lumbar puncture. How can you explain the differences in these two cases?
3. A 37-year-old man is seen because of a 6-month history of progressive weakness in his legs and loss of pain and thermal sensation to the level of his nipples. Based on your findings on physical examination and normal roentgenographic findings in the head and in the cervical, thoracic, and lumbar regions of the spinal column, you perform a lumbar puncture with the following results:
a. Hydrodynamics:
(1) Opening pressure of 80 mm H$_2$O
(2) Spontaneous pulsations
Respiratory: 10 to 20 mm H$_2$O
Cardiac: None
(3) Abdominal compression gives prompt increase of 70 mm H$_2$O with rapid decrease to 80 mm H$_2$O on release of pressure
(4) Jugular compression gives an increase of 50 mm H$_2$O over 20 seconds, with a return of 100 mm H$_2$O 50 seconds after release of pressure
b. Spinal fluid examination:

(1) Appearance: Slightly yellow, clear fluid
(2) Cells:
(a) White blood cells = 4 lymphocytes per microliter
(b) Red blood cells = 0
(3) Chemistry:
(a) Protein = 700 mg/dl
(b) Glucose = 65 mg/dl
(c) Blood sugar = 100 mg/dl
Based on these findings, answer the following questions:
a. What is the location of this lesion? (level? lateralization?) Is this a mass lesion? What is the cause?
b. How would you explain each of the hydrodynamic findings on the lumbar puncture?
c. What structures did the lumbar puncture needle penetrate before CSF began to drip from the needle?
d. What radiologic study might help you locate the lesion(s) accurately?
4. You are called to the emergency room to see a semicomatose elderly woman who responds to painful stimuli with movement of all four extremities. She was brought to the hospital by police ambulance after being found in her apartment by neighbors who had not seen her for 3 days. The physical examination reveals blood pressure 120/80 mm Hg, pulse 120 per minute, respiration 124 per minute, and temperature 39.5°C rectally. There is marked resistance to flexion but not to lateral rotation of the neck. Results of the remainder of the examination are normal. A lumbar puncture reveals an opening pressure of 270 mm H$_2$O.
a. CSF examination:
(1) Appearance before centrifugation:
Tube #1: 2+ pink; 2+ turbid
Tube #3: slightly pink; 2+ turbid
(2) Appearance after centrifugation:
All tubes clear and colorless
(3) Cell counts:
Tube #1: 300 white blood cells (90% polymorphonuclear leukocytes), 2,800 red blood cells
Tube #3: 320 white blood cells (90% polymorphonuclear leukocytes), 700 red blood cells

(4) Protein:
    Tube #1: 180 mg/dl
    Tube #3: 176 mg/dl

(5) Glucose:
    10 mg/dl in all tubes

Based on these findings, answer the following questions:

a. What is the location of this lesion? (level? lateralization?) Is this a mass lesion? What is the cause?

b. How do you explain the differences in appearance and cellular count of the CSF between tubes #1 and #3?

c. What would you expect to find on Gram's stain of the CSF? On culture of the CSF?

d. How would you explain the CSF glucose result?

e. Would you have performed jugular compression? Explain.

Suggested Reading

Coben, L. A. Pathophysiology of the Cerebrospinal Fluid. In S. Eliasson, A. L. Prensky, and W. B. Hardin, Jr. (eds.), *Neurological Pathophysiology* (2nd ed.). New York: Oxford University Press, 1978. Pp. 394–415.

Fishman, R. A. *Cerebrospinal Fluid in Diseases of the Nervous System*. Philadelphia: Saunders, 1980.

Oehmichen, M. *Cerebrospinal Fluid Cytology: An Introduction and Atlas*. Philadelphia: Saunders, 1976.

Wood, J. H. *Neurobiology of Cerebrospinal Fluid*. New York: Plenum, 1983.

The Sensory System

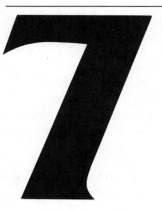

The information utilized by the central nervous system for reflex activity, decision making, and effecting behavioral change is derived from its internal and external environments. This chapter will describe how information is received, transmitted, and perceived by the human organism, and how this system may be altered by various disease states.

Impulses traveling toward the central nervous system are regarded as *sensory* and have been given the general term *afferent*. They may be utilized by the organism in many ways, each serving a different function. Sensory information may be transmitted (1) as largely unconscious data which, although utilized to modify behavior, remain unperceived by the organism; (2) as largely conscious data which are perceived by the organism and then utilized to modify behavior; and (3) in both a conscious and an unconscious manner.

Afferent impulses are functionally subdivided into the following:

1. General somatic afferent (GSA)—sensory information from skin, striated muscle, and joints.
2. General visceral afferent (GVA)—sensory information, largely unconscious in nature, from viscera and smooth muscle.
3. Special somatic afferent (SSA)—sensory information relating to vision, audition, and equilibrium.
4. Special visceral afferent (SVA)—sensory information relating to taste and smell.

Although introductory comments will be made in relation to each of these subdivisions, this chapter will be concerned primarily with the organization and function of the general somatic afferent sensory impulses.

Overview

The ability to detect and translate information from the environment is the function of the *receptor organs*. These specialized portions of the nervous system act like the transducers commonly employed in physiologic experiments; their function is to convert mechanical, chemical, photic, and other forms of energy into electrical potentials. Once converted into a form of information that can be utilized by the nervous system, impulses in the form of action potentials are transmitted by specific *pathways* to those regions of the central nervous system where they can be integrated and perceived.

Many but not all of the sensory pathways have the common features of sensory receptors and three orders of neurons:

1. The cell bodies of the first-order (primary order) neurons lie outside the central nervous system in a ganglion. The distal axon of each of these cell bodies receives information from the sensory receptor, and the proximal axon enters the spinal cord or brain stem via a dorsal root or cranial nerve.
2. The cell bodies of the second-order neurons lie within regions of the embryonic alar plate (dorsal gray matter of the spinal cord or analogous areas of the brain stem). The axons of these second-order neurons decussate (cross the midline) and continue cephalad. First- or second-order neurons, as they ascend in the spinal cord, are grouped into *tracts* (fasciculi), which are located primarily in the white matter (funiculi) of the spinal cord (Fig. 7-1). In the brain stem, the axons of second-order neurons continue to ascend in tracts (in this region, some are referred to as *lemnisci*) to reach the thalamus, where they terminate in *specific sensory nuclei.*
3. The cell bodies of the third-order neurons lie within the thalamus, and their axons pass via the thalamocortical radiation to the *sensory cortex.* The primary *somesthetic area* is located in the postcentral gyrus of the parietal lobe and is concerned with the reception and appreciation of somatic sensory impulses. Fibers terminating in this area are distributed over the postcentral gyrus in an organized fashion with the lower extremity represented in the parasagittal area; the arm and hand represented over the convexity; and the face, mouth, and tongue represented in the suprasylvian region (Fig. 7-2). Although the parietal sensory cortex is not concerned with the crude recognition of general somatic information (which enters awareness at the thalamic level), it is necessary for the discriminative aspects of sensation. Visual information is relayed to the occipital cortex, and auditory fibers terminate in the temporal lobe.

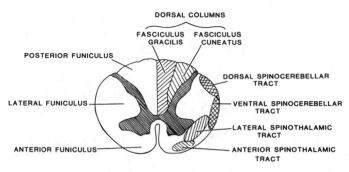

Fig. 7-1. Cross section of upper cervical spinal cord illustrating location of major ascending sensory pathways and their relationship to posterior, lateral, and anterior funiculi.

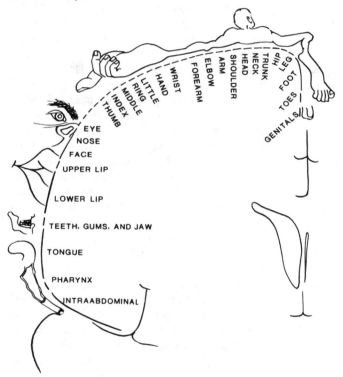

Fig. 7-2. Coronal section of a cerebral hemisphere showing the distribution of sensory fibers in the postcentral gyrus (sensory homunculus). (Redrawn from W. Penfield and T. Rasmussen. The Cerebral Cortex of Man: A Clinical Study of Localization of Function. New York: Macmillan, 1950.)

While information is generally relayed in a cephalad direction by these three orders of neurons, it is not simply transmitted but is processed and utilized by each order of neuron.

The pathways that this discussion will primarily be concerned with are those listed in Table 7-1. These pathways are of major importance in the understanding and interpretation of neurologic disease.

Lesions at different levels of the neuraxis will alter sensory function in different ways; by correlating the patient's signs and symptoms with the anatomic distribution of these pathways, it is possible to localize neurologic disorders. Abnormalities of peripheral nerves or spinal roots are distributed in segmental fashion, often involve all sensory modalities, and may be associated with the sensation of pain. Lesions involving the spinal cord may be associated with segmental sensory loss at the level of the lesion and varied

Table 7-1. Major General
Somatic Afferent Pathways

Pathway	Sensory modality
Lateral spinothalamic	Pain and temperature
Ventral spinothalamic	Simple touch
Dorsal column–medial lemniscal	Discriminative sensation; conscious proprioception, touch (vibration)
Spinocerebellar (dorsal and ventral)	Unconscious proprioception

sensory loss at all levels below the lesion. Lesions of the posterior fossa produce contralateral sensory loss over the trunk and extremities and may be associated with ipsilateral sensory disturbance in the face. Supratentorial lesions produce entirely contralateral sensory deficits.

Somatic Sensory Receptors

Sensory receptors are highly specialized structures that can respond to environmental change by producing action potentials for transmission to the nervous system. There are many types of receptors subserving different sensory functions.

Impulse Initiation in Somatic Sensory Receptors

Although the mechanism by which receptor potentials are produced varies with the receptor

Fig. 7-3. Rate of adaptation in sensory receptors to prolonged stimulus. Adaptation of receptor potentials and spike trains in primary afferent axons in rapid- and slow-adapting receptors is shown.

organ, certain general principles of receptor physiology are common to all. The application of a "specific stimulus" (one to which the receptor has a low threshold) will produce a *depolarization* or, as with the retina of the eye, a hyperpolarization in the receptor organ. This electrical event, caused by a membrane permeability change to multiple ions, produces a local potential, a *generator potential,* which is graded as a function of stimulus strength (see Chap. 5). If the generator potential is of sufficient magnitude, the associated electrotonic potential will induce a permeability change in the axon, innervating the receptor, and will produce an *action potential,* which is then propagated centrally. Receptor stimulation seldom induces a single action potential but rather produces a train of such discharges. Because all action potentials are of uniform amplitude, the stimulus intensity is coded by the frequency of these discharges (frequency modulation) and by the number of adjacent axons activated.

Receptor Adaptation

Adaptation is a characteristic of receptors in which the generator potential progressively decreases in response to a continuous stimulus. The receptor initiates action potentials in response to the stimulus, whose rate of discharge progressively decreases as long as the same stimulus is maintained. If there is a change in the stimulus or if the stimulus intensity is increased, the discharge rate increases again. There are rapid- and slow-adapting receptors; the rapid-adapting recep-

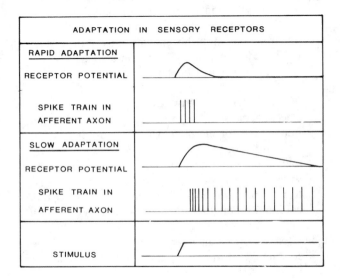

tors initiate potentials with a rapidly decreasing firing frequency, while the slow-adapting receptors have a more prolonged and gradual decrease in firing rates (Fig. 7-3). These different types of receptors transmit different types of information to the central nervous system.

Tonic receptors adapt slowly and continue to initiate impulses in the adjacent axon as long as the stimulus remains. These receptors, therefore, can best serve to keep the nervous system constantly apprised of the status of the body and its relation to its surroundings.

Phasic receptors adapt rapidly and respond primarily to a change in stimulus strength or intensity. Therefore they react maximally while change is actually taking place, and the number of action potentials initiated in the adjacent axon is related to their rate of change. This type of receptor thus serves to alert the nervous system to any change in the environment.

The excitability of the receptors is transiently abolished during *receptor fatigue*, when repetitive stimuli in a sensory receptor produce successively smaller amplitude generator potentials, to the point that the receptor no longer responds to the stimulus or change in the stimulus.

Receptor Specificity

A given receptor type is generally specialized so that it is more sensitive (that is, has a lower threshold) to one particular kind of stimulus. A number of factors may contribute to this specialization, including the position of the receptor in

Table 7-2. Types of Sensory Receptors

Type	Function
Mechanoreceptors	Touch
	Pressure
	Muscle stretch (muscle spindle)
	Joint movement (Golgi tendon organ)
	Labyrinthine function (hair cells in the ear)
Thermal receptors	Heat
	Cold
Chemoreceptors	Olfaction
	Taste
Nociceptors (pain)	Free nerve endings
	Mechanoreceptors
	Thermal receptors
	Polynodal receptors (mechanical, thermal, chemical)

the body, its anatomic structure, and the chemical composition of its surface membrane or of its organelles. Thus, somatic sensory receptors can be broadly classified into four main types: chemoreceptors (olfaction, taste), mechanoreceptors (touch and pressure receptors, muscle spindles, Golgi tendon organs, labyrinthine hair cells), thermal receptors, and nociceptive receptors (Table 7-2). Sensory discrimination could depend solely on the varied sensitivity of receptors to different forms of stimuli, as in the receptors found in the eye and ear. Such specificity is not usually true of the cutaneous receptors. For example, it was formerly believed that specialized cutaneous receptors, such as Krause's end bulbs, were exclusively responsible for the sensation of cold, while Ruffini's corpuscles mediated warmth. We now know that responses to changes in temperature are seen in areas of skin that have neither of these receptors present and that contain only free nerve endings. Furthermore, the various sensations of touch and pressure can be mediated by many cutaneous receptors.

Although certain types of receptors respond preferentially to specific stimuli, the receptor alone does not allow sensory discrimination. Sensory discrimination instead occurs as a result of a pattern of activity in various receptors, and the central nervous system has an important associated role in that it is capable of integrating the patterns of input from multiple receptors, which results in the appreciation of specific sensations.

The muscle spindle and Golgi tendon organ (receptors that signal information about the tension, length, and contraction of muscle) will be studied with the motor system; chemoreceptors and receptors for the special senses of vision, taste, audition, and equilibration also will be described further in Chapters 14 and 15.

Major Sensory Pathways

The general somatic afferent pathways of major importance for the diagnosis of neurologic disorders are those that conduct pain, temperature, touch, and proprioceptive sensations. These pathways transmit sensory information from the legs, trunk, and arms to higher centers via the spinal cord and brain stem. Pathways that carry sensory information from the head and face will not be discussed in detail at this time, but they will be considered further in Chapter 14 (The Posterior Fossa Level).

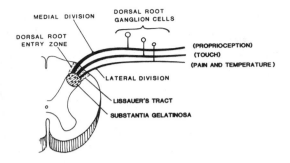

Fig. 7-4. Dorsal root entry zone. Largest, most heavily myelinated fibers mediating proprioception occupy the medial division. Medium-sized myelinated fibers mediating touch are centrally located, and finely myelinated fibers carrying pain and temperature sensation are located in the lateral division.

Sensory information from receptors is transmitted to the spinal cord by first-order neurons of the peripheral nerves. These are the distal axons of the primary sensory neurons. The cell bodies of these fibers are located in the dorsal root ganglia (spinal ganglia). Each ganglion cell possesses a single nerve process that divides into two branches in the dorsal root ganglion. A distal branch innervates the receptor, and a proximal branch enters the spinal cord through the dorsal root.* There are no synapses in a spinal ganglion. Afferent fibers enter the spinal cord in the posterolateral sulcus at the *dorsal root entry zone* (Fig. 7-4). The largest and most heavily myelinated fibers occupy the most medial position in this zone. Located next to these large-caliber proprioceptive fibers are the medium-sized fibers carrying tactile sense, and occupying a lateral position in the entry zone are the finely myelinated fibers that mediate pain and temperature sense. From this common entry, pathways for the different modalities of sensation diverge as they ascend the spinal cord to higher centers. In addition to these ascending sensory pathways, other descending axons from higher centers within the brain stem and telencephalon act on the afferent structures to determine what sensory information reaches conscious awareness by selecting, facilitating, or inhibiting the sensory modalities that enter the nervous system.

*Common usage has led to interchange of the terms *posterior* with *dorsal* and *anterior* with *ventral*. Although we freely use both conventions, with reference to the human, posterior and anterior are anatomically correct.

Pathways for Pain and Temperature (the Lateral Spinothalamic Tract)

Pain and temperature sensations travel a similar course through the nervous system, and therefore these two modalities of sensation will be considered together (Fig. 7-5). The complex sensation of "itch" appears to be closely related and travels via similar pathways.

The *peripheral receptors* for pain are free nerve endings, whereas those for temperature remain poorly defined, although they probably include similar receptors. Pain and temperature fibers, which have their primary neuron cell bodies located in dorsal root ganglia, enter the spinal cord in the lateral division of the dorsal root zone and divide into short ascending and descending branches that run longitudinally in the posterolateral fasciculus (Lissauer's tract) (see Fig. 7-4). Within several segments, they leave this tract to synapse with neurons located in the posterior or dorsal gray horn of the spinal cord. The pain fibers terminate in the substantia gelatinosa, where they release substance P, a peptide neurotransmitter for the pain fibers in the dorsal horn of the spinal cord. Axons arising from these second-order neurons in the dorsal horn either synapse locally or cross (decussate) to the opposite side in the *ventral white commissure* near the central canal. After crossing, the fibers that carry pain and temperature turn cephalad and form the *lateral spinothalamic tract*, which is located in the ventral portion of the lateral funiculus. Topographic organization is noted within this tract, with the sacral fibers laterally aligned, and the lumbar, thoracic, and cervical fibers aligned in more medial positions (Fig. 7-6). The tract extends without interruption through the spinal cord, medulla, pons, and midbrain. At the level of the midbrain, the spinothalamic tract runs within the lateral lemniscus. These second-order fibers terminate in the *ventral posterolateral nucleus* of the thalamus. Third-order neurons located in the thalamus give rise to *thalamocortical fibers*, which establish the final connection of this pathway with the postcentral gyrus of the parietal lobe.

Collateral fibers from this pathway, and from the other sensory pathways to be discussed, are given off at several levels of the neuraxis, but particularly in the brain stem, where they synapse with neurons contained within the centrally located reticular formation. These nonlemniscal

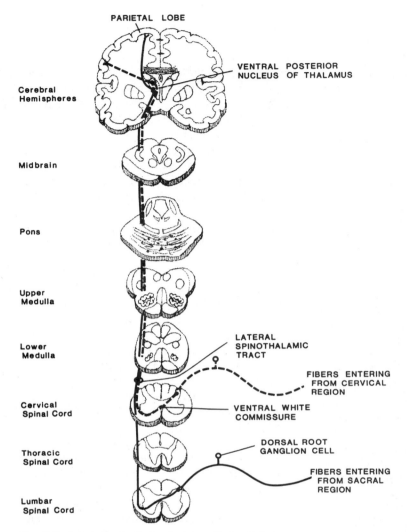

Fig. 7-5. Lateral spinothalamic tract. Pathway for pain and temperature.

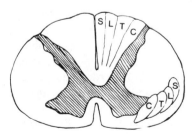

Fig. 7-6. Topographic organization of sensory fibers. In the lateral spinothalamic tract, cervical-originating fibers are medially located, while fibers carrying pain and temperature sensation from the sacral region are located near the periphery of the tract. In the dorsal columns, fibers from the lower extremities are located in the fasciculus gracilis, while those from the trunk and upper extremity are contained in the fasciculus cuneatus. (S = sacral; L = lumbar; T = thoracic; C = cervical.)

sensory pathways provide stimulation to the *ascending activating system,* which projects diffusely to wide areas of cortex, and are important in maintaining consciousness and alertness and in influencing the degree of conscious perception of each of the sensory modalities. They will be discussed further in Chapter 8 (The Consciousness System).

Two types of pain are recognized: (1) the sharp well-localized sense of pain induced by a pinprick or laceration and (2) a more diffuse aching type of discomfort or pain, which may outlast the actual stimulus. The former (referred to as *fast pain*) is carried peripherally by small myelinated fibers and transmitted by direct lemniscal pathways. The latter (referred to as *slow pain*) is mediated by slower conducting unmyelinated fibers in the periphery and transmitted by multisynaptic nonlemniscal pain pathways. The pain fibers project to various areas of the brain, including the reticular formation (a multisynaptic ascending and descending network within the brain stem), the periaqueductal gray matter of the midbrain, the periventricular gray matter of the diencephalon, the thalamus, the hypothalamus, the structures of the limbic system, and the cerebral cortex. Crude perception of painful stimuli may occur at the thalamic level without cortical participation; however, the localization of pain and the other disagreeable aspects that accompany this sensation are supplied by parietal and other areas of the cerebral cortex. These disagreeable aspects of pain can be accentuated or depressed by mental or emotional states, without any real change in the physiologic threshold for pain.

Pain fibers from the face are carried primarily in the trigeminal nerve (cranial nerve V) and have the cell bodies of their primary sensory neurons located in the gasserian (semilunar) ganglion (Fig. 7-7). On entering the brain stem in the pontine region, these fibers descend on the same side to the upper cervical spinal cord in the *descending* or *spinal tract of the trigeminal nerve.* Axons of this tract synapse with second-order neurons in the adjacent nucleus of the spinal tract of the trigeminal nerve and then cross to the opposite side of the neuraxis and ascend to the ventral posteromedial nucleus of the thalamus. Third-order neurons project from the thalamus to the parietal lobe via the posterior limb of the

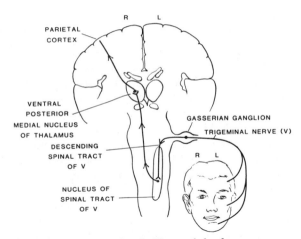

Fig. 7-7. Pathway of pain fibers of the face.

internal capsule. This slightly divergent pathway for pain provides the neuroanatomic basis for the frequent observation that lesions located in the lower part of the brain stem may alter pain perception over the face on the side of the lesion (ipsilateral) and trunk and extremities on the side opposite the lesion (contralateral).

Pain perception is not determined solely by this afferent system. The central nervous system can regulate and modify the transmission and perception of noxious and painful stimuli at various levels. Stimulation of the peripheral nerve fibers can suppress pain at the peripheral level by blocking the conduction of afferent fibers. Another site is the dorsal horn of the spinal cord, where local segmental mechanisms, other incoming sensory stimuli, and descending pathways from higher centers can interact and alter the transmission of noxious and painful stimuli. The brain-stem reticular formation, with its influence on ascending afferent pathways, has a significant role in regulating the conscious appreciation of pain and other sensory modalities. Stimulation of diencephalic and brain-stem areas, such as the periventricular and the periaqueductal gray matter, can block the synaptic transmission in the afferent pain pathways. The limbic system and cortical structures are involved with the affective and emotional responses to pain. Stress, for example, can inhibit the awareness of pain.

Pharmacologic agents, such as the opiates (for example, morphine), endorphins (an endogenous morphine-like substance within the nervous system), and enkephalins (an endogenous peptide substance within the nervous system) also can inhibit pain. The binding sites for these substances, the opiate receptors, are located in areas of the nervous system concerned with pain, including the limbic system, the periaqueductal and the periventricular gray matter, the thalamus, the brain stem, and the substantia gelatinosa of the spinal cord. These analgesic agents bind to the opiate receptors within the spinal cord and central nervous system and inhibit the afferent pain neurons, thus reducing or blocking the transmission of painful impulses.

The clinical manifestations of involvement of the pain and temperature pathways vary according to the level of the neuraxis involved. Lesions located outside the nervous system frequently will stimulate pain-sensitive free nerve endings and produce the subjective sensation of pain. This symptom is most important in calling attention to pathologic processes that occur in many organ systems. The parenchyma of internal organs, including the brain itself, is not supplied with pain receptors. However, the walls of arteries, all peritoneal surfaces, pleural membranes, and the dura mater may all be sources of severe pain, especially when they are subjected to inflammation or mechanical traction. In addition, abnormal contraction or dilation of the walls of hollow viscera causes pain. Pain of visceral origin is likely to be poorly localized, and at times it is felt in a surface area of the body far removed from its actual source (a phenomenon known as *referred pain*). For example, the pain of coronary artery disease may be felt in the chest wall, left axilla, or down the inside of the left arm; and irritation of the peritoneum covering the diaphragm may be felt in the shoulder. In each case, neurons conducting the painful stimuli from the visceral organ enter the central nervous system at a segment that corresponds not to the anatomic location of the organ but to the area in which the pain is felt.

One of the possible explanations of referred pain is that the visceral and somatosensory afferents enter the spinal cord via the same dorsal nerve roots and are transmitted together to the same pool of neurons and fiber pathways in the dorsal horn and spinothalamic tracts, respectively. As a consequence of this, the visceral impulses reaching the cortex are interpreted as coming formt he surface of the body at the level of this entry zone, resulting in a "misinterpretation" of

the location and true origin of the pain by the sensory cortex. (Further illustration and discussion are found in Chap. 10.)

Lesions that involve the peripheral level may cause either the sensation of pain or some loss of pain and temperature in the distribution of the affected nerves. Lesions of the central nervous system seldom produce pain unless associated pain-sensitive structures are involved, but the lesion results in an inability to perceive painful stimuli and to discriminate hot from cold in the areas below it. At the spinal level, a lesion involving the lateral spinothalamic tract results in contralateral loss of pain and temperature. At the posterior fossa level, contralateral loss of pain and temperature also is found in the trunk and extremities, but because of associated involvement of the pain fibers in the descending tract of the trigeminal nerve, there may be ipsilateral loss of pain and temperature in the face. Supratentorial level lesions produce contralateral loss of pain and temperature. Because pain is perceived at the thalamic level, suprathalamic lesions may leave crude pain perception intact, but precise localization of a painful stimulus is impaired.

Pathways for Conscious Proprioception and Discriminative Function (the Dorsal Column–Medial Lemniscal Pathway)

For motor function to proceed normally, the nervous system must receive sensory information from muscles, joints, and tendons; this information is referred to as *proprioceptive* and is of two types: conscious and unconscious.

Fibers conveying conscious proprioceptive information have their first-order primary neuron cell bodies located in the dorsal root ganglia. The distal axons receive information from sensory receptors in muscle, connective tissue, and joints (these receptors are discussed in more detail in Chap. 9). The proximal axon enters the dorsal root entry zone in its medial division and turns cephalad, without synapse, in the posterior funiculus, usually called the *dorsal* or *posterior columns* (Fig. 7-8). Fibers from the lower extremity ascend adjacent to the dorsal median septum and form the *fasciculus gracilis*. The *fasciculus cuneatus,* which contains fibers primarily from the thorax and upper extremity, is not present in the lumbar spinal cord but is found only in the upper thoracic and cervical regions,

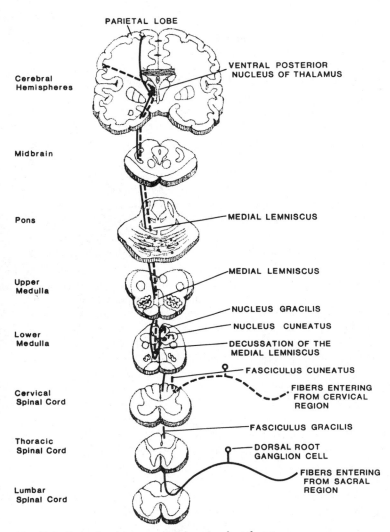

Fig. 7-8. Dorsal column–medial lemniscal pathway. Conscious proprioception and discriminative sensation.

where it is located just lateral to the fasciculus gracilis in the posterior funiculus. Thus, at the upper spinal level, topographic organization is also found in this pathway, with sacral and lumbar fibers medially and thoracic and cervical fibers laterally located in the dorsal columns (see Fig. 7-6). First-order axons contained in the fasciculus gracilis and cuneatus ascend to the lower medulla, where they terminate in the *nucleus gracilis* and *nucleus cuneatus,* respectively. Second-order axons from neurons in these nuclei cross to the opposite side in the lower medulla as the *internal arcuate fibers* (decussation of the medial lemniscus). They then ascend as the *medial lem-*

niscus to the thalamus and terminate in the *ventral posterolateral nucleus*. Third-order thalamo-cortical fibers from this relay center project to the postcentral gyrus of the parietal lobe via the posterior limb of the internal capsule. This band of cortex has been designated as the *somesthetic area* and displays a topographic organization, with the lower extremity represented in the parasagittal region and the upper extremity and head lying over the surface above the sylvian fissure (see Fig. 7-2). The conscious recognition of body and limb position requires cortical participation.

In addition to conscious proprioception, fibers concerned with the sense of touch also travel in the dorsal column–medial lemniscal pathway. (Other pathways for touch will be discussed later in this chapter.) This pathway is necessary for tactile discrimination: the ability to distinguish two separate points applied to the skin simultaneously; to recognize the size, shape, and texture of objects in the hand; and to identify letters and figures drawn on the skin. The ability to perform these discriminative tasks is called *stereognosis;* its absence is designated as *astereognosis.*

The ability to perceive vibration as tested clinically with a tuning fork has traditionally been associated with fibers traveling in this pathway as well. Recent evidence suggests this may not be true, and although frequency discrimination travels via this pathway, the gross recognition of vibration may ascend like touch-pressure via multiple divergent routes. From the standpoint of practical clinical diagnosis, however, vibratory perception is so often altered along with posterior column function that it may be considered to be associated with this pathway.

As with pain sensation, there is a descending system from higher centers and the brain-stem reticular formation that acts to control and modify neuronal transmission within the dorsal column–medial lemniscal pathway.

The clinical manifestations of lesions that damage the dorsal column–medial lemniscal pathway are expressed mainly as defects in joint position sense and stereognosis. The symptoms are most prominent with diffuse damage to peripheral nerves or the posterior funiculi, but they also may occur with lesions of the nucleus gracilis and nucleus cuneatus, the medial lemniscus, the thalamus, and the postcentral gyrus. Patients with bilateral lesions affecting the primary sensory neurons in these pathways also will have signs of *ataxia,* a loss of muscular coordination, and a severe disturbance of gait. Unless the patients can watch the movement of limbs and voluntarily correct their errors, they stumble, stagger, and fall. Whether these abnormalities are due solely to the involvement of this pathway or to associated involvement of unconscious proprioceptive (spinocerebellar) pathways is unclear. In summary, the clinical signs of injury to this pathway are an inability to recognize limb or joint position, astereognosis, loss of two-point discrimination, diminished vibratory sense, and ataxia that is improved by visual cues.

Pathways for Unconscious Proprioception (the Spinocerebellar Tracts)

Fibers conveying unconscious proprioceptive in-

formation have their primary neuron cell bodies located in the dorsal root ganglia. The distal axons innervate sensory receptors located in muscle, primarily the muscle spindles and Golgi tendon organs. The proximal axons enter the dorsal root entry zone in its medial division.

Some of the proprioceptive fibers from muscle spindles course directly through the dorsal gray matter into the ventral gray horn. These are the afferent fibers of the two-neuron muscle-stretch reflex arc that is the anatomic basis for the *muscle-stretch* (deep tendon) *reflexes* commonly tested in clinical neurology. A sudden pull on the muscle (by the reflex hammer) stretches the muscle and stimulates the muscle spindle receptors. This in turn produces action potentials which traverse the afferent fibers that enter the spinal cord and synapse on the anterior horn motor cells. These anterior horn cells in turn initiate action potentials that travel back to the muscle of origin and cause the muscle to contract. This is the classic example of a *local segmental reflex* and will be discussed further in Chapter 9. This reflex will be lost whenever disease involves the primary proprioceptive axon or other components of the reflex arc at that segment.

The spinocerebellar pathways transmit information about the activity of muscles and limbs to the cerebellum, where it is integrated and processed. The cerebellum is then capable of modifying the action of these and associated muscle groups so that movements are performed smoothly and accurately. The information carried by these pathways does not directly reach consciousness, and hence it is referred to as *unconscious proprioception.*

Two pathways convey this information to the cerebellum (Fig. 7-9): the ventral and the dorsal spinocerebellar tracts. Axons of first-order neurons entering the lumbar and sacral levels of the cord carry information from the lower extremities. They enter the spinal cord with conscious proprioceptive fibers but synapse at the level of entry in the dorsal gray horn. Axons from second-order neurons cross to the opposite side and proceed cephalad in the lateral funiculus as the *ventral* (anterior) *spinocerebellar tract.* These fibers ascend through the spinal cord, medulla, and pons and enter the cerebellum via a circuitous route through the superior cerebellar peduncle (brachium conjunctivum). Within the posterior fossa, some of these fibers may again cross

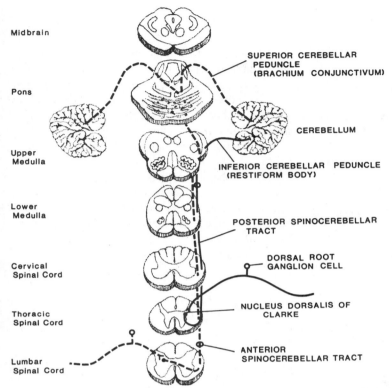

Fig. 7-9. *Ventral (anterior) (dotted line) and dorsal (posterior) (solid line) spinocerebellar tracts carrying unconscious proprioception. Refer to the text for variations in dorsal spinocerebellar pathways at levels above and below the location of the nucleus dorsalis of Clarke.*

to the ipsilateral side, providing the cerebellum with a bilateral representation of activity in the lower extremities.

First-order proprioceptive fibers entering the thoracic cord synapse in the dorsal gray matter in a nucleus called the *nucleus dorsalis of Clarke (Clarke's column)*. Second-order axons from this nucleus enter the ipsilateral lateral funiculus to form the *dorsal (posterior) spinocerebellar tract* located in the lateral margins of the spinal cord just dorsal to the anterior spinocerebellar tract. Fibers ascend in this location and, at the level of the medulla, enter the cerebellum via the inferior cerebellar peduncle (restiform body). Because the nucleus dorsalis of Clarke is found only between the T-1 and L-1 spinal cord segments, two modifications of the basic organization of this pathway occur above and below these levels.

1. The posterior spinocerebellar tract (in contrast to the anterior spinocerebellar tract) has a very small representation from the lower extremity, but fibers carrying unconscious proprioceptive information bound for the dorsal spinocerebellar tract, which enter the spinal cord *below* L-1 spinal level, ascend in the posterior columns until they reach a segment where they may synapse in Clarke's column. At that point, secondary axons from Clarke's column form the tract. Thus, there is no dorsal spinocerebellar tract in the lumbosacral spinal cord.

2. Proprioceptive fibers entering *above* T-1 (that is, in the cervical spinal cord) also do not have direct access to Clarke's column. Therefore, they also ascend in the posterior columns to the lower medulla, where they synapse in a nucleus analogous to Clarke's column, the *lateral cuneate nucleus*. Second-order neurons from this nucleus give rise to axons that form the cuneocerebellar tract and enter the ipsilateral restiform body along with the fibers from the dorsal spinocerebellar tract.

The clinical manifestation of disease involving these pathways is motor incoordination (ataxia) involving the extremities. Although these pathways are of great physiologic importance, clinically it is extremely difficult to identify abnormalities from damage to these pathways, which are commonly involved along with the dorsal columns.

Pathways for Touch

Tactile sensation is complex and involves the blending of a number of elementary components. Two different forms of touch sensibility are recognized: *simple touch*, consisting of the sensations of light touch, touch pressure, and a crude sense of tactile localization, and *tactile discrimi-*

nation, consisting of the sensations of deeper pressure, spatial localization, and the perception of the size and shape of objects.

The pathway for tactile discrimination already has been described as the *dorsal column–medial lemniscal pathway*. Some fibers for simple touch may ascend via this pathway as well. The remaining touch fibers ascend via the *anterior* (ventral) *spinothalamic tract*, which runs a course similar to that of the lateral spinothalamic tract (Fig. 7-10).

The peripheral receptors for touch include several of the receptor organs previously described. The myelinated fibers that convey sensory impulses from these endings have their cell bodies in the dorsal root ganglia and enter the spinal cord by way of the dorsal roots. The axons of

Fig. 7-10. Dorsal column–medial lemniscal pathway (solid line) *for tactile discrimination and anterior spinothalamic tract* (dotted line) *mediating simple touch. Since sensation of touch ascends on both sides of spinal cord, loss of touch is seldom noted with unilateral spinal cord lesions.*

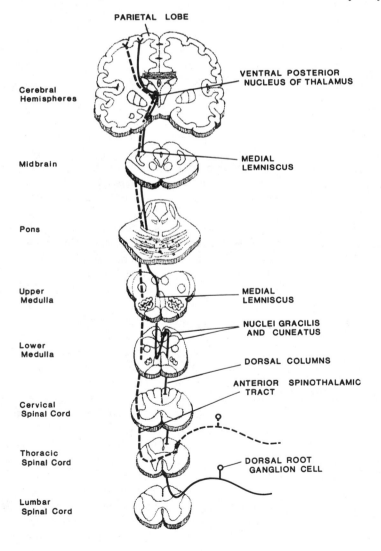

PARIETAL LOBE

VENTRAL POSTERIOR
NUCLEUS OF THALAMUS

Cerebral
Hemispheres

MEDIAL
LEMNISCUS

Midbrain

Pons

Upper
Medulla

MEDIAL
LEMNISCUS

NUCLEI GRACILIS
AND CUNEATUS

Lower
Medulla

DORSAL COLUMNS

ANTERIOR SPINOTHALAMIC
TRACT

Cervical
Spinal Cord

Thoracic
Spinal Cord

DORSAL ROOT
GANGLION CELL

Lumbar
Spinal Cord

these first-order neurons synapse with cells located in the central part of the dorsal gray horn, but they do not do so until a considerable amount of longitudinal dispersion has taken place and the axons have spread over several spinal cord segments. The axons of second-order neurons arise from this region and cross to the opposite side in the anterior white commissure and turn cephalad as the *anterior spinothalamic tract.* This tract is smaller and more diffuse than the lateral spinothalamic tract and is located near the periphery of the anterior funiculus. The tract takes a direct, upward course through the spinal cord and brain stem and ends in the ventral posterolateral nucleus of the thalamus. Third-order thalamocortical fibers then relay sensory impulses to the postcentral gyrus of the parietal lobe via the posterior limb of the internal capsule. The tract in its course through the brain stem is indistinct. At the level of the medulla, it is probably located in a

Fig. 7-11. The optic pathways. The visual field defects produced by lesions in these pathways are shown at the left. The visual field of the left eye is shown in the left circle, that of the right eye in the adjacent circle. Lesions anterior to optic chiasm (A) produce monocular visual loss. Lesions at optic chiasm (B) produce bitemporal hemianopia due to involvement of nasal-retinal crossing fibers. Unilateral lesions behind optic chiasm affecting optic tract (C), lateral geniculate body, optic radiations (D), or occipital cortex produce contralateral homonymous hemianopia.

region between the medial lemniscus and the lateral spinothalamic tract.

The clinical manifestation of disease involving this pathway is primarily an inability to perceive light touch. However, because of the dual pathway for the transmission of touch (that is, the dorsal columns on one side and the ventral spinothalamic tract on the other), this sensation is frequently not altered unless there is bilateral spinal cord disease, damage to all touch fibers entering the dorsal root entry zone at a particular segment of the spinal cord, or damage to peripheral nerves.

Pathways for Other Senses

The pathways discussed previously mediate the major general somatic afferent sensations. Sensation from visceral structures (general visceral afferent sensations) will be discussed further in Chapter 10. The special visceral afferent sensations of taste and smell, as well as the special somatic afferent sensations of hearing and balance, will be discussed in association with the posterior fossa (Chap. 14) and supratentorial (Chap. 15) levels. Because of the importance of the special somatic afferent sensation of vision in clinical neurologic diagnosis, discussion of this pathway will be introduced now.

The visual pathways are located entirely at the supratentorial level (Fig. 7-11). The receptors and primary neurons are located in the retina. Fibers

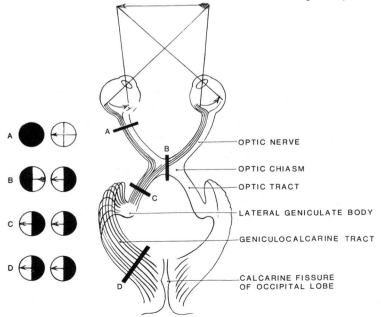

OPTIC NERVE

OPTIC CHIASM

OPTIC TRACT

LATERAL GENICULATE BODY

GENICULOCALCARINE TRACT

CALCARINE FISSURE
OF OCCIPITAL LOBE

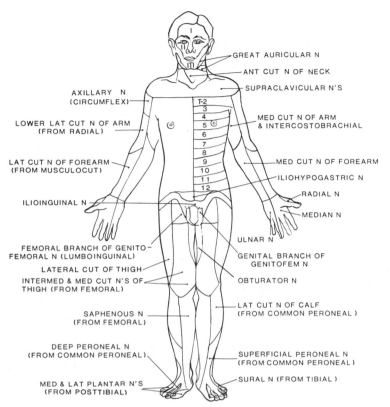

GREAT AURICULAR N

ANT CUT N OF NECK

SUPRACLAVICULAR N'S

AXILLARY N
(CIRCUMFLEX)

T-2
3
4
5
6
7
8
9
10
11
12

MED CUT N OF ARM
& INTERCOSTOBRACHIAL

LOWER LAT CUT N OF ARM
(FROM RADIAL)

LAT CUT N OF FOREARM
(FROM MUSCULOCUT)

MED CUT N OF FOREARM

ILIOHYPOGASTRIC N

RADIAL N

MEDIAN N

ILIOINGUINAL N

ULNAR N

FEMORAL BRANCH OF GENITO-
FEMORAL N (LUMBOINGUINAL)

GENITAL BRANCH OF
GENITOFEM N

LATERAL CUT OF THIGH

INTERMED & MED CUT N'S OF
THIGH (FROM FEMORAL)

OBTURATOR N

SAPHENOUS N
(FROM FEMORAL)

LAT CUT N OF CALF
(FROM COMMON PERONEAL)

DEEP PERONEAL N
(FROM COMMON PERONEAL)

SUPERFICIAL PERONEAL N
(FROM COMMON PERONEAL)

MED & LAT PLANTAR N'S
(FROM POSTTIBIAL)

SURAL N (FROM TIBIAL)

Fig. 7-12. Cutaneous distribution of the major peripheral nerves. (Redrawn from W. Haymaker and B. Woodhall, Peripheral Nerve Injuries: Principles of Diagnosis *[2nd ed.]. Philadelphia: Saunders, 1953.)*

from the retina travel through the *optic canal* as the *optic nerve.*

The optic nerves from the right and left eyes join at the *optic chiasm,* where a partial decussation (crossing) of fibers occurs. The fibers from the nasal half of each retina cross to the opposite side, whereas the fibers from the temporal half of each retina remain on the same side. After the decussation in the chiasm, the fibers from the nasal half of the right eye and the temporal half of the left eye form the left *optic tract,* and similarly, the fibers from the nasal half of the left eye and temporal half of the right eye form the right optic tract. Because the lens reverses the projection of images of the visual field on the retina, the right visual field projects to the nasal half of the retina of the right eye and temporal half of the left eye, while the images of the left visual field project to the nasal retina of the left eye and temporal retina of the right eye. As a consequence of the partial decussation of fibers at the chiasm, the images from the right visual field

travel in the left optic tract and the images of the left visual field travel in the right optic tract. The optic tracts project to the thalamus and synapse in the right and left *geniculate nuclei,* where they give rise to fibers that project to the *occipital cortex* as the *optic radiations.* Thus, the visual images of the right half of the visual field project to the left occipital cortex, while the images of the left visual field project to the right occipital cortex.

Lesions located anterior to the optic chiasm in the optic nerves interfere with vision only in the ipsilateral eye (monocular visual loss). Lesions in the center of the optic chiasm interfere only with the nasal crossing fibers, producing a loss of function of the nasal retina and of temporal vision in both eyes (bitemporal hemianopia). Lesions that are located behind the optic chiasm in the optic tracts, lateral geniculate body, optic radiations, or occipital cortex produce a loss of vision in the contralateral visual fields of both eyes (homonymous hemianopia).

Clinical Correlations

Disease processes involving the sensory system produce various symptoms including pain, hypes-

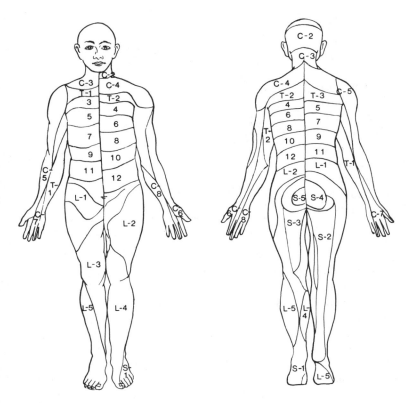

Fig. 7-13. Cutaneous distribution of spinal nerve roots. Note considerable overlap between segments, and note that the distribution differs from that of peripheral nerves. (Redrawn from F. R. Ford. Diseases of the Nervous System: In Infancy, Childhood and Adolescence [3rd ed.]. Springfield, Ill.: Thomas, 1952.)

thesia (reduced sensation), anesthesia (a complete loss of cutaneous sensibility), dysesthesia (an altered or perverted interpretation of sensation, such as a burning, tingling, or painful feeling in response to touch), and paresthesia (spontaneous sensation of prickling or tingling). In some instances, sensory stimuli are more keenly felt than normal (hyperesthesia). It is extremely important in every case of pain or sensory loss to determine its exact distribution.

Lesions at the Peripheral Level
The distal axons of the primary sensory neurons mediating all types of afferent input are gathered together, along with motor and autonomic fibers, in peripheral nerves. Thus, a lesion that affects peripheral nerves would be expected to produce a variable sensory loss for all modalities and a loss of muscle-stretch reflexes in the anatomic distribution of that nerve. Some motor or autonomic

deficit usually can be found if such fibers are present in the involved nerve. This type of deficit may occur in a focal distribution when only a single peripheral nerve is involved (such as might occur from trauma) and is called *mononeuropathy*. When these symptoms and signs occur in a diffuse distribution, the deficit is called *polyneuropathy*. Pain, paresthesias, or dysesthesias are common accompaniments of peripheral nerve lesions. Figure 7-12 shows the cutaneous distribution of the major peripheral nerves.

Lesions at the Spinal Level
Disease processes located within the spinal canal typically produce (1) a *segmental* neurologic deficit limited to one level of the body and usually caused by involvement of the nerve roots or spinal nerves, and (2) an *intersegmental* sensory deficit involving all the body below a particular level and caused by interruption of the major ascending sensory pathways.

Mechanical compression or local inflammation of a dorsal nerve root or spinal nerve produces pain along the anatomic distribution of the affected root. The area of skin supplied by one dorsal root is known as a *dermatome* (Fig. 7-13);

pain due to nerve root involvement in the distribution of one or more dermatomes is known as *radicular pain*. This type of pain, which may vary in intensity, is often lancinating (a sharp, darting type of pain). Maneuvers that increase intraspinal pressure (and presumably increase the traction on irritated nerve roots), such as coughing, sneezing, and straining, produce a characteristic increase in this type of pain. In addition to producing radicular pain, lesions of the dorsal root or spinal nerve produce areas of paresthesia, hyperesthesia, or loss of cutaneous sensation in a dermatomal distribution. At appropriate levels, segmental loss of muscle-stretch reflexes, weakness, and autonomic disturbances can be seen.

COMMISSURAL SYNDROME.   A special type of segmental deficit can result from a lesion involving the central regions of the spinal cord, usually over several segments. This deficit is characterized by a loss of pain and temperature sensation from interruption of the second-order axons as they are decussating to form the spinothalamic tracts (Fig. 7-14). The sensory loss is bilateral (because fibers from both sides are interrupted by such a lesion), and it involves the crossing fibers of several adjacent segments. Thus, a lesion involving the central regions of segments T-2 through T-5 produces loss of pain and temperature only in those segments. The commissural syndrome can be produced only by a lesion in the substance of the spinal cord. As the lesion en-

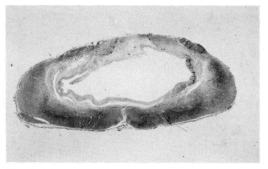

Fig. 7-15. Syringomyelia. Transverse section of cervical spinal cord showing central cavity lined by thickened glial membrane and associated with degeneration of surrounding tissue. (H & E; ×4.)

larges, other adjacent sensory tracts become involved. This type of lesion may result from trauma (hematomyelia), neoplasm, or other conditions including syringomyelia.

Syringomyelia is a common cause of the commissural syndrome and consists of cavitation occurring within the central area of the spinal cord (Fig. 7-15). Whether the cavity develops as a result of dilatation of the primitive central canal (hydromyelia) or as a result of some other destructive process in the central region of the cord, such as an intramedullary neoplasm, is not always clear. Although initially the cavity is centrally located, expansion of the cavity and surrounding gliosis tends to extend the syrinx irregularly throughout the gray matter and at times into the white matter of the dorsal and lateral columns. The lesion most commonly occurs in the cervical area.

SPINOTHALAMIC TRACT SYNDROME.   A lesion involving the spinothalamic tract causes a loss of pain and temperature sensation on the opposite side of the body, involving all segments below the level of the lesion. Pain and temperature fibers enter through the dorsal root branch and extend rostrally in Lissauer's tract for up to two segments above their entry zone before synapsing with the spinothalamic tract neurons of the dorsal horn. Therefore, the sensory level on the side opposite a spinothalamic tract lesion is usually at least two segments below the level of the actual lesion. Within the spinothalamic tract, the fibers are arranged in a laminar fashion, with the sacral fibers near the periphery and fibers from higher levels more toward the center. Hence, lesions

Fig. 7-14. Commissural syndrome. Distribution of loss of pain and temperature sensations, with a lesion in the location shown on the left.

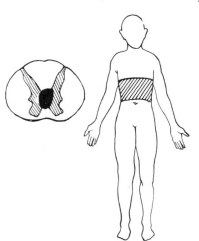

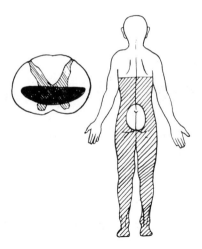

POSTERIOR VIEW

Fig. 7-16. Sensory loss with sacral sparing due to the intramedullary lesion shown on the left, involving lateral spinothalamic tracts bilaterally. (Note that figure in diagram is a view from behind.)

arising within the substance of the spinal cord (intramedullary lesions) may involve only the central portions of the tract and spare the peripheral fibers, to produce a loss of pain and temperature in all levels below the lesion except the sacral level. This is referred to as *sacral sparing.* When present, sacral sparing is an important clue to an intramedullary spinal cord lesion (Fig. 7-16).

In certain instances of intractable pain involving the lower extremity, pain may be relieved by

placing a lesion in the spinothalamic tract (spinothalamic tractotomy). It is usually done by surgically cutting the ventral portion of the lateral funiculus in the cervical area. While there is probably some damage to the anterior spinocerebellar tract, no permanent symptoms are produced, except loss of pain and temperature sensibility on the contralateral side.

BROWN-SÉQUARD'S SYNDROME. This syndrome is seen in pure form with hemisection of the spinal cord. In clinical practice, the syndrome is often partial and incomplete; however, the findings of ipsilateral motor deficit, ipsilateral dorsal column deficit, and contralateral loss of pain and temperature usually are present and are characteristic of a unilateral spinal cord lesion (Fig. 7-17).

Lesions at the Posterior Fossa Level
Disease processes affecting the posterior fossa level are characterized by a contralateral intersegmental loss of sensory function in the trunk and limbs because of interruption of the major ascending pathways. However, there is frequently also a loss of sensory function (primarily pain and temperature) over the ipsilateral face because of segmental involvement of the trigeminal nerve or its descending tract and nucleus (Fig. 7-18).

Lesions at the Supratentorial Level
At this level, all major sensory pathways have

Fig. 7-17. Brown-Séquard's syndrome. Sensory loss produced by damage to one-half of the spinal cord by lesion shown on the left. A motor deficit would also be present (see Chap. 9).

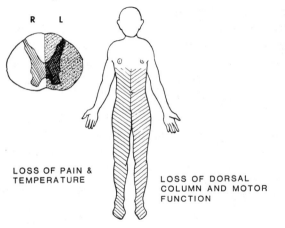

LOSS OF PAIN & TEMPERATURE

LOSS OF DORSAL COLUMN AND MOTOR FUNCTION

Fig. 7-18. Distribution of pain and temperature sensation loss characteristic of lesions at the posterior fossa level, as shown on the left.

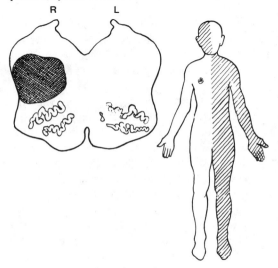

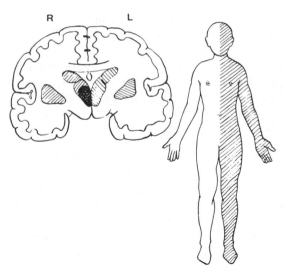

Fig. 7-19. Thalamic syndrome. Loss of all modalities of sensation contralateral to the lesion.

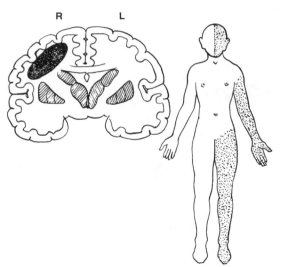

Fig. 7-20. Suprathalamic syndrome. Loss of cortical sensory functions contralateral to the lesion.

crossed to the contralateral side; therefore, lesions at this level alter sensory function over the entire contralateral side of the body.

Two important variations of sensory loss may be encountered with lesions at this level.

THALAMIC SYNDROME.   The thalamus functions as an important integrating and relay station for sensory perception. A lesion affecting the specific sensory nuclei of the thalamus causes a relatively complete loss of all forms of general somatic afferent sensation in the contralateral face, trunk, and limbs (Fig. 7-19). If the portion of the thalamus related to vision is also involved, a contralateral homonymous hemianopia is produced. After a localized lesion of the thalamus, perhaps due to faulty integration of sensory information, a severe burning (dysesthetic) pain in the area of sensory loss sometimes is produced.

SUPRATHALAMIC SYNDROME.   Lesions that involve sensory pathways from the thalamus to the cortex or in the cortex itself also alter all forms of general somatic afferent sensation on the contralateral side of the body. However, in contrast to the dense loss of sensation found with thalamic lesions, suprathalamic involvement is characterized by only minimal involvement of pain, temperature, touch, and vibratory sensibility and a severe deficit in the discriminative sensations that require cortical participation (Fig. 7-20). These

sensations are joint position sense, two-point discrimination, touch localization, and the recognition of objects placed in the hand (stereognosis), and suggest that discriminative sensations require intact thalamocortical pathways for their full appreciation, whereas the primary modalities of superficial sensation are perceived and integrated at the thalamic level. This type of discriminative sensory loss is often found with lesions of the parietal lobe and is commonly referred to as a *cortical sensory deficit.* If the optic radiations are also involved, a contralateral visual field defect is produced. In the absence of a visual field defect or other signs of supratentorial involvement, this type of sensory deficit may be confused with the findings of dorsal column disease. A severe deficit in conscious proprioception, bilateral involvement, and associated alteration in vibratory sense all favor a lesion of the dorsal columns. When the deficit is unilateral, the distinction between a suprathalamic and a high-cervical spinal cord lesion can be extremely difficult unless other signs and symptoms are present to aid with localization.

Irritative lesions located in the region of the postcentral gyrus may initiate seizures. The clinical manifestations of seizures in this area consist primarily of a feeling of tingling (paresthesias) on the opposite side of the body. As the localized neuronal discharge spreads from its focus of origin, these sensations may be experienced as

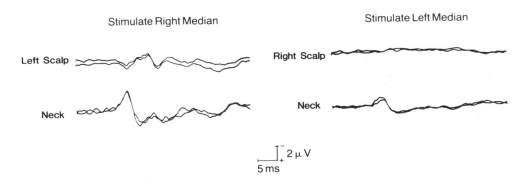

Stimulate Right Median   Stimulate Left Median

Left Scalp   Right Scalp

Neck   Neck

$2\,\mu V$
5 ms

Fig. 7-21. Somatosensory evoked responses recorded from the neck and scalp in a patient with multiple sclerosis.

moving in an orderly fashion dictated by the topographic organization of the gyrus. Further spread to the adjacent precentral gyrus may produce associated motor activity, and spread to subcortical structures may produce a loss of consciousness.

Somatosensory Evoked Response

The somatosensory evoked response is an electrodiagnostic test that is used to evaluate the sensory system (Fig. 7-21). Evoked responses are electrical potentials that occur with a fixed latency in response to a stimulus. Since these potentials are very small, a number of successive responses need to be averaged and amplified to be seen. The somatosensory evoked responses are potentials occurring in response to stimulation of a peripheral nerve which can be recorded from the nerve, the plexus, the sensory pathways within the spinal cord and brain stem, the thalamocortical pathways, and the somatosensory cortex. Abnormalities of the somatosensory evoked responses occur with lesions or disease processes involving the sensory pathways at any of these levels and are manifested either by an increase in latency or by a reduced amplitude or an absent response. The somatosensory evoked responses are used to document or diagnose multiple sclerosis, degenerative processes, traumatic lesions, and other structural lesions affecting the peripheral or central sensory system.

The Differential Diagnosis of Ataxia

DEFINITION.   Sensory information is vital to the smooth, harmonious production of motor activity. A failure to produce normally smooth motor acts is referred to as *ataxia*. Ataxia may be manifest in individual limb motions, but it more commonly is evident during walking. With ataxia, movements become jerky and uncoordinated. The central nervous system must be constantly apprised of the position, tone, and movement of the limbs and trunk. It accomplishes this task by integrating (primarily in the cerebellum) proprioceptive input and information from the receptors for equilibrium, which are located in the labyrinths of the ear, and by relaying these data back to the appropriate motor effectors. Visual input may be utilized in part to compensate for a defect in this integrating mechanism.

TYPES OF ATAXIA.   *Sensory ataxias* include conditions in which motor performance is faulty when the motor pathways and the cerebellum are intact. This occurs because there is a defect in transmitting proprioceptive or equilibratory information to higher centers. This type of ataxia frequently can be compensated for by utilizing visual input to guide limb position, and hence the ataxia is often worse in the dark or when the eyes are closed. *Motor ataxias* include conditions in which the sensory pathways are intact but motor performance is faulty and there is a defect in the integration and processing of proprioceptive information. Motor ataxia is usually due to a disease in the cerebellum. This type of ataxia is often poorly compensated for by visual input.

DIFFERENTIATION.   The Romberg test is a quick and convenient method of distinguishing between these two types of ataxias. The patient who shows no unsteadiness when standing with feet together and eyes open but who displays unsteadiness with the eyes closed has a *positive* Romberg test, indicating that the patient has a sensory ataxia. The patient with a motor (cerebellar) ataxia may or may not be unsteady in the Romberg position but shows little or no increase in unsteadiness when he closes his eyes and thus has a negative Romberg test.

Patients who have a sensory ataxia generally have difficulty either with vestibular function or with proprioception, as a result of peripheral nerve or spinal cord disease. Ataxic patients with a negative Romberg test will often show abnormalities in cerebellar function.

Neurologic Examination: Sensory System

A complete sensory examination includes the evaluation of touch, pain, temperature, joint position, and vibratory senses, as well as various discriminatory modalities. Comparison of one side of the body with the other, and with the examiner's own sensory abilities, is useful for establishing normal and abnormal. Much of the sensory examination is best performed with the patient's eyes closed to eliminate visual cues. Examination of sensation consists of three portions: (1) qualitative, to determine the elements of sensation that are affected; (2) quantitative, to determine the degree of involvement when sensation is impaired; and (3) anatomic, to map out the areas of sensory impairment.

Sensation is tested in the following manner:

1. *Touch.* Lightly place a piece of cotton on the face, trunk, and extremities and ask the patient to respond when it is felt.
2. *Pain.* Gently prick the patient with a pin. A more accurate determination can be made by randomly touching the patient with the point or head of a pin and noting whether the patient can appreciate "sharp" and "dull" sensations.
3. *Temperature.* Randomly apply warm and cool objects to the skin and note the patient's ability to distinguish between them.
4. *Vibration Sense.* Place a vibrating tuning fork over bony prominences and note whether the patient can detect the sensation and can determine when the vibration ceases. (In patients more than 50 years of age, vibratory sense is often reduced in the feet.)
5. *Joint Position Sense.* Firmly grasp the sides of the great toe, or of a finger, and ask the patient to detect and respond to movements in an upward or downward direction.

6. *Two-Point Discrimination.* A two-point caliper is used. This sensation is normally examined only on the fingertips, by asking the patient to respond to the tactile stimulus of one or two points. The threshold (minimal recognizable separation) is determined and compared on the two sides of the body.
7. *Tactile Localization.* Touch the patient, and request that the point of contact be identified.
8. *Graphesthesia.* Ask the patient to identify numbers or letters traced on the palm of his hand with a blunt object.
9. *Stereognosis.* Ask the patient to close his eyes and identify objects of different sizes, shapes, and textures (such as a coin, key, clip, or safety pin) placed in the hand.

In the absence of any sensory symptoms or the patient's subjective sensation of pain, a brief screening examination consisting of a test of touch, pain, joint position, and vibratory sense in both hands and both feet and of a test of pain and touch perception on the face is all that is required. When a sensory deficit is suspected or identified, the examiner must determine the modalities of sensation involved and map its distribution to see if it conforms to that found with lesions of the peripheral nerve, spinal nerve or dorsal root, spinal cord, posterior fossa, or supratentorial region.

Objectives

1. Define receptor potential, receptor adaptation, and receptor specificity.
2. Define in physiologic terms the differences between slowly adapting (tonic) receptors and rapidly adapting (phasic) receptors.
3. List the types of somatic sensory receptors.
4. Name the function of the following pathways and trace their paths:
   a. Dorsal (posterior) spinocerebellar tract
   b. Ventral (anterior) spinocerebellar tract
   c. Dorsal column-medial lemniscal tracts
   d. Lateral spinothalamic tract
   e. Anterior (ventral) spinothalamic tract
5. Describe the roles of endorphins, enkephalins, and substance P as they relate to pain.
6. Describe the regulation of pain sensation.
7. List the clinical manifestations of lesions involving the five pathways in question 4, and

list the differences that may be encountered when the lesion is located at the peripheral, spinal, posterior fossa, and supratentorial levels.

8. Define sacral sparing, cortical sensory loss, and Brown-Séquard's syndrome, and describe the anatomic basis for these conditions.
9. Describe the pathologic changes in syringomyelia.
10. Differentiate between sensory and motor ataxia.
11. Given a patient problem, list the aspects of the history and physical examination that point to a disturbance of the sensory system, localize the area of disturbance to a particular portion of the neuraxis, and state the likely pathologic nature of the responsible lesion.

Clinical Problems

Each of the following clinical problems illustrates some aspect of dysfunction within the sensory system. For each problem, determine the anatomic-pathologic diagnosis (as outlined in the objectives in Chap. 4) and answer the related questions.

1. A 48-year-old woman experienced the abrupt onset of pain, followed by paresthesia and loss of feeling in a rather circumscribed area along the lateral aspect of her right thigh. Examination revealed a localized area of decreased perception of pinprick, temperature, and touch in this region only. Results of the remainder of the examination were normal.
   a. What is the anatomic-pathologic diagnosis?
   b. What specific anatomic structure is involved?
   c. How would the distribution of symptoms differ if the lesion involved the median nerve at the wrist?
2. A 40-year-old man had the onset of neck pain and paresthesias over the occipital region of the head 6 months ago. These symptoms were aggravated by coughing and sneezing. Three months ago, his symptoms became worse and he noted a tingling sensation up and down his spinal column whenever he bent his neck. One month ago, he noted progressive difficulty in

walking in the dark. On examination, he was found to have decreased perception to touch and pinprick over the posterior scalp region, reduced position sense in his arms and legs bilaterally, decreased vibratory sensation in both upper and lower extremities, and decreased ability to perceive discriminative tactile sensation bilaterally.
   a. What is the anatomic-pathologic diagnosis?
   b. What segmental structures provide sensory innervation to the posterior scalp region?
   c. What sensory structures are involved by the lesion?
   d. What is the precise level of the responsible lesion?
   e. What are the most likely precise pathologic lesions responsible for this clinical syndrome?
   f. How would the symptoms and signs differ if the lesion were located at the T-6 spinal level?
3. A 41-year-old woman noted a painless, slowly progressive loss of sensation in an area involving the back of her head, neck, shoulders, and both upper extremities. Neurologic examination revealed a sensory loss involving only pain and temperature in this area. Specific testing of all other modalities of sensation in the affected areas and elsewhere revealed no abnormalities, and there were no changes in motor performance, strength, or deep tendon reflexes.
   a. What is the anatomic-pathologic diagnosis?
   b. What sensory structure(s) is involved by the lesion?
   c. What is the most likely pathologic lesion responsible for this clinical syndrome?
4. A 21-year-old soldier returned from the war after receiving a gunshot wound in his spinal column. On examination, you note that he has weakness of the left lower extremity. In addition, he has loss of pain and temperature perception on the right side from about the level of his navel downward. Vibration, joint position sense, and discriminatory function are reduced in the left leg. Touch is normal.
   a. What is the anatomic-pathologic diagnosis?
   b. What is the precise level of the lesion?
   c. What is the name given to this type of syndrome?

d. Why was the sensation of touch preserved in this patient?

e. Where in the nervous system would you expect to find evidence of wallerian degeneration?

5. A 68-year-old hypertensive woman awoke one morning noting that she was unable to feel anything over the entire left side of her body. On examination, motor strength and reflexes were normal, as were the visual fields; however, she did not respond to pinprick, temperature, or touch over the left side of her face, trunk, and extremities, and she could not perceive joint motion or vibration in her left arm and leg.

a. What is the anatomic-pathologic diagnosis?

b. What specific sensory system structure(s) is most likely involved?

c. Where in the nervous system would you expect to find evidence of wallerian degeneration?

6. A 31-year-old man noticed the gradual onset of headaches. On several occasions during the past month, he experienced spells consisting of a curious tingling, burning sensation that began in the left thumb and the left corner of his mouth. This gradually became more intense and spread to involve his left hand and the left side of his face and then extended up his arm, trunk, and leg. In 5 minutes, the spell would cease and he would feel tired and sleepy. Examination reveals a striking inability to perceive joint position, motion, and other discriminative testing over the left side. Touch, pain, temperature, and vibratory sense were preserved.

a. What is the anatomic-pathologic diagnosis?

b. What is the nature of the spell experienced by the patient?

c. Why were some forms of sensation involved and others not?

Suggested Reading

Cannon, J. T., Liebeskind, J. C., and Frenk, H. Neural and Neurochemical Mechanisms of Pain Inhibition. In R. A. Sternbach (ed.), *The Psychology of Pain*. New York: Raven, 1978. Pp. 27–47.

Carpenter, M. B. *Human Neuroanatomy* (7th ed.). Baltimore: Williams & Wilkins, 1976.

Chiappa K. H. *Evoked Potentials in Clinical Medicine*. New York: Raven, 1983. Pp. 203–312.

Guyton, A. C. *Basic Human Neurophysiology* (3rd ed.). Philadelphia: Saunders, 1981.

Jones, E. G., and Powell, T. P. S. Anatomical Organization of the Somatosensory Cortex. In A. Iggo (ed.), *Handbook of Sensory Physiology*. Vol. 2: *The Somotosensory System*. New York: Springer-Verlag, 1973. Pp. 579–620.

Kandel, E. R., and Schwartz, J. H. *Principles of Neural Science*. New York: Elsevier–North Holland, 1981.

Kerr, F. W. L., and Wilson, P. R. Pain. *Annu. Rev. Neurosci.* 1:83, 1978.

Mayer, D. J., and Price, D. D. Central nervous system mechanisms of analgesia. *Pain* 2:379, 1976.

Monnier, M. *Functions of the Nervous System*. Vol. 3: *Sensory Functions and Perception*. New York: Elsevier, 1975.

Mountcastle, V. B. (ed.). *Medical Physiology* (14th ed.). St. Louis: Mosby, 1980. Vol 1.

Sinclair, D. *Mechanisms of Cutaneous Sensation*. New York: Oxford University Press, 1981. Pp. 106–151.

Snyder, S. H., and Childers, S. R. Opiate receptors and opioid peptides. *Annu. Rev. Neurosci.* 2:35, 1979.

Willis, W. D. and Coggeshall, R. E. *Sensory Mechanisms of the Spinal Cord*. New York: Plenum, 1978. Pp. 1–8; 129–166; 197–259.

The Consciousness
System

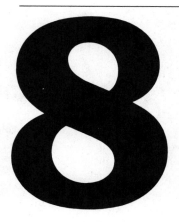

The previous chapter described the major afferent pathways that provide the central nervous system with direct access to information about its external environment. Running parallel with those pathways is another ascending system, which we will call the *consciousness system,* that allows one to selectively attend to and perceive isolated stimuli and to maintain varied levels of wakefulness, awareness, and consciousness.

Although both ascending systems transmit sensory information to the cortex, the primary afferent pathways do so by way of relatively direct pathways and through specific thalamic nuclei that project primarily to the sensory cortex. In contrast, the pathways of the consciousness system transmit via indirect, multineuronal pathways to nonspecific thalamic nuclei, which project to all areas of the cortex.

In this chapter the normal anatomy and physiology of the consciousness system, its role in the regulation of sleep, and the pathologic states of altered consciousness which are a reflection of deranged activity within the system will be described.

Overview

The consciousness system is a multineuronal, polysynaptic system located in the brain stem, diencephalon, and cerebral hemispheres. Structures in the system are (1) portions of the brainstem reticular formation, (2) the ascending projectional system, (3) nonspecific thalamic nuclei, (4) diffuse projections from the nonspecific thalamic nuclei to the cortex, and (5) widespread areas of cerebral cortex. The first four of these are collectively called the Ascending Reticular Activating System (ARAS).

The *reticular formation* is a diffuse aggregate of neurons that receives and integrates information from many areas of the neuraxis, including the sensory system, cerebral cortex, hypothalamus, cerebellum, and brain-stem nuclei, and projects to diffuse areas of the cerebral cortex (via the nonspecific thalamic nuclei) as well as to the motor and visceral systems. Thus, the reticular formation can modify a wide variety of neural activities and, through the thalamus, can selectively modulate the activity of the cortex.

Proper functioning of this system, and hence the regulation of consciousness and awareness, is predicated on a continuous interaction between the cortex and the ascending reticular activating system. The electrical activity of a neuronal aggregate such as the cerebral cortex is a reflection of its own intrinsic activity and of ascending influences primarily from the thalamus and ascending reticular activating system.

The *electroencephalogram* (EEG) is a means of recording cortical activity. The waveforms that are seen represent summations of the postsynaptic, dendritic potentials generated near the surface in response to the intrinsic, neuronal electrical activity of the cerebral cortex as modified by input from subcortical structures. The EEG thus can provide information not only about cortical functioning but also about activity throughout the consciousness system.

Consciousness is an awareness of environment and self and is achieved through the action of the ascending reticular activating system on the cortex. The process of *attention* by which normal persons can focus their thoughts on specific information is achieved by the modulation of neuronal input to the cortex through the ascending reticular activating system, which permits a person to direct his attention to specific aspects of the environment without being continually distracted by multiple simultaneous stimuli.

Sleep is a normal cyclic physiologic alteration of consciousness, which is readily reversed by appropriate stimuli. It has been divided into two stages, rapid eye movement and nonrapid eye movement sleep. *Rapid eye movement* (REM) *sleep* depends on activity in the locus ceruleus and release of norepinephrine. It is characterized by rapid eye movements, increased body movement, decreased muscle tone, dreaming, and an EEG pattern resembling that of a waking recording. *Nonrapid eye movement* (non-REM) *sleep* depends on the raphé nuclei and the release of serotonin. It is characterized by the absence of rapid eye movements, reduced body movements, and an EEG pattern showing the characteristic waveforms of the sleep state.

Pathologic processes that destroy or depress function of the reticular formation, of the ascending projectional pathways, or of both cerebral hemispheres produce alterations in consciousness. Unilateral lesions of the cerebral hemispheres will not alter consciousness unless there is associated involvement of the ascending reticular activating system. Examples of states of altered conscious-

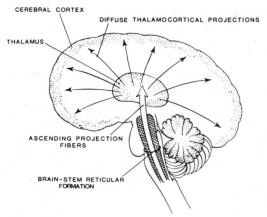

Fig. 8-1. Lateral view of the brain showing the components of the consciousness system.

ness include *coma,* a state of extended unconsciousness from which the patient cannot be aroused; *concussion,* a brief loss of consciousness after a blow to the head from which the patient recovers without neurologic sequelae; *seizure,* a transient alteration in brain function due to excessive neuronal discharge which, when generalized and involving the consciousness system, results in loss of consciousness; and *syncope,* a transient loss of consciousness due to widespread neuronal ischemia.

Fig. 8-2. Input pathways to brain-stem reticular formation.

Evaluation of a patient with a disorder of consciousness requires analysis of associated neurologic signs to determine whether the responsible lesion is (1) located at the supratentorial level, (2) located at the posterior fossa level, or (3) diffusely distributed at both levels.

Anatomy of the Consciousness System

Structures of the consciousness system include portions of the brain-stem reticular formation, the ascending projectional system, nonspecific thalamic nuclei, diffuse thalamocortical projections, and widespread areas of the cortex (Fig. 8-1).

Reticular Formation

The reticular formation is a complex aggregate of large multipolar and small round neurons and their axons, diffusely distributed in cellular clusters throughout the central tegmental portions of the brain stem and extending from the decussation of the pyramids in the medulla to the thalamus. Phylogenetically older than the surrounding structures, the reticular formation consists of poorly organized nuclei and fiber tracts. The diffuse arrangement of its multipolar neurons and many interconnections allows a single reticular neuron to make synaptic contact with many afferent fibers and gives rise to the term *reticular* (forming a network). With phylogenic advancement, this centrally located network became sur-

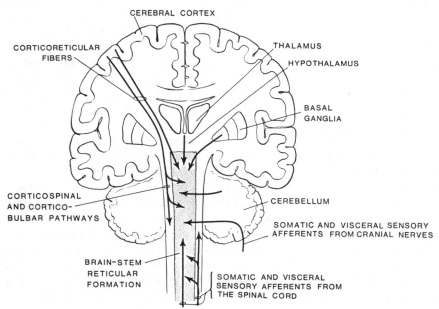

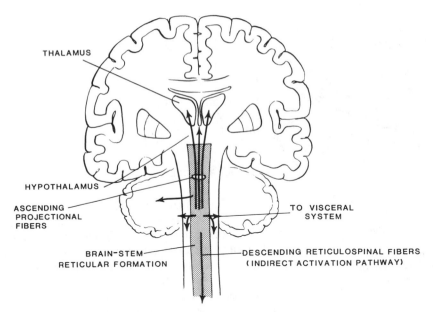

THALAMUS

HYPOTHALAMUS

ASCENDING
PROJECTIONAL
FIBERS

TO VISCERAL
SYSTEM

BRAIN-STEM
RETICULAR FORMATION

DESCENDING RETICULOSPINAL FIBERS
(INDIRECT ACTIVATION PATHWAY)

Fig. 8-3. Output pathways of brain-stem reticular formation.

rounded by structures serving specific functions within the motor and sensory systems. Functionally, the reticular formation can be divided into a *lateral receptive area,* which receives collateral branches from ascending sensory pathways, and a *medial projectional area,* from which efferent pathways arise.

Afferent pathways to the reticular formation (Fig. 8-2) consist of (1) collateral branches from the primary ascending tracts of the sensory system (spinothalamic and lemniscal pathways), which synapse with cells in the reticular formation, (2) fibers from the cerebral cortex, consisting of corticoreticular fibers from widespread cortical areas as well as collateral branches from the corticospinal and corticobulbar tracts of the motor system, (3) fibers from other structures, including the cerebellum, basal ganglia, hypothalamus, cranial nerve nuclei, and the colliculi, and (4) visceral afferents from the spinal cord and cranial nerves. In addition to the ascending projections of the reticular formation in the consciousness system, other projections convey information to the motor and visceral systems (Fig. 8-3). By means of these multiple connections and pathways, the reticular formation can integrate information from various levels of the neuraxis and thereby can regulate and modify the activities of the nervous system.

Ascending Projectional System
The ascending projectional system consists of fibers of the reticular formation that project diffusely to the hypothalamus and to the nonspecific nuclei of the thalamus (Fig. 8-3). They are not located in specific tracts but are found throughout the pons, midbrain, and diencephalon.

Nonspecific Thalamic Nuclei
Functionally, the thalamic nuclei are subdivided into (1) *specific thalamic nuclei,* which are associated with the sensory and motor systems and which project to localized areas of cortex, and (2) *nonspecific thalamic nuclei,* which receive afferents from the reticular formation, the cortex, and other thalamic nuclei and project to all areas of the cortex via the diffuse thalamic projection system. The nonspecific nuclei include the *midline nuclei,* located near the massa intermedia, the *intralaminar nuclei,* located along the internal medullary lamina—a band of myelinated fibers separating the anterior, medial, and lateral thalamic nuclei—and the *reticular nuclei,* located on the lateral margin of the thalamus (Fig. 8-4).

The reticular formation, ascending projectional system, the nonspecific thalamic nuclei, and the diffuse thalamocortical projections also are referred to collectively as the *Ascending Reticular Activating System* (ARAS), and many textbooks use this term rather than the one we are using, the consciousness system.

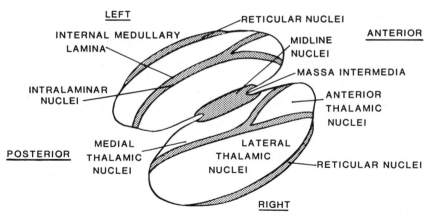

Fig. 8-4. *Dorsolateral view of the thalamus with nonspecific thalamic nuclei* (stippled). *(Redrawn from F. H. Netter.* The Ciba Collection of Medical Illustrations. *Volume I:* The Nervous System. *Summit, N.J.: Ciba Pharmaceutical Products, 1962. P. 48.)*

Diffuse Thalamocortical Projections

Diffuse projections from the nonspecific thalamic nuclei connecting the ascending reticular activating system to widespread areas of cortex have been designated as the *thalamocortical reticular system* (Fig. 8-5). They have a critical role in regulating the electrical activity of the cerebral cortex and in modifying the states of consciousness and alertness.

Cerebral Cortex

Although many specific functions, such as somatic sensation and vision, are relayed and inte-

Fig. 8-5. *Diffuse thalamocortical projections of the consciousness system.*

grated in specific areas, no single area of cortex is responsible for the maintenance of consciousness. Indeed, because of the widespread interconnections between the nonspecific thalamic nuclei and the cortex, all areas of cortex appear to participate in consciousness and are therefore considered to be part of the consciousness system.

Physiology of the Consciousness System

Neurophysiology of Single Cells

As described in Chapter 5, neurons generate two types of potentials, synaptic potentials and action potentials.

SYNAPTIC POTENTIAL (DENDRITIC POTENTIAL). The *synaptic* or *dendritic potential* is a local po-

Fig. 8-6. *Diagram of a cortical neuron showing synaptic potentials generated in the dendrite and action potentials generated in the axon.*

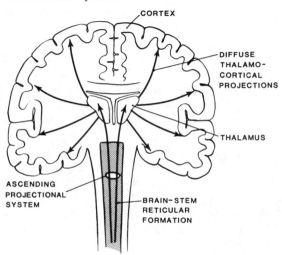

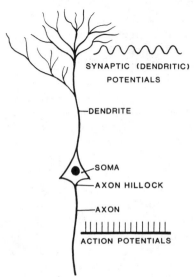

tential generated in the dendritic portion of the nerve cell as a result of a neurotransmitter interacting with the cell membrane (Fig. 8-6). Synaptic potentials are localized, nonpropagated, graded fluctuations of the dendritic membrane potential and can be excitatory (EPSPs) when the neurotransmitter causes a depolarization in the cell membrane, or inhibitory (IPSPs) when the neurotransmitter causes a hyperpolarization of the cell membrane. The duration of these potentials is usually 15 to 20 msec, and they do not have a refractory period.

ACTION POTENTIAL.   The action potential usually arises from the axon hillock of the neuron and propagates along the axon (Fig. 8-6). (In some instances, it can also arise from the dendrite or cell body.) The action potential occurs only when the neuronal membrane is depolarized beyond a critical (threshold) level. The spike discharge is brief (usually less than 1 msec). It is an all-or-none phenomenon that is propagated down the axon and is followed by a temporary refractory period (Fig. 8-6).

Neurophysiology of Neuronal Aggregates
Neurons in the central nervous system and cortex do not function in isolation but function as part of neuronal aggregates. These neurons have rich synaptic interconnections, and the electrical activity of the aggregate reflects the summated effect of all the dendritic potentials and action potentials occurring within that aggregate. This activity is recorded as complex waveforms rather than as the simple spikes of single cells. The cortex generates these electrical waves in response to local activity within the neuronal aggregate and to input from both the specific and the nonspecific nuclei of the thalamus. Since the thalamic nuclei have widespread connections with the cerebral cortex, they can exert a strong influence on cortical activity. They can act to excite, inhibit, or promote widespread synchronization of cortical neuronal activity.

The electrical activity of the cortex can be detected by the EEG, which records cortical activity from electrodes placed on the scalp. This brain-wave activity consists of continuous rhythmic or arrhythmic oscillating waveforms that vary in frequency, amplitude, polarity, and shape. These electrical potentials are usually in the range

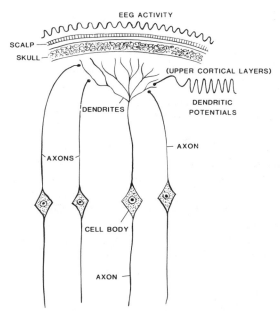

Fig. 8-7. The electroencephalogram (EEG) is a recording of the dendritic potentials in the upper cortical layers as they appear on the scalp.

of 20 to 50 μV. The activity seen on the EEG (Fig. 8-7) reflects the summation of synaptic potentials of many dendrites lying near the surface of the cortex. The fluctuation of the EEG is due to varied excitatory and inhibitory synaptic potentials impinging on the dendritic membranes.

Cortical neuronal activity is modulated, in part, by synaptic input from other cortical neurons, but the most important regulatory influences come from the thalamus. Thalamic influences determine the intrinsic resting frequencies of the brain waves because structures in the thalamus serve as the "pacemakers" in producing widespread synchronization and rhythmicity of cortical activity over the cerebral hemispheres.

Electrical stimulation of the thalamus alters the EEG pattern. A low-frequency stimulus produces a more rhythmic and synchronized EEG pattern, whereas a high-frequency stimulus results in a low-amplitude, arrhythmic, desynchronized pattern. Electrical stimulation of different nuclei of the thalamus results in different EEG patterns. Stimulation of the specific sensory nuclei causes a diphasic evoked response, the *augmenting response,* which is localized to the corresponding sensory area of the cortex. Stimulation of the midline nonspecific thalamic nuclei causes a waxing and waning response, the *recruiting response,* which occurs in a widespread distribution over the cortex.

Functions of the Consciousness System

The consciousness system is responsible for the maintenance of consciousness, alertness, attention, and regulation of the sleep state.

CONSCIOUSNESS. This is a subjective state defined as an "awareness of environment and self." It implies an awake and alert condition in which the person is capable of perceiving his internal and external environments and, if the motor system is intact, of responding in an appropriate manner to input stimuli. There are two aspects of consciousness: (1) the *content of consciousness,* representing cognitive mental functions that reflect the activity of the cerebral cortex, and (2) *arousal* and *wakefulness,* which are dependent on the ascending reticular activating system and which in turn are activated by direct stimulation, sensory stimuli, or cortical influences.

Direct electrical stimulation of the reticular formation in a sleeping animal results in a state of behavioral arousal, indicated by opening of the eyes, turning of the head, and movement of the limbs. Associated with this is a change in the EEG from a synchronous slow-wave sleep pattern to the low-voltage, fast pattern of the waking state.

The reticular formation receives sensory input via collateral branches from every major sensory pathway, which keeps the ascending reticular activating system in an excited state and in turn activates the cortex to maintain wakefulness. The importance of sensory influences in maintaining a wakeful state is illustrated by the progressive decrease in the degree of wakefulness that occurs with loss or reduction in sensory input. If the consciousness system is intact, then stimulation of the ascending reticular activating system results in an arousal response; however, if a portion of the consciousness system is destroyed, particularly the rostral part of the brain stem and thalamus, a permanent "sleep" state ensues.

The consciousness system is activated by input from the cortex as well as by sensory activity. Almost all areas of the cerebral cortex send corticoreticular fibers to the reticular formation. Electrical stimulation of certain cortical areas, such as the orbitofrontal area and superior temporal gyrus, evokes an arousal response. Emotional stimuli such as anger and fear also act as powerful stimulants to the consciousness system.

The state of wakefulness and alertness thus is achieved by the consciousness system through the action of the ascending reticular activating system on the cerebral cortex; the ascending reticular activating system, in turn, is activated by activity in the sensory pathways and by fibers from the cerebral cortex.

ATTENTION. The consciousness system not only determines the state of alertness and wakefulness but also influences the degree of overall attentiveness to the environment and perception of specific sensory modalities. By facilitating or inhibiting transmission of neural impulses through sensory pathways, the consciousness system enhances or attenuates responses to incoming stimuli, directing attention to a specific input while other incoming signals are suppressed. Electrical activity reaching the cortex via specific sensory pathways is not perceived unless it is followed by activity via the diffuse projection paths. For example, when reading a book, a person is absorbed by the words on the page and is not aware of body contact with a chair or outside noises. The consciousness system, in response to corticoreticular direction, selectively sends "alerting" signals to the cortex receiving the visual input and suppresses sensory input in auditory or somatic pathways. The consciousness system thus acts in an adaptive manner to prevent the cortex from being overwhelmed and to permit selective attention to specific external or internal stimuli.

SLEEP STATES. Consciousness may be altered by a number of conditions. One normal physiologic alteration is that associated with *sleep,* which is defined as a cyclic, temporary, and physiologic loss of consciousness that is readily, promptly, and completely reversed by appropriate stimuli.

Sleep results from an interaction between the reticular formation and the hypnogenic (sleep-producing) centers of the brain. Originally, sleep was considered to be primarily due to a passive deafferentation of the cortex, caused by a decrease in sensory input, loss of the facilitative effects of the ascending reticular activating sys-

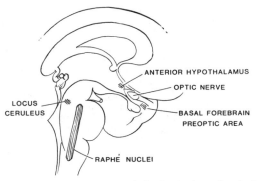

Fig. 8-8. Sleep centers of the brain (crosshatched areas).

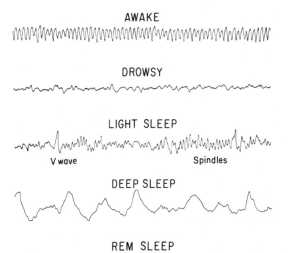

Fig. 8-9. EEG patterns of wakefulness and different levels of sleep. The awake EEG is recorded from occipital areas with eyes closed. With the eyes open, the EEG resembles the REM sleep pattern.

tem, and a consequent decrease in cortical responsiveness. However, more recent studies have shown that sleep is an active phenomenon in which hypnogenic areas of the brain and neurochemical substances actively promote sleep and inhibit the arousal system.

The sleep centers of the brain include the raphé nuclei in the upper medullary and lower pontine areas of the reticular formation of the brain stem, the locus ceruleus in the lateral portion of the upper pons and lower midbrain, the anterior portion of the hypothalamus, and the basal forebrain preoptic area (Fig. 8-8). Stimulation of any of these areas can induce sleep by producing excita-

tion of other areas of the brain associated with sleep and by actively inhibiting areas of the ascending reticular activating system that are responsible for maintaining a wakeful state. Destruction of these areas can result in decreased sleep.

Two distinctive patterns of sleep are seen in normal persons: rapid eye movement (REM) sleep and nonrapid eye movement (non-REM) sleep (Table 8-1). *REM sleep* is sleep in which there are rapid conjugate eye movements; fluctuations of body temperature, blood pressure, heart rate, and respiration; a decrease in muscle tone; an increase in body movements; muscle twitches; and penile erection. This is also the stage of sleep in which dreams occur. An EEG recorded during this time shows a low-amplitude fast pattern resembling that of an alert state with eyes open (Fig. 8-9). Because of the above characteristics, REM sleep is also known as *paradoxical, active,* or *dream* sleep.

Non-REM sleep is sleep during which there are no rapid eye movements. Vital signs are more stable, and less body movement is apparent. During non-REM sleep, the EEG shows different patterns, depending on the depth of sleep (Fig. 8-9). During drowsiness, the EEG shows a low-amplitude background with an attenuation of rhythmic activity. During light-to-medium levels

Table 8-1. Characteristics of the Two Major Patterns of Sleep (REM and non-REM)

Sleep activity	REM sleep	non-REM sleep
Eye movements	Rapid	None
Body movements	Muscle twitches	Muscle relaxation
Muscle tone	Decreased	Some tone in postural muscle groups
Vital signs	Fluctuating	Stable
Penile erection	Positive	Negative
Dreams	Common	Rare
EEG	Low-voltage pattern	Spindles, V waves, K complexes, slow waves
Percentage in adults	20	80
Percentage in infants	50	50

of sleep, specific EEG waveforms (sleep spindles, V waves, and K complexes) are present. *Sleep spindles* are sinusoidal waveforms ranging from 10 to 14 hertz (Hz) and are usually present over the frontal head regions. *V waves* (vertex waves) are high-amplitude, sharp waveforms occurring over the frontal and parietal regions. *K complexes* are a combination of V waves and spindle activity and often signify a partial arousal response in the EEG. During deep levels of sleep, widespread high-amplitude slow waves are present.

Non-REM sleep is the predominant type of sleep in adults and accounts for 80 percent of the nocturnal sleep pattern while REM sleep accounts for only 20 percent. In newborn infants, however, 50 percent of sleep is REM sleep. During a night's sleep in adults, non-REM sleep occurs first and generally lasts for 60 to 90 minutes. It is then interrupted by a REM period, which may last from several minutes to one-half hour and which is subsequently followed by another non-REM period. A total night's sleep usually consists of four to six such cycles of alternating non-REM and REM sleep.

Experimental data have shown that non-REM and REM sleep are produced by different anatomic and physiologic systems. Non-REM sleep has been associated with a group of neurons, the *median raphé nuclei,* which are rich in serotonin and which lie in the midline tegmentum of the pons and medulla (Fig. 8-10A). REM sleep has been associated with the dorsal lateral portion of the pontine reticular formation and the locus ceruleus. The *locus ceruleus,* a group of melanin-pigmented cells rich in norepinephrine, is located in the lateral portion of the tegmentum of the upper pons and lower midbrain (Fig. 8-10B).

The current theory of sleep suggests that the serotonergic neurons of the raphé nuclei are primarily involved with non-REM sleep, while the REM state is mediated by the noradrenergic neurons located in the locus ceruleus and the cholinergic neurons in the reticular formation of the pontine tegmentum. The exact mechanisms governing sleep, however, are still undefined. The mechanisms of initiating REM and non-REM sleep and the transitions between sleep and wakefulness are believed to occur as a sequence of a reciprocal activation and deactivation of neuronal

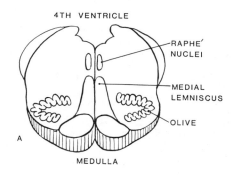

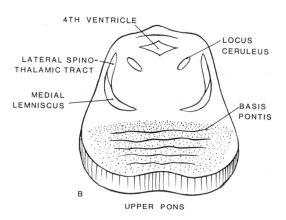

Fig. 8-10. Location of raphé nuclei at level of medulla (A) and locus ceruleus at level of the upper pons (B).

populations of the brain stem, including the reticular formation, the raphé nucleus, and the locus ceruleus, and the interaction of neurotransmitter substances, including serotonin, peptides, and possibly hypnogenic factors.

Clinical Correlations

Sleep Disorders

Narcolepsy is a disorder of sleep control mechanisms characterized by excessive sleepiness. In this disorder, the patient spontaneously and precipitously falls asleep at any time during the day. These episodes of sleepiness are most frequent during monotonous situations and after meals. In addition, the patient also may have cataplexy, sleep paralysis, or hypnagogic hallucinations. *Cataplexy* is a sudden loss of muscle tone, which may cause the patient to suddenly fall to the ground. Cataplexy is often precipitated by emotional events such as laughter, fright, or excitement. *Sleep paralysis* occurs during the transition between wakefulness and sleep and is a temporary state of paralysis and inability to move. *Hypnagogic hallucinations* are false visual or auditory perceptions that occur just before the patient falls asleep; often they occur in conjunction with sleep paralysis. Most patients with narcolepsy have no known structural lesion, and the neurologic examination usually reveals no abnormality.

Sleep apnea is a condition in which the patient stops breathing when asleep. After a period of apnea, which may range up to a minute or more, the changes in levels of oxygen and carbon dioxide cause the patient to arouse from sleep, with noisy, gasping respirations. When the patient goes back to sleep, the cycle repeats. As a result, he or she awakens with a reduced amount of sleep and is excessively drowsy when awake.

Nocturnal enuresis (bed wetting), *somnambulism* (sleepwalking), and *night terrors* are other types of sleep disorders. They have been shown to occur predominantly during deep levels of non-REM sleep.

Prolonged sleep deprivation can result in decreased vigilance, decreased attention span, poor performance of tasks, increased irritability, diplopia, unsteadiness, slurring of speech, hallucinations, illusions, and psychotic behavior.

Disorders of Consciousness

Consciousness is a function of the combined activity of the ascending reticular activating system and the cerebral cortex. Major damage to, or depression of, either of these parts of the consciousness system results in a pathologic alteration in consciousness, or *loss of consciousness*. The loss of consciousness may be transient or prolonged, and it may vary from mildly increased sleepiness to deep coma.

Lesions that alter consciousness are located at the supratentorial or posterior fossa levels. Interruption of the ascending reticular activating system produces different effects on consciousness and on the states of sleeping and wakefulness, depending on the level of involvement (Fig. 8-11).

If nonfatal destruction of the high cervical spinal cord or cervicomedullary junction occurs, leaving the consciousness system intact, then both wakeful and sleeping states will still be

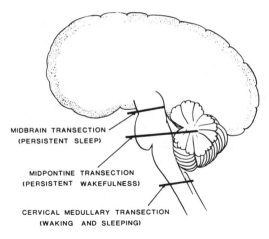

MIDBRAIN TRANSECTION
(PERSISTENT SLEEP)

MIDPONTINE TRANSECTION
(PERSISTENT WAKEFULNESS)

CERVICAL MEDULLARY TRANSECTION
(WAKING AND SLEEPING)

Fig. 8-11. Levels of lesions in the brain stem, producing different effects on wakefulness and sleep.

present clinically and electrographically. Arousal occurs in response either to sensory stimuli from the cranial nerves or to stimulation of the reticular formation.

If damage occurs at the midpontine pretrigeminal level, just rostral to the trigeminal nerve entry zone and above the medullary and pontine sleep centers, there will be a persistent EEG pattern of wakefulness, consisting of low-voltage fast activity characteristic of an awake state.

A lesion at the midbrain level results in a "sleep state" in which neither sensory stimuli nor direct stimulation of the reticular formation or thalamus will produce an arousal response.

Bilateral lesions that affect the ascending projectional pathways in the region of the diencephalon (thalamus and hypothalamus) produce a state of sustained somnolence, with the EEG showing diffuse slow-wave activity.

Focal or unilateral lesions of the cerebral hemispheres do not result in loss of consciousness as long as the projections of the consciousness system to at least one cerebral hemisphere are intact. However, if there is bilateral destruction of the cerebral hemispheres, there is no longer a substratum for the appreciation of consciousness, and unconsciousness ensues.

Thus, the more rostral portions of the consciousness system, in particular the area above the trigeminal nerve entry zone, are critical for maintaining alertness and consciousness. However, portions of the reticular system of the lower pons and medulla seem to have important influences on certain stages of sleep, though they do not seem to be directly required for the maintenance of consciousness.

DEGREES OF ALTERED CONSCIOUSNESS. Regardless of the cause, various degrees of altered consciousness result from lesions affecting this system. *Coma* is a state of extended unconsciousness in which the patient is unarousable and shows little or no spontaneous movement and little or no alerting response to extremely painful or noxious stimuli. Often the muscle-stretch reflexes, the plantar responses, and the pupillary and light reflexes are depressed or absent. Vital signs are usually altered, particularly with lesions affecting the brain stem; the patient has a slow and variable pulse rate and a periodic respiratory pattern.

In *stupor,* the patient often shows a moderate amount of spontaneous movement and can be aroused to respond purposefully to afferent stimuli. If sufficiently aroused, the patient can give a brief response to questions or simple commands.

Obtundation is a state in which alertness of the patient is mildly to moderately decreased. When left undisturbed, the patient falls asleep; when aroused, he or she shows a slowed or reduced response to all forms of stimuli.

In *somnolence,* the patient is easily aroused and shows appropriate verbal and motor responses to sensory stimuli. When the stimulus stops, the patient drifts back to sleep.

Confusion is a transient state, distinct from dementia, in which there is a progressive decline in cognitive functions in the presence of normal consciousness. Level of attention is decreased and the ability to think clearly is impaired. Responses to verbal stimuli are slowed, and the patient is less able to recognize and understand what is going on in the environment.

Delirium is an agitated state of confusion associated with *illusions* (false interpretations or misrepresentations of real sensory images), *hallucinations* (false sensory perceptions for which there are no external bases), and *delusions* (false beliefs or misconceptions that cannot be corrected by reason).

Sleep, in contrast to the pathologic alterations previously described, is a normal physiologic state, but one that also can be associated with pathologic involvement of the consciousness system. The sleeping person, as compared with one in coma, is fully aroused by appropriate stimuli. During sleep, the eyes are closed, the muscles are relaxed, and the cardiac output, pulse rate, blood pressure, and respiration decrease.

CAUSES OF LOSS OF CONSCIOUSNESS. The consciousness system may suffer either from physiologic alterations of function that produce a transient loss of consciousness or from structural lesions that result in a persistent loss of consciousness. A transient disturbance of consciousness occurs as a result of (1) concussion, (2) a generalized seizure, (3) syncope, or (4) a metabolic encephalopathy.

Concussion is a brief loss of consciousness, usually occurring after a sudden blow to the head. Although the patient is unconscious, arousal by vigorous stimuli is often possible. After return of consciousness, there is some confusion and *amnesia* (loss of memory) which persist for a variable period afterward, but usually there are no permanent neurologic sequelae. Mechanisms postulated to cause the transient loss of consciousness include (1) a sudden increase in pressure in the region of neurons critical for consciousness, (2) cerebral ischemia, (3) sudden depolarization or hyperpolarization (or both) of neurons, and (4) transient alteration in neuronal functioning secondary to mechanical distortion of neurons or axons. Although no gross neuropathologic change is usually apparent, diffuse axonal injury and individual neuronal alteration have been found on microscopic examination, especially in the region of the brain-stem reticular formation.

Seizures (convulsions) are transient episodes of supratentorial origin in which there is an abrupt and temporary alteration in cerebral function. Seizures may consist of abnormal movements (such as tonic or clonic movements), an abnormal sensation (such as paresthesias or visual hallucination), or a disturbance in behavior or consciousness. They are caused by a spontaneous, excessive discharge of cortical neurons, which may occur as a result of an increase in neuronal excitability, an excessive excitatory synaptic input impinging on the nerve cells, or a decrease in normal inhibitory mechanisms.

Seizures can be either focal or generalized. A

focal seizure, also called *partial* seizure, involves only a localized area of the cortex. Partial seizures have been subdivided into simple partial seizures, in which there is no loss of consciousness, and complex partial seizures, in which there is some alteration of consciousness. A *generalized* seizure involves widespread and bilateral areas of both hemispheres simultaneously. It may have some spread to the thalamus and reticular activating system and, therefore, is associated with a loss of consciousness.

Syncope (fainting) is a transient loss of consciousness due to a decrease in cerebral blood flow and ischemia of the entire brain. This occurs as a result of decreased cardiac output, slowing of the heart rate, or pooling of blood in the periphery. The loss of consciousness is usually brief (a matter of seconds to minutes) and is preceded by light-headedness, weakness, giddiness, sweating, and dimming of vision. During this time, the patient is pale and sweaty; his pulse is weak, and his blood pressure is reduced.

A number of systemic disorders produce a *metabolic encephalopathy* which diffusely affects the consciousness system and causes a transient alteration in consciousness, often without localizing signs. Hypoglycemia, hyponatremia, and drug overdosage are commonly encountered causes of metabolic encephalopathy.

Structural lesions can result in persistent impairment of consciousness or in coma. Although we will use the general term *coma* in this discussion, stupor and somnolence are also produced by identical disease processes. Coma results from lesions that involve the reticular formation and its projectional systems or the cerebral hemispheres bilaterally.

Direct damage or depression of the consciousness system in the posterior fossa or diencephalon may occur from infarction, hemorrhage, neoplasia, trauma, metabolic disturbances, and anesthetic agents and drugs. Unilateral lesions of the cerebral hemispheres do not cause coma if the consciousness system is intact. However, coma does result from bilateral lesions that diffusely affect the cerebral hemispheres, such as encephalitis, meningitis, subarachnoid hemorrhage, metabolic disturbances (such as hypoglycemia), hypoxia, some degenerative diseases, and certain drugs.

Indirect involvement of the consciousness system also can result in coma. This involvement is usually the result of mass lesions which, although extrinsic to the consciousness system, compress or distort the diencephalon and brain stem. Common examples are mass lesions of the posterior fossa (for example, a cerebellar neoplasm) or expanding unilateral cerebral masses that result in herniation of the brain contents and secondary compression of diencephalic or midbrain structures (see Chap. 14 for further discussion).

In summary, coma can be produced by:

1. Focal lesions of the posterior fossa that *directly* involve the brain stem.
2. Focal lesions of the posterior fossa that *indirectly* result in depression of consciousness.
3. Focal supratentorial lesions, if they are of such magnitude as to directly or indirectly involve the deep midline diencephalic structures necessary for the maintenance of consciousness.
4. Diffuse lesions, generally of an anoxic, toxic-metabolic, or inflammatory nature, capable of causing widespread depression.

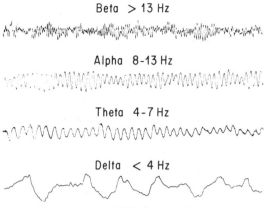

Fig. 8-12. *Four basic EEG frequencies.*

Beta > 13 Hz

Alpha 8-13 Hz

Theta 4-7 Hz

Delta < 4 Hz

The Electroencephalogram
The EEG is a useful adjunct to neurologic diagnosis. Electrical activity recorded by the EEG from the cerebral cortex is classified into four main types, depending on the frequency or number of waveforms per second (hertz) (Fig. 8-12).

1. *Beta activity* is low-amplitude fast activity occurring at a frequency of more than 13 Hz. This type of activity is usually seen over the anterior head regions.

2. *Alpha activity* is rhythmic waves at a frequency of 8 to 13 Hz. These rhythms occur in the posterior head regions and are the predominant background activity during the relaxed waking state when the eyes are closed (Fig. 8-13). With eye opening or with attention, there is attenuation of the rhythmic alpha background and replacement by a low-voltage pattern.

3. *Theta activity* ranges from 4 to 7 Hz and may be normal when present in a child or in an adult in a drowsy state, but when present in a fully awake adult, it is abnormal.

4. *Delta activity* is the slowest wave form, occurring at a frequency of less than 4 Hz. This activity is normal when present in an infant or in a sleeping adult but is abnormal under any other circumstances.

The EEG is helpful in studying normal physiologic activities; however, it attains its greatest usefulness in detecting abnormalities of cerebral functioning. The EEG reflects the intrinsic cortical activity as modified by subcortical structures (the thalamus and the ascending projections of the ascending reticular activating system). An EEG abnormality therefore occurs as a result of a

Fig. 8-13. Normal EEG pattern during wakeful state, showing presence of alpha activity in the posterior head region. (In each EEG illustration, electrical activity is a bipolar recording of the potential difference between electrodes, indicated by letters and numbers to the left of each line. Location of each electrode is shown on the schematic diagram of the head.)

disturbance of (1) cortical neuronal activity, (2) subcortical structures that regulate cortical neuronal activity, and (3) the thalamocortical projection pathways.

The two main types of EEG abnormalities are slow-wave abnormalities and epileptiform abnormalities; both can be either focal or generalized. A focal EEG abnormality indicates a localized disturbance of cortical functioning, while a generalized EEG abnormality indicates a bilateral and diffuse disturbance of cortical functioning or a disturbance that is projected to the surface from subcortical structures. The EEG thus helps distinguish between a focal and a generalized disturbance of cerebral function and in determining the level of the brain involved.

In coma secondary to diffuse cortical disease, the EEG shows widespread, generalized slowing (Fig. 8-14), with the degree of slowing often paralleling the degree of coma. When there is dysfunction of subcortical structures, the EEG shows different types of abnormalities, depending on the level of the neuraxis involved. With diencephalic or midbrain involvement, the EEG shows intermittent, rhythmic slow waves occurring bilaterally and synchronously over both hemispheres. This is often referred to as a *projected rhythm* because it is projected to the surface from subcortical structures. If the pons or lower brain stem is involved, the EEG may contain alpha activity and resemble a normal waking record, but unlike the normal alpha rhythm in an alert person, this activity does not show normal reactivity to light, noise, or noxious stimuli. In addition, there may be cyclic sleep patterns consisting of sleep spindles, V waves, and delta waves. When there are

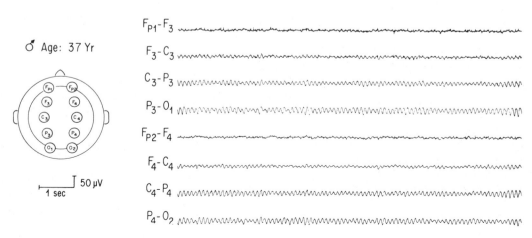

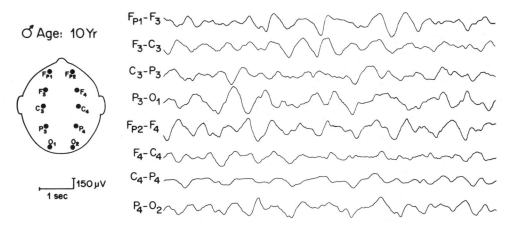

Fig. 8-14. *EEG of a comatose patient with encephalitis, showing widespread delta slowing.*

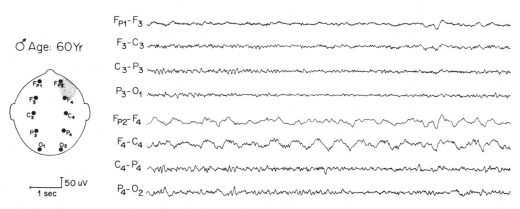

Fig. 8-15. *EEG showing focal delta waves over the right frontal area (stippled in diagram) due to right frontal tumor.*

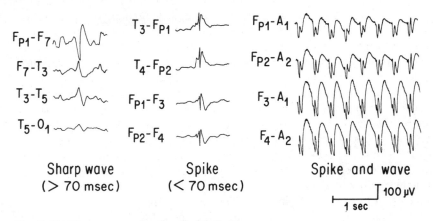

Fig. 8-16. *Three types of epileptiform discharges. The sharp-wave discharge (left) was recorded from the left temporal region. The spike (center) and spike and slow-wave discharges (right) were recorded from widespread areas of cortex.*

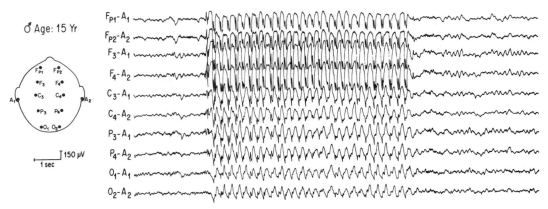

♂ Age: 15 Yr

⌐ 150 µV
⊢━━┤
1 sec

Fig. 8-17. Generalized 3-Hz spike and wave discharge with an absence seizure, during which the patient was unresponsive.

focal cerebral lesions, focal slowing is seen on the EEG (Fig. 8-15). If the primary cerebral lesion is large enough to distort or cause a pressure effect on the diencephalic or mesencephalic structures, the EEG shows a "projected" abnormality in addition to the focal slow-wave abnormality.

In the diagnosis of seizure disorders, the EEG shows epileptiform abnormalities consisting of sharp waves, spikes, or spike and slow-wave discharges (Fig. 8-16). During an actual seizure, these occur in a sustained repetitive and rhythmic fashion (Fig. 8-17).

A patient with nonorganic disease may appear to be unconscious. In these circumstances, the EEG shows a normal waking pattern that is reactive to afferent stimuli.

Brain Death
Brain death occurs when neural damage is irreversible and, although cardiac activity may be present, there is no longer evidence of cerebral or brain-stem function. The patient is unresponsive and shows no spontaneous movement or behavioral response to external stimuli. The absence of brain-stem function is manifested by loss of respiratory activity and all brain-stem reflexes. Absence of cerebral function can be confirmed by the EEG, which shows a flat pattern with no sign of electrocerebral activity. Since brain function is markedly depressed by certain anesthetic agents and other drugs, these can also result in a flat EEG. These should be excluded before concluding that irreversible brain death is present.

Neurologic Examination of the Consciousness System
Examination of the patient with altered consciousness represents a challenge to the physician. The situation is often emergent, and the patient is frequently uncooperative. Furthermore, assessment of the functions of the consciousness system alone seldom provides sufficient information for anatomic-pathologic diagnosis, and one must rely on other associated clues from the history and results of physical examination to determine the location and cause of the responsible lesion.

Assessment of the Consciousness System
Involvement of the consciousness system is evaluated by noting the patient's ability to perceive and attend to the external environment. The degree of coma is determined by the patient's response to stimuli, such as touch, pinprick, calling the patient's name, a handclap, or some other form of loud noise. If the patient is unresponsive to milder forms of stimulation, then noxious or painful stimuli, such as pinching or deep pressure in sensitive areas, are utilized. The patient's response is observed to define the presence of delirium, confusion, somnolence, stupor, or coma (as previously described), any of which would suggest some involvement of the consciousness system. However, from this evaluation one cannot determine the site or nature of the involvement.

Anatomic-Pathologic Diagnosis
Lesions affecting the consciousness system are located at the supratentorial or posterior fossa (or both) levels; therefore one must seek clues that suggest involvement at these levels by noting the

vital signs (pulse, blood pressure, respiration, temperature) and examining motor, sensory, and cranial nerve functions. Precise anatomic localization is seldom necessary, but some attempt should be made to apply the general principles of anatomic diagnosis described in Chapter 3 to decide whether the responsible lesion is (1) located at the supratentorial level, (2) located at the posterior fossa level, or (3) diffusely distributed at both levels.

This seemingly crude localization is actually extremely useful in the clinical setting and, when combined with information about the temporal evolution of the illness, it is used (as described in Chap. 4) to establish a cause (vascular, inflammatory, toxic-metabolic, traumatic, neoplastic, or degenerative). Judicious selection of appropriate ancillary studies such as x-rays, blood studies, CT scan, radioisotope brain scan, EEG, and CSF examination is often required to establish a precise anatomic-pathologic diagnosis.

Objectives

1. Describe the anatomy of the consciousness system, with special reference to the reticular formation, the nonspecific thalamic nuclei, the ascending projectional system, and the cerebral cortex.
2. List the major input and output connections of the reticular formation.
3. Describe and differentiate the electrical activity of single neurons and neuronal aggregates.
4. Name the two main types of sleep patterns, describe the differences between them, and outline the current anatomic-pathologic-pharmacologic theory for the production of sleep cycles.
5. Describe the effects on sleep of a transection of the brain at the level of the high cervical cord, the midpons, and the midbrain.
6. Define narcolepsy, delirium, confusion, somnolence, stupor, coma, concussion, seizure, and syncope, and list the characteristics of each.
7. State the anatomic locations of lesions that result in loss of consciousness, and give examples of specific disease processes that affect each area.
8. Describe the neurophysiologic basis of the EEG and the fundamental waking and sleeping

patterns, and describe how the EEG is useful in evaluating the patient with disorders of consciousness.

Clinical Problems

1. A 56-year-old diabetic man became confused and then unresponsive over a period of several hours. He had given himself his usual injection of insulin on awakening in the morning. Because of an upset stomach, he failed to eat anything during the day. When brought to the emergency room, he was comatose but was without localizing neurologic signs.
   a. What is the anatomic-pathologic diagnosis?
   b. What portions of the consciousness system are involved?
   c. What is the precise etiologic diagnosis?
   d. What changes might be found in the EEG?
2. A 74-year-old woman with a history of hypertension had a sudden onset of a severe, right-sided headache, followed by weakness of the left side of her face and body and somnolence. When hospitalized 1 hour later, she had severe weakness on the left side of the body and face and decreased sensation on the left side of the body and face. During the next few hours, she became progressively less responsive and finally comatose.
   a. Prior to the patient's entering the hospital, what would be the most appropriate anatomic-pathologic diagnosis?
   b. What is the nature of the pathologic lesion?
   c. What is the mechanism for her becoming comatose?
   d. What changes would be expected in the EEG?
3. A 38-year-old woman had a 3-year history of generalized grand mal seizures. On the day of admission to the hospital, she was found unresponsive on the floor of her living room. When brought to the emergency room, she was stuporous, with continuous bilateral convulsive movements of the face and upper and lower extremities. These subsided and, within 24 hours, the results of the neurologic examination were normal.
   a. What is the anatomic-pathologic diagnosis?

b. What changes might be seen in the EEG during the seizure?

c. List six types of conditions that cause generalized seizures.

d. If focal seizures were also present in this patient, would that influence your choice as to their possible cause?

Suggested Reading

Ajmone Marsan, C., and Gumnit, R. J. Neurophysiological Aspects of Epilepsy. In P. J. Vinken and G. W. Bruyn (eds.), *Handbook of Clinical Neurology*, Vol. 15. Amsterdam: North Holland, 1974. Pp. 30–59.

Browne, T. R., and Feldman, R. G. *Epilepsy: Diagnosis and Management*. Boston: Little, Brown, 1983.

Cartwright, R. D. *A Primer on Sleep and Dreaming*. Reading, Mass.: Addison-Wesley, 1978.

Delafresnaye, J. F. (ed.). *Brain Mechanisms and Consciousness: A Symposium*. Oxford, Engl.: Blackwell, 1954.

Guilleminault, C., and Baker, T. L. Sleep and electroencephalography: Points of interest and points of controversy. *J. Clin. Neurophysiol.* 1:275, 1984.

Guyton, A. C. *Basic Human Neurophysiology* (3rd ed.). Philadelphia: Saunders, 1981.

Jasper, H. H., et al. *Reticular Formation of the Brain*. Boston: Little, Brown, 1958.

Jouvet, M. The Role of Monoaminergic Neurons in the Regulation and Function of Sleep. In O. Petre-Quadens and J. D. Schlag (eds.), *Basic Sleep Mechanisms* (NATO Advanced Study Institute, Bruges, 1971). New York: Academic, 1974. Pp. 207–236.

Kales, A. *Sleep: Physiology & Pathology: A Symposium*. Philadelphia: Lippincott, 1969.

Kandel, E. R., and Schwartz, J. H. *Principles of Neural Science*. New York: Elsevier–North Holland, 1981.

Kiloh, L. G., et al., *Clinical Electroencephalography* (4th ed.). Boston: Butterworth, 1981. Pp. 1–38; 64–131.

Magoun, H. W. *The Waking Brain* (2nd ed.). Springfield, Ill.: Thomas, 1963.

Plum, F., and Posner, J. B. *The Diagnosis of Stupor and Coma* (3rd ed.). Philadelphia: Davis, 1980.

The Motor System

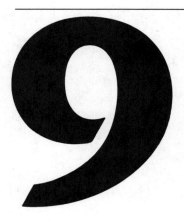

Abnormalities in the afferent pathways that carry information into the nervous system produce impairment of sensation, as described in Chapters 7 and 8. Disorders involving efferent pathways produce impairment of movement. Many diseases are encountered in all specialties of medicine in which movement or motor function is impaired. Common motor symptoms include weakness, paralysis, twitching, jerking, staggering, wasting, shaking, and stiffness, and such terms as "spastic" and "incoordinated" have been used to describe patients' behavior. All these and many other symptoms point to involvement of the *motor system,* the neuroanatomic structures that control movement. Motor disorders may involve movement of the arms, the legs, the trunk, the eyes, or the muscles involved in speech.

All body movements, whether visceral or somatic, result from the contraction of muscle. The neural structures that control muscle are classified by the embryologic origin of the muscle they innervate:

1. General somatic efferent structures that innervate muscles derived from somites—striated muscle in the trunk, limbs, and head.
2. Special visceral efferent structures that innervate muscles derived from branchial arches—most striated muscle of the head and neck.
3. General visceral efferent structures that innervate muscles derived from visceral mesoderm—smooth muscle.

In this chapter, only the disorders that impair function of the striated or skeletal muscles that have general somatic efferent and special visceral efferent functions will be considered. The smooth muscle of the viscera, controlled by the visceral system, will be considered in Chapter 10.

The motor system, like the sensory system, includes a complex network of structures and pathways at all levels of the nervous system and is organized to mediate many types of activity. An understanding of this organization, and the integration of the motor system with the sensory system, is necessary for the accurate localization and diagnosis of disease involving the nervous system.

Overview

The motor system includes all structures that are directly involved in the performance of motor activity by striated somatic and visceral musculature. It includes four major divisions:

1. The final common pathway
2. The direct activation pathway
3. The indirect activation pathway
4. The control circuits

Each of these receives information from the sensory system described in Chapter 7. The sensory input initiates or modifies the activity in the motor system to obtain the appropriate motor action. The interrelationships of these major divisions are diagrammed schematically in Figure 9-1.

Sensory-Motor Integration

Motor activity is generally initiated in response to sensory input. As illustrated in Figure 9-1, the sensory information can reach the motor system at a number of levels and through a number of pathways. The pathways utilized and the structures involved in conveying the sensory information are represented in the center of the figure. Pathway 1 represents the sensory fibers that produce activity by local synapses within the spinal cord. Pathway 2 includes the ascending pathways to the cerebral hemispheres for pain, touch, temperature, position, and vibration sensations (spinothalamic pathways and the posterior columns). Pathway 3 is composed of the spinocerebellar pathways to the cerebellum. Pathway 4 is composed of branches from the spinothalamic pathway and medial lemniscal pathway that make synapses with the reticular formation in the brain stem. Disease in the sensory portion of this integrated system results in disorders that are manifest as motor abnormalities. One example of this—sensory ataxia—was discussed in Chapter 7.

The integration of sensory and motor pathways to provide an appropriate response to particular sensory stimuli is best demonstrated by reflexes. A *reflex* is a stereotyped response to a specific sensory stimulus. In a reflex, the action potentials from the sensory pathways activate cells in the motor system, which then initiate a specific motor response. One of the most familiar examples

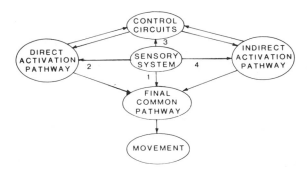

Fig. 9-1. *Organization of major divisions of motor system. The four numbered pathways indicated in the diagram are those in the sensory system that act on the motor system. The structures in the four pathways are: local spinal cord connections (1), posterior columns and spinothalamic pathways (2), spinocerebellar pathways (3), and sensory input to reticular formation (4).*

of a reflex is the *knee jerk,* in which the leg moves involuntarily in response to tapping of the quadriceps tendon. This reflex is a simple reflex involving only the primary sensory neuron, a localized portion of the spinal cord, and the final common pathway. Other reflexes are more complex and involve structures at many levels.

Final Common Pathway

The somatic musculature performs the work involved in moving the parts of the body. Each muscle is designed to perform particular movements, but each may be involved in a wide variety of complex motor activities. The skeletal muscles are all under the direct control of neurons known as the *lower motor neurons* and contract only in response to activation by these neurons. These neurons, located in the anterior horn of the spinal cord and brain stem, control the activities of groups of fibers in a muscle. A lower motor neuron and the muscle fibers under its control make up a *motor unit.* The *final common pathway* consists of many motor units through which all other components of the motor system must act.

The motor unit includes the *alpha motor neuron,* a single cell in the anterior horn of the spinal cord, its axon, which leaves the spinal cord and travels peripherally in a nerve to a specific muscle where it subdivides into a number of terminal axons, and each of the muscle fibers with which these terminal axons make contact. The alpha motor neuron integrates activity from a number

of sources (Fig. 9-1) and transmits the resultant activity to the muscle in order to produce contraction. A disease process impairing the function of the motor unit prevents the normal activation of muscle fibers in that motor unit and is manifest as an inability of the muscle to contract fully (weakness or paralysis). Abnormal discharges may occur in the motor unit and produce involuntary activity.

The final common pathway receives input from three major sources: the sensory system directly, the direct activation pathway, and the indirect activation pathway. The lower motor neurons integrate these inputs to produce the required motor action.

The first of these inputs arises locally from the sensory system and produces simple, stereotyped reflex responses like the knee jerk. Such activity is involuntary, specific, and localized to limited areas of the body, such as one muscle, one leg, or both legs. This source of input is lost if there is damage to the sensory pathways. This damage could result in the loss of a reflex, just as damage to the final common pathway itself could. The inputs to the lower motor neuron from direct and indirect activation pathways descend from higher centers.

Direct Activation Pathway

The second major input to the final common pathway is the direct activation pathway. This, like other pathways, is known by different names, including the *pyramidal tract* and the *corticospinal tract.* The *direct activation pathway* is a direct route by which information can travel from the cerebral cortex to the spinal cord without an intervening synapse. Its major function is to effect voluntary activity, in particular skilled movements under conscious control. These may occur in response to a specific sensory input, as in turning off the hot water when a bath feels too hot, but they are not called reflexes because they are not stereotyped.

The direct activation pathway descends from the cerebral cortex through the white matter of the cerebral hemispheres, the brain stem, and the spinal cord to end on the final common pathway on the opposite side of the body. The effectiveness of this pathway obviously depends on an intact final common pathway to carry information to the end organ, that is, muscle. Damage to the direct activation pathway results in a loss of voluntary movements, especially fine, skilled movements, with preservation of other forms of movement such as segmental reflexes.

Indirect Activation Pathway

The third major input to the final common pathway is the indirect activation pathway, sometimes called the *extrapyramidal pathway*. This group of tracts and nuclei is more complex than the direct activation pathway and is composed of a number of short pathways and of structures between the cerebral hemispheres and the anterior horn cells in the spinal cord. These pathways mediate the enormous number of automatic activities involved in normal motor function. For example, the maintenance of erect posture when sitting or standing requires the coordinated contraction of many muscles. This coordination is under subconscious control and is mediated by the indirect activation pathway. The performance of many voluntary actions also requires the integration of activity in a multitude of supporting muscles. Such activities also are mediated in large part by the indirect activation pathways.

The major extrapyramidal pathways include the reticulospinal, vestibulospinal, and rubrospinal tracts. Disease affecting extrapyramidal pathways is manifested in many ways, depending on the location and structures involved. In particular the abnormalities are those of abnormal muscle tone and reflexes.

Control Circuits

The fourth major division of the motor system does not have a direct input to the final common pathway but rather serves to integrate the activity in the diverse structures involved in the performance of motor action. There are two major control circuits: (1) the cerebellum and its connections with other components of the motor system and (2) the basal ganglia and their connections with the other components of the motor system. Each receives input from the other divisions of the motor system, as well as from the sensory system, and each provides information to the direct and indirect activation pathways via the cortex to modulate their activities in accordance with activities in other structures. The *basal ganglia* are concerned primarily with learned, automatic behavior and with preparing and maintaining the background support or posture for motor activity. The *cerebellum* accomplishes the coordination and correction of movement errors of muscles during active movements. Abnormalities in the control circuits result in disorders of posture or coordination, at times accompanied by abnormal involuntary movements, though not by weakness. (It should be noted that the basal ganglia are often classified as part of the extrapyramidal pathways, and they may be listed as such in some textbooks. We will consider them as a control circuit.)

Final Common Pathway

The final common pathway is the peripheral effector mechanism by which all motor activity is mediated. It includes motor neurons in the anterior horn of the spinal cord and their axons extending peripherally via nerves to innervate muscles. These motor neurons are called *alpha motor neurons* or *alpha efferents*. The alpha efferents innervate the muscle fibers that are responsible for skeletal muscle contraction.

Anatomy

The basic functional component of the final common pathway is the motor unit. The concept of the *motor unit,* that is, an anterior horn cell (alpha motor neuron), together with the muscle fibers innervated by it, is a physiologic one, developed largely as a result of the work of Sir Charles Sherrington and his colleagues on the reflex activity of the spinal cord. By definition, each unit consists of the cell body of a motor neuron, its single axon (which leaves the spinal cord in the ventral root and extends through the peripheral nervous system before ramifying to innervate the muscle fibers in a particular muscle), and all the muscle fibers innervated by the terminal axons (Fig. 9-2).

ANTERIOR HORN CELLS. The cell bodies of lower motor neurons lie in the anterior horn of the spinal cord. These cells are relatively large (50 to 80 μm) and are arranged in well-defined columns that extend through many spinal segments and the brain stem. These are called *alpha motor neurons*. There are other smaller neurons in the anterior horns which are more diffusely arranged, the interneurons and gamma motor neurons. *Gamma motor neurons* innervate muscle

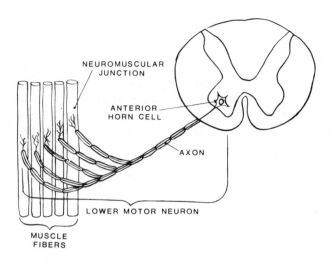

NEUROMUSCULAR
JUNCTION

ANTERIOR
HORN CELL

AXON

LOWER MOTOR NEURON

MUSCLE
FIBERS

Fig. 9-2. A single motor unit and its component parts: the lower motor neuron and muscle fibers innervated by it. The final common pathway contains hundreds of thousands of such units innervating skeletal muscle.

spindles, and *interneurons* interconnect other neurons. The motor units of craniofacial muscles have their motor neurons in the brain stem. Destruction of the anterior horn cell of a motor unit results in degeneration of the axon and a loss of innervation of the muscle fibers of that motor unit. The muscle becomes weak or paralyzed, and the muscle fibers atrophy.

MOTOR AXONS.   Motor axons (nerve fibers) are large, myelinated fibers, 6 to 20 μm in diameter, located in the peripheral nerves. The large myelinated motor nerve fibers of most nerves innervating muscle have axons of two sizes because of the presence of two distinct fiber types in these nerves. Nearly half of the fibers are the large alpha motor fibers that innervate muscle fibers (extrafusal muscle fibers), whereas the remainder are the gamma motor fibers to the muscle spindles (intrafusal muscle fibers). The gamma motor axons to the muscle spindles originate in the smaller neurons in the anterior horn of the spinal cord and are of smaller caliber (6 to 10 μm) than the alpha motor axons.

Branching of motor nerve fibers occurs along the course of nerves at the nodes of Ranvier and is greatest distally in the muscle. As they branch, the nerve fibers become greatly reduced in diameter (1 to 3 μm), and at their termination they are unmyelinated. Each terminal ramification of a

nerve fiber ends on a *neuromuscular junction*, a motor end plate on a single muscle fiber. In most muscles, these are located in a narrow zone across the muscle near the entry of the motor nerve into the muscle. The nerves that go to muscle also contain many sensory fibers arising mainly from the muscle spindles. Mild damage to the motor axons in the peripheral nerve can block the conduction of action potentials to the muscle, whereas severe damage can produce wallerian degeneration of the axon distal to the site of the lesion. In either instance, there will be loss of function of the muscle.

THE NEUROMUSCULAR JUNCTION.   The points of contact between the terminal ramifications of the motor axons and the muscle fibers innervated by them are known as *motor end plates* or the *neuromuscular junction*. Each motor end plate is a composite structure belonging partly to the motor nerve and partly to the muscle fiber. The terminal axon loses its myelin sheath a few microns from the end plate and is covered only by an attenuated Schwann cell. The *endomysium* is a connective tissue sheath that surrounds the muscle fiber and extends over the end-plate region. The terminal axon lies in a hollow indentation of the surface of the muscle fiber, the *synaptic gutter*. The membrane of the nerve terminal and that of the muscle fiber are separated by only a narrow space, the *synaptic cleft*. The nerve terminal holds many vesicles which contain a neurotransmitter, acetylcholine. There are high concentrations of the enzyme cholinesterase situated in the postsynaptic *subneural apparatus* of the end plate, where it degrades acetylcholine after its release from the nerve terminal.

ORGANIZATION OF MUSCLE FIBERS IN A MOTOR UNIT. The nerve terminals of a single motor axon innervate muscle fibers that may be distributed widely throughout the muscle, intermingling with muscle fibers innervated by other neurons. A muscle may contain from 50 to 1,000 motor units.

The size of a motor unit is determined by the number of extrafusal fibers innervated by a single motor neuron. This is expressed as the *innervation ratio,* the number of muscle fibers per axon. Muscles concerned with fine movements have smaller innervation ratios than do those that perform cruder movements. The motor units of the powerful limb muscles, for example, each contain from 500 to 2,000 muscle fibers. In contrast, motor units in intrinsic hand muscles have innervation ratios of only 10 to 50, and eye muscles have ratios of 3 to 10.

After destruction of isolated anterior horn cells, as occurs for example in poliomyelitis, reinnervation of some of the denervated fibers may occur by branching of the remaining motor nerve fibers. These new collateral sprouts of intact axons form new motor end plates on the denervated muscle fibers, resulting in an increase in the number of muscle fibers in the remaining motor units and, thus, an increase in the innervation ratio.

MUSCLE FIBER STRUCTURE. *Muscle fibers* of skeletal muscles are long, cylindrical structures, each of which is a syncytium containing hundreds of nuclei. These nuclei are situated near the surface of the fiber adjacent to the sarcolemmal sheath. In transverse sections, the fibers are seen as rounded or polygonal structures. The cytoplasm of the muscle fiber contains mitochondria, sarcoplasmic reticulum, and *myofibrils,* the contractile elements of the muscle. The myofibrils have a banded structure that subdivides them into units called sarcomeres. A *sarcomere* is the distance between two well-defined cross striations on the muscle fiber, the Z *bands.* On electron microscopic examination, the myofibrils are found to consist of filaments of the proteins actin and myosin, whose arrangement in the myofibrils is responsible for the cross striation.

Each muscle fiber is enclosed in a *sarcolemmal sheath,* which consists of the cell membrane of the muscle fiber, a basement membrane, and collagen and reticulin fibers called *endomysial connective tissue.* This delicate connective tissue framework contains an abundant network of capillary blood vessels.

Individual muscle fibers may be several centimeters long. They may run from one end of the muscle to the other, or they may be attached to tendinous insertions within the muscle. The fibers are arranged in groups or *fasciculi,* each of which is a bundle of parallel fibers bound together and surrounded by connective tissue containing blood vessels and nerves. Adult muscle fibers range from 30 to 90 μm in diameter. Differences in fiber diameter between different muscles and between the muscles of different people occur because of differences in build and muscular development. The size of muscle fiber also depends on the activity of the muscle and on undefined *trophic factors* released from the nerve terminals. Lack of use causes muscle fibers to shrink, but they do so more severely and rapidly with immobilization or with loss of innervation. In cases of loss of innervation, this loss of size, or *atrophy,* of the fiber is limited to the muscle fibers that were innervated by the damaged neuron. In abnormalities of the muscle itself, atrophy involves all fibers in the muscle.

Muscle fibers can be classified into two or more types on the basis of their histochemical character and appearance. These are often called red or white (type I or type II) and are intermingled in each muscle. These are discussed further in Chapter 12 (The Peripheral Level).

Physiology

The motor unit is the physiologic unit of reflex and voluntary contraction. Under normal conditions, the motor unit behaves in an all-or-none manner, which means that an impulse in the motor nerve fiber produces an action potential in, and a synchronous contraction of, all the muscle fibers it supplies. The resulting contraction of the motor unit is thus the sum of the mechanical responses of the component muscle fibers.

Activation of a lower motor neuron in the spinal cord or brain stem by any of the three sources of input produces an action potential that spreads to each of the terminal branches of the motor axon in the muscle. Each of these axons releases the neurotransmitter *acetylcholine,* which diffuses rapidly across the synaptic cleft and acts on the postsynaptic membrane of the muscle fiber to produce an end-plate potential. The end-plate potential initiates an action potential in the muscle fiber which then spreads along the entire length of the muscle fiber. The electrical currents generated by the muscle action potential invade the depths of the muscle fiber via a tubular system to "turn on" the contractile mechanism which produces the actual twitch of the muscle.

In the normal activation of lower motor neurons, the neurons discharge repetitively at rates of 5 to 20 per second. At these rates, the twitch of slow muscles is not completed before the next action potential arrives, so that smooth movements or steady contractions can be obtained from repetitive action potentials. Normal movements involve the coordinated activity of hundreds to thousands of motor units in many muscles. The speed and strength of a movement are controlled by the number of motor units active, their rate of firing, and the characteristics of the motor units activated.

Units with low innervation ratios are needed for some tasks. For example, extrinsic ocular muscles, which must fixate accurately, need very fine control and therefore have low innervation ratios. The number of muscle fibers in a motor unit is also related to the load that it must move. For example, to move the mass of the lower limb

Fig. 9-3. Anatomic basis of stretch reflex. This reflex is a two-neuron reflex mediated by stretch receptors in the muscle spindle, sensory axons with their cell bodies in the dorsal root ganglion, a synapse in the spinal cord, and an anterior horn cell innervating the striated muscle.

even slightly requires the simultaneous action of many muscle fibers, and consequently in the muscles responsible for such movements, high innervation ratios are found. Since activation of a normal anterior horn cell results in contraction of all the muscle fibers in the motor unit, gradation of contraction is accomplished by varying the frequency of firing of single motor units and the number of motor units activated. When effort is increased, more motor units are brought into action.

In general, the motor units in limb muscles may be divided into two groups according to their speed of contraction, which generally corresponds to the muscle fiber type, fast twitch (type II) and slow twitch (type I). The distinction is based on the differences in time from the start of the contraction to the time at which the motor unit develops its peak tension in response to a single stimulus. In a typical fast-twitch motor unit, this contraction time is approximately 25 msec, while in a slow-twitch unit, the time is approximately 75 msec. The relaxation times are comparable to the contraction time in each case. Present evidence suggests that the motor nerve innervating the muscle fibers of the motor unit determines the twitch time. How this influence comes about is not known: It may be by some trophic (chemical) substance liberated at the nerve endings independently of acetylcholine, by the pattern of nerve impulses reaching the motor end plate, or by some other means.

Slow-twitch motor units tend to be found in certain muscles, for example, the soleus muscle. This has led to the use of the term *slow muscle.* Other muscles containing predominantly fast-twitch motor units are designated *fast muscles.* The slow-twitch muscles tend to have a deeper

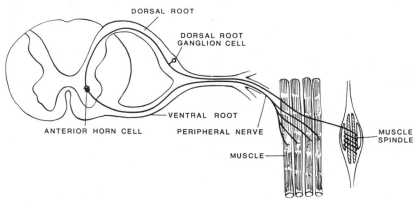

DORSAL ROOT

DORSAL ROOT GANGLION CELL

ANTERIOR HORN CELL   VENTRAL ROOT

PERIPHERAL NERVE   MUSCLE SPINDLE

MUSCLE

red color than the fast-twitch muscles. The segregation of more motor units of a particular speed into certain muscles is of functional significance. It is generally agreed that slow limb muscles, like the soleus muscle, subserve a predominantly postural role, while the fast limb muscles are concerned more with phasic, voluntary movements. However, fast- and slow-twitch motor units are intermingled in most muscles.

Local Reflexes

Three local reflexes involving the final common pathway are of particular importance: stretch reflexes, the lengthening reflex, and Renshaw inhibition. Of these, the stretch reflex is of the most clinical importance because it is the basis of the neurologic testing of tendon reflexes. The *stretch reflex* is a simple two-neuron reflex arising by stimulation of a muscle spindle and ending with activation of the motor unit (Fig. 9-3).

Fig. 9-4. Muscle spindle. A. Entire spindle with axons innervating it. B. Detailed longitudinal view of spindle at its center and at one end. C. Cross-sectional view of spindle at middle (A-A) and end (B-B).

THE MUSCLE SPINDLES.   Striated muscles are rich in sensory receptors, containing muscle spindles, Golgi tendon organs, and bare nerve endings. Of these sensory organs, the muscle spindles are by far the most complex and best understood. The *muscle spindle* is a group of specialized muscle fibers with two types of sensory receptors, the *primary* and *secondary endings,* which measure the length and velocity of stretch in a muscle. The muscle spindle fibers are referred to as intrafusal fibers (inside the muscle spindle) in contrast to the extrafusal fibers that make up the bulk of the muscle.

The muscle spindles are arranged parallel with the extrafusal muscle fibers. Each spindle is surrounded by a connective tissue capsule that connects the spindle to the origin and insertion of the muscle. Within the connective tissue capsule are two types of intrafusal muscle fibers, the large-diameter, longer *nuclear bag* fibers and the smaller *nuclear chain* fibers. The former have a number of nuclei close together in the middle, while in the latter, the nuclei are distributed evenly throughout the length of the muscle fiber (Fig. 9-4).

The *primary sensory ending* or *annulospiral*

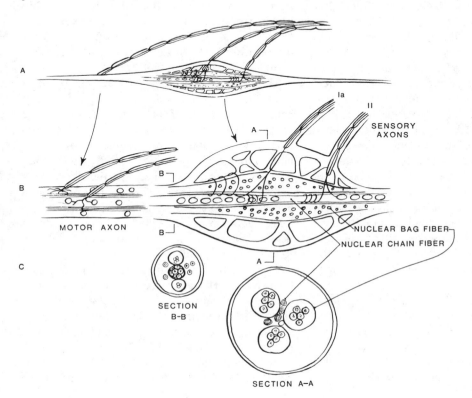

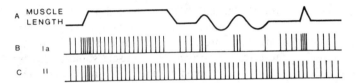

Fig. 9-5. Responses of afferent fibers from muscle spindle. A. Length of muscle-containing spindle. Muscle length is changed with various waveforms of stretch. B. Response of type Ia afferent fibers from primary ending of spindle. C. Response of type II afferent fibers from secondary ending of spindle. Type Ia afferents respond to rapid stretch; type II afferents respond to length.

ending of the muscle spindle forms a spiral around both the nuclear bag fibers and the nuclear chain fibers. This sensory ending gives rise to large-diameter, fast-conducting afferent nerve fibers (type Ia) which end monosynaptically in the spinal cord on the motor neurons of the muscle of origin and synergistic muscles. Collateral branches from the primary afferent fibers pass up the posterior columns to other levels and also connect via interneurons to the motor neurons of antagonistic muscles. The spindle *secondary sensory endings* or *flower spray endings* are almost exclusively on nuclear chain fibers. They give rise to smaller-diameter and therefore slower-conducting (type II) afferent axons which connect with motor neurons only via interneurons. Primary and secondary afferents from the muscle spindle make up a large proportion of the direct sensory input to the final common pathway.

Both primary and secondary sensory endings are sensitive to stretch in the intrafusal fibers. They may be activated by stretch of the skeletal muscle containing the spindle or by contraction of the intrafusal muscle fibers in the spindle. Because of differences in viscosity, the two types of intrafusal fibers differ in their response to stretch, and their discharges are divided into dynamic (phasic) and static (tonic) phases. The former occurs during the period of stretching; the latter occurs while the sensory endings are held stretched (Fig. 9-5).

The action potentials from the type Ia muscle spindle afferents are excitatory to the anterior horn cells that innervate synergistic muscles and are inhibitory to antagonistic muscles (Fig.9-6). Thus, sudden activation of the spindles in a muscle results in a brisk muscle contraction. The re-

sponse of the primary endings in the muscle spindle to a quick stretch is the basis of stretch reflexes, called *myotatic reflexes,* in which the physician taps a tendon with a reflex hammer and produces a stretch of the muscle. The resulting discharge of a large number of type Ia afferents is sufficient to activate the anterior horn cells on which these afferents end and to cause a muscle twitch. Therefore, a loss of either the afferent fibers or the lower motor neuron results in a loss of myotatic reflexes.

A common clinical test is to gauge the resistance of a muscle to passive movement. Normally, when the examiner moves a limb and a muscle is stretched, there is a mild resistance to the passive movement, referred to as *muscle tone.* Tone is due in part to the intrinsic elasticity of the tissue, but it is also a result of the activation of motor units with stretching of the muscle spindles. An increase in the input to the alpha or gamma motor neurons results in an increase in muscle tone (hypertonia). A reduction in either the afferent input from the muscle spindles or the efferent activity of the lower motor neurons results in a decrease of muscle tone (hypotonia).

The central connections of the type II axons from the secondary spindle endings are more complex than those of the primary endings. Like the type Ia endings, they have monosynaptic, excitatory connections with synergistic muscles and have inhibitory connections with antagonistic muscles so that they may participate in the myotatic reflexes. However, they also have more widespread, polysynaptic connections that have a longer duration of action, which may be part of flexion reflexes in which a limb is withdrawn from noxious stimuli.

The type II axons also participate in the clasp-knife reflex. The increased tone in patients with upper motor neuron lesions decreases with passive stretch of the muscle. This reduction in tone has been likened to the rapid snapping shut of a pocket knife (clasp knife). The reduction in hypertonia with muscle stretching is length dependent, that is, the tone decreases in direct

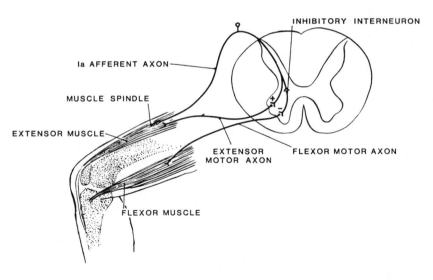

INHIBITORY INTERNEURON

Ia AFFERENT AXON

MUSCLE SPINDLE

EXTENSOR MUSCLE

EXTENSOR MOTOR AXON

FLEXOR MOTOR AXON

FLEXOR MUSCLE

Fig. 9-6. Central connections of a type Ia afferent fiber from muscle spindle. Spindle activity activates the muscle and inhibits the antagonist.

proportion to the increase in muscle length. Muscle length is signaled by the secondary muscle spindle endings, which therefore mediate the clasp-knife reflex.

For a muscle spindle to respond appropriately to a stretch or change in muscle length, the spindle length must be adjusted as the length of the muscle changes. This is accomplished through a separate motor innervation of the spindle fibers. The motor innervation of the intrafusal muscle fibers is known as the *fusimotor system* (and comes from gamma motor neurons) (Fig. 9-7). The neuromuscular terminations of the fusimotor system are of two types: *plate endings* and *trail*

endings. The former are discrete single endings, while the latter are diffuse multiple endings. These endings can preferentially increase either the phasic (changing) discharge from the muscle spindle or the tonic (maintained) discharge. The independent motor control of the two types of intrafusal muscle fibers allows independent control of the spindle's phasic and tonic discharges. Such control is of considerable importance in maintaining stability of the stretch reflex during movements.

During a muscle contraction, the type Ia fiber discharge would be completely suppressed by "unloading" if the gamma motor neuron were not simultaneously active. Therefore, gamma motor neurons are coactivated with the alpha motor neurons to a muscle in order to maintain the spindle receptor sensitivity to unexpected movements (Fig. 9-8).

Muscle spindles are not equally distributed throughout the muscles. More are present in slow muscles, such as the soleus, than in fast muscles, such as the gastrocnemius. Within the spinal

Fig. 9-7. Gamma motor system. Contraction of intrafusal fibers by gamma motor neurons can maintain a muscle spindle at proper length to respond to muscle stretch, even though the muscle changes length.

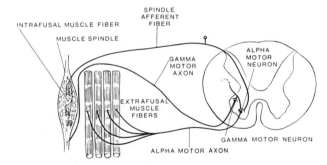

INTRAFUSAL MUSCLE FIBER

MUSCLE SPINDLE

SPINDLE AFFERENT FIBER

GAMMA MOTOR AXON

ALPHA MOTOR NEURON

EXTRAFUSAL MUSCLE FIBERS

GAMMA MOTOR NEURON

ALPHA MOTOR AXON

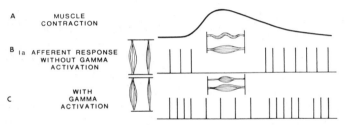

Fig. 9-8. Effect of gamma motor neuron activation. A. Length of muscle (muscle contraction) as it actively contracts. B. Action potential discharges in type Ia afferent fibers during muscle contraction without gamma motor neuron activation. C. Type Ia afferent firing during muscle contraction with gamma motor neuron activation.

cord, there is a concentration of monosynaptic spindle afferents on the synergistic slow motor neurons. The spindle mechanism is thus of greater importance in control of the tonic activity of slow muscles.

Another important sensory structure in muscle is the *Golgi tendon organ*, a sensory receptor with type Ib axons that is sensitive to tension and is located in the tendon. Because it is in series with the extrafusal muscle fibers, the Golgi tendon organ increases its discharge rate in response to an increase in tension, whether generated by passive stretch or active muscle contraction (Fig. 9-9). This is in contrast to the muscle spindle, which is in parallel with the extrafusal muscle fibers and increases its discharge rate with passive stretch of the muscle, but not with muscle contraction (Fig. 9-10).

Through interneurons, the Golgi tendon organ

inhibits the motor neurons to the same muscle and synergistic muscles and excites motor neurons to antagonistic muscles (Fig. 9-10). The Golgi tendon organ thereby provides a direct tension feedback mechanism for either increases or decreases in tension.

Renshaw loops originate as collateral branches from the axons of alpha motor neurons. The axon branches synapse with interneurons (the Renshaw cells) that inhibit the motor neurons of synergistic muscles. Activity in such a loop temporarily inhibits the motor neurons. The function of the Renshaw loop is probably to stabilize the discharge frequency of motor neuron pools and generally to prevent the neurons from discharging at excessive rates. The Renshaw loops originate mainly from the motor neurons innervating fast-

Fig. 9-10. Muscle spindle and Golgi tendon organ. A. Central connections of types Ia and Ib afferents. On left, the type Ia connections produce excitation (+) of synergistic muscles (myotatic reflex) and inhibition (−) of antagonistic muscles through inhibitory interneurons. On right, the type Ib connections produce inhibition of synergistic muscles through an inhibitory interneuron (−). B. Effects of passive muscle stretch (1) and active muscle contraction (3) on action potential firing in type Ia axons from muscle spindle and type Ib axons from tendon organ.

Fig. 9-9. Golgi tendon organ. A. Schematic diagram. B. Action potentials in afferents from Golgi tendon organ are shown as muscle is passively stretched. C. Afferent activity with active muscle contraction.

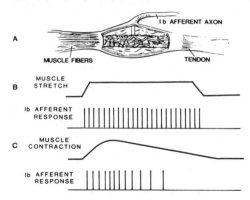

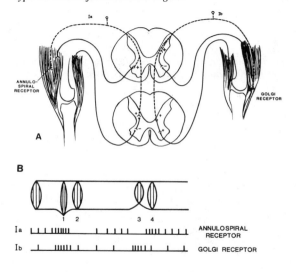

twitch motor units, but act primarily on the smaller alpha motor neurons that innervate slow-twitch skeletal muscle fibers. The primary function of slow motor units is to subserve static postural functions, and the primary function of the fast motor units is to produce phasic movements. The asymmetric Renshaw inhibitory distribution thus also acts to subdue the postural stretch reflexes in slow muscle during the activity of phasic motor neurons.

Integration in the Final Common Pathway

We have just discussed some of the input that impinges on the motor neuron: afferent activity from the muscle spindles, the Golgi tendon organs, and the Renshaw cells. In addition to sensory input, the anterior horn cell receives input from three other major sources: the direct activation pathway, the indirect activation pathway, and other segments of the spinal cord. Each of these sources may transmit excitatory or inhibitory impulses to the final common pathway, which are integrated by the anterior horn cells before they respond. Figure 9-11 is a schematic diagram of the major descending pathways that act on the final common pathway and their relationship to one another. These will be described in the remainder of this chapter.

Clinical Correlations

Diseases may affect the final common pathway at the anterior horn cell, the axon, or the muscle fiber. However, damage to all these sites has common clinical features that permit the clinician to identify disease of the motor unit. These include weakness, atrophy, loss of reflexes, and loss of tone. Other features that may indicate abnormal function of the motor unit include fasciculations, cramps, and excessive contraction.

In the weakness or paralysis due to final common pathway disease, there is an inability to obtain voluntary contraction, a loss of involuntary movements, and a loss of reflex contraction of the muscle. The weakness occurs either because the action potentials cannot be transmitted to the muscle owing to disease of the lower motor neuron, or because diseased muscle fibers cannot respond to the action potentials of the lower motor neurons.

The strength of a muscle is generally proportional to its size: a little old lady has less strength than a young weight lifter, though both have normal muscle function. A physician must evaluate strength in proportion to size. The loss of muscle bulk in disease is referred to as *atrophy* and is often found with weakness due to disease of the final common pathway. Two types of atrophy must be differentiated. The first, *neurogenic atrophy,* occurs with loss of innervation, when a muscle undergoes atrophy and is weak (out of proportion to its size). The second, *disuse atrophy,* occurs with lack of use of the muscle. In disuse atrophy, strength is appropriate to the size of the muscle. Disuse atrophy is not a sign of disease of the neuromuscular system, whereas neurogenic atrophy is. Atrophy may also occur in muscle disease.

In general, if the lower motor neurons are lost, reflexes, in particular the tendon reflexes, are also

Fig. 9-11. Descending pathways and major areas in the brain that act on final common pathway.

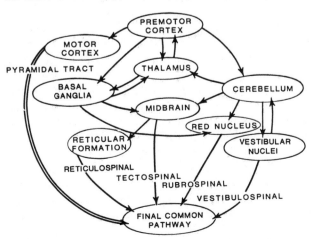

lost. They are most consistently lost if the disease process damages the afferent fibers of the reflex arc. Disruption of the reflex arc also results in loss of the normal tone or response to passive movement. This state is called *flaccidity,* and the weakness with disease of the final common pathway is *flaccid paralysis*.

Weakness, flaccidity, and atrophy also occur in the face, tongue, and pharyngeal muscles, with disease of the lower motor neurons in the brain stem. This results in a characteristic breathy, imprecise, nasal speech called *flaccid dysarthria* (dysarthria = abnormal utterances).

Diseases of the motor unit also may be associated with excessive activity or spontaneous firing, with a low threshold for discharge. This may take the form of a single, spontaneous discharge of a motor unit, a *fasciculation*. A fasciculation can be seen on the surface of the skin as a brief, localized twitch. A continuous, high-frequency discharge of fascicles of muscle fibers is a cramp. Both may be manifestations of disease, or may be due simply to "physiologic irritability," such as can occur after excessive exertion. After destruction of the lower motor neuron, the muscle fibers that have lost their innervation will generate slow repetitive action potentials and contract regularly, a process called *fibrillation*. Fibrillations are not visible through the skin.

Direct Activation Pathway

Anatomy and Physiology

The direct activation pathway is the second of the three major influences on the final common pathway. It is a direct route without synapses from the cerebral cortex in each hemisphere to the ventral horn on the opposite side of the spinal cord and to the motor nuclei in the brain stem. The fibers in the direct activation pathway are corticospinal and corticobulbar. Those traveling to the spinal cord are called the *corticospinal tract* or the *pyramidal tract*. Those ending on brain-stem nuclei are corticobulbar fibers. The neurons from which these tracts arise are known as upper motor neurons (Fig. 9-12). The major function of the direct activation pathway is to initiate and control skilled voluntary activity.

Each corticospinal tract arises primarily from cells in the cortex of the frontal lobe of one hemisphere and descends through the corona radiata into the internal capsule. The tract passes from the internal capsule via the cerebral peduncles to the base of the brain stem, where it forms the medullary pyramids. At the caudal end of the pyramids, most of the tract from each side decussates to the opposite side to lie in the lateral funiculus of the spinal cord as the lateral corticospinal tract.

The name corticospinal tract is based on its origin and termination. The pyramidal tract is so named because of its association with the *medullary pyramids,* the large, paired fiber tracts on the ventral surface of the medulla. Properly speaking, only the corticospinal fibers, in contradistinction to corticobulbar fibers, pass through the pyramids; but it is common to include in the pyramidal tract both the upper motor neurons to the spinal cord (corticospinal) and similar (so-called supranuclear) fibers to the brain-stem motor nuclei (corticobulbar). It was formerly believed that the fibers of the pyramidal tract originated in the giant Betz cells of the fifth layer of the motor cortex in the precentral gyrus (area 4 in Brodmann's numbering system), but only a small percentage (about 2%) so originate. The bulk of the fibers arise from other cells in the precentral cortex (area 4 and probably area 6 in Brodmann's system) and a few from the postcentral gyrus. The remaining fibers are believed to originate in the prefrontal, parietal, and possibly even the occipital and temporal lobes.

MOTOR CORTEX. The motor cortex occupies the anterior lip of the central sulcus of Rolando and the adjacent precentral gyrus (area 4) (Fig. 9-13). It has a somatotopic organization with the contralateral body represented upside down just as in sensory cortex (see Fig. 7-2): the head area is located above the fissure of Sylvius, the upper extremity next with the thumb and index finger in proximity to the face, the trunk interposed between the shoulder and hip areas high on the convexity, and the lower limb representation extending onto the paracentral lobule in the longitudinal fissure. The size of the cortical representation varies with the functional importance of the part represented. Thus, the lips, jaw, thumb, and index finger have a large representation; the forehead, trunk, and proximal portions of the limbs have a small one. As in other areas

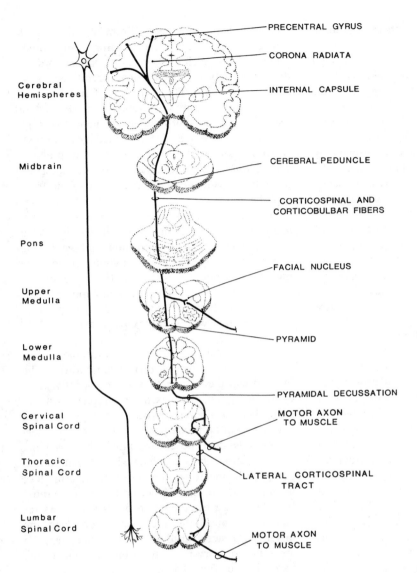

PRECENTRAL GYRUS

CORONA RADIATA

INTERNAL CAPSULE

Cerebral
Hemispheres

Midbrain

CEREBRAL PEDUNCLE

CORTICOSPINAL AND
CORTICOBULBAR FIBERS

Pons

FACIAL NUCLEUS

Upper
Medulla

PYRAMID

Lower
Medulla

PYRAMIDAL DECUSSATION

MOTOR AXON
TO MUSCLE

Cervical
Spinal Cord

Thoracic
Spinal Cord

LATERAL CORTICOSPINAL
TRACT

Lumbar
Spinal Cord

MOTOR AXON
TO MUSCLE

Fig. 9-12. Corticospinal tract. Course of fibers in tract is shown descending through cerebral hemispheres, brain stem, and spinal cord. The tract is composed of axons extending the entire length, as shown schematically for a single neuron on the left.

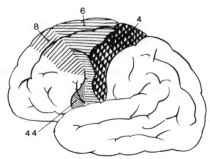

Fig. 9-13. Lateral view of cerebral hemisphere with motor areas (Brodmann's numbering) indicated. Area 4 is motor cortex; area 6 is premotor cortex; area 8 includes the frontal eye fields; area 44 is motor cortex for speech (Broca's area).

of the central nervous system, there are more neurons in the areas subserving delicate and complex functions. The cortical areas in the frontal lobe anterior to the precentral gyrus are also concerned with motor function, but at a higher level. They may be considered areas of cortical programming of voluntary activity. Area 6 is an area controlling the performance of background activity in support of the direct activity initiated by the cell columns in area 4. Inferiorly, near the face area is *Broca's area* (area 44) where speech is formulated. Higher, in area 8, voluntary eye movements are controlled.

Within the motor cortex, topographic localization is not as strict as in other areas (for example, sensory and visual). The motor cortex, however, is functionally subdivided into vertical columns or cells which are concerned with types of movements. These functions, however, can be readily subsumed by other columns. This functional flexibility of the motor cortex is exemplified in several ways. For example, ablation of a small area leads to temporary rather than permanent paralysis, and the result of electrical stimulation varies with the parameters of stimulation. The result of electrical activation also varies with the antecedent set of the area, as determined by previous activity. Thus, repetition of a stimulus after a conditioning shock may elicit a larger (facilitation) or a smaller (inhibition) response, or the opposite response, as when flexion results from a stimulus that previously yielded extension. The activity induced by electrical stimulation of the cortex may continue for some time after cessation of the stimulus. This *afterdischarge* has been attributed to reverberation within cortical circuits, and its peripheral manifestations of tonic (maintained contractions) or clonic (alternating contractions) movements are the experimental equivalent of the corresponding phases of a seizure.

Experimentally, individual muscle contractions have been elicited from cortical stimulation of motor neurons that are organized in columns. Such contractions are fragments of movement, the pieces out of which it is built by the cortical interconnections. The neurons that give rise to the corticospinal tracts generate action potentials in response to sensory input, and these are relayed to individual muscles. The input to these cells in the motor cortex includes a multitude of excitations and inhibitions. Thus, a given area of cortex may be regarded as a reflex center on

which afferents impinge and from which efferents project. Motor cortical areas differ from simpler reflex centers, such as those in the spinal cord, in the complexity of the neuronal circuits and synaptic connections. The synthesis of fragments of movement into useful movements is effected in the motor cortex, but complex behavior, with its sequences of movement, is mediated through wider areas of cortex than the motor strip alone. The voluntary initiation and control of motor activity includes much of the convexity of the frontal lobe.

Other cortical motor areas exist besides the primary motor area previously described. These also have a somatotopic organization and lie in the upper lip of the fissure of Sylvius (secondary motor area) and on the medial surface of the cerebral hemisphere (supplementary motor area). Epileptic involvement of these areas can produce motor seizures with complex patterns.

INTERNAL CAPSULE. Axons from the motor cortex converge in the corona radiata toward the internal capsule, where they are compactly gathered. Here, too, there is a topographic localization. The corticobulbar fibers occupy a more anterior location in the posterior limb of the internal capsule than the corticospinal fibers, so that the projection fibers are located from anterior to posterior in the following order: face, arm, leg, bladder, and rectum. Anterior to the pyramidal tract fibers are frontopontine fibers and fibers reciprocally connecting the frontal lobe and the thalamus; posterior to the pyramidal fibers are the ascending sensory tracts from the thalamus to the parietal lobe (Fig. 9-14).

BRAIN STEM. The pyramidal fibers remain grouped together as they pass from the internal capsule to the cerebral peduncle in the midbrain. In the midbrain, the corticospinal and corticobulbar fibers occupy the middle two-thirds of the cerebral peduncle, with the corticobulbar fibers being more medial. During their course in the brain stem, the corticobulbar fibers leave the pyramidal pathway at several levels, some crossing the midline and some remaining uncrossed. These connect with the motor nuclei of the cranial nerves—oculomotor, trochlear, abducens, trigeminal, facial, vagus, spinal accessory, and hypoglossal.

In the pons, the descending pyramidal fibers

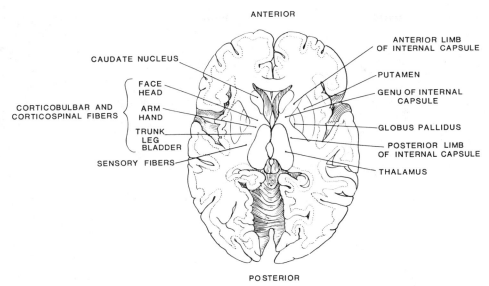

Fig. 9-14. Horizontal section of cerebral hemisphere showing somatotopic representations of motor function in internal capsule.

are split into small bundles by the interspersed pontine nuclei. The topographic localization persists with the face medially, leg laterally, and the upper limb in the intermediate position. The fibers reunite in the medulla to form the medullary pyramids. At the lower border of the medulla, the main pyramidal decussation occurs, and about 80 percent of the fibers cross over to the opposite side of the spinal cord.

SPINAL CORD.   In the spinal cord, the crossed pyramidal fibers occupy the lateral column (the lateral corticospinal tract) (Fig. 9-15), and the much smaller number of uncrossed pyramidal fibers descend in the anterior column (the anterior corticospinal tract) to the cervical and thoracic levels. There is doubt whether the anterior corticospinal fibers ultimately cross or remain un-

Fig. 9-15. Somatotopic representation of motor function in lateral corticospinal tract. (C = cervical, Th = thoracic, L = lumbar, S = sacral.)

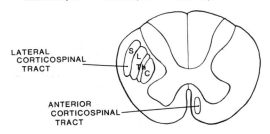

crossed; it is likely that some of them remain uncrossed and are responsible for the ipsilateral innervation of certain muscle groups.

Crossed Innervation

Because of the decussation of most of the fibers of the pyramidal tracts, the voluntary movements of one side of the body are under the control of the opposite cerebral hemisphere. However, there are some exceptions to this rule which are of importance in clinical diagnosis. In general, muscle groups of the two sides of the body that habitually act in unison tend to have a bilateral cortical innervation, whereas muscle groups that act alone in isolated, delicate, and especially in learned movements tend to have a unilateral representation from the opposite hemisphere. Thus, paraspinal muscles are innervated by both hemispheres, as are the muscles in the upper half of the face (Fig. 9-16). Because of this arrangement, a massive lesion of one hemisphere will cause severe weakness of the opposite side of the body but not of upper facial or paraspinal muscles. These principles do not apply in all cases, however. Even in muscles such as those of the tongue and the palate, which might be expected to work in unison, there is a greater innervation from the contralateral hemisphere.

Effect on Final Common Pathway

The action potentials descending in the pyramidal tracts travel to the ventral horn of the spinal cord, where they may synapse directly on motor neurons or, more commonly, act on them through

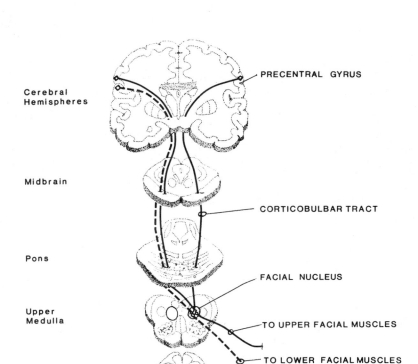

Cerebral
Hemispheres

PRECENTRAL GYRUS

Midbrain

CORTICOBULBAR TRACT

Pons

FACIAL NUCLEUS

Upper
Medulla

TO UPPER FACIAL MUSCLES

TO LOWER FACIAL MUSCLES

Lower
Medulla

Fig. 9-16. Crossed innervation of motor neurons to the facial muscles on one side. The upper facial muscles have bilateral control; lower facial muscles have unilateral control from contralateral hemisphere.

interneurons. The corticospinal fibers act on all motor neuron pools but particularly on distal muscles of the arm and hand. They have relatively little tonic effect, although there is some tonic excitation of arm extensors and leg flexors.

Clinical Correlations

Knowledge of the clinical manifestations of disease of the direct activation pathway comes equally from experimental studies and from observation of clinical disorders. For example, the pattern of clinical seizures and results of cortical stimulation have done much to reveal the functional anatomy of the brain. Similarly, planned, discrete ablations in the experimental laboratory and therapeutic ablations by surgery have filled out the knowledge gained from the study of random lesions of disease.

Disturbances of the corticospinal system may be irritative or paralytic (positive or negative). These two types of disturbance are clinically ex-

emplified by seizures and paralysis and experimentally exemplified by the results of stimulation and ablation. John Hughlings Jackson, from his study of the attacks that now bear his name (jacksonian seizures), surmised that there must be somatotopic representation of motor function in the brain. Focal motor seizures are likely to start in the cortical areas governing the thumb and index finger, the corner of the mouth, or the great toe, because of the relatively large extent of those areas. The spread (march) of the attack is determined by the pattern of cortical localization. Thus, a seizure starting in the thumb and index finger may spread to involve the wrist, elbow, shoulder, trunk, and lower limb, spreading from hip to foot.

While the terminations of the corticospinal pathways act on all the cells of the ventral horn, including alpha and gamma motor neurons, they seem to have their major influence on the motor neurons in the lateral portions of the ventral horns, that is, on those controlling the distal movements of the extremities. Lesions limited to the pyramidal pathways will therefore result in a characteristic clinical pattern. There is weakness or paralysis of muscles, especially the distal muscles of the extremities. The impairment is greatest for fine movements, skilled movements, and movements under voluntary control. The paralysis is not associated with atrophy, and reflexes may be preserved, although they are often mildly reduced. The muscles are flaccid, with a reduced tone, because of loss of excitatory input to the gamma motor neurons.

The distribution of the weakness is a function of the site of the lesion. If the lesion is localized in a limited area of cortex, then a single limb or one side of the face only may be involved. If the lesion involves only the pyramidal tract fibers in the pyramids of the medulla, then one side of the body below the level of the lesion will be affected. The distribution also depends on whether innervation is unilateral or bilateral. For example, the upper part of the face is spared when corticobulbar lesions involve facial fibers. If the lesion involves the frontal eye fields, there will be paralysis of conjugate eye movements to the opposite side.

In addition to the weakness, hypotonia, and reduction in reflexes, certain specific signs occur with lesions of the corticospinal pathway. The abdominal and cremasteric reflexes are segmental reflexes that depend on an intact pyramidal tract. With a pyramidal lesion, these reflexes will be lost on one side. Some abnormal reflexes become manifest after a corticospinal tract lesion. The response to uncomfortable stimulation of the sole of the foot when the pyramidal pathway is damaged is a dorsiflexion of the great toe and a spreading of the other toes. This is *Babinski's sign* and is a fractionated withdrawal reflex mediated by local spinal cord mechanisms akin to a nociceptive withdrawal reflex. In the normal adult, the corticospinal pathway suppresses this withdrawal response, and the toes are immobile or curl down. With damage to the corticospinal tract, this suppression is lost and Babinski's sign appears. In a similar fashion, gentle stroking of the palm elicits an abnormal grasping response, the *grasp reflex,* when there is motor cortex damage.

The occurrence of this pattern of a distal flaccid paralysis with Babinski's sign is unusual and occurs *only* with small lesions in the medullary pyramids or in the primary motor cortex. In other areas, such as the internal capsule and the spinal cord, these pyramidal pathways (direct activation)

are intermingled with fibers of the indirect activation pathways (the extrapyramidal system). The results of combined damage to these systems are significantly different from the flaccid hemiplegia previously described. As will be described in detail in the next section, damage to indirect pathways adds increased tone and spasticity to the list of clinical findings.

Lesions involving anterior portions of the frontal lobe may spare the primary motor cortex and produce no weakness. However, such lesions can result in impairment of the voluntary activation of the motor system. The loss of the ability to perform skilled motor acts by will when they can still be elicited automatically or reflexly is called *apraxia.* Apraxia may be considered the highest-level abnormality of motor function in which the initiation of complex movements is lost. Apraxia may involve any of the motor activities, including speech and movements of the arms, legs, or eyes. Apraxia of *speech* is characterized by an inability to say a word at will, while still being able to think of it and to utter it correctly, automatically or reflexly. Motor apraxia of speech is sometimes referred to as a type of aphasia (loss of speech).

The localization of lesions along the pyramidal pathways is relatively straightforward. Widespread cortical lesions may involve all of one side of the body, but a facial, arm, or leg monoplegia is more likely with a lesion of the cerebral cortex. Occasionally, the arm and face are involved together because of their proximity (often with apraxia of speech if the lesion is in the dominant hemisphere). More anterior lesions of the frontal cortex may result in impaired voluntary eye movements or apraxia of motor activity. Lesions in the internal capsule or cerebral peduncles typically produce weakness of the opposite arm and leg and opposite side of the face.

Cortical lesions also may have positive manifestations such as focal seizures. However, seizures do not occur with a lesion of the direct activation pathway at lower levels, for example in the internal capsule or below, where the findings are those of a loss of function such as weakness.

The level of lesions along the pathway sometimes can be identified by the associated segmental involvement of other structures, such as one of the cranial nerves in the case of a brain-stem lesion or one of the spinal nerves in cases of cord lesions.

MOTOR NEURON DISEASE. Some diseases seem to selectively affect the motor system. One of these is *amyotrophic lateral sclerosis* or *motor neuron disease.* It is a progressive, degenerative disease of unknown cause. Pathologically, this condition is characterized by degeneration of the motor cells in the spinal cord, brain stem, and cerebral cortex, associated with secondary axonal degeneration in the peripheral nerves and in the lateral funiculus of the spinal cord (corticospinal tract).

Motor neuron disease expresses itself with varying degrees of involvement in the final common pathway and the direct and indirect activation pathways. Damage to the final common pathway results in diseased anterior horn cells, which are initially irritable, producing frequent, widespread fasciculations. After death and degeneration of the lower motor neurons, there is a combination of flaccid weakness and atrophy of muscle. The denervated muscle fibrillates, although this is not seen clinically. Involvement of the descending pathways may produce Babinski's sign and hyperactive reflexes as well.

Indirect Activation Pathways

Anatomy and Physiology
The third major division of the motor system is also a source of input to the final common pathway. It consists of axons from the cerebral hemispheres to the red nucleus and reticular formation and three fiber tracts from these nuclei and the vestibular nuclei to the lower motor neuron: the vestibulospinal, the reticulospinal, and the rubrospinal tracts. The indirect pathways maintain posture, tone, and the associated activities needed to provide the framework on which the direct activation pathway can accomplish its specific skilled actions. The indirect pathways extending from the brain stem to the spinal cord are sometimes called *extrapyramidal pathways* because they are not in the medullary pyramids. Since clinicians sometimes use *extrapyramidal* to refer only to the basal ganglion, the term *indirect activation pathways* will be used for the descending motor pathways to the lower motor neurons that are not in the pyramids.

The greatest amount of suprasegmental (or supraspinal) reinforcement of the motor neurons controlling posture comes from projection systems that originate in the reticular formation and vestibular nuclei (group A descending pathways). Group A fibers facilitate extensor muscle activation and flexor muscle inhibition. In the normal person, these systems are balanced by activity from the cerebral cortex and other forebrain structures, which inhibits extensor muscle contraction and facilitates flexor activation via corticoreticular pathways. If these cortical controls are rendered nonfunctional, the unchecked pontine-medullary pathways make the extensor motor neurons hyperexcitable, a condition manifested clinically as increased tone or spasticity. Which muscles will manifest spasticity depends on the level of the lesion. Motor control by group A fibers is particularly strong to axial and proximal muscles.

DESCENDING INFLUENCES FROM THE RETICULAR FORMATION. The reticular formation is a field of dispersed cells or small nuclei in between large nuclei and tracts throughout the medulla and the pontine and mesencephalic tegmentum. In addition to mediating ascending sensory activity and consciousness as described in Chapters 7 and 8, it has complex and mixed effects on spinal cord motor neurons. Two major areas of the reticular formation produce relatively consistent and contrasting motor effects.

The *excitatory dorsolateral reticular formation* extends from the midbrain through the rostral medulla. Activity in this part of the reticular formation produces excitation of extensor motor neurons and inhibition of flexor motor neurons, which are manifest as postural tone. Pontine reticulospinal fibers originating from cells in the excitatory, dorsolateral reticular formation descend uncrossed in the medial part of the anterior funiculus of the spinal cord as the medial reticulospinal tract. They terminate in the ventral medial portion of the ventral horn mainly on gamma motor neurons (Fig. 9-17).

The *inhibitory ventromedial reticular formation* is situated in the caudal portion of the medulla. Activity in this region produces mixed effects, most frequently inhibition of extensor motor neurons and excitation of flexors. This region depends on descending stimulation from supratentorial motor structures; that is, inhibition by reticulospinal pathways requires their excitation by rostral motor areas. Medullary reticulospinal fibers are crossed and uncrossed and descend in

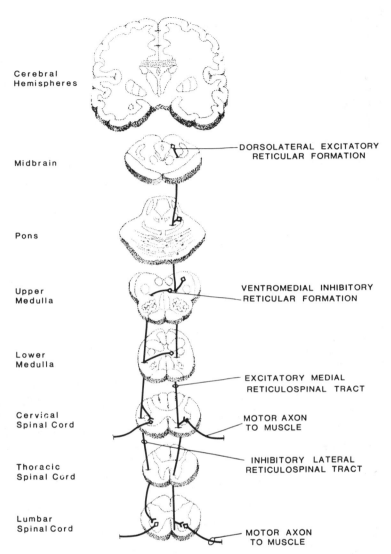

Cerebral
Hemispheres

Midbrain

DORSOLATERAL EXCITATORY
RETICULAR FORMATION

Pons

Upper
Medulla

VENTROMEDIAL INHIBITORY
RETICULAR FORMATION

Lower
Medulla

EXCITATORY MEDIAL
RETICULOSPINAL TRACT

Cervical
Spinal Cord

MOTOR AXON
TO MUSCLE

Thoracic
Spinal Cord

INHIBITORY LATERAL
RETICULOSPINAL TRACT

Lumbar
Spinal Cord

MOTOR AXON
TO MUSCLE

Fig. 9-17. Reticulospinal pathways. Both tracts are present bilaterally but are shown only on one side. The medial reticulospinal tract arising from the excitatory dorsolateral reticular formation is shown on the right. The lateral reticulospinal tract arising from the inhibitory ventromedial reticular formation is shown on the left.

the spinal cord in the anterior part of the lateral funiculus as the lateral reticulospinal tract. They terminate in the dorsolateral part of the ventral horn, in the same areas where the corticospinal tracts terminate (Fig. 9-17).

DESCENDING INFLUENCES FROM THE VESTIBULAR NUCLEI. The vestibular system consists of a group of brain-stem nuclei receiving sensory in-

put from the vestibular apparatus and the cerebellum and projecting in turn to brain-stem, cerebellar, and spinal cord terminations. Ascending and descending brain-stem projections of the vestibular nuclei run in the medial longitudinal fasciculus. These projections modulate motor neuron activity of eye and neck muscles and will be considered in greater detail in Chapter 14 (The Posterior Fossa Level).

The lateral vestibular nucleus is the source of the major vestibular projection to spinal motor neurons. This nucleus receives primary afferent input from the vestibular nerve, as well as other input from the cerebellum. Activity in the nucleus produces excitation of extensor motor neurons, while the effects on flexor motor neurons

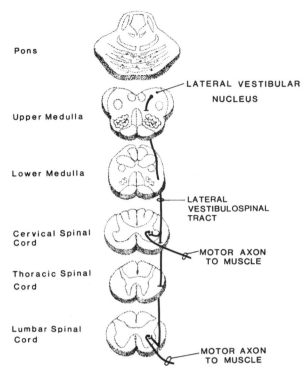

Pons

LATERAL VESTIBULAR
NUCLEUS

Upper Medulla

Lower Medulla

LATERAL
VESTIBULOSPINAL
TRACT

Cervical Spinal
Cord

MOTOR AXON
TO MUSCLE

Thoracic Spinal
Cord

Lumbar Spinal
Cord

MOTOR AXON
TO MUSCLE

Fig. 9-18. The vestibulospinal tract arising from the lateral vestibular nucleus is bilateral but is shown on only one side.

are generally insignificant. Descending discharges through this system are seen in the tendency to fall after rapid whirling. The *vestibulospinal tract,* which originates from cells in the lateral vestibular nucleus, descends mostly uncrossed in the anterior funiculus of the spinal cord. These fibers terminate in the ventromedial portion of the ventral horn on both alpha and gamma motor neurons, which also receive terminals of the pontine reticulospinal tract. Additional, less important vestibulospinal fibers descend crossed in the anterior funiculus of the spinal cord as a caudal extension of the medial longitudinal fasciculus to the rostral portions of the spinal cord (Fig. 9-18).

OTHER DESCENDING INFLUENCES ON SPINAL NEURONS.   The *rubrospinal tract* originates in the *red nucleus,* and the fibers immediately decussate in the ventral tegmental decussation to descend on the opposite side. The tract occupies about the same position as the lateral corticospinal tract with which its fibers intermingle in the spinal cord. The sites of termination are much the same, but few *rubrospinal fibers* reach the lower spinal

cord, so that the main rubrospinal influence is upon flexor muscles of the upper extremities (Fig. 9-19).

The red nucleus receives cortical projections that retain somatotopic organization and provides another indirect path from the cortex to the spinal cord. Other input (cerebellum and basal ganglia) can modify the descending activity in the red nucleus. The rubrospinal tract is not well defined in humans; although some authors consider that it is rudimentary, others think that it projects through the length of the spinal cord. It is constituted mainly of small fibers. The rubrospinal tract, unlike the other indirect pathways, has different effects on the motor neurons to the arms and the legs. It facilitates the activity in arm flexors but has little effect on leg muscles.

There is little consensus as to the functional significance of other brain-stem projections to the spinal cord. The *tectospinal tract* is believed to be important in mediating reflex movements of the head and eyes in response to visual or auditory stimuli. This tract originates from cells in the superior colliculus, crosses in the brain stem, and descends near the medial longitudinal fasciculus. In the spinal cord, the tract travels in the anterior funiculus and does not extend below the cervical levels. Fibers terminate in the ventrome-

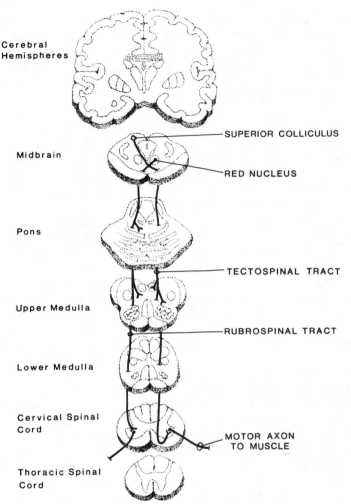

Cerebral Hemispheres

Midbrain

SUPERIOR COLLICULUS

RED NUCLEUS

Pons

TECTOSPINAL TRACT

Upper Medulla

RUBROSPINAL TRACT

Lower Medulla

Cervical Spinal Cord

MOTOR AXON TO MUSCLE

Thoracic Spinal Cord

Fig. 9-19. Rubrospinal and tectospinal pathways, though both bilateral, are shown unilaterally. Rubrospinal tract is shown descending on the left. It arises in red nucleus on opposite side. Tectospinal tract is shown descending on right after arising in colliculus on left.

dial regions along with the pontine reticulospinal and vestibulospinal tracts (Fig. 9-19).

Effects on the Final Common Pathway

In general, the response of a gamma motor neuron to a particular stimulus is the same as that of the corresponding alpha motor neuron; that is, both gamma and alpha neurons innervating extensor muscles are excited by the vestibulospinal tract and the pontine reticulospinal tract. However, gamma motor neurons have lower response thresholds to all forms of stimulation than do alpha motor neurons, so that stimuli insufficient to produce alpha motor neuron discharge may be sufficient to discharge the gamma motor neurons, whereas a stimulus just adequate to discharge the alpha motor neurons may exert a pronounced effect on the gamma motor neurons.

As has been true with other inputs to the anterior horn cells, the effects differ for flexor and extensor neurons, as well as for neurons innervating the arm and leg. A lesion that damages most or all the corticoreticular fibers above the midbrain and red nucleus results in increased extensor tone in the legs and increased flexor tone in the arms (decorticate posture) because of loss of inhibition of all descending pathways. Such a lesion at the level of the midbrain below the red nucleus removes arm flexor excitation and results in excitation of all extensor muscles and a generalized increase in extensor tone (decerebrate posture). Such a lesion below the medulla results in loss of all the descending input (generalized flaccidity).

Clinical Correlations

The clinical effects of damage to the descending indirect pathways are in large part a function of two complicating factors. First, the fibers of these pathways are not in well-defined bundles and therefore are not damaged selectively; they are widespread enough so that significant effects occur only with large lesions, which will almost always also cause damage to the corticospinal pathways. Second, the clinical findings with major damage to these or other pathways change with time because of the development of *denervation hypersensitivity*. The loss of all or most of the afferent input to a cell or groups of cells gradually results in an increased response to stimuli that normally would evoke a lesser response. This is best exemplified in major, acute lesions of the spinal cord.

If the spinal cord is transected, all long descending pathways to the alpha and gamma motor neurons are destroyed. A large proportion of the input to these cells is lost, and they become inactive; clinically, all motor activity is markedly reduced or lost, along with all reflexes. Tone is flaccid. But these changes persist for only a few weeks or months. There remain significant inputs to the motor neurons in the spinal cord, including the local sensory input from the periphery and from other parts of the spinal cord. With time the neurons recover their excitability and become hyperexcitable. Postural and voluntary activity remains lost, but local tendon reflexes and other cord reflexes are preserved and become overactive. At times, more complex reflexes, like the withdrawal of a limb from pain, occur, mediated by local spinal cord connections.

Lesions in the lower brain stem that are severe enough to damage the reticular formation and vestibular nuclei are not compatible with life, and specific syndromes of destruction of the descending indirect pathways at this level are not seen. However, with major damage at higher levels to the descending pathways from the cerebral hemispheres, the patient will manifest findings that depend on the indirect pathways. Loss of forebrain control of the inhibitory reticular formation, which inhibits extensor neurons and excites flexor neurons, results in overactivity of the extensor neurons under the drive of the excitatory reticular formation and vestibular nuclei. The clinical findings are those of increased extensor tone and increased reflexes. The importance of the vestibular nuclei in this increase in extensor tone can be shown by destruction of the vestibular nuclei, which results in a marked reduction in extensor hyperactivity. In addition to increased tone and reflexes, patients with indirect pathway damage have *spasticity,* an increase in resistance to passive movement of an extremity, which subsides with continued pressure. The reduction in tone is the clasp-knife response.

Bilateral damage to the indirect activation pathways from the cortex to the brain stem in the midbrain below the red nucleus produces extensor spasticity of all extremities. This condition has been called a *decerebrate posture* and occurs in humans with massive cerebral trauma, anoxic damage, or midbrain destructive lesions. Lesions large enough to produce decerebrate posture will also produce coma. Decerebrate posture is due to the release of reticulospinal and vestibulospinal excitation when the inhibitory drive of forebrain structures on the medullary reticular formation is lost. If damage occurs above the level of the red nucleus, the excitatory drive of the red nucleus on the flexor neurons of the upper extremity with inhibition of the extensor neurons results in flexor rather than extensor spasticity in the arms. Flexor spasticity in the arms with extensor spasticity in the legs is called *decorticate posture.* Decorticate posture occurs with indirect activation pathway (upper motor neuron) damage above the level of the red nucleus.

HEMIPLEGIA AND HEMIPARESIS. Lesions of the motor pathways of the cerebral hemispheres are common and are called *upper motor neuron lesions.* Because of the intermingling of the direct and indirect pathways (pyramidal and extrapyramidal), they are only rarely damaged selectively. The clinical findings, therefore, are usually a combination of the effects already described for lesions of the direct and indirect activation pathways. The combined paralytic and release phenomena are exemplified by a lesion in the internal capsule. Such a lesion produces a characteristic pattern of impaired motor activity on one side of the body. If paralysis is severe, the pattern is called a *hemiplegia.* If mild, it is called a *hemi-*

paresis. The typical findings of hemiparesis are as follows:

Movement. Motor activity is slowed, and weakness is present in a characteristic distribution: the upper portion of the face is spared, while the lower portion is weak contralateral to the lesion. Volitional facial movements are weak, while emotional and associated movements such as smiling are spared or exaggerated. There may be slight weakness of the palate contralateral to the lesion and a tendency for the tongue to deviate on protrusion to the side of the hemiplegia. In the upper extremity, the weakness affects the extensor muscles more than the flexors, whereas in the lower extremity the flexors are weaker than the extensors. Skilled, delicate, precision movements are chiefly affected. The fingers, therefore, are particularly involved. There is also greater weakness of extension of the wrist and elbow and of abduction and elevation of the shoulder. In the lower limb, the weakness involves chiefly the dorsiflexors of the toes and ankle, the flexors of the knee, and the flexors of the hip.

Movements tend to be massive and crude. The patient may be unable to carry out selective movements; for instance, he or she may be able to flex and extend all the fingers together but not individually, and on an attempt to dorsiflex the ankle, may also flex the knee. The patient walks with a characteristic circumduction of the affected leg. Movements that the patient is unable to carry out voluntarily may occur reflexly; when the patient yawns or is tickled, the paretic upper limb may elevate and the fingers extend and abduct. Involuntary associated movements also occur in the paralyzed limb when powerful movements are carried out on the nonparalyzed side.

Muscle Tone and Posture. There is myotatic hyperreflexia with an upper motor neuron lesion, which is expressed as increased muscle stretch reflexes and an increased resistance to passive movement (spasticity). There is overactivity of the spinal reflexes that maintain upright posture and a corresponding increase of tone in the antigravity muscles. In humans, the *antigravity muscles* are the flexors in the upper limb and the extensors in the lower limb. Lesions of the upper motor neuron result in a characteristic posture: The upper limb is adducted and flexed at the elbow, wrist, and fingers; the lower limb is adducted and extended at the hip and knee. The

response to passive movement includes the clasp-knife response, in which the increased resistance to passive movement, present with initial stretch, subsides with continued stretch. Large, acute, supratentorial lesions may produce a transient flaccid paralysis.

Impaired speech also occurs with upper motor neuron lesions. Because of bilateral innervation of bulbar muscles, these findings are most common with bilateral disease. They are referred to as *spastic dysarthria*, characterized by a harsh, labored, slow, monotonous, and weak speech with poor articulation.

Reflexes. The stretch reflexes in upper motor neuron disease differ from normal in that the threshold is lowered and the response is exaggerated and more protracted (hyperreflexia). When the stretch reflexes occur in series, *clonus* or repeated jerking of the muscle occurs, each relaxation initiating another contraction. (Clonus must be distinguished from the clonic, jerking movement in a seizure.) The abdominal and cremasteric reflexes are impaired or lost, while Babinski's sign appears.

The sources of these phenomena are listed in Table 9-1.

Control Circuits

The execution of motor activity requires the integration of a large amount of sensory information from the peripheral cutaneous, joint, and muscle receptors and the coordination of the activity in the direct and indirect activation pathways. Simple integration and coordination occur at the level

Table 9-1. Origins of Signs with an Upper Motor Neuron Lesion

Direct activation pathway damage	Indirect activation pathway damage
Hypotonia	Clonus
Loss of fine, skilled movement	Increased tone of arm flexors and leg extensors
Distal weakness	Spasticity (with clasp-knife response)
Absent abdominal reflexes	Decorticate or decerebrate posture
Babinski's sign	Hyperactive stretch reflexes
Hyporeflexia	

of the spinal cord and the brain stem via the pathways already described. However, these are inadequate to effect the wide range of complex motor activities seen in vertebrate species, and two additional groups of nuclei and pathways have evolved to control these activities. Neither of the control circuits have any significant direct output to the descending pathways. Their major function is the integration and coordination of impulses at the cerebral level, acting through the cortex for the generation of efficient, smooth motor performance. The two control circuits are the cerebellum and its connections and the basal ganglia and their connections. (In some textbooks the basal ganglia are considered part of the extrapyramidal pathway.)

The *basal ganglia* may be considered as the structures that plan and program motor activity, in particular the activity needed for the maintenance of normal posture and background static muscle contraction. The *cerebellum* integrates and coordinates activity in the execution of the movements for muscle contraction in smooth, directed movements. The activities of the control circuits also must be coordinated with each other—coordination that is carried out by the anatomic connections. Each of these control circuits will be discussed separately.

The Basal Ganglia Control Circuit

ANATOMY AND PHYSIOLOGY. The basal ganglia include the caudate nucleus, the putamen, and the globus pallidus. The substantia nigra and subthalamic nucleus are closely related to the basal ganglia and will be considered with them. The term *striatum* refers to the combination of the caudate nucleus and putamen, the largest subcortical masses of gray matter, which act as a single functional unit. The basal ganglia are sometimes classified as extrapyramidal structures. Since the term originally meant "outside the medullary pyramids," this is, strictly speaking, correct. However, by this logic, the cerebellum is also extrapyramidal, though never considered as such. For our purposes, the basal ganglia are better considered as one of the two control circuits for motor activity and not as a major descending pathway for motor activity.

The basal ganglia are derived embryologically from the telencephalon, and anatomically they are closely related to the cerebral cortex. Yet, despite their location, anatomic connections, and large size, current knowledge does not permit us to describe the specific functions of the individual components of the basal ganglia. Much of our knowledge comes from a consideration of how the brain functions when these nuclei are not working normally. Specific motor dysfunctions are known to accompany histopathologic or chemical changes in the basal ganglia. Lesions in certain structures closely related to the basal ganglia, such as the substantia nigra and the subthalamic nucleus, also produce pathologic motor symptoms. In general, the basal ganglia control the background tone and posture for movements initiated in the cerebral cortex and participate in automatic movements such as walking and in learning new motor behavior.

PATHWAYS. The striatum receives input primarily from the cerebral cortex but also from the intralaminar thalamic nuclei and the substantia nigra and sends efferents to the substantia nigra and globus pallidus. The major efferent pathways from the basal ganglia originate in the globus pallidus. Its major input comes from the striatum, though some input arises from other sources. It sends fibers to a number of areas: to the thalamus for relay back to the cerebral cortex, to the subthalamic nucleus and neighboring areas including the region of the red nucleus, and to the reticular formation of the brain stem. Of these pallidal efferents, only those to the reticular formation and perhaps those to the area of the red nucleus reach descending pathways to the spinal cord. The bulk of the pallidal efferents project to the nucleus ventralis anterior to the thalamus via the ansa lenticularis and fasciculus lenticularis (Fig. 9-20). Basal ganglia pathways thus are made up of a number of loops, in particular: (1) striatum to globus pallidus to thalamus to cortex to striatum, (2) striatum to substantia nigra to striatum, and (3) globus pallidus to subthalamus to globus pallidus.

The striatum is the structure in the brain richest in two important central nervous system neurotransmitters, acetylcholine and dopamine, and in enzymes associated with their metabolism. Most of the axons of cells in the striatum are short and terminate within the nuclei in which they lie. Acetylcholine is the synaptic transmitter for most of these neurons. The dopamine in the striatum is

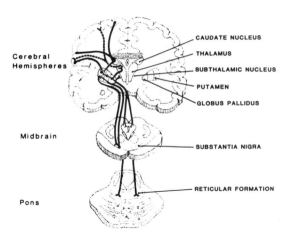

Fig. 9-20. *Basal ganglia pathways. The major outflow pathway is from globus pallidus to cortex via nucleus ventralis anterior in the thalamus.*

manufactured within the substantia nigra and is transmitted to the striatum along the nigrostriatal axons to act as a neurotransmitter in the striatum. Destruction of neurons in the substantia nigra results in lowering of the dopamine content in the striatum. Most efferents from the striatum to the globus pallidus and from the globus pallidus to the substantia nigra release an inhibitory neurotransmitter, gamma-aminobutyric acid (GABA).

CLINICAL CORRELATIONS. The basal ganglia control system is a damping or modulating system. Excess discharge in the basal ganglia produces slowing; a lack of discharge produces hyperactivity. Lesions in the striatum produce deficits in the ability to perform complex motor responses. Pathologic symptoms and signs with disease of the basal ganglia may be classified into two types: abnormal movements and changes in tone. The abnormal movements may be a reduction in mobility (hypokinesia) or involuntary movements (hyperkinesia).

With hypokinesia, there is usually an increase in tone, without the clasp-knife reaction seen in spasticity. This increased resistance to passive movements occurs through direct effects on the alpha motor neuron and is known as *rigidity*. Movements are slow, stiff, and initiated or stopped with great difficulty. Abnormal postures are often assumed, which may involve the entire body, one-half of the body, or single limbs. Hypokinesia is often due to disease in the substantia nigra.

Involuntary movements may arise with excessive activity in the dopaminergic fibers. These may be slow and writhing (athetosis) or may involve abnormal posturing of the trunk or an extremity (dystonia). Rapid involuntary movements also can occur. These may be gross, rapid, flinging movements in the presence of lesions of the subthalamic nucleus (hemiballismus), brief rapid jerks in striatal disease (chorea), or regular alternating tremor in substantia nigra disease (parkinsonism). The tremor seen with parkinsonism, the most common form of basal ganglia disease, is characteristic in its 3 to 4 per second, regular alternation *at rest*. It is diminished with voluntary activity.

Speech in basal ganglia disease has various manifestations but can be classified as a *hypokinetic dysarthria* or a *hyperkinetic dysarthria*. The former is much more common and is characterized by a quiet, weak, monotonous voice with poor articulation, short rushes of words, and a breathy quality. A hyperkinetic dysarthria is recognizable as sudden changes in speech, such as bursts of loudness, elevation of pitch, voice stoppages, distortion of vowels, and disintegration of articulation.

Examples of hypokinetic and hyperkinetic basal ganglia disorders, with paucity of movement and excessive movement, are parkinsonism and Huntington's chorea. Patients suffering from *Parkinson's disease* have lesions of the substantia nigra with lowered striatal dopamine levels. The dopamine of the substantia nigra acts to inhibit the firing of cells of the striatum. In its absence, the cells fire action potentials more rapidly under the drive of the acetylcholine-secreting neurons. This disordered striatal output results in loss of the normal modifying influence of the basal ganglia on the motor activities of the pyramidal and extrapyramidal pathways. Patients with Parkinson's disease typically have gradually progressive rigidity, akinesia (slow movement), and tremor. Parkinsonism may occur after encephalitis, carbon monoxide poisoning, manganese poisoning, or toxicity from some psychoactive drugs. In most patients with this relatively common disorder, there is no apparent cause, and the disease is said to be idiopathic. The pathologic changes in the brain include cellular degeneration in the substantia nigra, whose cells may have hyaline inclusion bodies (Lewy bodies).

Huntington's chorea is a chronic, progressive, dominantly inherited disease with onset in adult life. It is a diffuse degenerative disease, with widespread loss of cholinergic and GABA-nergic neurons and secondary cerebral atrophy. This is most marked in the basal ganglia, especially in the caudate nucleus, which is severely shrunken, producing a characteristic dilatation of the lateral ventricle. There is also atrophy of the cerebral cortex. These degenerative changes underlie the generalized mental deterioration, chorea, and decreased tone. *Chorea* is the random, continuous occurrence of brief, abrupt, jerky movements of any part of the body due to overactivity of dopaminergic neurons. Reflexes and sensation are generally normal.

Another form of chorea, *Sydenham's chorea*, has a subacute onset in children with rheumatic fever. Sydenham's chorea is an immunologic disorder in which the body produces antibodies to the streptococcal bacteria. The protein structure of the streptococcal antigen is similar to that of proteins in the membrane of striatal neurons, so that the antibodies to these antigens also attack basal ganglia neurons and produce chorea. The disorder is usually a transient one with full recovery.

The Cerebellar Control Circuit

ANATOMY AND PHYSIOLOGY.   The cerebellum and its connections comprise the second major control circuit. It is concerned with the coordination of muscle groups during phasic motor activity. The cerebellum regulates or controls movements, especially skilled movements. This regulation, carried out in conjunction with the motor regulation by the basal ganglia, depends on cerebellar inputs from proprioceptive, somatic, vestibular, visual, and auditory sense organs, and from motor and nonmotor portions of the cerebral cortex. In turn, the cerebellum sends outputs to brain-stem neurons and to the motor cortex. The pathway to the latter involves a relay in the ventral lateral nucleus of the thalamus. In the thalamus, cerebellar and striatal outputs can interact before reaching the cerebral cortex.

GROSS STRUCTURE.   The cerebellum may be divided from anterior to posterior or from side to side (Fig. 9-21). From anterior to posterior, the cerebellum is made up of the *anterior lobe,* the *posterior lobe,* and the *flocculonodular lobe.* From side to side, it is divided into midline

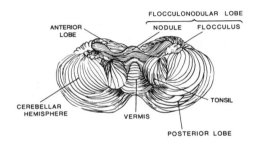

Fig. 9-21. Gross anatomic subdivisions of cerebellum.

structures and lateral structures. The midline of the anterior and posterior lobes is called the *vermis,* while the lateral portions are the *cerebellar hemispheres.* The midline of the flocculonodular lobe is the nodulus; the lateral portion is the *flocculus.* The flocculonodular lobe is sometimes called the *archicerebellum,* the anterior lobe is called the *paleocerebellum,* and the posterior lobe is called the *neocerebellum.* In animals low on the phylogenetic scale, only the archicerebellum is found. It is the primary connection with the vestibular apparatus for coordination of location in space and motion. The paleocerebellum is a more recent development, found in reptiles and amphibia. It serves as the projection area for spinocerebellar proprioceptive information in regulating primitive motor acts such as postural reflexes. The neocerebellum is the most recent development and is primarily concerned with coordination of voluntary muscle activity and muscle tone.

HISTOLOGY.   The cerebellar cortex has three layers: an outer molecular layer, the layer of Purkinje cells, and an inner granular layer. The most prominent neurons of the cerebellum are the *Purkinje cells* (see Fig. 4-1). These are large flask-shaped neurons with extensive dendritic arborizations in the molecular layer of the cerebellum. Axons of Purkinje neurons are the sole output neurons of the cerebellar cortex and leave via the granular layer to synapse on cells of the deep cerebellar nuclei.

PATHWAYS.   Nerve fibers enter or leave the cerebellum in three structures: the inferior, middle, and superior cerebellar peduncles. These are also known as the *restiform body,* the *brachium pontis,* and the *brachium conjunctivum,* respectively.

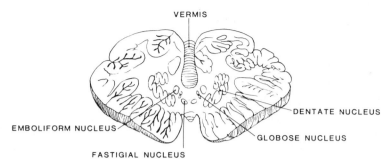

Fig. 9-22. Cerebellar nuclei in horizontal section through cerebellum.

Most of the output of the cerebellum exits after synapse in the deep cerebellar nuclei: the dentate, the globose, the emboliform, and the fastigial nuclei (Fig. 9-22). Axons of Purkinje cells carrying efferent activity from the cerebellum synapse in these nuclei, which then send axons out via the superior or inferior cerebellar peduncles.

The cerebellar pathways form three loops. The first is via the dentate nucleus to the opposite red nucleus, and the thalamus to the cerebral cortex (Fig. 9-23). The loop is completed by axons from the frontal lobe through the internal capsule and cerebral peduncles to the pontine nuclei (fronto-pontine fibers). Pontine nuclei send axons across the midline via the middle cerebellar peduncle

Fig. 9-23. The three cerebellar pathways. Cerebello-dentato-rubro-thalamo-cortico-ponto-cerebellar loop is represented by a solid line, cerebello-rubro-olivo-cerebellar loop by a dashed line, and cerebello-vestibulo-cerebellar loop by a dotted line.

back into the cerebellum. This loop—the longest—modulates voluntary activity. The second loop is also from the dentate nucleus to the opposite red nucleus. It is completed via connections with the inferior olive, which projects back across the midline into the cerebellum via the inferior cerebellar peduncle (Fig. 9-23). This loop coordinates extrapyramidal and cerebellar functions. The third loop interconnects the cerebellum with the ipsilateral vestibular nuclei.

The following generalizations about the cerebellar inputs and outputs are important:

1. The middle cerebellar peduncle is an afferent pathway. Its inflow decussates in the pons.
2. The superior cerebellar peduncle is mostly an efferent pathway, with the exception of the ventral spinocerebellar tract. The superior cerebellar peduncle outflow decussates in the decussation of the brachium conjunctivum.
3. The inferior cerebellar peduncle is mostly afferent, with a strong vestibular and reticular efferent path.

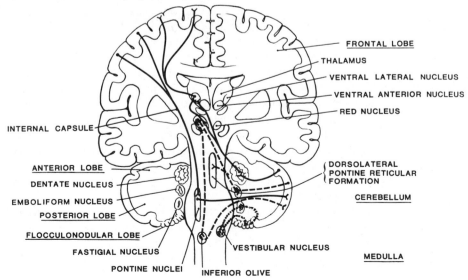

Table 9-2. Cerebellar Afferents and Efferents

From	Via	To
Input (afferent)		
1. Vestibular nerve and nuclei	Inferior cerebellar peduncle	Flocculonodular lobe
2. Spinal cord (dorsal spinocerebellar tract)	Inferior cerebellar peduncle	Anterior lobe and vermis
3. Basal ganglia (rubroreticulo-olivocerebellar pathway)	Inferior cerebellar peduncle	Posterior lobe
4. Cerebral cortex (pontine nuclei)	Middle cerebellar peduncle	Posterior lobe
5. Spinal cord (ventral spinocerebellar tract)	Superior cerebellar peduncle	Anterior lobe
Output (efferent)		
1. Flocculonodular lobe	Fastigial nucleus and inferior cerebellar peduncle	Vestibular nuclei Reticular formation
2. Anterior lobe and vermis	Emboliform and globose nuclei and superior cerebellar peduncle	Red nucleus and reticular formation
3. Posterior lobe	Dentate nucleus and superior cerebellar peduncle	Red nucleus, thalamus, and cortex

4. Each cerebellar hemisphere is connected to the opposite thalamus and cerebral cortex and controls the ipsilateral extremities.

The major connections of the cerebellum are listed in Table 9-2.

FUNCTIONAL ASPECTS OF THE CEREBELLUM. The physiology of the cerebellar cortex has certain distinguishing features: The Purkinje cells and other cerebellar neurons spontaneously fire at high rates and are generally inhibitory in their action; that is, the axonal outputs of Purkinje and other neurons depress activity in the cells of the deep cerebellar nuclei. Most of the neurons in the cerebellar nuclei have excitatory effects on their synaptic targets.

Activity in proprioceptive, exteroceptive, visual, auditory, and vestibular end organs or pathways produces responses in the cerebellum. There is a somatotopic representation of these sensations on the cerebellar cortical surface. In addition, the cerebral cortex projects in a similar topographic pattern on the cerebellum. This topographic patterning of inputs to the cerebellar cortex is similar to, although less detailed than, the motor and sensory representation in the cerebral cortex.

The cellular organization and pathway connec-

tions of the cerebellum are designed to modulate motor activities, including equilibration, posture and gait, and voluntary movements.

Equilibration. The flocculonodular lobe modulates equilibration and the orientation of the head and eyes. This lobe has connections with the vestibular nuclei. Lesions in the flocculonodular lobe produce inability to stand or sit without swaying or falling (truncal ataxia) and abnormalities of head and eye movements (nystagmus).

Posture and Gait. The anterior lobe is concerned mainly with posture, gait, and truncal tone. Lesions produce unsteady walking, staggering (gait ataxia), and hypotonia.

Voluntary Movements. The posterior lobe, in particular the large lateral hemispheres, provides a servomechanism for coordination of skilled action. Lesions in the posterior lobe produce irregular movements of the limbs (limb ataxia), loss of muscle coordination (dyssynergia), loss of ability to measure range of motion (dysmetria), and tremor with voluntary activity (intention tremor). In general, movements become clumsy and uncoordinated.

CLINICAL CORRELATIONS. Three major patterns of cerebellar pathophysiology can be distinguished.

Flocculonodular syndrome occurs, especially

in midline tumors in children, and produces truncal ataxia wtih disturbances in standing, with unsteadiness, falling, and disturbances of gait, and usually with associated nystagmus of the eyes.

Anterior lobe syndrome is most commonly due to degenerative disease in adults and ·is manifested as a severe gait ataxia without ataxia of the upper limbs and mild ataxia of the legs when they are tested individually.

Cerebellar hemisphere disease produces symptoms of limb ataxia with hypotonia, intention tremor, dyssynergia, and dysmetria ipsilateral to the side of the lesion.

Disorders of speech also occur in cerebellar disease, particularly when it involves the vermis. These disorders are manifested as irregularities of pitch, loudness, and rhythm and are known as *ataxic dysarthria.* Speech is slowed, with excess stress on some words or syllables and random breakdown of articulation.

Certain diseases affect the nervous system widely and have effects on all the components of the motor system. One of these was originally considered to be a degenerative disorder and is now known to be metabolic in origin. *Wilson's disease* or hepatolenticular degeneration is a disorder of copper metabolism in which there is excessive deposition of copper in many areas. This

Table 9-3. Findings on Neurologic Examination of Motor Function Related to the Divisions of the Motor System at the Four Levels of the Nervous System

	Level of damage			
	Peripheral	Spinal	Posterior fossa	Supratentorial
Final common pathway	Weakness, atrophy, hyporeflexia, hypotonia, absent abdominal reflexes, cramp, and fasciculation	Weakness, atrophy, hyporeflexia, hypotonia, absent abdominal reflexes, cramp, and fasciculation	Weakness, atrophy, and fasciculation	
Direct activation pathway		Weakness, loss of abdominal reflex, and Babinski's sign	Weakness, loss of abdominal reflex, Babinski's sign, hyporeflexia, and hypotonia	Weakness, loss of abdominal reflex, Babinski's sign, seizure, apraxia, hyporeflexia, and hypotonia
Indirect activation pathway		Hyperreflexia, clonus, spasticity, and clasp-knife reflex	Hyperreflexia, clonus, spasticity, clasp-knife reflex, and decerebrate posture	Hyperreflexia, clonus, spasticity, clasp-knife reflex, apraxia, decorticate posture
Cerebellar control circuit			Ataxia, dysmetria, dyssynergia, intention tremor, past pointing, rebound, hyporeflexia, and hypotonia	Ataxia
Basal ganglia control circuit				Rigidity, athetosis, dystonia, chorea, hemiballismus, hyperkinesia, and resting tremor

results in a typical brown stain at the edge of the cornea (Kayser-Fleischer ring) and damage to the liver. The deposition of copper in the cortex, cerebellum, and basal ganglia results in a combination of motor manifestations from one or more of these structures. The involved areas show loss of neurons, gliosis, atrophy, and if severe, cavitation. This is most prominent in the putamen and globus pallidus. Because of the widespread involvement, the clinical findings can vary widely and may include tremor, rigidity, bizarre movements, dystonia, spasticity, and Babinski's sign.

Motor System Examination
Movement in the normal person involves the simultaneous, coordinated activities of all four of the major divisions of the motor system. These four are therefore tested together in the neurologic examination. The examination is best organized into separate evaluation of strength, reflexes, coordination, gait, tone, and muscle bulk and observation for abnormal movements. The changes in each of these with disease in each division of the motor system are outlined in Table 9-3.

Strength
Strength testing evaluates the power of muscle groups in performing specific actions. Strength depends on age, occupation, physical activity, and muscular development. It may be apparently reduced in patients with bone deformity, pain, or a lack of understanding of the test. Since the object of strength testing is to detect disease of the neuromuscular system, these extraneous factors must be excluded. Strength cannot be graded as abnormal on the basis of an absolute measure of force. It must be judged for each person on the basis of age and all the other variables noted.

Strength is tested by having the patient resist pressure initiated by the examiner. The position of the extremity during testing is of great importance in isolating the action of specific muscle groups and in providing optimal leverage. Each muscle group should be tested in the position that best isolates its function and puts it at a relative mechanical disadvantage (partially contracted position). Force should not be applied suddenly but should be applied gradually to a maximum.

There are a number of systems for grading strength (or weakness). A simple and universally understood one uses a verbal description:

Normal. Level of strength expected for that person.
Mild weakness. Level of strength less than expected but not sufficient to impair any daily function.
Severe weakness. Strength sufficient to activate the muscle and move it against gravity, but not against any added resistance.
Complete paralysis. No detectable movement.

The following muscle groups are tested as part of a general neurologic examination. The individual muscles participating in these functions will be discussed in Chapter 12.

FACIAL MUSCLES.   Upper and lower facial muscles are tested separately by having the patient wrinkle the forehead, squeeze the eyes shut, and show the teeth.

NECK MUSCLES.   The patient resists attempts by the examiner to flex and extend the neck by exerting pressure on the occiput and forehead, respectively.

ARM ABDUCTORS.   The patient holds the arms laterally at right angles to the body while the examiner pushes down on the elbows.

ELBOW FLEXORS AND EXTENSORS.   With the elbow bent at a right angle, the patient resists attempts to straighten it out (flexing to prevent extension) and to bend it (extending to prevent flexion).

WRIST EXTENSORS.   The patient holds the wrist straight with knuckles up, while the examiner attempts to depress it.

FINGER FLEXORS.   The patient resists attempts to straighten the fingers of a clenched fist (or squeezes two of the examiner's fingers in his or her hand).

TRUNK FLEXORS.   The patient attempts to do a sit-up from a supine position with the legs extended.

HIP FLEXORS.   In a sitting position, the patient holds the knee up off the chair against resistance; supine, the patient keeps the knee pulled up to the chest.

HIP EXTENSORS. Prone, the patient holds the bent knee off the examining table; supine, the patient resists attempts to lift the leg straight off the examining table; these are the major muscles used in arising from a squatting position (with knee extensors).

KNEE FLEXORS. The patient resists attempts to straighten the knee from a 90-degree angle position.

KNEE EXTENSORS. The patient resists attempts to bend the knee from a 90-degree angle position; these are major muscles used in arising from squatting.

ANKLE PLANTAR FLEXORS. The patient's ability to rise onto the toes of one foot or to walk on toes is assessed. This ability is too powerful to test by hand unless it has been severely weakened.

ANKLE DORSIFLEXORS. The patient holds the ankle in a resting 90-degree angle position against attempts to depress it.

Reflexes

Two major types of reflexes are tested in the neurologic examination: stretch reflexes and superficial (cutaneous) reflexes. The former depend on a rapid, brisk stretch of the muscle, whereas the latter depend on an uncomfortable stimulus to the skin. Correct positioning and application of the stimulus are extremely important in eliciting reflexes. There are also significant variations among patients, and even of a reflex in a single patient on repeated testing. Therefore, much experience with normal reflexes is required before the presence of abnormality can be assessed.

The jaw, biceps, triceps, knee, and ankle reflexes are the most important muscle-stretch reflexes. The patient must be completely relaxed in the testing of all these reflexes.

JAW JERK. The examiner's index finger is placed lightly on the patient's mandible below the lower lip. It is then tapped briskly with the reflex hammer. The reflex is a brisk jaw closure.

BICEPS JERK. The patient's elbow is bent to 90-degree angle position with the forearm resting on the lap or on the examiner's arm. The examiner's

thumb is placed on the patient's biceps tendon with slight pressure. The thumb is then tapped firmly and briskly with the reflex hammer. The reflex is a quick biceps muscle contraction with tendon (and forearm) movement.

TRICEPS JERK. The patient's elbow is bent to 90-degree angle position with the forearm hanging limply, supported at the elbow by the examiner's hand. A firm, brisk tap is applied directly to the tendon of the triceps, 1 to 3 cm above the olecranon. The elbow extends in this reflex.

KNEE JERK. The patient's knee is bent to 90 degrees in the sitting position. A firm, brisk tap is applied to the quadriceps tendon 0.5 to 1.0 cm below the patella. The knee extends in this reflex.

ANKLE JERK. The patient's ankle is passively bent to 90 degrees and held by the examiner in that position. The examiner gives a firm, brisk tap to the Achilles tendon 2 to 3 cm above the heel. The foot plantar flexes in the reflex.

ABDOMINAL REFLEX. The patient lies supine with the abdomen relaxed. By means of a sharp object, the skin of the patient's abdomen is scraped quickly and lightly in each quadrant along a line toward the umbilicus. The umbilicus moves toward the stimulus.

PLANTAR RESPONSES. The sole of the patient's foot is scratched firmly with a blunt instrument such as a key. The stimulus is begun at the heel and smoothly carried forward along the lateral border of the sole to the base of the toes and then medially to the base of the great toe. A normal response is a curling of the toes. Babinski's sign is extension of the great toe and fanning of the other toes.

Coordination

The ability to coordinate the movements of multiple muscle groups can be observed during ordinary activity, such as shaking hands, talking, dressing, and writing. Specific tests allow assessment of coordination in localized areas. All may be done with the patient sitting or supine, and each should be done individually for all four extremities.

FINGER-TO-NOSE TESTING. The patient is asked

to alternately touch his or her own nose and the examiner's finger with the tip of his or her own index finger. The examiner's finger should be far enough away so that the patient must fully extend the arm. Test this with the patient's eyes both open and closed.

HEEL-TO-SHIN TESTING. The patient places the heel carefully on the opposite knee and slides it slowly along the edge of the tibia to the ankle and back up to the knee again.

RAPID ALTERNATING TESTING. The patient pats each hand or foot as rapidly and regularly as possible against a firm surface. A more difficult variation requires alternately patting the front and back of the hand on the knee as rapidly and regularly as possible.

Gait and Station
Tests of gait and station involve all areas of the motor system, and a wide variety of patterns of gait abnormality occur with different disorders. The test of gait and station is perhaps the single most useful motor system test and should be observed in all patients.

GAIT. The patient walks normally back and forth at a moderate rate; he or she then walks on heels, toes, and tandem along a straight line, touching heel to toe; the patient then hops on each leg.

STATION. The patient is asked to stand with the feet together, first with the eyes open and then with the eyes closed. There should be little or no sway.

Muscle Tone
The elbows, wrists, and knees are passively flexed and extended with the patient completely relaxed. There should be only a minimal smooth resistance to the movement.

Muscle Bulk
All major muscle groups should be examined for signs of focal atrophy. The diameters of the extremities may be measured and compared with each other.

Abnormal Movements
Because many motor disorders are manifest as abnormal involuntary movements, the patient should be examined undressed, both sitting and supine and fully relaxed for such movements. Fasciculations in particular require careful observation of each area under good lighting.

Objectives
1. Draw the pathways and name the major nuclear structures in the direct and indirect activation pathways, the final common pathway, and the control circuits.
2. Describe the function of each of the four major divisions of the motor system. Identify those pathways acting on the motor unit and describe their effects.
3. Describe the reflex arc and its function in the motor system.
4. Name the symptoms and signs resulting from disease of the motor system and identify the major division of the motor system in which a lesion causing them would be located.
5. Describe the mechanisms by which each of the signs of motor dysfunction occurs.

Clinical Problems
1. A 26-year-old housewife began having infrequent, brief episodes of twitching of her left hand 10 months ago. These ceased 4 months ago, but she then noted clumsiness when using her left hand. This progressed to moderate weakness and a "peculiar" feeling in her hand. In the past month, she began having headaches.

   On examination, she was lethargic but otherwise mentally intact. There was mild swelling of the optic disks bilaterally. She had a mild droop of the lower part of her face on the left, moderate weakness and slowing of rapid alternating movements of the left hand, and a circumduction gait on the left. Reflexes were hyperactive in the left arm and leg, with Babinski's sign on the left. Muscle tone was increased on the left. Sensation was normal except for inability to recognize some objects in her left hand.
   a. Identify the level, side, and type of lesion.
   b. Which spinal cord tracts would show wallerian degeneration?
   c. How does the firing rate of the gamma motor neurons to left-side extremity mus-

cles compare with normal?

d. What were the transient episodes?

e. Would the jugular compression test be useful?

2. A 23-year-old woman has a slowly progressive disorder that first began in high school when she was noted to be "fidgety." She did well in school and worked as a secretary for 3 years. During this time, she experienced gradually increasing jerking movements of her arms and face, and her speech became slurred, to the point that she was no longer able to work. During the past 2 years, her gait has become unsteady and her movements have slowed. She also has had occasional, uncontrollable, flailing movements of her arms. During the past year, her memory has been poor and her intellectual capabilities have deteriorated.

On neurologic examination, she had occasional, coarse, asymmetric jerks of the upper extremities and neck, with some grimacing. Sensation, strength, and reflexes were unremarkable. Her tone was increased, with rigidity in all extremities. She had a coarse intention tremor of both arms.

a. Identify the level, side, and type of disease.

b. What major divisions of the motor system are involved?

c. What two general types of cause must be considered in this disorder?

d. Name the structures in the diseased pathways.

e. What are the signs of basal ganglia disease?

3. A 21-year-old single woman was found lying unresponsive in bed by her girlfriend, who had stopped off in the morning to drive her to work. She called for an ambulance and brought the patient to the hospital. The following facts were obtained from the friend on questioning. The patient had been in good health. She was well the evening before. She was apparently on no medications, and no empty or partially filled bottles were in evidence. There were no signs of a struggle or violence and no suicide note. She was in bed as though she had been asleep. There were no unusual findings about the patient: no blood, urine, feces, or injuries. But her skin had a

peculiar pink appearance.

On examination she was unresponsive to all but painful stimuli, to which she responded with decerebrate posturing, with her arms, legs, and neck stiffly extended. Her eyes apparently did not respond to threatening stimuli but appeared to close randomly. Her jaw was tightly clenched. There were bilateral extensor plantar responses. Her respirations were irregular. Tone was generally increased with some lengthening reaction. Reflexes were generally hyperactive. All other aspects of the examination were within normal limits.

a. Identify the level, side, and most likely type of disease.

b. What other types of disorders can have this temporal profile?

c. There is evidence of involvement of which divisions of the motor system?

d. How is decerebrate rigidity produced?

e. Which sensory receptors are responsible for a clasp-knife reflex?

4. A 9-year-old boy developed a mild "cold," which a day later was associated with a fever and severe aching muscle pains, especially in his back. He was generally weak, but by the fourth day, he noted an inability to move his right leg and the fingers of his left hand. Lumbar puncture revealed that the CSF was clear and colorless, with a sugar level of 68 mg per deciliter, a protein level of 86 mg per deciliter, and 46 lymphocytes per microliter. His generalized symptoms cleared over the next week.

On examination at 3 weeks, there was almost complete paralysis of his right leg, moderate weakness of his left arm, and mild weakness of other muscles, including the facial muscles. Results of sensation and coordination tests were normal—where he was able to perform them. Reflexes were hypoactive in the right leg, which was flaccid. There was atrophy of all muscles, most strikingly in the right leg and left arm.

a. Identify the level, side, and type of disease.

b. Are the spinal fluid findings of any help in identifying the disease?

c. Which division of the motor system is involved?

d. What are the signs of disease in this division?

e. List the major inputs to the final common pathway.

5. A 58-year-old banker suddenly lost the ability to speak, and within a few minutes he was unable to move his right arm. On examination later in the day, there had been no progression in symptoms. He appeared to understand what he was told, but he could not answer questions. In attempting to speak, he uttered nonsense words or garbled words. A very few words came out correctly, such as "hello." His right arm was paralyzed, and the right cheek and right side of his mouth drooped. Forehead movements were normal. Leg strength was normal. Deep tendon reflexes were hypoactive in his right arm but normal elsewhere. He seemed to recognize sensations everywhere. Results of coordination tests were normal, except in the right arm. His gait was normal. Optic fundi were normal.

a. Identify the level, side, and type of lesion.
b. Specifically, what division and what site in the motor system are involved?
c. How do plantar responses and abdominal reflexes change with lesions in this division?
d. What term is used to describe this speech disorder?
e. Why was forehead movement on the right normal?

6. A 7-year-old boy with a history of chronic recurrent otitis media awoke one morning complaining of a headache. At school, he was noted to be awkward and to have trouble using his right hand. By the next day, he was unable to hold a glass of milk in his right hand without spilling it, and he veered to the right when walking.

On examination, his neck was slightly stiff, though his fundi were normal. He had an intention tremor of his right arm and leg, with marked dysmetria of these extremities on finger-to-nose and heel-to-shin testing. Reflexes on the right were slightly hypoactive. Sensation was normal.

a. Identify the level, side, and type of lesion.
b. Why should you hesitate to do a lumbar puncture?

c. Which division of the motor system is involved?
d. Which fiber pathways in this division decussate?
e. What are the functional subdivisions of this division of the motor system?

Suggested Reading

Bird, E. D., and Spokes, E. G. S. Huntington's Chorea. In T. J. Crow (ed.), *Disorders of Neurohumoural Transmission.* New York: Academic, 1982. Pp. 145-182.

Brodal, A. *Neurological Anatomy in Relation to Clinical Medicine* (3rd ed.). New York: Oxford University Press, 1981.

Evarts, E. V. Role of Motor Cortex in Voluntary Movements in Primates. In V. B. Brooks (ed.), *Handbook of Physiology,* Section 1, Vol. II, Part 2. Bethesda, Md.: American Physiological Society, 1981. Pp. 1083–1120.

Ferrendelli, J. A., and Landau, W. M. Movement Disorders. In S. Eliasson, A. L. Prensky, and W. B. Hardin, Jr. (eds.), *Neurological Pathophysiology* (2nd ed.). New York: Oxford University Press, 1978. Pp. 156–167.

Hornykiewicz, O. Parkinson's Disease. In T. J. Crow (ed.), *Disorders of Neurohumoural Transmission.* New York: Academic, 1982. Pp. 121–143.

Kuypers, H. G. J. M. Anatomy of the Descending Pathways. In V. B. Brooks (ed.), *Handbook of Physiology,* Section 1, Vol. II, Part 1. Bethesda, Md.: American Physiological Society, 1981. Pp. 597–666.

Lance, J. W., and McLeod, J. G. *A Physiological Approach to Clinical Neurology* (3rd ed.). Boston: Butterworth, 1981. Pp. 30–218.

Landau, W. M. The Upper Motor Neuron Syndrome. In S. Eliasson, A. L. Prensky, and W. B. Hardin, Jr. (eds.), *Neurological Pathophysiology* (2nd ed.). New York: Oxford University Press, 1978. Pp. 139–155.

Newsom-Davis, J. Myasthenia. In T. J. Crow (ed.), *Disorders of Neurohumoural Transmission.* New York: Academic, 1982. Pp. 7–43.

Thach, W. T. Pathophysiology of Cerebellar Disorders. In S. Eliasson, A. L. Prensky, and W. B. Hardin, Jr. (eds.), *Neurological Pathophysiology* (2nd ed.). New York: Oxford University Press, 1978. Pp. 167–172.

Towe, A. L., and Luschei, E. S. *Motor Coordination (Handbook of Behavioral Neurobiology,* Vol. 5). New York: Plenum, 1981.

The Visceral System

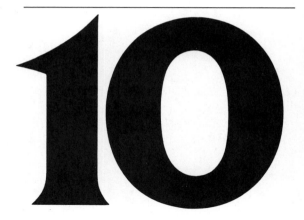

The somatic sensory and motor systems establish contact with the external world through the appreciation of environmental stimuli and the control of movements that adapt to the environment. The visceral system, in contrast, deals with the inner world by responding to stimuli from the internal environment and by regulating the function of the visceral glands and organs. The visceral system has an organization similar to that of the somatic systems. It has longitudinal sensory (afferent) and motor (efferent) components, which interact at each level of the nervous system to provide the wide range of reflex responses needed to maintain a suitable internal environment, that is, *homeostasis*. The visceral efferent structures are referred to as the *autonomic nervous system*.

The visceral system differs from the somatic system in three major respects, which gives the viscera a measure of independence from neural control:

1. *Autonomy* of the effector organs. Unlike somatic muscle, many of the organs and glands regulated by the visceral system can function without external control.
2. *Peripheral reflex connections*. Unlike the somatic systems, in which all reflexes are mediated in the central nervous system, visceral reflexes can occur in the periphery.
3. *Neurohumoral control*. Many viscera are regulated by hormones secreted into the blood by endocrine glands under neural control.

The functions of endocrine glands and visceral structures (gastrointestinal, cardiovascular, pulmonary, and renal) are subjects beyond the scope of this book, but a discussion of their neural control will be presented.

Overview

The visceral system has longitudinal motor and sensory pathways with major representations at each level. The limbic system and hypothalamus are at the supratentorial level; the reticular formation and preganglionic parasympathetic neurons are at the posterior fossa level. The preganglionic sympathetic and parasympathetic neurons are at the spinal level. The ganglia, receptors, and effectors are at the peripheral level (Fig. 10-1).

Visceral Sensory Pathways

Visceral receptors are found throughout the body and are of two major types: *mechanoreceptors* and *chemoreceptors*. The former respond to tension, stretch, and pressure, while the latter signal changes in the chemical environment, such as changes in pH and O_2 levels. The impulses generated by these receptors are transmitted via plexuses to autonomic ganglia either in or near the visceral organs. The visceral afferent fibers may synapse in the ganglia to initiate local reflexes or may proceed to the central nervous system.

Visceral afferent information can reach the central nervous system by two routes: (1) Sensory information may go directly to the brain stem via the cranial nerves or (2) it may enter the spinal cord via the splanchnic and pelvic nerves and then be relayed to the brain stem. Sensations can travel via both of these routes; however, discrete, localized, reflex activities are carried via the cranial nerves while activity eliciting diffuse responses (including painful stimuli) enters the central nervous system via the splanchnic nerves.

Both the ascending afferent input from the spinal cord and the input directly to the brain stem make relay connections in the reticular formation of the brain stem, where vital functions such as respiration and cardiovascular control as well as other visceral functions are regulated. Visceral afferent information also ascends to the hypothalamus, thalamus, and cerebral cortex at the supratentorial level, where areas in the insula and on the medial surface of the hemispheres provide conscious perception of visceral sensations. At the supratentorial level, the visceral sensory input is joined by the special visceral afferent sensation of olfaction. The olfactory afferents project to areas at the base of the brain known as the *rhinencephalon*.

The extensive afferent input to the central nervous system from the viscera provides pathways for reflex activity of increasing complexity at each major level of the nervous system, and for the integration of this activity with that of the somatic systems. Visceral and somatic afferent and efferent activity is integrated and coordinated at the supratentorial level by a group of cortical and subcortical structures known as the *limbic system*. Affective and emotional responses are generated in the limbic system.

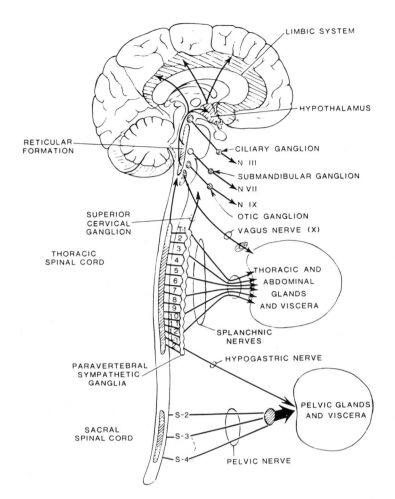

Fig. 10-1. Major components of the visceral system.

Central Visceral Control

The *hypothalamus* provides the major control of reflex responses of the visceral and endocrine systems. Afferent activity reaches the hypothalamus from all visceral structures. The efferent activity of the hypothalamus travels to the periphery over two routes: the neural pathways in the brain stem and spinal cord, and the humoral pathways of the pituitary gland and endocrine glands. The neural pathway is more direct, faster, and more specific, while the humoral pathway is more generalized and longer acting.

The functions of the hypothalamus include maintenance of a stable internal environment or *homeostasis*. Examples of this function include regulation of the levels of normal blood constituents, regulation of functions that restore or rejuvenate the body (such as eating and digestion),

and control of activities that prepare an individual for interaction with the external environment (such as aggressive behavior). The restorative activities, called *parasympathetic*, are regulated by the anterior portions of the hypothalamus and are concerned with specific, localized visceral activities. The preparative activities, called *sympathetic*, are mediated by posterior hypothalamic areas, and are more diffuse responses as shown in Table 10-1.

Visceral Efferent Pathways

The sympathetic and parasympathetic efferent neural outflows of the hypothalamus descend to the reticular formation where a number of functional centers regulate specific activities such as respiration and heart rate. The efferent activity from the hypothalamus and reticular formation can travel via either of two pathways, the sympathetic or the parasympathetic. Parasympathetic

Table 10-1. Longitudinal Subdivisions of Visceral Efferent Pathways

	Parasympathetic	Sympathetic
Function	Build, restore	Prepare
Responses	Local, specific	Diffuse, less specific
Location		
Supratentorial	Limbic system	Limbic system
	Anterior hypothalamus	Posterior hypothalamus
Brain stem	Reticular formation	Reticular formation
Preganglionic neuron	1. Cranial nerve nuclei (nerves III, VII, IX, and X)	1. Thoracic cord, T-1 through T-12
	2. Sacral cord, S-2 through S-4	2. Lumbar cord, L-1 and L-2
Postganglionic neuron	Ganglion in or near organ	Paravertebral or prevertebral ganglion
Preganglionic neurotransmitter	Acetylcholine	Acetylcholine
Postganglionic neurotransmitter	Acetylcholine	Norepinephrine or acetylcholine

activity passes out through the nuclei and axons of cranial nerves III, VII, IX, and X to the head and trunk, down the lateral funiculus of the spinal cord to neurons and efferent axons in the sacral spinal cord which control parasympathetic activity in the pelvic organs. These parasympathetic efferents are known as the *craniosacral division* of the visceral efferents.

The parasympathetic neurons in the brain stem and spinal cord that give rise to the efferent axons leaving the central nervous system are called *preganglionic*. They all secrete the neurotransmitter acetylcholine and are therefore called *cholinergic*. The craniosacral, visceral efferent preganglionic neurons have long axons that terminate in ganglia in or near the effector organs. They act on postganglionic neurons in the ganglia, which are also cholinergic. Short axons of the postganglionic parasympathetic neurons innervate the visceral effectors.

The sympathetic efferent pathway from the hypothalamus and reticular formation travels via the lateral funiculus of the spinal cord to neurons in the thoracic and upper lumbar cord which mediate sympathetic activity to the entire body. These sympathetic visceral efferents are known as the *thoracolumbar division*. The preganglionic sympathetic neurons are cholinergic and have relatively short axons that terminate in the paravertebral or prevertebral ganglia on postganglionic neurons. From these ganglia, long postganglionic axons travel to the visceral effectors. Most (but not all) of these postganglionic neurons secrete norepinephrine and are therefore called *adrenergic*. The sympathetic division also sends preganglionic fibers to the adrenal gland where they can stimulate the release of epinephrine from the adrenal medulla to produce widespread sympathetic effects.

Visceral Sensory Pathways

Healthy persons are ordinarily unaware of their viscera except for feeling fullness of the stomach, bladder, or rectum. In contrast, visceral sensations such as pain or nausea may be overwhelming during illness. Visceral symptoms are of major importance in the recognition and diagnosis of diseases of the visceral organs, but perception of them is restricted by four factors: (1) Only a limited number of visceral sensations reach the level of consciousness; (2) the sensation perceived may be unrelated to the type of stimulus; for example, a burning sensation is not due to stimulation of thermal receptors; (3) the same sensation may be generated by a number of stimuli, for example, compression, stretch, or ischemia; and (4) a sensation arising in one site may be felt in or referred to an entirely different area.

The limited ability to recognize or localize visceral sensation, in contrast to the wide range of sensibilities in the somatic system, is even more surprising in view of the many sensory fibers in the visceral system. The vagus nerve, one of the largest nerves in the body, is entirely visceral and more than 80 percent afferent in composition. In fact, most major nerves in the visceral system have more sensory than motor fibers. The magnitude of sensory input that does not reach the level of consciousness indicates that these signals are involved in reflexes mediated at a subconscious level.

Visceral Sensory Receptors

The visceral system has two general types of receptors: the mechanoreceptors and the chemoreceptors. Each of these is further specialized to perform very limited functions. Some mechanoreceptors are slowly adapting receptors that signal stretch or tension, and thereby reflect the size of or pressure in such organs as the stomach, intestines, and bladder. Other rapidly adapting mechanoreceptors indicate pressure, movement, or flow in visceral organs or arteries. The baroreceptors in the atria and ventricles of the heart and the carotid baroreceptors, for example, signal the pulsatile variation in blood pressure (Fig. 10-2).

Fig. 10-2. Mechanoreceptors in carotid sinus and aortic arch respond to blood pressure changes. Chemoreceptors in carotid and aortic bodies respond to changes in PaO_2 and $PaCO_2$ in the blood.

The lung also has pressure receptors sensitive to inflation or deflation and other receptors sensitive to stimuli that initiate coughing.

The second major type of visceral receptor, the chemoreceptor, is not found in the somatic afferent system. It is the receptor type for both the special visceral afferents of taste and smell and for some general visceral afferents. The chemoreceptors are specialized to measure chemical changes such as pH in the stomach, osmotic pressure in the intestinal tract, or PaO_2 and $PaCO_2$ in the carotid and aortic bodies of the carotid artery and aorta (Fig. 10-2).

Less is known about the sources and mechanisms of pain in the viscera. Excessive stimulation of both mechanoreceptors and chemoreceptors, although not painful or even reaching consciousness at low levels of stimulation, reaches consciousness and produces pain with strong or prolonged activation. Whether there are additional sensory endings that function purely to signal the presence of damage (nociceptor endings) has not been determined. Nonetheless, irritation, torsion, traction, strong contractions, or distention of viscera will be perceived as pain.

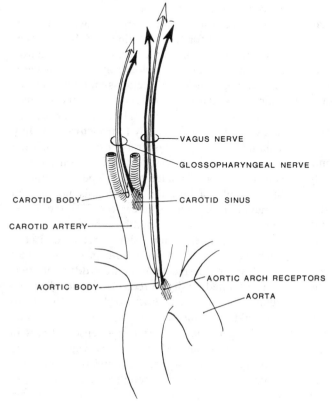

VAGUS NERVE

GLOSSOPHARYNGEAL NERVE

CAROTID BODY

CAROTID SINUS

CAROTID ARTERY

AORTIC BODY

AORTIC ARCH RECEPTORS

AORTA

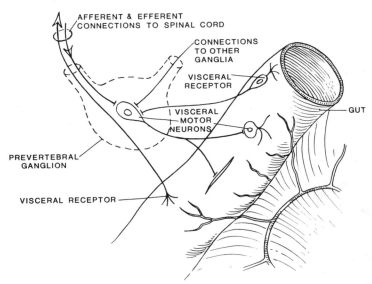

AFFERENT & EFFERENT
CONNECTIONS TO SPINAL CORD

CONNECTIONS
TO OTHER
GANGLIA

VISCERAL
RECEPTOR

VISCERAL
MOTOR
NEURONS

GUT

PREVERTEBRAL
GANGLION

VISCERAL RECEPTOR

Fig. 10-3. Peripheral visceral sensory connections. Electrical activity arising in visceral receptors may terminate in peripheral ganglia to mediate local reflexes or may travel to the spinal cord.

There are also visceral sensory receptors located within the central nervous system, particularly in the hypothalamus and the reticular formation, which respond to changes in blood osmolality, blood sugar level, and serum electrolytes.

The afferent signals generated in the peripheral sensory receptors follow four routes: (1) Some remain in the periphery, mediating local reflexes; (2) some enter the spinal cord, especially via the sympathetic chain of ganglia; (3) some enter the brain stem via cranial nerves VII, IX, and X; and (4) some enter the rhinencephalon via the olfactory nerve.

Visceral Afferents in the Periphery
The afferent fibers from visceral receptors are small and conduct slowly. Some are unmyelinated. The cell bodies of these fibers are in the innervated organ, in peripheral ganglia, or in dorsal root ganglia. Fibers entering the central nervous system have their cell bodies in the dorsal root ganglia or in ganglia of the cranial nerves. Fibers making local connections within a viscus or in a peripheral ganglion have their cell bodies in the periphery.

These visceral sensory neurons make synaptic connections with visceral motor neurons within

the viscera or in peripheral autonomic ganglia (Fig. 10-3). Although the number, extent, and specific function of these peripheral connections are as yet unknown, they could serve as important neural mechanisms providing local control of visceral organs, independent of the central nervous system.

Visceral Afferents Entering at the Spinal Level
Much of the visceral sensory input enters the nervous system at the spinal level (Fig. 10-4). These afferent fibers, like those in the somatic sensory system, have their cell bodies in the dorsal root ganglia. Distal fibers of the dorsal root ganglia reach the extremities by two pathways, (Fig. 10-5), either with the peripheral nerves or with the blood vessels. Axons associated with blood vessels pass through the sympathetic trunk in the paravertebral region and the rami communicantes to the spinal nerve.

The visceral sensory fibers entering the spinal cord make multiple connections at this level. First, they synapse either with visceral efferent neurons to mediate visceral reflexes or with somatic efferent neurons to produce related somatic activity, such as the spasm of abdominal muscles often associated with abdominal disease. Second, visceral sensory fibers make synaptic connections with sensory neurons in the dorsal horns that also receive sensory input from the primary sensory neurons of the somatic system (Fig. 10-6). This convergence of input on its way to the cerebral cortex is the basis of referred pain. Patients with

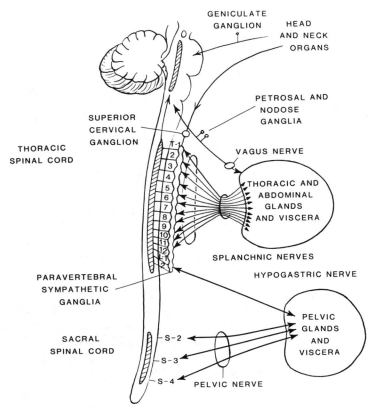

Fig. 10-4. Visceral afferent pathways to the central nervous system follow two routes, one to the spinal cord and the other to the brain stem. Cell bodies are in the dorsal root or in cranial nerve ganglia (geniculate, nodose, petrosal).

disease of visceral organs localize (refer) the pain to more superficial areas of the body that have the same segmental representation in the spinal cord as the viscera involved (Fig. 10-7). Third, visceral sensory fibers synapse with fibers that ascend in association with the lateral spinothalamic tract and dorsal columns to the reticular formation, the thalamus, and the hypothalamus.

Most of the visceral afferent activity entering the spinal cord does not reach the level of consciousness. That which does includes dull, diffuse, aching pain which enters through the sympathetic trunk; sharp, more localized pain which enters directly with peripheral nerves; and fullness from pelvic organs which enters directly via pelvic nerves.

Visceral Afferents Entering at the Posterior Fossa Level

Afferent visceral impulses also reach the central

nervous system via the cranial nerves (see Fig. 10-4). Cranial nerve X, the *vagus nerve*, carries afferent information from pulmonary, cardiac, and gastrointestinal receptors to the brain stem. The vagal fibers mediate reflexes for coughing, blood pressure, heart rate, vomiting, and hiccuping. The sensations of fullness, nausea, and movement in the body cavities reach the level of consciousness via this pathway. Pain is not carried by the vagus nerve. The glossopharyngeal (IX) and the facial (VII) cranial nerves carry the special visceral afferent sensation of taste from the tongue and pharynx. All these cranial nerves make connections in the brain stem which project to the reticular formation, the thalamus, and the hypothalamus. Table 10-2 summarizes afferent pathways.

Visceral Input to the Supratentorial Level
Olfaction, a special visceral afferent sensation from the olfactory nerves (cranial nerve I), enters the nervous system at the supratentorial level and passes to areas at the base of the brain known as the *rhinencephalon,* including the amygdala, the uncus on the medial surface of the temporal lobe,

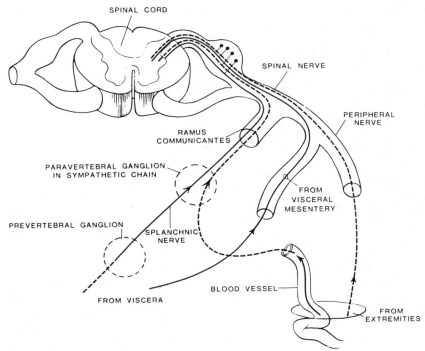

Fig. 10-5. *Visceral afferents reach spinal cord by multiple pathways. Afferents travel directly via peripheral nerves or indirectly through sympathetic paravertebral ganglia, whether coming from either the extremities or the viscera.*

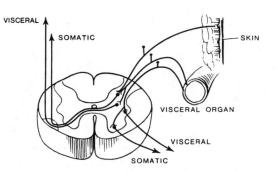

Fig. 10-6. *Visceral afferents make multiple spinal cord connections. Local reflexes are mediated via visceral and somatic motor neurons. Synapses with secondary neurons carry information to the brain in association with the spinothalamic tract. Some of the visceral afferents may end on secondary neurons in the somatosensory system as well, to result in referred pain.*

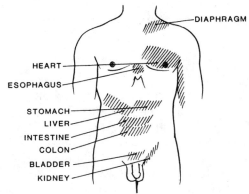

Fig. 10-7. *Shading shows dermatomal areas in which pain is felt when there is disease in visceral organs (referred pain).*

and cortical areas on the medial and basal frontal lobe.

The central projections of some visceral afferents, including the vagus, project to supplementary sensory areas in the insula and on the medial surface of the cerebral hemispheres. The cingulate, orbital, and insular cortex of the frontal lobes also receive visceral afferent activity which ascends from the hypothalamus via the dorsomedial nucleus and from the mammillary bodies via the anterior nucleus of the thalamus.

Despite these cortical connections, the major destination of visceral afferent activity is the hypothalamus. The hypothalamus, as the major integrator of visceral information, receives input from the cerebral cortex, thalamus, rhinencephalon, and reticular formation. It also contains re-

Table 10-2. Visceral Afferent Pathways
to the Central Nervous System

Extremities and trunk	Peripheral and spinal nerves directly to dorsal roots
	Along blood vessels to sympathetic trunk and then to dorsal roots
Viscera	Peripheral nerves in mesentery directly to spinal nerves and dorsal roots (sharp pain)
	Pelvic and splanchnic nerves to sympathetic trunk (dull pain)
	Vagus nerve to brain stem (fullness and nausea)

ceptor cells that can directly sense chemical changes in the blood, such as changes in osmolality. The multiple afferent inputs are integrated with activity from cortical areas by the hypothalamus to provide central visceral control of neural and endocrine activities. The hypothalamus acts as the neuroendocrine transducer, coordinating the functions of neural and endocrine visceral activities.

Clinical Correlations
Because of the multiple pathways for visceral sensation and the limited conscious perception of visceral activity, there are no clinical disorders except for loss of olfaction (see Chap. 15) in which a specific loss of visceral sensation is manifest. The loss of reflex alterations in blood pressure or heart rate in some neuropathies is partly due to damage to visceral sensory fibers. In addi-

tion, the painful, posttraumatic syndrome of causalgia has been attributed to altered function in visceral afferent fibers. In some types of seizures, there is spread of epileptic activity into areas that mediate visceral sensory activity, so that the patients describe odors, or peculiar sensations in their chest or abdomen.

Central Visceral Control
Central visceral control occurs in three areas: the cortex and hypothalamus at the supratentorial level and the reticular formation in the brain stem. The hypothalamus is the major supratentorial area concerned with visceral function. The cerebral cortex, in contrast, has only a minor role in the regulation of visceral organs. The cortical and subcortical structures in the cerebral hemispheres that are active in visceral and emotional activity are known collectively as the *limbic system*. The reticular formation contains a number of centers controlling specific visceral activities, such as respiration and heart rate. They are under the more general control of the hypothalamus.

Cerebral Cortex
Two types of cerebral cortex participate in visceral function: frontal cortex and the rhinencephalic cortex on the medial surface of the frontal and temporal lobes. The cortical sensory areas that receive visceral afferent activity project via intracortical connections to frontal cortex and rhinencephalon. Activation of an area of frontal cortex that controls somatic activity in a specific structure also elicits a visceral response in the same structure. For instance, activity in the lip and tongue area may result in salivation. These visceral responses are *secondary* or *auxiliary functions* coordinated with the primary somatic activity. Visceral efferent projections

Fig. 10-8. Limbic areas on the medial surface of the brain.

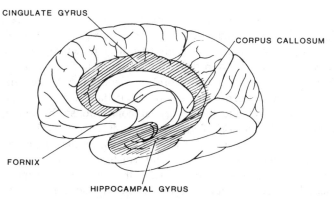

CINGULATE GYRUS

CORPUS CALLOSUM

FORNIX

HIPPOCAMPAL GYRUS

from neocortical areas end in the hypothalamus, mammillary bodies, and brain-stem reticular formation. There are no known cortical-visceral efferent projections directly to the spinal cord.

The rhinencephalic cortex receives input from the thalamus, other cortical areas, and the hypothalamus. It mediates some visceral functions such as bladder control and participates strongly in a person's emotional responses by coordinating feelings and their visceral manifestations, such as blushing and crying. These cortical areas are also called the *limbic lobe* and are part of the limbic system (Fig. 10-8). The limbic system coordinates visceromotor and somatic motor activity and is particularly important in the emotional responses associated with anger or fright. It is probably a major element in emotional disorders in humans.

Fig. 10-9. A. Medial surface of hemisphere showing hypothalamus in wall of third ventricle (shaded). B. Coronal section of brain showing hypothalamus at base of brain.

The afferent pathways that carry visceral and somatic input to the limbic system from all other areas of the cortex permit it to synthesize sensory perceptions and affective responses for storage in *memory* (see Chap. 15). The visceral functions of these areas are also evident in seizures originating in them. For example, medial temporal lobe seizures produce visceral sensations, chewing movements, pupillary dilatation, and breath-holding.

The Hypothalamus

The primary integration of affective, visceral, and humoral activities occurs in the hypothalamus. This organ is derived from the basal plate but serves both afferent and efferent functions in regulating the neural and humoral efferents of the visceral system. It receives input from all areas in the periphery, from the cerebral cortex, and from receptors lying within it. The hypothalamus has multiple functions which can be classified into three types:

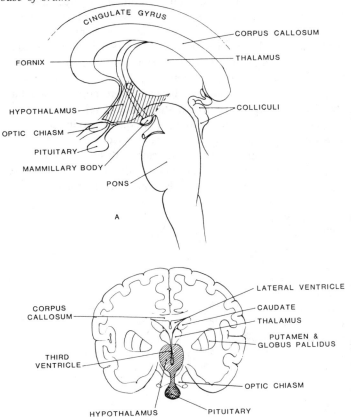

1. Those that act to *maintain* the physicochemical environment necessary for viability of the body tissues, including homeostatic mechanisms such as thermoregulation and electrolyte balance.
2. Those that act to *restore,* rebuild, or regenerate energy and body stores, such as digestion, menstruation, and sleep.
3. Those that improve the reactivity of or *prepare* the somatic motor system for external stress: the vasodilatation of blood vessels needed for increased physical performance or self-protection is one example.

The preparative activities are integrated in the posterior hypothalamus and are mediated by humoral mechanisms and a sympathetic neural pathway. The restorative activities are controlled largely by the anterior hypothalamus via humoral mechanisms and a parasympathetic neural pathway. The homeostatic mechanisms are regulated by the medial ventral hypothalamus via the posterior pituitary.

The hypothalamus makes up the ventral half of the diencephalon and includes a group of small, ill-defined nuclei and fibers (Fig. 10-9). It forms the lateral walls of the third ventricle and is below and anterior to the thalamus, from which it is separated by the hypothalamic sulcus. The pituitary gland (hypophysis) lies just beneath the hypothalamus in the pituitary fossa. Below and anterior to the hypothalamus is the *optic chiasm,* a useful landmark. The hypothalamus is divided into four regions: preoptic, ahead of the chiasm; supraoptic, over the chiasm; tuberal, connected with the hypophyseal stalk; and the mammillary bodies. The supraoptic nuclei and the posterior pituitary gland are homeostatic, the preoptic and anterior nuclei are mainly restorative, while the paraventricular and posterior nuclei are mainly preparative.

The hypothalamus, in addition to receiving afferent information from many other areas, also has receptors within it. *Receptors for body temperature,* which can evoke compensatory temperature changes by directing sweating, piloerection, or change in blood vessels, have been identified in the hypothalamus. Other *receptors for osmolality* of the blood are active in the control of salt and water metabolism, thirst, and kidney function.

Hypothalamic fiber tracts are shown schematically in Figure 10-10. Two major fiber tracts are the *fornix,* which travels from the hippocampus on each side to the mammillary bodies, and the *mammillothalamic tracts,* which travel from the mammillary bodies to the anterior nucleus of the thalamus. Descending fibers from the hypothalamus to the reticular formation, cranial nerve nuclei, and spinal cord are not localized in a single bundle, although they are more concentrated laterally in the brain stem and spinal cord.

The hypothalamus is unique in having the highest concentration of a number of neuropeptides, a group of neurotransmitters whose function in the brain is currently under study (Table 10-3). These peptides include the hypothalamic-releasing hor-

Fig. 10-10. Afferent and efferent connections of hypothalamus.

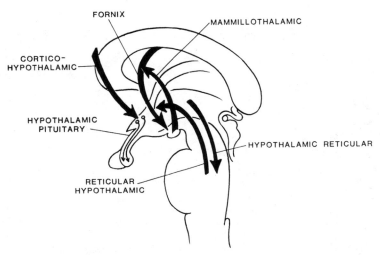

FORNIX

MAMMILLOTHALAMIC

CORTICO-HYPOTHALAMIC

HYPOTHALAMIC PITUITARY

HYPOTHALAMIC RETICULAR

RETICULAR HYPOTHALAMIC

Table 10-3. Peptides Found in the Brain*

Hypothalamic-releasing hormones	Gastrointestinal peptides
Corticotropin-releasing hormone	Bombesin
Gonadotropin-releasing hormone	Cholecystokinin
Growth-hormone–releasing hormone	Gastrin
Somatostatin	Glucagon
Thyrotropin-releasing hormone	Insulin
	Leucine-enkephalin
Neurohypophyseal hormones	Methionine-enkephalin
Neurophysin	Motilin
Oxytocin	Neurotensin
Vasopressin	Secretin
	Substance P
Pituitary peptides	Vasoactive intestinal polypeptide
Adrenocorticotropic hormone	
Beta-endorphin	Others
Growth hormone	Angiotensin II
Luteinizing hormone	Bradykinin
Alpha-melanocyte–stimulating hormone	Calcitonin
Prolactin	Carnosine
Thyrotropin	Neuropeptide

*These peptides are also found in the regions under which they are classified in this table, which are the areas in which they were first identified.

mones and many peptides that were originally identified in the pituitary and nonneural tissue, such as the gut. Some of these peptides have been found in the same neurons as other, better known, transmitters, such as acetylcholine, and may be released together with them.

While different pathways of synthesis of these peptides have been identified in diverse areas, propiomelanocortin (POMC), the prototype precursor molecule from which many of the peptides are derived by proteolysis, is found predominantly in cells of the hypothalamus. The diverse character of the peptides listed in Table 10-3 shows the multiplicity of their functions, but their importance in the brain is only beginning to be defined. They have already been shown to be of

importance in pain mechanisms (substance P, enkephalins, and opioid peptides) and in memory, learning, and behavior (beta-endorphins, corticotropin, vasopressin, and oxytocin). Significant alterations in brain peptides have been reported in Alzheimer's disease and Huntington's chorea, two degenerative brain diseases with dementia; peptides also may be important in psychiatric diseases.

Recognition of the importance of the brain peptides occurred at the same time as the identification of a wide range of neurotransmitter receptors for peptides and other transmitters in the brain, many of which are integral in the visceral system. The categories of receptor types are listed in Table 10-4. Some individual neurons in

Table 10-4. Neurotransmitter Receptor Types

Category	Example
Opiate	Morphine and enkephalin selective
Calcium antagonist	Verapamil selective
Adenosine	Alpha-1 and alpha-2 (stimulates adenylate cyclase)
GABA	Alpha and beta (baclofen) selective
Dopamine	Dopamine-1 and dopamine-2 (extrapyramidal actions)
Serotonin	5-hydroxytryptamine-1 and 5-hydroxytryptamine-2
Alpha-adrenergic	1 (sympathetic postsynaptic) and 2 (sympathetic nerve terminals)
Beta-adrenergic	1 and 2 (epinephrine more potent than norepinephrine)
Cholinergic	Muscarinic-1 (sympathetic ganglia)

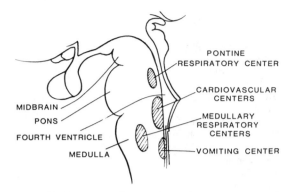

Fig. 10-11. Visceral centers in brain-stem reticular formation.

the visceral system have multiple types of such receptors, permitting a variety of responses to different inputs. The action of many drugs in clinical medicine is through interaction with these receptors.

Reticular Formation

The reticular formation is a diffuse accumulation of small to medium-sized multipolar cells surrounding the central core of the brain stem from the medulla through the midbrain. The reticular formation receives visceral input from widespread areas, including all of the periphery and the hypothalamus. In addition, some cells in the reticular formation are sensitive to humoral or metabolic changes in the blood and act as receptors, for instance to elevation of carbon dioxide levels or to epinephrine.

The reticular formation is not organized into specific nuclei, but certain areas called *centers* are related to specific visceral activities (Fig. 10-11). Stimulation or destruction of some areas in the medulla produces changes in heart rate, blood pressure, and peripheral circulation. These cardiovascular centers have been subdivided into *pressor* and *depressor centers,* which constrict or dilate blood vessels to elevate or lower blood pressure. Closely associated with the bulbar pressor areas in the medulla are other areas that speed or slow the heart rate.

Another reticular formation center controls respiration. *Respiration* is a complex interaction of the visceral and somatic systems. The afferent activity controlling the respiratory centers is entirely visceral in origin from receptors in the lungs and blood vessels. The efferent activity is

carried in part by somatic efferents that control the muscles of the chest and diaphragm and in part by visceral efferents that control the size of the bronchioles and pulmonary blood vessels. Three respiratory centers have been identified in the pontine and medullary reticular formation. An *apneustic center* in the pons is responsible for prolonged deep inspiration. Ventral inspiratory and dorsal expiratory centers in the medullary reticular formation modify the frequency and depth of inspiratory and expiratory movements. Each of these centers is modified by afferent neural activity and by carbon dioxide levels. Destructive lesions in the medulla and pons, therefore, result in abnormal patterns of respiration, hiccups, or total loss of breathing.

Gastrointestinal activities such as peristalsis and secretion also are modified by the brain-stem reticular formation; however, the only identifiable "center" is the *vomiting center,* located in the dorsolateral part of the medullary reticular formation just beneath the fourth ventricle. This area may be activated by peripheral stimuli in gastrointestinal disease, by descending activity in psychogenic vomiting, by circulating drugs that induce vomiting, and by direct local stimulation due to a lesion in the region of the center. The efferent activity from the vomiting center utilizes both somatic and visceral efferent pathways so that transection of neither the vagus nerves nor the somatic nerves alone abolishes vomiting.

Visceral Efferent Pathways

Introduction

Central visceral structures control the peripheral glands and organs via three distinct pathways: humoral, parasympathetic, and sympathetic. The hypothalamus controls the pituitary by the *humoral pathway.* The parasympathetic and sympathetic are neural paths extending through the brain stem and spinal cord to the periphery. These provide dual innervation to mediate the dual functions of restoration (parasympathetic) and preparation (sympathetic). Since there are dual paths, and since some activities can be controlled entirely in the periphery, there is no final common pathway in the visceral system. The visceral efferent structures are summarized in Table 10-5.

Humoral Efferent Pathway

The hypothalamus regulates the pituitary gland

Table 10-5. Visceral Efferent Structures

Structure	Location	Termination
Cerebral cortex	Orbital frontal and medial temporal	Hypothalamus
Hypothalamus	Diencephalon	1. Reticular formation 2. Pituitary gland
Reticular formation	Brain stem	1. Cranial nerve nuclei (nerves III, VII, IX, and X) 2. Intermediolateral column of spinal cord
Preganglionic parasympathetic neurons	1. Cranial nerve nuclei (nerves III, VII, IX, and X) 2. Spinal cord, S-2 through S-4	Ganglia in or near organs
Preganglionic sympathetic neurons	Spinal cord, T-1 through L-2	Paravertebral or prevertebral ganglia
Postganglionic neurons	Peripheral ganglia	Effector organs

and thereby the endocrine system. The hypothalamus exerts both a neural and a humoral control over the pituitary. The neural pathway is formed by fibers from the supraoptic and paraventricular nuclei that descend through the infundibulum into the posterior pituitary gland and end in relation to a capillary network into which they secrete the polypeptides oxytocin and vasopressin. These, in turn, regulate uterine contraction, milk ejection, and diuresis. These pathways are shown in Figure 10-12.

The humoral pathway from the hypothalamus to the hypophysis is a complex network of veins, the *hypophyseal portal system,* which extends from the hypothalamus to the anterior pituitary. Blood flowing through it supplies the anterior pituitary gland. At the upper end of this network, the hypothalamus secretes polypeptides, called *releasing factors,* into the blood, which act on the cells in the anterior pituitary gland at the lower end. The releasing factors modulate the production of hormones by the anterior pituitary gland (see Table 10-3). The interrelationships of the hypothalamus and endocrine system are diagrammed in Figure 10-13. Lesions in the hypothalamus can produce endocrine disorders with disturbances in growth, feeding, temperature control, water balance, and other visceral activities.

Parasympathetic Efferent Pathway

The descending, parasympathetic, restorative activity follows two routes to the peripheral effectors, one via cranial nerves to viscera in the head and trunk, and the other via the sacral spinal cord and pelvic nerves to pelvic organs. Descending fibers from the hypothalamus and reticular formation are diffusely distributed in the lateral areas of the brain stem and spinal cord. They terminate on either cranial nerve nuclei III, VII, IX, and X, or neurons in the lateral gray matter of the spinal cord. The parasympathetics are therefore called the *craniosacral division.*

The visceral efferent neurons of cranial nerves III, VII, IX, and X are all parasympathetic and originate from the general visceral efferent column. They give rise to long, preganglionic

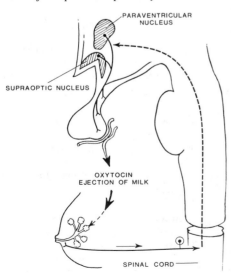

Fig. 10-12. Combined neural and humoral control of milk ejection is result of neural stimuli arising from sucking reflex traveling over neural pathways to hypothalamus, which forms oxytocin for release into circulation from posterior pituitary.

PARAVENTRICULAR NUCLEUS

SUPRAOPTIC NUCLEUS

OXYTOCIN EJECTION OF MILK

SPINAL CORD

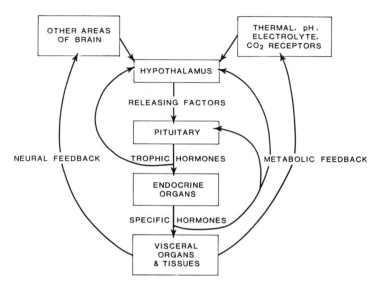

Fig. 10-13. Interactions of hypothalamus and endocrine system. Direct arrows indicate control, while
loops show feedback pathways.

fibers that secrete acetylcholine and terminate on
neurons in ganglia in or near the effector organ.
The postganglionic neurons have short, cholinergic fibers which innervate smooth muscle and
glands. These parasympathetic neurons send
fibers to visceral structures in the head and the
abdominal and chest cavities (Table 10-6 and Fig.
10-14). They innervate the pupils via the oculomotor nerve, the salivary glands via the facial
and glossopharyngeal nerves, and the viscera via
the vagus nerve.

The parasympathetic neurons in the second
through the fourth sacral cord segments are located in the lateral gray matter, but not as a well-
defined column. These neurons are preganglionic
and give rise to long, cholinergic axons that leave
the cord via the sacral spinal nerves, but then
branch from them as the pelvic nerves. The parasympathetic axons in the pelvic nerves terminate
on postganglionic neurons in ganglia near the rectum, bladder, and genital organs. These neurons
control defecation, micturition, erection, and
uterine contraction. There is a reflex center for

Table 10-6. Cranial Efferent Parasympathetic Innervation

Brain stem	Nucleus	Nerve	Ganglion	Organ	Effect of stimulation
Midbrain	Edinger-Westphal	Oculomotor (III)	Ciliary	Eye	Accommodation, miosis
Pons	Facial	Facial (VII)		Blood vessels	Vasodilatation
	Salivatory		Submaxillary	Salivary gland, submandibular	Secretion
Medulla	Salivatory	Glossopharyngeal (IX)	Otic	Parotid gland, sublingual	Secretion
	Nucleus dorsalis	Vagus (X)	Cardiac plexus	Heart	Inhibition of coronary blood flow
	Nucleus dorsalis		Intramural	Bronchi	Constriction, secretion
	Nucleus dorsalis		Intramural	Stomach and intestines	Enhanced peristalsis
	Nucleus dorsalis		Mesenteric plexus	Proximal colon	Vasodilatation, secretion

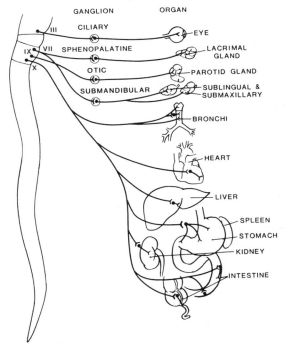

Fig. 10-14. Visceral efferents arising in brain stem.

micturition and erection in the sacral cord. The sacral parasympathetic efferents are listed in Table 10-7.

Sympathetic Efferent Pathway

The descending sympathetic fibers from the hypothalamus and reticular formation are located in the lateral areas of the brain stem and spinal cord. They terminate on preganglionic visceral efferent neurons in the intermediolateral cell column of the thoracic and upper lumbar spinal cord. Neurons in these lateral projections of the gray matter

between the first thoracic and the second lumbar level give rise to the *preganglionic sympathetic fibers*. These fibers are cholinergic, relatively short, and extend only to the paravertebral or prevertebral ganglia, where they synapse with the postganglionic neurons (Fig. 10-15). Each preganglionic sympathetic fiber synapses with many postganglionic neurons to produce widespread effects. The preganglionic neurons are cholinergic, while most postganglionic neurons are adrenergic. There are some postganglionic cholinergic sympathetic fibers to blood vessels and to sweat glands.

The preganglionic sympathetic fibers leave the thoracic and lumbar spinal cord via the ventral roots, but branch from the spinal nerve as the white rami communicantes shortly after they pass out of the vertebral column (Fig. 10-16). These fibers either synapse in the immediately adjacent paravertebral ganglion of the sympathetic trunk or pass through it to the prevertebral ganglia around the aorta. The postganglionic neurons in these ganglia provide sympathetic innervation to the entire body (Table 10-8). The sympathetic efferents in general produce constriction of blood vessels, sweating, and piloerection.

Lesions involving the spinal cord produce autonomic dysfunction that is determined by the level of the lesion. Lesions interrupting the descending sympathetic pathways result in loss of blood pressure control and, in particular, hypotension in the erect position (orthostatic). Lesions in the sacral cord impair bladder function.

Visceral Ganglia

The visceral nervous system is organized periph-

Table 10-7. Sacral Efferent Parasympathetic Innervation

Spinal cord	Ganglion	Organ	Effect of stimulation
S-2 through S-4	Intramural	Distal colon	Enhanced peristalsis, secretion, defecation, inhibition of anal sphincter
	Hypogastric plexus		
S-2 through S-4	Intramural (vesical plexus)	Urinary bladder	Contraction of vesical muscle
	Hypogastric plexus		Inhibition of urethral sphincter
S-2 through S-4	Hypogastric plexus (pelvic plexus)	Male genitals	Vasodilatation, erection
S-2 through S-4	Hypogastric plexus	Female genitals	Vasodilatation

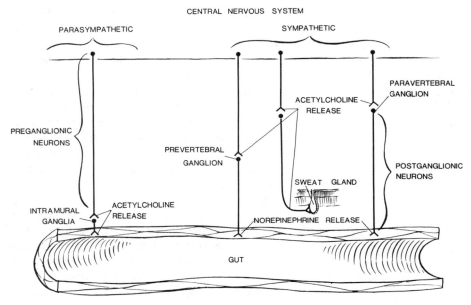

Fig. 10-15. Anatomic and pharmacologic differences between sympathetic and parasympathetic neurons.

erally in ganglia and plexuses. A *ganglion* is a group of nerve cells in a connective tissue capsule. A *plexus* is a complex network of axons traveling from one area to another. The most distal motor neuron in the visceral system, the postganglionic neuron, is located either in a ganglion or in a neural plexus within an organ.

The visceral neurons arise from the neural crest during development and migrate peripherally. Some of the visceral neurons are found in the dorsal root ganglia as visceral sensory neurons, some in the paravertebral ganglia, some in the

Fig. 10-16. Pathway of sympathetic visceral efferents arising from thoracolumbar spinal cord.

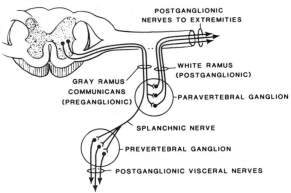

prevertebral ganglia, and others in ganglia in or near specific organs. Different types of neurons are intermingled during development so that the large *visceral plexuses* such as the celiac plexus contain postganglionic sympathetic neurons, preganglionic parasympathetic axons, and afferent fibers from the viscera.

The ganglia consist of large round cells with multiple short dendrites in complex arborizations, some of which form cups or glomeruli. Their cytoplasm has a relative lack of Nissl substance, and each cell is encased in a thin capsule. The entire ganglion is embedded in a dense connective tissue capsule, but there is not a blood-neuron barrier in the ganglion of the type found in the central nervous system. The complex dendritic processes provide each ganglion cell with multiple inputs from the spinal cord, from other levels of the visceral system, and from afferent

Table 10-8. Efferent Sympathetic Innervation

Spinal cord	Ganglion	Site	Effect of stimulation
T-2 through T-6	Stellate	Upper limbs	Vasoconstriction, sweating, piloerection
T-5 and T-6	Stellate	Cardia	Contraction
T-6 through T-9	Celiac plexus	Stomach	Inhibition of peristalsis and secretion, vasoconstriction
T-9 and T-10	Celiac plexus	Intestine	Inhibition of peristalsis and secretion, vasoconstriction
T-6 through T-9	Celiac plexus	Liver	Vasoconstriction
T-6 through T-10	Celiac plexus	Pancreas	Vasoconstriction, possible secretion
T-12 and L-1	Superior mesenteric plexus	Proximal colon	Inhibition of peristalsis and secretion, vasoconstriction
T-12 and L-1	Celiac plexus	Kidney	Vasoconstriction, inhibition of secretion
T-10 through L-1	Chromaffin cells	Adrenal gland	Secretion
T-12 and L-1	Hypogastric plexus	Urinary bladder	Inhibition of vesical muscle, contraction of internal sphincter, contraction of prostate and spermatic vein
T-12 and L-1	Hypogastric plexus	Uterus	Contraction of uterus
L-1 and L-2	Inferior mesenteric plexus, hypogastric plexus	Distal colon, rectum	Inhibition of peristalsis
T-11 through L-2	Lumbosacral sympathetic trunk	Lower limbs	Vasoconstriction, sweating, piloerection

fibers, and permit single ganglion cells to integrate activity from multiple sources. Some of the cells in the ganglia are interneurons called *chromaffin cells* whose axons remain within the ganglion.

Specific Ganglia

The visceral ganglia in the periphery are the location of the postganglionic neurons in the sympathetic and parasympathetic pathways. Since the central connections of the sympathetic and parasympathetic neurons are separated into the thoracolumbar and craniosacral divisions, the ganglia in the head, the pelvis, and near organs contain parasympathetic neurons, whereas those along the vertebral column and the aorta contain sympathetic cells. While many of these ganglia, such as those in the sympathetic trunk, contain only one of these types of fiber, some of the parasympathetic ganglia contain postganglionic sympathetic axons that pass through without synapse on their way to the effector glands and organs.

The parasympathetic ganglia that innervate cra-

nial structures include the ciliary, the submandibular, the sphenopalatine, and the otic ganglia, which provide parasympathetic innervation for the pupil, salivary glands, lacrimal glands, and blood vessels of the face.

The *superior cervical ganglion* provides the sympathetic supply to cranial structures. It lies behind the internal carotid artery high in the neck at the level of the angle of the jaw at the upper end of the sympathetic trunk (Fig. 10-17) and gives rise to the postganglionic sympathetic axons, which travel to their destination via plexuses around blood vessels. Preganglionic fibers innervating this ganglion leave the spinal cord in the T-1 spinal nerve and ascend to the ganglion in the sympathetic trunk. The postganglionic fibers to the sweat glands are cholinergic; all others are adrenergic. Stimulation of these fibers causes vasoconstriction, sweating, and piloerection.

The *inferior cervical ganglion* or *stellate ganglion* in the sympathetic trunk lies anterior to the transverse process of the seventh cervical vertebra and sends postganglionic sympathetic fibers

Fig. 10-17. Sympathetic nerves and ganglia innervating the head. Additional axons follow blood vessels widely to all other areas of the head.

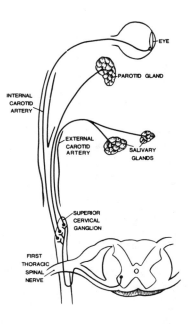

*Fig. 10-18. Sympathetic nerve supply to the upper extremity from stellate ganglion in paravertebral sympathetic trunk. (*Dashed lines *represent postganglionic axons.)*

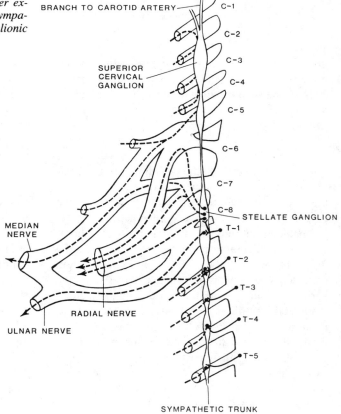

to the cervical spinal nerves via the gray rami. These fibers are distributed to the upper extremity (Fig. 10-18) and the heart. Like other sympathetic ganglia, they produce vasoconstriction, sweating, and piloerection of the extremity, and an increased heart rate.

The *paravertebral* or *chain ganglia* in the sympathetic trunk are the sites of many of the postganglionic sympathetic neurons that provide innervation for the viscera of the chest and abdominal cavity and for the lower extremities. Each of these ganglia gives rise to a gray ramus to the corresponding spinal nerve, which provides sympathetic efferent innervation in the distribution of that nerve. Other branches join blood vessels to reach their destinations, but the major branches of the paravertebral ganglia join to form three splanchnic nerves: the superior, middle, and inferior. The splanchnic nerves enter the chest and abdominal cavities, where they join the parasympathetic fibers to form the major plexuses. The cardiac and pulmonary plexuses lie in the chest cavity, and the celiac, mesenteric, and hypogastric plexuses lie in the abdominal cavity. Another plexus, the myenteric plexus, lies within the wall of the intestinal tract. The celiac plexus

is the largest of these lying at the level of the last thoracic vertebra, anterolateral to the aorta. Some of the components of a celiac ganglion are illustrated in Figure 10-19. Activity in the sympathetic fibers generally results in inhibition of activity in the abdominal viscera and increased cardiac activity.

The postganglionic sympathetic neurons to the lower extremities are in the caudal end of the paravertebral chain ganglia. The axons reach the spinal nerves and the blood vessels to the legs via the gray rami. Branches from the lumbar sympathetic ganglia also enter the abdominal cavity to join parasympathetic and afferent fibers in the hypogastric and sacral plexuses to the bladder, rectum, and genital organs. Activity in the sympathetic fibers inhibits defecation, partially inhibits the bladder wall, and produces ejaculation in the male and uterine contraction (during parturition) in the female.

The hypogastric plexus also contains parasympathetic ganglia with postganglionic neurons that provide innervation to the bladder, rectum, and genitals via the pelvic splanchnic and hypogastric nerves. Activity in the parasympathetic nerves enhances peristalsis in the rectum, defecation, contraction of the bladder wall, relaxation of the internal sphincter (micturition), and hyperemia of the genital organs. Vasodilatation of the erectile tissue occurs with activity in cholinergic para-

Fig. 10-19. Visceral fibers in celiac plexus to intestine. Afferents are shown as broken lines, efferents as solid lines.

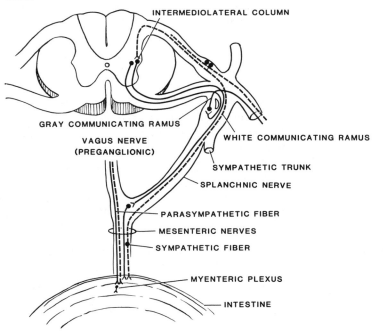

INTERMEDIOLATERAL COLUMN

GRAY COMMUNICATING RAMUS

VAGUS NERVE
(PREGANGLIONIC)

WHITE COMMUNICATING RAMUS

SYMPATHETIC TRUNK

SPLANCHNIC NERVE

PARASYMPATHETIC FIBER

MESENTERIC NERVES

SYMPATHETIC FIBER

MYENTERIC PLEXUS

INTESTINE

Table 10-9. Autonomic Effects on Various Organs of the Body

Organ	Effect of sympathetic stimulation	Effect of parasympathetic stimulation
Eye (pupil)	Dilated	Contracted
Glands		
Lacrimal	Vasoconstriction	Stimulation of thin,
Parotid		copious secretion containing many enzymes
Skin sweat glands	Copious sweating (cholinergic)	None
Piloerector muscles	Excited	None
Skin blood vessels	Constricted (adrenergic) Dilated (cholinergic)	None
Heart		
Muscle	Increased rate	Slowed rate
Coronary vessels	Vasodilated	Constricted
Lungs		
Bronchi	Dilated	Constricted
Blood vessels	Mildly constricted	None
Gut		
Lumen	Decreased peristalsis and tone	Increased peristalsis and tone
Sphincter	Increased tone	Decreased tone
Bladder		
Detrusor	Inhibited	Excited
Trigone	Excited	Inhibited
Ureter	Inhibited	Excited
Penis and clitoris	Ejaculation (penis)	Erection
Systemic blood vessels		
Visceral	Constricted	None
Muscle	Constricted (adrenergic) Dilated (cholinergic)	None

sympathetic fibers. The extremities receive no known parasympathetic innervation.

The visceral efferent (autonomic) dual pathways (sympathetic and parasympathetic) have widespread effects, which are summarized in Table 10-9.

Visceral Effectors

The visceral system contains efferent axons that innervate the organs and glands of the body, including all of the secretory glands, the gastrointestinal tract, the heart, blood vessels, lungs, kidneys, bladder, skin, eyes, salivary glands, and genital organs. There are, however, important general principles pertaining to all these effector organs that should be understood.

The effector organs of the visceral system are smooth muscles and glands. The sensory receptors are located in the glands or organs. The visceromotor structures are the smooth muscle fibers. These have unique properties that make

them different from the striated muscle of the somatic motor system. *Smooth muscle* has excitability and contractility, as does somatic muscle, but it also has three other features that distinguish it: automatism, adaptation, and intramural conduction. Smooth muscle that is isolated from any innervation will continue to contract in an organized and often rhythmic fashion in response to natural stimuli—that is, it is *automatic*. The automatism is often due to rhythmic generation of impulses in a pacemaker area, which then spread to other areas. The pacemakers may shift from one region to another. Temperature, oxygen concentration, and ionic balance all have major effects on the amount and pattern of the automatic activity.

Smooth muscle also can *adapt* to different situations. For instance, the rhythmicity of contractions and the amount of contraction are altered without neural influence by the stretch or distention of an organ. The smooth muscle response to neural stimuli is also greatly influenced by chemical and humoral factors.

The third property of smooth muscle is *intramural conduction*. If a local area of a visceral organ, such as intestine, is stimulated, local contraction will ensue that will then travel slowly along the length of the gut. The mechanism of spread involves local intramural neural connections and transmission of impulses through the syncytium that smooth muscle cells form. Although most syncytial muscle is spontaneously active, some smooth muscle is organized into units similar to striated muscle, which are not active without neural input. This is a much less common arrangement but is seen, for instance, in walls of the vas deferens and in the intrinsic eye muscles. Smooth muscle has no cross striations, and the nerve terminal, although in close contact, does not form a direct connection of the type found in somatic neuromuscular junctions.

All smooth muscle cells alter their activity in response to neurotransmitters, especially acetylcholine and norepinephrine, which are released at

the endings of the postganglionic sympathetic and parasympathetic fibers to produce an enhancement, inhibition, or alteration in smooth muscle activity. This variability of response to transmitters forms the basis for the clinical effects of many medications and toxins.

Activity in the visceral system may also result in a change in the activity of glands. The salivary glands, the sweat glands, and glands in the intestinal tract may increase, decrease, or change the character of their secretion in response to neural activity. Like smooth muscle, some glands may continue to function in the absence of innervation. This ability to function autonomously permits the visceral effectors independence from nervous control, and, as a result, with neural lesions, altered visceral system function is often less apparent than altered somatic function.

Visceral Neurotransmission

The physiologic and pharmacologic properties of neurons in ganglia are of importance in understanding the response of the body to drugs and medications, many of which act at visceral efferent synapses. The postganglionic neurons are of two types: cholinergic and adrenergic. The syn-

Fig. 10-20. Synthesis of norepinephrine and epinephrine.

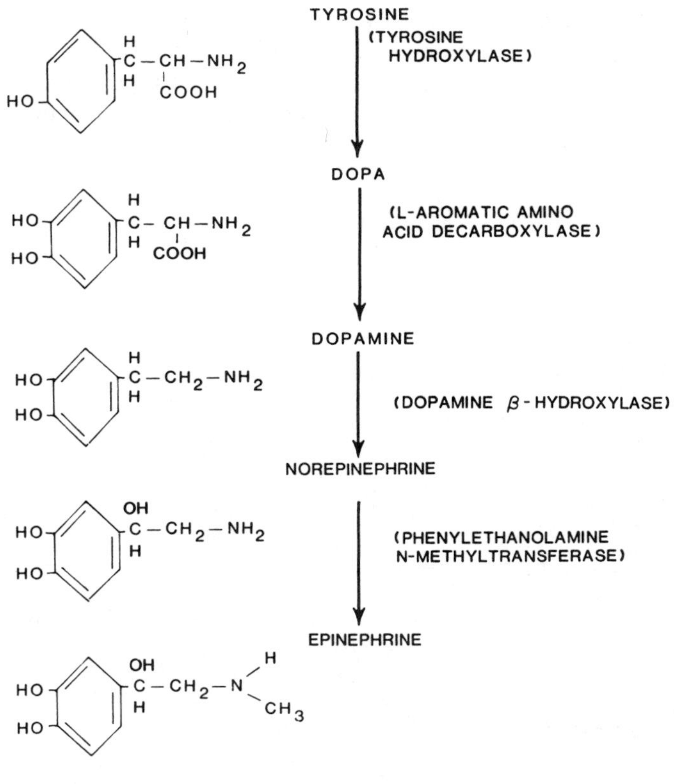

thesis of acetylcholine and norepinephrine in both cholinergic and adrenergic neurons occurs in the nerve terminals, is catalyzed by enzymes transported down the axon from the cell body, and is similar to formation of these substances elsewhere in the nervous system. The synthesis of each will be considered in detail.

Norepinephrine

The first step in the formation of norepinephrine is the conversion of tyrosine to dopa (dihydroxyphenylalanine) by reaction with the enzyme tyrosine hydroxylase, a reaction that is localized to adrenergic nerves in the periphery (Fig. 10-20). Dopa decarboxylase reacts with dopa in the presence of pyridoxal phosphate (vitamin B$_6$) to yield dopamine. Dopamine is converted to norepinephrine by the addition of a hydroxyl group on the alpha carbon of the side chain. This is done by reaction with the enzyme dopamine-beta-hydroxylase, which is a copper-containing enzyme employing ascorbate and fumarate as cofactors. Norepinephrine may be converted to epinephrine by methylation of the terminal amino group. This is accomplished by reaction with the enzyme phenylethanolamine-*N*-methyltransferase in the adrenal medulla.

Fig. 10-21. Release of norepinephrine (NE) at nerve terminals for alpha- and beta-adrenergic receptors. (COMT = catechol-O-methyltransferase, VMA = deaminated derivative.)

The enzymes are synthesized in the cell body and transmitted to the nerve terminals by axonal transport. At the nerve terminal, the first two steps take place in the cytoplasm. The final step, conversion of dopamine to norepinephrine, takes place inside the catecholamine storage vesicle. These vesicles, which correspond to the dense core vesicles seen in adrenergic nerves under the electron microscope, contain the active dopamine-beta-hydroxylase. An active transport system brings dopamine into the vesicle and hence into contact with dopamine-beta-hydroxylase. Changes in the rate of synthesis of norepinephrine in response to changes in demand for the transmitter occur by end-product inhibition of tyrosine hydroxylase, the rate-limiting step in the synthesis of norepinephrine.

After synthesis, norepinephrine is stored in the vesicle in a complex with adenosine triphosphate (ATP). The storage vesicle serves the dual functions of protecting the neurotransmitter from intraneuronal degradation by enzymes and of maintaining the neurotransmitter in a package suitable for release to the exterior of the cell. Release of catecholamines from both the adrenal medulla and the sympathetic nerve terminals takes place by a calcium-dependent exocytosis that is initiated by an action potential (Fig. 10-21). The storage vesicle moves to the surface of the membrane and fuses with it so that part or all of the soluble contents are discharged to the exterior. The process of neurotransmission, therefore,

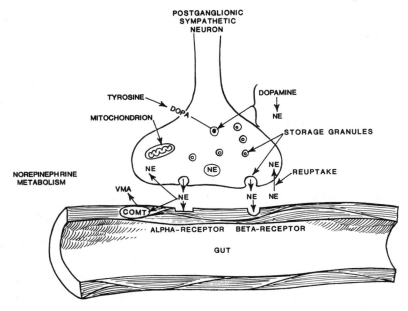

involves not only the release of chemical transmitter but also (in the case of adrenergic nerves) the release of ATP, proteins, and other substances that can mediate the trophic influences of nerves on their effector cells. Catecholamines also can be released from nerves by drugs such as tyramine which displace them from their binding sites within the storage vesicle. In this type of drug-induced release, other substances are not released with the transmitter.

Enzymatic degradation of catecholamines is accomplished by two enzymes: monoamine oxidase (MAO) and catechol-O-methyltransferase (COMT). Eighty percent of the metabolites produced are either the O-methylated derivatives (metanephrine and normetanephrine) or the deaminated derivative (VMA). Monoamine oxidase is present in high concentration inside the nerve terminal, apparently associated with the outer membrane of the mitochondria. However, COMT is not found within the nerve, but is associated with the postsynaptic effector cells. The different tissue distribution of these two enzymes corresponds to different metabolic roles. MAO degrades ingested intraneuronal catecholamines. COMT degrades catecholamines released from the nerve terminal. However, the inhibition of MAO and COMT does not increase the duration of action of norepinephrine, since it is taken up into the terminals of adrenergic nerves by an active carrier-mediated process that requires metabolic energy and operates against a concentration gradient. In addition to terminating the action of released norepinephrine, the process of neuronal uptake may have another function, that of conservation of transmitter. Norepinephrine, which is taken up in adrenergic nerve endings and reaccumulated in the vesicles, represents transmitter that does not have to be replaced by synthesis. The chromaffin cells (interneurons in ganglia) release dopamine as neurotransmitter which is synthesized by the same metabolic pathway.

The neurons that synthesize and release the catecholamines (dopamine, norepinephrine, and epinephrine) are found in several brain areas and are the sites of action of a number of drugs that alter behavior. Dopamine-producing neurons are more numerous than the other two types and are found largely in the midbrain and diencephalon, projecting to the diencephalon and telencephalon (especially the substantia nigra and ventral tegmen-

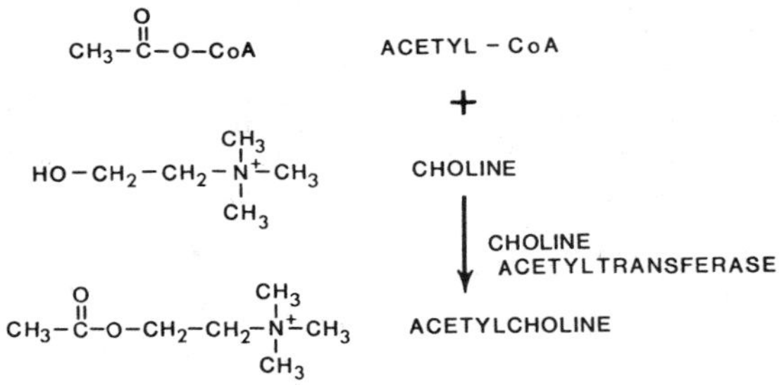

Fig. 10-22. Synthesis of acetylcholine.

tum). Norepinephrine neurons are mainly in the medulla and pons (especially the locus ceruleus and lateral tegmentum). Epinephrine neurons are not limited to specific areas.

Acetylcholine

The synthesis of acetylcholine (ACh), the choline ester of acetic acid, in nerves is less complex than that of norepinephrine (Fig. 10-22).

In a single-step reaction, acetyl-CoA and choline are combined to form ACh in a reaction catalyzed by choline acetyltransferase (choline acetylase). The source of acetyl-CoA for this reaction is either acetate or citrate in mitochondria. Choline is taken up from plasma by cholinergic nerves with an efficient mechanism that is greatly stimulated by nerve activity. Even so, the supply of choline probably limits the rate of synthesis of ACh. Wherever ACh synthesis takes place, ACh is stored within vesicles inside the nerve terminal.

The release of acetylcholine from nerve terminals occurs by a calcium-dependent exocytosis initiated by an action potential, just as with norepinephrine. The action of acetylcholine released from nerves is terminated exclusively by the degradative enzyme *acetylcholinesterase* (AChE). This enzyme catalyzes the hydrolysis of acetylcholine into acetate and choline.

Neurotransmitter Action

A single transmitter may have different actions on different areas of a cell membrane (different receptors). These receptors can be identified with microelectrode recordings of their electrical potentials, but can be distinguished more readily by their responses to blocking agents. The neurotransmitter receptors on visceral neurons and peripheral effectors can be differentiated into four

Table 10-10. Receptor Types

Receptor	Usual transmitter	Effect and site of action	Blocking agent
Alpha-adrenergic	Norepinephrine	Depolarization and smooth muscle contraction	Phenoxybenzamine
Beta-adrenergic	Epinephrine	Hyperpolarization and smooth muscle relaxation	Dichloroisoproterenol
Nicotinic	Acetylcholine	Short-duration EPSP at striated muscle or ganglia	Curare
Muscarinic	Acetylcholine	Slow depolarization of smooth or cardiac muscle	Atropine

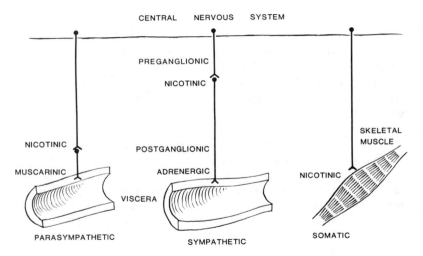

Fig. 10-23. Usual locations of nicotinic and muscarinic acetylcholine receptors.

types according to their responses to pharmacologic agents: alpha-adrenergic, beta-adrenergic, nicotinic, and muscarinic (Table 10-10 and Fig. 10-23).

Norepinephrine may act on some neurons, but its primary site of action is on alpha-adrenergic receptors of smooth muscle. It is generally excitatory, resulting in contraction of smooth muscle in blood vessels, kidneys, and other areas and in enhancement of glycogenolysis. Other catecholamines such as epinephrine have similar effects. The alpha-adrenergic receptors respond to a neurotransmitter with an increased permeability to sodium ions, depolarization, and an increased cell discharge frequency.

In contrast, beta-adrenergic receptor activation results in relaxation of contracting muscle and in vasodilatation of bronchioles and intestine. The beta-adrenergic receptors are particularly sensitive to isoproterenol (epinephrine with a propyl group), but they are activated by epinephrine released from the adrenal medulla into the general circulation by splanchnic nerve activity. Beta-adrenergic receptor activation results in increased cellular metabolism, increased sodium pump activity with hyperpolarization, and reduced cell firing rates.

The receptors for acetylcholine are also of two types and can be differentiated by electrical response or their response to nicotine and muscarine, both of which, like acetylcholine, produce a depolarization of cholinergic receptors. Nicotine produces a depolarization that is sustained

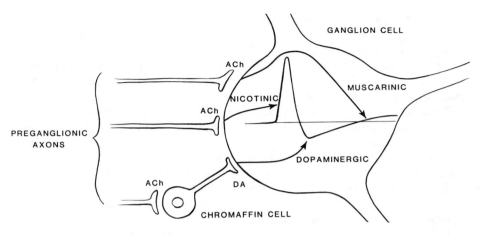

Fig. 10-24. Responses of postganglionic cell to pre-ganglionic activity: acetylcholine (ACh), dopamine (DA). The direction and relative duration of the membrane potential change from each type of synapse are shown to the right of the synapse. An upward deflection indicates depolarization.

with high doses and results in inactivation of the receptor. This action is blocked by curare but not by atropine and is typical of the response (nicotinic) to acetylcholine seen at striated muscle and at most ganglionic synapses. The action of acetylcholine on smooth muscle and heart is more like that of muscarine. It can be blocked by atropine, and depolarization is transient, even at high doses.

There may be more than one type of receptor present on a single neuron, each producing distinct electrical changes. Nicotinic and muscarinic receptor excitations both result in excitatory postsynaptic potentials (EPSPs); however, they are of differing durations. The nicotinic receptor gives a fast EPSP of a few milliseconds in duration,

whereas a slow depolarization occurs at the muscarinic receptor. Ganglionic neurons in ganglia also exhibit slow IPSPs due to norepinephrine release by chromaffin cells. Figure 10-24 illustrates different receptors on a single neuron in a sympathetic ganglion. Long-duration potential changes (10 to 20 seconds) can result from metabolic alterations rather than from a membrane conductance change.

Recently, a third type of transmission has been demonstrated in the visceral system in the gastrointestinal tract. Some postganglionic sympathetic fibers do not end near the smooth muscle cells but act through small interneurons that have short axons in the wall of the intestine. These neurons, the third in the peripheral sympathetic pathway, release ATP and are referred to as *purinergic neurons*. They inhibit smooth muscle activity. A number of other neurotransmitters are known in the central nervous system and may be active in visceral neurotransmission.

Table 10-11. Comparison of Neurotransmitter and Hormonal Transmitter Action

Characteristic	Synaptic transmission	Neurohormonal communication
Avenue	Between contiguous cells in synaptic contact	Between remote cells without synaptic contact
Distribution	Limited by axonal connections	Limited by receptors on target cells
Substance	Acetylcholine, amino acid, catecholamines, peptide	Peptide
Release	Synaptic terminals	Neurocirculatory terminals
	Ca^{2+} dependent	Ca^{2+} dependent
Receptors	At synapse	Extrasynaptic
Actions	Rapid acting	Rapid and slow acting
Function	Regulation of single neuron	Regulation of multiple cells

Neurotransmitters, one of the major forms of chemical transmission, are all synthesized in cell bodies, rapidly transported down axons, and released at a synapse; they act rapidly on single postsynaptic cells and are metabolized by enzymes. The other group of transmitters of the visceral system, neurohumoral transmitters, are also synthesized in cell bodies, transported to nerve terminals, and destroyed by enzymes. However, they are all peptides, are released into the circulation, have slow but long-lasting action, act on many cells, and, as such, are hormones (Table 10-11).

While the receptor response to these neurotransmitters may be a direct change in the membrane conductance in some cases (e.g., acetylcholine on nicotinic receptors), in others, a "second messenger" transduces the effect of the neurotransmitter on the cell membrane or cell metabolism. The second messengers in the membranes of visceral system neurons include the well-known cyclic adenosine monophosphate (AMP) and the recently identified calcium-linked polyphosphoinositide.

Ganglionic neuronal receptor responses to drugs and toxins underlie the signs and symptoms associated with some intoxications. Poisoning with some types of mushrooms is due to the effects of muscarine and produces salivation, small pupils, wheezing, diarrhea, slow pulse, and delirium. It is treated by atropine, which blocks cholinergic activity at muscarinic receptors. In contrast, the "deadly nightshade" mushroom contains belladonna, an atropine-like drug that produces dilated pupils; hot, dry, red skin; dry mouth; rapid pulse; rapid respiration; and urinary retention. This poisoning has no adequate antidote, and symptomatic treatment is used.

Loss of function in the visceral nervous system may occur because of a lesion in the peripheral effector, but this cause is uncommon. Functional loss also may occur from damage to the postganglionic neuron. Loss of this neuron and its neurotransmitter results in an alteration of the effector cell membrane, so that it has an increased sensitivity to the neurotransmitter, known as *denervation hypersensitivity*. The presence of denervation hypersensitivity can be used as evidence that a lesion involves the postganglionic neuron rather than the more proximal portions of the visceral system.

Clinical Correlations

The activities of the visceral nervous system are involved in virtually all functions of the body and, therefore, have a broad range of clinical significance. Lesions at the supratentorial level can interfere with any of the hypothalamic-hypophyseal functions and, through them, the endocrine system. Lesions at the posterior fossa level often affect the visceral efferents at that level or the visceral centers in the brain stem, especially the respiratory centers. Lesions at the spinal cord level can alter cardiovascular and bladder function in particular. A number of peripheral disorders can result in diffuse autonomic failure.

The degenerative disorder of idiopathic orthostatic hypotension (Shy-Drager syndrome) is due to degeneration of cells in the intermediolateral cell column of the spinal cord and may be associated with degenerative changes in other systems. The major symptoms are those of postural hypotension, impotence, loss of sweating, and sphincter disturbances. Diffuse peripheral nerve disease, such as that with diabetes, can also produce diverse autonomic disturbances of the pupils, sweating, hypotension, impotence, sphincter disturbance, diarrhea, and other cardiovascular disturbances. Another diffuse visceral system disorder, botulism, is due to the toxin of *Clostridium botulinum*, which binds to the nerve terminal to block the release of acetylcholine. Weakness, blurred vision, dry mouth, constipation, hypotension, nausea, and vomiting are common symptoms. The pupils are unreactive; there may be urinary retention; and weakness, especially of eye muscles, is common.

In addition to these generalized disorders, specific disorders of the pupil, cardiovascular system, bladder, and sweat glands are of clinical importance.

Localized lesions in four areas of the nervous system produce visceral system syndromes. Damage to the hypothalamus produces a wide variety of disorders of metabolism—eating, drinking, temperature regulation, growth, and endocrine disorders. Localized brain-stem lesions can produce ipsilateral deficit of cranial parasympathetic functions and descending sympathetic pathways. Spinal lesions can produce sympathetic or parasympathetic disturbances at the appropriate levels. Peripheral damage can result in loss of

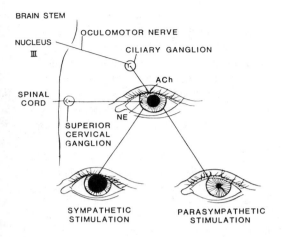

*Fig. 10-25. Effects of sympathetic and parasympathetic activity on pupil size. (*ACh = *acetylcholine,* NE = *norepinephrine.)*

sympathetic function in the extremities or of both functions in the viscera.

Although many symptoms, signs, and tests relate indirectly to function in the visceral system, the clinician has available only a limited number of procedures for directly testing visceral neural functions. The visceral afferent sensations of olfaction and taste can be directly tested but will be considered with the functions of the posterior fossa and cerebral hemispheres in subsequent chapters.

Pupil

The pupil of the eye changes its size automatically under control of the visceral nervous system in response to environmental illumination and other afferent or emotional stimuli. The pupil is

controlled by two sets of muscles: the constrictors (a circular band of muscle) and the dilators (a radial band of muscle). The constrictors are innervated by preganglionic parasympathetic fibers arising in the Edinger-Westphal nucleus and traveling in the *oculomotor nerve* to the ciliary ganglion in the orbit. The postganglionic fibers pass directly from the ganglion into the eye. The dilator fibers are innervated by the postganglionic sympathetic fibers arising in the *superior cervical ganglion,* which receive their innervation from cells in the intermediolateral column of the upper thoracic cord via the first and second thoracic nerves and the sympathetic chain (Fig. 10-25).

The size of the pupils is a function of the relative activity in these two systems. A large pupil may result from overactivity of the sympathetic fibers or from underactivity of the parasympathetic fibers. Lesions that produce such alterations may occur at any level and involve preganglionic or postganglionic fibers. The light reflex, in which the pupil constricts in response to a flash of light, and the accommodation reflex, in which the pupil constricts during near vision, are of particular interest to the clinician who is looking for disease of the nervous system. The former depends on afferent fibers from the retina, which travel via the optic nerves to the upper midbrain, where synapses are made bilaterally so that stimuli in either eye will constrict both pupils. The pattern of pupillary responses with lesions at different sites is listed in Figure 10-26.

The miosis (small pupil) seen with damage to the sympathetic efferents to the pupil often occurs in combination with an absence of sweating and ptosis (drooping) of the eyelid. These occur because of the loss of innervation of the sweat glands and loss of innervation of the tarsal muscle that aids in maintaining the eyelids open. This combination is known as *Horner's syndrome* and

Fig. 10-26. Pupil size with and without light stimulation in presence of lesions at different sites.

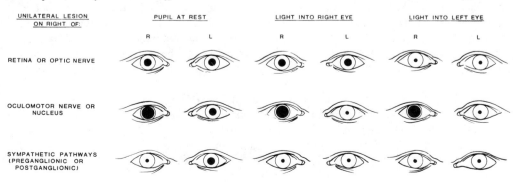

UNILATERAL LESION ON RIGHT OF:	PUPIL AT REST		LIGHT INTO RIGHT EYE		LIGHT INTO LEFT EYE	
	R	L	R	L	R	L
RETINA OR OPTIC NERVE						
OCULOMOTOR NERVE OR NUCLEUS						
SYMPATHETIC PATHWAYS (PREGANGLIONIC OR POSTGANGLIONIC)						

is seen with lesions of the descending sympathetic fibers in the brain stem or the spinal cord, lesions of the first and second thoracic spinal nerves, or lesions of the postganglionic fibers in the sympathetic trunk or carotid sheath. Damage to the third cranial nerve produces a mydriasis (dilated pupil). This is an important sign in diagnosing herniation of the brain stem. The differentiation of preganglionic from postganglionic lesions often can be made by placing drugs that act on the pupil on the conjunctiva. With a postganglionic lesion, axons may degenerate and the pupil muscle fibers become denervated. The pupil then becomes sensitive to low concentrations of drugs that act like norepinephrine or acetylcholine because of denervation hypersensitivity. Within a preganglionic lesion, the postganglionic fibers remain intact, and drugs that displace the neurotransmitter from the nerve terminal can activate the paralyzed muscle fibers. This differentiation can be made for sympathetic or parasympathetic lesions.

Skin
The skin receives sympathetic innervation to the sweat glands, to the piloerector muscles, and to the blood vessels. Sympathetic fiber activity results in constriction of the blood vessels, sweating, and erection of the hair and is the mechanism by which cold, clammy skin occurs with fear or anxiety. There is no parasympathetic innervation to the skin, so that the loss of the sympathetic innervation will result in warm, dry skin. This occurs after surgical removal of a portion of the sympathetic trunk and with damage to peripheral nerves. The former is sometimes performed to improve blood supply to a limb. Anhydrosis (lack of sweating) is also one of the characteristic features of Horner's syndrome.

Sympathetic innervation of the skin is tested by determining the patient's ability to sweat. The changes that occur in skin resistance with sweating and vasoconstriction in response to emotional stimuli are a major part of the recordings made in lie detector tests.

Circulation
The visceral system controls circulation through its modulation of both blood vessel size and cardiac rate. The former is partially mediated by sympathetic fibers, the latter by both sympathetic and parasympathetic nerves. Both respond to visceral sensory input from cardiac receptors, blood vessels, and receptors in the central nervous system. These reflexes can selectively alter blood flow to individual organs. A number of diseases may alter these responses, with the most striking abnormality being an inability to maintain normal blood pressure. For example, generalized disorders of peripheral visceral nerve fibers cause a loss of adjustment in blood pressure with changes in posture—orthostatic hypotension. The patient's blood pressure decreases on standing, with lightheadedness and fainting. This hypotension is tested by measuring the heart rate and blood pressure during changes in position.

Bladder
Micturition (the passage of urine) is primarily under the control of the visceral system. The neural supply to the bladder is of three types—sympathetic, parasympathetic, and somatic—all arising from the upper lumbar or sacral spinal cord (Fig. 10-27), and all under control of descending motor and incoming sensory information.

The preganglionic sympathetic fibers leave the spinal cord as white communicating rami in the region of the lower thoracic and upper two lumbar segments. They proceed to the paired sympathetic chains and pass through them to the aortic plexus where they synapse with postganglionic fibers. The lower portion of the aortic plexus is the hypogastric plexus which divides into right and left halves, each of which forms a hypogastric nerve. The hypogastric nerve passes deeply in the pelvis and joins the pelvic plexus, from which fibers pass to smaller plexuses around to the bladder, prostate, seminal vesicles, and proximal portion of the urethra.

The parasympathetic nerves arise as preganglionic branches from the second, third, and fourth sacral spinal nerves. They join to form the pelvic nerve. These fibers proceed to the pelvic plexus, where they join the sympathetic fibers. They may form synapses in the pelvic plexus or pass through it and synapse with postganglionic cells in the wall of the bladder. They initiate bladder contraction for voiding.

The *pudendal nerve* contains both somatic motor and sensory fibers. It arises from the second, third, and fourth sacral nerves and divides into the dorsal nerve of the penis or the clitoris and

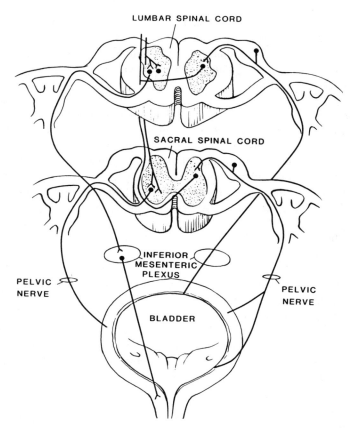

Fig. 10-27. Nerve supply to bladder. Afferents are shown on left, efferents on right.

the perineal nerve. The muscular branches of the perineal nerve supply the muscles of the perineum (including the external urethral sphincter, which stops the flow of urine when closed).

Afferent sensory fibers are present in the sympathetic, parasympathetic, and somatic nerves. The sensory pathways from the bladder are not clearly understood, but the afferent fibers associated with parasympathetic nerves (pelvic nerves) carry most of the clinically important afferent fibers from the bladder and adjacent structures. The pudendal nerves furnish sensory innervation to the perineum and urethra. The sympathetic nerves carry no more than vague bladder sensations. Sensations of pain, temperature, and bladder fullness ascend to the cerebral hemispheres via the spinothalamic tracts and posterior columns.

The genital organs of the male have their main parasympathetic supply through the pelvic nerves from the third and fourth sacral segments. Stimulation of these nerves produces increased secretion of prostatic fluid and penile erection by vasodilation in the corpora cavernosa. The sympathetic innervation of the genital organs is via the sympathetic trunk and the pelvic plexus. Stimulation of the sympathetic nerves produces contraction of the musculature of the seminal vesicles and ejaculation and, in addition, causes contraction of the internal urethral sphincter. Sensory nerves from the genitalia are found in both the sympathetic and the parasympathetic pathways.

The reflex center for micturition is in the sacral portion of the spinal cord. Most bladder activity is mediated in this center, initiated by sensory input from the pelvic and pudendal nerves. However, it is modulated through visceral efferent tracts from the brain. These descending fibers are in the direct and indirect activation pathways. The areas in the brain concerned with micturition are on the medial surface of both frontal lobes.

Disorders of bladder function may occur with various types of neural damage. Although bladder dysfunction is manifested by different symptoms and signs, the following functions are commonly impaired:

1. *Sensory.* The feeling of fullness or desire to void can be lost. Specific modalities of sensation are not normally recognizable.
2. *Motor.* The ability to initiate or stop voiding can be lost. Inability to prevent voiding results in urinary incontinence; inability to initiate voiding results in urinary retention.
3. *Reflexes.* Intrinsic bladder reflexes cannot be readily tested clinically. However, the bulbocavernosus reflex and anal reflex are mediated via the conus medullaris and are of value in evaluating bladder disturbances. To test these reflexes, the contraction of the anal sphincter is palpated by a finger in the rectum. The bulbocavernosus reflex is elicited by squeezing the glans penis, the anal reflex by pricking the perianal skin with a pin. Both actions should result in a brisk contraction of the anal sphincter.
4. Other important features of a bladder with neurogenic dysfunction are the frequency of void-

Fig. 10-28. Sites of lesions producing different disturbances of bladder function. A. Reflex bladder. B. Autonomous bladder.

ing, the amount voided, the capacity of the bladder (the amount of liquid it will hold), and the residual urine (the amount left after voiding). The latter two are determined by catheterization.

Disorders producing bladder dysfunction may destroy the reflex arc for micturition by damaging the sensory fibers, motor fibers, or the reflex center in the conus. However, they may also leave the reflexes intact by damaging the descending pathways or higher centers. These are called *nonreflex* and *reflex neurogenic bladders,* respectively, and can be subdivided into five groups, each of which has been given a number of names.

NONREFLEX, AUTONOMOUS BLADDER.　A nonreflex, autonomous bladder, also called *nuclear* or *infranuclear,* results from damage to the sacral spinal cord, the nerve roots, or the peripheral nerves to the bladder. The reflex arc for micturition has been interrupted by destruction of the conus, the cauda equina, or the pelvic nerves that carry both the motor (parasympathetic) and sensory fibers that control the bladder.

In this disorder, bladder sensation is abolished and the desire to urinate is gone, although there

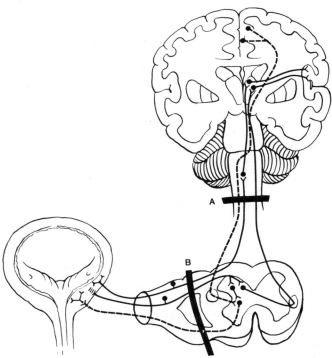

may be some vague sensations of fullness in the suprapubic or perineal areas. There is no voluntary control (ability to inhibit or initiate urination) and little or no activity of muscle in the bladder wall. There may be minor rhythmic bladder contractions of the smooth muscle initiated in the ganglia of the bladder wall. These contractions are insufficient to empty the bladder, producing only irregular, intermittent jets or spurts. If the abdominal muscles are intact it may be possible for the patient to express some urine by means of abdominal straining or manual compression. The bulbocavernosus and anal reflexes are impaired or lost. The amount of residual urine usually is large, and the capacity of the bladder is variable. The bladder has reduced tone (atonic) (Fig. 10-28).

NONREFLEX, SENSORY PARALYTIC (OR SENSORY ATONIC) BLADDER.   If only the sensory fibers from the bladder are damaged, sensation is lost and the normal emptying reflexes do not occur. The bladder becomes distended, and urine dribbles out (overflow incontinence). Bladder capacity and residual are large. Anal and bulbocavernosus reflexes are often lost as well. This is an uncommon form of neurogenic bladder occurring mainly in tabes dorsalis, a form of neurosyphilis.

NONREFLEX, MOTOR PARALYTIC (OR MOTOR ATONIC) BLADDER.   If only the motor fibers to the bladder are lost, sensation remains intact but voluntary control and all reflexes are lost. The bladder becomes distended with overflow incontinence. This form of neurogenic bladder is rare, occurring with motor polyradiculopathies.

REFLEX, AUTOMATIC (OR SUPRANUCLEAR) BLADDER.   A supranuclear lesion is located above the sacral segment of the spinal cord so that the reflex arc for micturition remains intact and an automatic reflex bladder is the result. In the classic automatic reflex bladder with spinal cord destruction, the patient is incontinent, with involuntary evacuation of urine generally occurring at regular intervals. The interval is determined by the bladder volume, and the voiding is initiated by sensory activity from the distended bladder. The automatic reflex bladder may function efficiently if the interval between evacuations

of urine is substantial (one or several hours) (Fig. 10-28).

Patients have no sensation of bladder filling and no knowledge of the desire to void, but may have sensations that warn them of impending micturition in sufficient time to procure a urinal. Examples of such sensations are sweating, headache, or sensations of abdominal discomfort. Patients may be able to find trigger areas in the region supplied by nerves served by the sacral segments so that tapping, stroking, or pinching the skin around the anus, perineum, inner surfaces of the thighs, vulva, penis, or scrotum may induce micturition. The bulbocavernosus and anal reflexes are intact.

Residual urine can result from the bladder's inability to expel its contents completely and is the underlying difficulty that is responsible for most of the problems associated with automatic reflex bladders. It is impossible, from present knowledge, to decide which is the greater factor responsible for residual urine, the resistance to the outflow of urine or the inefficient expulsion of the urine. Both factors probably are involved.

The amount of residual urine present in an automatic reflex bladder is the best measure of the efficiency of the bladder. The volume of urine that an automatic reflex bladder can hold may be much less than normal, and such a bladder has been called *hypertonic* or *spastic*. In some persons, the bladder capacity becomes so small that the short interval between voidings simulates the intermittent spurts of the nonreflex autonomous bladder. The frequent, irregularly spaced evacuation of urine is one of the most troublesome forms of bladder involvement in spinal cord disease. There are several contributing causes to this annoying situation, including (1) loss of the reservoir function of the bladder because of the relatively small difference between residual urine and bladder capacity amounts; (2) loss of the suprasegmental control; (3) nonbladder reflexes, such as flexion of the lower extremities and spasm of the abdominal muscles, which may act as a trigger mechanism to initiate bladder contraction; and (4) local irritation within the bladder itself, from infection, bladder stones, or obstruction, which also may trigger contraction of the bladder.

REFLEX, UNINHIBITED BLADDER.   In some cerebral disorders, normal sensation, tone, and reflexes are present. Bladder capacity and residual are usually also normal. Yet the patient is unable to voluntarily inhibit voiding. This often occurs with less severe, incomplete spinal cord lesions or with supratentorial lesions and is the type of bladder present in children before they become toilet trained.

Examination of Visceral Function

The visceral nervous system encompasses all the major organ systems, and therefore complete evaluation would require examination of each of these systems. Such examinations are not germane to this presentation. A number of visceral functions are carried via cranial nerves and will be considered in detail in Chapter 14. A limited but important number of specific functions should be tested as part of the neurologic examination of visceral function.

Pupil

The size and equality of the pupils and their reaction to light depend on the balance of sympathetic and parasympathetic input. They must be carefully noted. Normal pupils are between 2 and 4 mm in diameter, are equal, and react briskly on both sides to light in each eye.

Skin

Skin temperature and moisture are directly controlled by the sympathetic fibers. A search should be made for the localized absence of sweating and asymmetric skin temperature or color, as well as for the presence of normal oral and conjunctival moisture.

Cardiovascular

Pulse and blood pressure can reflect alterations in neural input and must be part of each examination. A pronounced decrease in blood pressure while the patient is standing (orthostatic hypotension) and an alteration in the blood pressure and heart rate responses to the Valsalva maneuver may be signs of neurovisceral impairment.

Bladder

The bladder cannot be examined directly, but palpation and percussion of the bladder can provide evidence of abnormal bladder distention. The anal and bulbocavernosus reflexes test the integrity of the sacral reflex arc.

Pharmacologic

The eye and skin can be tested with cholinergic and adrenergic drugs to determine if there is denervation hypersensitivity (excessive response) or loss of response, in an attempt to distinguish preganglionic from postganglionic lesions.

The visceral system makes up a major part of the control systems for normal function, mediating all the unconscious activities of the viscera and organs. It makes use of a duality of pathways and overlapping of function, providing much more autonomy and resistance to disorders of the central or peripheral nervous system. Its sensory and motor components are organized at multiple levels, with a multiplicity of outflow pathways, both neural and humoral.

Objectives

1. List the major components including motor and sensory and their connections in the visceral system at the supratentorial, posterior fossa, spinal, and peripheral levels.
2. Describe the location and visceral function of the hypothalamus, reticular formation, cranial parasympathetic nuclei, intermediolateral cell column, and peripheral ganglia.
3. Differentiate sympathetic and parasympathetic pathways by their location, cellular features, function, and pharmacology.
4. List three reasons why damage to somatic and visceral systems differs in severity and type of alteration in function.
5. Describe the clinical effects of a lesion of the hypothalamus, medullary reticular formation, oculomotor nerve, superior cervical and stellate ganglia, and conus medullaris.
6. List sites at which lesions could produce pupil abnormalities and describe the type of abnormality seen with each.
7. List the sites at which lesions could produce bladder disorders, and the type of disorder seen with each.

Clinical Problems

1. A 52-year-old man was referred for evaluation because of blackouts. The spells had begun a year before admission and were becoming more frequent. They occurred only when he arose from a supine or sitting position to a standing one and were most severe in the morning. This change in position precipitated

a giddy feeling in his head and dimness of vision and often was followed by complete loss of consciousness. No convulsive movements were observed and shortly after hitting the floor he regained consciousness, only to pass out again if he got up too quickly.

In addition to this primary symptom, the patient complained that, during the past 3 years, he had also gradually become sexually impotent. He also noted that he felt very uncomfortable in hot weather and did not perspire as he had before. On occasion, fever would develop during hot weather, with no evidence of infection.

On examination, blood pressure was recorded at 130/70 mm Hg when the patient was supine. When he sat up, it decreased to 110/50 mm Hg and when he stood, it was 70/30 mm Hg, and he began to complain of faintness. The pulse rate was 82 to 90 per minute during the entire episode. The skin was warm and dry and remained so after many minutes in a hot examining room. Results of the remainder of the physical examination were normal.

a. What is the site of the pathology?

b. What is the type of pathology?

c. Which of the patient's symptoms could be due to a disorder of sympathetic efferents?

d. What effect would pilocarpine (which directly stimulates sweat glands) have on this patient?

e. Which of the following may result in hypotension?

(1) Spinal cord lesion at T-2

(2) Fear

(3) Peripheral nerve disease

(4) Micturition

2. A 51-year-old tree trimmer had gradually experienced difficulty with urination during a 6- to 9-month period. He felt less urge to urinate, had difficulty in starting, and voided only small amounts. Recently, he had also developed incontinence and a urinary tract infection.

On examination, he had reduced anal sensation with absent anal and bulbocavernosus reflexes. His bladder was distended, but he was unable to empty it.

a. What is the location of the pathology?

b. What is the type of pathology?

c. What type of bladder disturbance is this?

d. What abnormalities of sexual function might be expected?

3. A 37-year-old man who had had a thyroid carcinoma completely resected had a 2-month progressive history of left shoulder pain, with no motor or sensory symptoms.

Examination revealed drooping of the left eyelid, the left pupil smaller than the right (though both reacted normally to light), and dry skin on the left side of his face.

a. What is the location of the pathology?

b. What is the type of pathology?

c. What structure is most likely involved?

d. Does the lesion involve sympathetic or parasympathetic fibers?

e. List the structures where these pathways could be damaged to result in a similar syndrome.

f. In this patient, a drug that releases norepinephrine from nerve terminals has no effect. What does this indicate?

g. If a drug that causes the release of norepinephrine from nerve terminals evokes a pupillary dilatation, where is the lesion most likely to be located?

4. An elderly, retired oil tycoon was brought to the emergency room complaining of severe, cramping abdominal pain, vomiting, diarrhea, and shortness of breath. He was able to relate that he became ill about half an hour after ingestion of a hearty meal served to him by his young bride of only a month. The meal consisted of steak smothered in mushrooms, mashed potatoes, and home-canned green beans. His spouse had complained of not feeling well before dinner and had not eaten at all.

Examination revealed marked tearing. The pupils were pinpoint in size. The patient was salivating profusely. Pulse rate was 50 per minute. Examination of the chest revealed diffuse rales in inspiration and wheezing in expiration. Auscultation of the abdomen revealed markedly active bowel sounds, and the examination was frequently interrupted by the patient's urgent need for a bedpan.

a. What is the location of the pathology?

b. What is the type of pathology?

c. Is the disorder due to an abnormality in the sympathetic or parasympathetic pathways?

d. What is the most likely cause of the disorder?

e. What would be the effect of a cholinergic blocking agent on the pupils?

f. Give examples of situations in which emotional activity in the limbic system alters function in the following organs:
 (1) Heart
 (2) Gastrointestinal tract
 (3) Urinary tract
 (4) Skin
 (5) Lacrimal glands

5. A 14-year-old boy was examined because of a complaint of a discharge over a 4-month period from his nipples. Additional questioning also elicited a 2-year history of some headaches when supine, a 20-lb weight gain, and recently some lethargy and irritability.

   Examination revealed mild obesity and sallow skin. The patient moved slowly, and his voice was deep. He had a clear discharge from both nipples. He had no secondary sexual characteristics. Examination of the cranial nerve showed only a partial loss of vision in the temporal fields bilaterally.

   a. What is the level and site of the lesion?
   b. What is the type of pathology?
   c. Which neural structures are involved?
   d. What are the major efferent and afferent pathways to this area?
   e. What receptors are found in this area?
   f. By what mechanism are most of the symptoms occurring?

Suggested Reading

Appenzeller, O. *The Autonomic Nervous System* (3rd rev. ed.). New York: Elsevier, 1982.

Boyarsky, S. Pathophysiology of the Bladder. In S. Eliasson, A. L. Prensky, and W. B. Hardin, Jr. (eds.), *Neurological Pathophysiology* (2nd ed.). New York: Oxford University Press, 1978. Pp. 134–138.

Cooper, J. R., Bloom, F. E., and Roth, R. H. *The Biochemical Basis of Neuropharmacology* (2nd ed.). New York: Oxford University Press, 1974. Pp. 65–174.

De Vivo, D. C. The Autonomic Nervous System. In S. Eliasson, A. L. Prensky, and W. B. Hardin, Jr. (eds.), *Neurological Pathophysiology* (2nd ed.). New York: Oxford University Press, 1978. Pp. 109–121.

De Vivo, D. C. Some Hypothalamic Disturbances. In S. Eliasson, A. L. Prensky, and W. B. Hardin, Jr. (eds.), *Neurological Pathophysiology* (2nd ed.). New York: Oxford University Press, 1978. Pp. 121–134.

Eadie, M. J., and Tyrer, J. H. *Biochemical Neurology.* New York: Liss, 1983.

Guttman, L. The Neurogenic Bladder: Vesical Pathophysiology. In E. S. Goldensohn and S. H. Appel (eds.), *Scientific Approaches to Clinical Neurology*, Vol. II. Philadelphia: Lea & Febiger, 1977. Pp. 1927–1940.

Lance, J. W., and McLeod, J. G. *A Physiological Approach to Clinical Neurology* (3rd ed.). Boston: Butterworth, 1981. Pp. 263–285.

McLeod, J. G. Peripheral Autonomic Failure. In T. J. Crow (ed.), *Disorders of Neurohumoural Transmission.* New York: Academic, 1982. Pp. 45–82.

The Vascular System

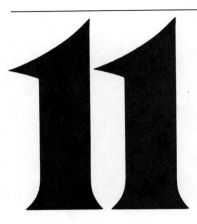

The blood vessels to an organ provide it with a relatively constant supply of oxygen and other nutrients and a means for removal of metabolic wastes. Failure to meet these vital requirements results in disease in that organ. Because of the unique structure and organization of the nervous system, localized abnormalities in blood supply may produce devastating alterations in neural function. In this chapter, the normal anatomy and physiology of the vascular supply to neural tissue and the clinical manifestations of pathologic processes affecting this system will be described.

Of all neurologic diseases likely to be encountered, cerebrovascular disease (stroke) is among the most common. Cerebrovascular disease represents a major cause of disability and death throughout the world. In the United States, stroke ranks third as a cause of death (heart disease is first; cancer is second; accidents are fourth). Because the majority of stroke victims survive the acute phase of their illness and may live for years thereafter in a disabled condition, the social and economic impact of stroke is immeasurable. It is estimated that more than $440 million is spent annually on diagnosis, treatment, and rehabilitation of stroke victims.

Vascular disease involving cerebral vessels is no different from vascular disease involving other organ systems. The processes of atherosclerosis and thromboembolism differ little whether they involve the cerebral, peripheral, or coronary circulation. However, understanding the clinical problems in patients with cerebrovascular disease depends on a more detailed understanding of activities that are unique to the nervous system.

In the other longitudinal systems already discussed, the manifestations of disease are a direct result of damage to neural tissue within that system. The vascular system, however, is a supporting system, and diseases of the vascular system will be manifest as secondary alterations in function in other neural systems. The vascular cause of disease is identified by the characteristic temporal profile of sudden onset and rapid evolution of symptoms involving other systems.

Overview

In order to sustain aerobic metabolism, the brain is supplied by two major arterial systems. Much of the cerebral hemispheres is supplied by the carotid arterial system, while the entire posterior fossa, occipital lobes, and portions of the temporal lobes are supplied by the vertebrobasilar system. A series of anastomotic channels, including the circle of Willis located at the base of the brain, interconnect these two systems. Lesions involving the carotid arterial system may alter function in the distribution of any or all of its three clinically important branches: ophthalmic artery, anterior cerebral artery, and middle cerebral artery. Therefore the various combinations of hemiparesis, hemisensory deficit, monocular visual loss, homonymous hemianopia, and aphasia are suggestive of a lesion in this system. Lesions involving the vertebral and basilar arteries may alter function in the distribution of any or all of their clinically important branches, which include those to the brain stem, to the cerebellum, and to the occipital and temporal lobes via the posterior cerebral artery. The various combinations of diplopia, dysarthria, dysphagia, and disequilibrium, associated with hemiparesis, hemisensory deficit, or homonymous hemianopia, are suggestive of a lesion in the vertebrobasilar system.

The blood supply to the spinal cord is via the anterior spinal artery and paired posterior spinal arteries (branches of the vertebral arteries and descending aorta), and the vascular supply to the peripheral nerves is usually via nutrient vessels from accompanying major arterial channels.

Cerebral blood flow is normally maintained at a relatively constant rate of approximately 50 to 55 ml/100 g brain tissue per minute by a process of *autoregulation* and can thereby compensate for fluctuations in perfusion pressure and cerebrovascular resistance. Reduction in blood flow below a critical threshold level results in ischemia and infarction.

The clinical pattern seen with disease in the cerebrovascular system is distinctive. The cardinal identifying feature is its *acute* onset. The symptoms produced are a reflection of the location and nature of the pathologic process. The symptoms of vascular disease may be either focal or diffusely distributed and result from parenchymal dysfunction secondary to the primary pathologic change in the blood vessels or circulatory system. The parenchymal lesions, which are the result of either occlusive-ischemic or hemorrhagic disease processes, may be of a mass or a nonmass type (Table 11-1).

Table 11-1. Correlation of Vascular and Parenchymal Disease

Type of vascular disease	Resultant parenchymal lesion	
	Focal	Diffuse
Occlusive-ischemic	Infarct (nonmass)	Anoxic encephalopathy
Hemorrhagic	Intracerebral hemorrhage (mass)	Subarachnoid hemorrhage

Occlusive-Ischemic Vascular Disease

When a portion of neural tissue is deprived of its blood supply, *ischemia* develops. If the normal protective mechanisms are insufficient to compensate for this deprivation, death of tissue, *infarction,* results. The clinical symptoms will reflect tissue damage in the regions of ischemia and infarction. Disease of a blood vessel may result in local thrombus formation, which may progress to occlusion, *thrombosis,* of the vessel; or a portion of the thrombus (embolus) may break loose and lodge in a more distal portion of the circulation. Both processes may result in localized areas of neural tissue being deprived of blood supply, and both may produce a focal destructive lesion (infarct). Atherosclerosis is by far the most important disease process responsible for thromboembolic disease; it is not, however, the only disease process responsible for it. Ischemia also may occur without occlusive disease if there is hemodynamic failure of the circulatory system (as might be seen with cardiac disease or profound hypotension). This type of ischemia also may result in infarction, but the defect is usually diffusely distributed throughout the brain as *anoxic encephalopathy.*

Hemorrhagic Vascular Disease

A diseased blood vessel may rupture and leak, producing *hemorrhage.* Depending on the site of accumulation of the blood, focal or diffuse neurologic symptoms may result. Blood that extravasates throughout the subarachnoid space is a *subarachnoid hemorrhage* and results in diffuse neurologic signs. Subarachnoid hemorrhage is commonly the result of trauma, rupture of an intracranial aneurysm, or bleeding from an arteriovenous malformation. Blood that accumulates within the substance of the brain is an *intracerebral hemorrhage* and results in signs of a focal, mass lesion. Intracerebral hemorrhage is commonly the result of hypertensive arteriolar disease or bleeding from an arteriovenous malformation.

Roentgenographic examination of the cerebral blood vessels by injection of a radiopaque substance into the arterial system (cerebral angiography) and computed tomography are important neurodiagnostic techniques that are utilized to identify vascular and other intracranial disease processes.

Anatomy of the Vascular System

Blood Supply to the Brain

All the arteries that supply the supratentorial and posterior fossa levels arise from the aortic arch (Fig. 11-1). The innominate (brachiocephalic) artery divides into the right common carotid and the right subclavian arteries. The left common carotid artery arises directly from the apex of the aortic arch. The right and left common carotid arteries ascend in the neck lateral to the trachea. Slightly below the angle of the jaw each vessel bifurcates into the internal and external carotid arteries.

The *internal carotid* artery on each side enters the skull, without branching, through the carotid canal located in the petrous portion of the temporal bone. After entering the cranium, each internal carotid artery forms an S-shaped curve, the carotid siphon, and lies within the cavernous sinus. As it leaves the cavernous sinus to enter the subarachnoid space at the base of the brain, it gives rise to the *ophthalmic artery,* an important anastomotic communication with branches of the external carotid artery. Each internal carotid artery then divides into an anterior cerebral artery and a middle cerebral artery (Fig. 11-2).

The *vertebral arteries* arise as the first branches of the right and left subclavian arteries. Each artery ascends through foramina in the transverse processes of the upper six cervical vertebrae, curves behind the articular process of the atlas, pierces the dura, and enters the subarachnoid space at the level of the upper cervical spinal cord. The vertebral arteries enter the cranial cavity through the foramen magnum. The verte-

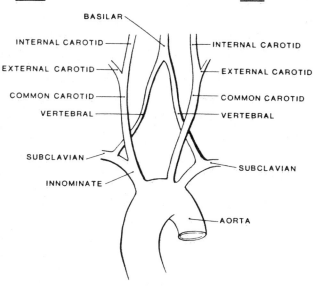

Fig. 11-1. Major arteries supplying supratentorial and posterior fossa levels.

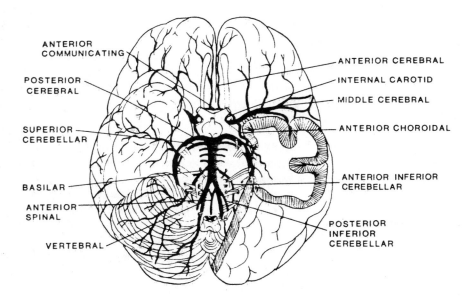

Fig. 11-2. Principal arterial vessels on basal aspect of brain. Portions of the left temporal lobe and the left cerebellar hemisphere have been removed. (Redrawn from B. Pansky and E. L. House. Review of Gross Anatomy [3rd ed.]. New York: Macmillan, 1975.)

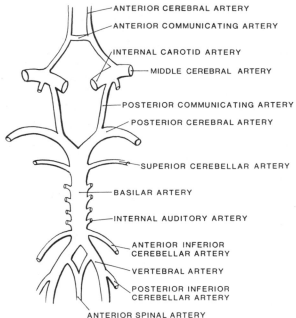

ANTERIOR CEREBRAL ARTERY

ANTERIOR COMMUNICATING ARTERY

INTERNAL CAROTID ARTERY

MIDDLE CEREBRAL ARTERY

POSTERIOR COMMUNICATING ARTERY

POSTERIOR CEREBRAL ARTERY

SUPERIOR CEREBELLAR ARTERY

BASILAR ARTERY

INTERNAL AUDITORY ARTERY

ANTERIOR INFERIOR
CEREBELLAR ARTERY

VERTEBRAL ARTERY

POSTERIOR INFERIOR
CEREBELLAR ARTERY

ANTERIOR SPINAL ARTERY

Fig. 11-3. Major intracranial arteries and circle of Willis (anterior cerebral, anterior communicating, posterior communicating, and posterior cerebral arteries).

bral arteries are subject to normal anatomic variation; the left vertebral artery frequently arises directly from the arch of the aorta. In addition, the two vertebral arteries are often of unequal caliber.

The vertebral arteries enter the cranium and ascend on the anterior lateral surface of the medulla oblongata (Fig. 11-2). At the lower border of the pons, they unite to form the *basilar artery.* At the level of the midbrain, the basilar artery divides into the right and left posterior cerebral arteries.

CIRCLE OF WILLIS.   At the base of the brain, surrounding the optic chiasm and pituitary stalk, anastomotic connections occur between the internal carotid and vertebrobasilar arterial systems. This ringlike series of vessels is called the circle of Willis (Fig. 11-3) and consists of the *anterior communicating artery,* which unites the two anterior cerebral arteries, and the *posterior communicating arteries,* which join the internal carotid arteries with the posterior cerebral arteries. The circle of Willis is subject to frequent anatomic

variation, and a "normal" circle is seen in only approximately 50 percent of the population. Common variations in the circle occur when the posterior cerebral arteries arise directly from the internal carotid via an enlarged posterior communicating artery, when one or both posterior communicating arteries are absent, and when there are multiple small anterior communicating arteries.

BLOOD SUPPLY TO THE CEREBRAL HEMISPHERES. The supratentorial level is provided with blood from the anterior, middle, and posterior cerebral arteries (Fig. 11-4). The *anterior cerebral artery* supplies the medial surface of the cerebrum and the superior border of the frontal and parietal lobes. The *middle cerebral artery* supplies most of the lateral surface of the cerebral hemispheres, including the lateral portions of the frontal lobe, the superior and lateral portions of the temporal lobes, and the deep structures of the frontal and parietal lobes. The *posterior cerebral artery* supplies the entire occipital lobe and the inferior and medial portions of the temporal lobe. The deeper structures of the cerebral hemispheres are supplied by penetrating branches of the larger arteries. Of notable importance are the perforating *lenticulostriate arteries,* which supply the basal ganglia and internal capsule, and the perforating branches of the posterior cerebral artery, which supply the thalamus (Fig. 11-5).

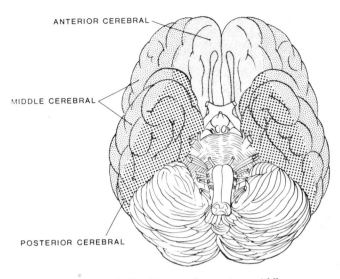

ANTERIOR CEREBRAL

MIDDLE CEREBRAL

POSTERIOR CEREBRAL

Fig. 11-4. Areas of distribution of anterior, middle, and posterior cerebral arteries to the base of the brain.

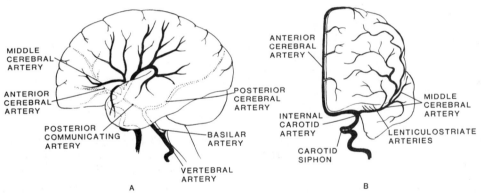

MIDDLE CEREBRAL ARTERY

ANTERIOR CEREBRAL ARTERY

POSTERIOR COMMUNICATING ARTERY

POSTERIOR CEREBRAL ARTERY

BASILAR ARTERY

VERTEBRAL ARTERY

A

ANTERIOR CEREBRAL ARTERY

INTERNAL CAROTID ARTERY

CAROTID SIPHON

MIDDLE CEREBRAL ARTERY

LENTICULOSTRIATE ARTERIES

B

Fig. 11-5. Course and distribution of major supratentorial arteries in a lateral view (A) and an anteroposterior view (B).

ANASTOMOSES AND COLLATERAL CIRCULATION. Extensive communications exist between the arterial systems that supply the brain. Because of the potential for additional circulation through these alternate channels, occlusion of one or more intracranial or extracranial vessels may occur at times, with few or no resultant neurologic signs and symptoms. The major anastomotic channels are (1) the circle of Willis; (2) corticomeningeal anastomoses—communications of the three major cerebral vessels on the surface of the hemispheres at the junctional zones of the areas supplied by these vessels; and (3) anastomoses between extracranial and intracranial arteries. The most significant in the last group occur in the regions of the face and orbit where the ophthalmic artery, a branch of the internal carotid artery, communicates with the superficial temporal and facial branches of the external carotid artery. Occasionally, anastomoses between the external carotid and vertebral arteries occur in the neck.

BLOOD SUPPLY TO THE POSTERIOR FOSSA. The structures contained in the posterior fossa (midbrain, pons, medulla, and cerebellum) are supplied by branches of the vertebral and basilar arteries (see Fig. 11-2). Although there are numerous branches from these vessels, the pattern of blood supply from these branches is relatively constant (Fig. 11-6). At each level of the brain stem, short *median* and *paramedian perforating branches* arise and supply a zone on either side of

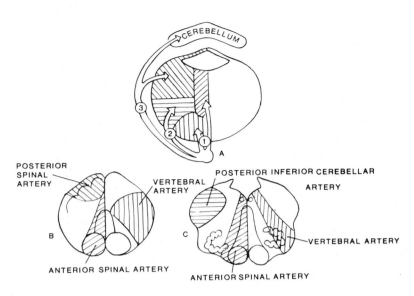

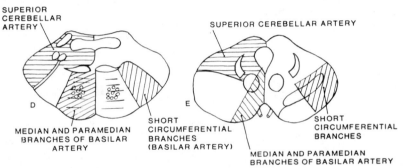

Fig. 11-6. Blood supply to posterior fossa. A. General pattern of blood supply. Arising from the basilar artery are (1) short median and paramedian branches supplying blood to the medial tegmentum and base of the brain stem, (2) short circumferential branches supplying blood to the ventrolateral tegmentum, and (3) long circumferential branches supplying blood to the dorsolateral tegmentum and the cerebellum. The areas of distribution of specific arteries are shown in the caudal medulla (B), medulla (C), rostral pons (D), and mesencephalon (E).

ferior cerebellar arteries arise from the vertebral arteries and supply the lateral medulla and posterior inferior aspect of the cerebellum. The *anterior inferior cerebellar artery* is a branch of the basilar artery and supplies the lateral aspect of the pons and the anterior inferior cerebellum. The *superior cerebellar artery* is a branch of the basilar artery and supplies the lateral midbrain and superior surface of the cerebellum.

FUNCTIONAL ANATOMY OF THE CEREBRAL VASCULATURE. Clinically, the distribution of a presumed arterial lesion can be inferred by relating the observed signs and symptoms to the anatomy of the cerebral vessels. Although precise localization to a specific blood vessel is at times desirable, it is *essential* to be able to determine whether a lesion lies in the distribution of either the carotid or the vertebrobasilar arterial systems.

Lesions involving the internal carotid artery may alter function in the distribution of any or all of its three clinically important branches: (1) the

the midline. The paramedian area of the caudal medulla is supplied by the *anterior spinal artery,* which arises from the union of branches from each vertebral artery. The paramedian area at higher levels is supplied by penetrating branches of the basilar artery. An intermediate zone, situated more laterally at each level, is supplied by *short circumferential branches* of the vertebrobasilar system. The lateral areas of the brain stem and the cerebellum are supplied by three pairs of *long circumferential arteries.* The *posterior in-*

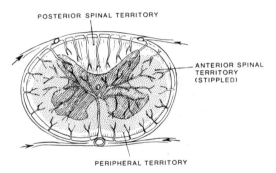

POSTERIOR SPINAL TERRITORY

ANTERIOR SPINAL TERRITORY (STIPPLED)

PERIPHERAL TERRITORY

Fig. 11-7. Schematic transverse section of spinal cord illustrating the areas of supply of the anterior and posterior spinal arteries and the peripheral zone supplied by the circumferential vessels.

ophthalmic artery, producing ipsilateral monocular loss of vision; (2) the anterior cerebral artery, producing contralateral weakness and sensory loss primarily in the leg; and (3) the middle cerebral artery, producing contralateral weakness and sensory loss maximal in the face and arm and to a lesser degree in the leg. If the optic pathways are involved, a contralateral homonymous hemianopia may be produced. With dominant hemisphere lesions, there may be involvement of speech areas, which will result in aphasia.

The various combinations, therefore, of hemiparesis, hemisensory deficit, monocular visual loss, homonymous hemianopia, and aphasia are suggestive of a lesion in the carotid arterial system.

Lesions involving vertebral and basilar arteries may alter function in the distribution of any or all of their clinically important branches: (1) branches to the brain stem itself, resulting in loss of brain-stem function, cranial nerve abnormalities with or without hemiparesis, and hemisensory deficits; (2) branches to the cerebellum, resulting in ataxia and disequilibrium; and (3) posterior cerebral artery, resulting in unilateral or bilateral hemianopia.

The various combinations, therefore, of diplopia, dysarthria, dysphagia, and disequilibrium associated with hemiparesis, hemisensory deficit, and homonymous hemianopia are suggestive of a lesion in the vertebrobasilar arterial system.

Blood Supply to the Spinal Cord
The spinal cord is supplied with arterial blood by one anterior and two posterolateral vessels that run along the length of the cord and by an irregular plexus of segmentally arranged vessels that encircle the cord and interconnect the major vessels (Fig. 11-7). The *anterior spinal artery* is a single vessel lying in the ventral median fissure. It arises from a pair of small branches of the vertebral arteries that fuse along the caudal medulla and descend along the cervical spinal cord (see Fig. 11-2). A series of six to eight ventral radicular arteries arising from the intercostal, lumbar, and sacral arteries connect with the anterior spinal artery at various levels along the length of the spinal cord (Fig. 11-8). The largest of these radicular arteries enters at the low thoracic or upper lumbar region. Because of this uneven blood supply, the spinal cord is most vulnerable to ischemia at the midthoracic and upper lumbar levels, as shown by the stippled areas in Figure 11-8. Sulcal branches of the anterior spinal artery pass alternatively to the right and left at each segment to supply blood for the interior of the spinal cord (see Fig. 11-7).

The *posterior spinal arteries* are paired structures that run along the posterolateral aspect of the cord near the dorsal roots. They receive contributions from the posterior radicular arteries (Fig. 11-9) and supply the dorsal funiculus and dorsal gray horns (see Fig. 11-7).

Vascular diseases of the spinal cord are less common than similar processes in the posterior fossa or cerebrum. When ischemic disease occurs, however, it is most often confined to the distribution of the anterior spinal artery, where it produces loss of motor function and loss of pain and temperature sensation below the lesion; the functions associated with the dorsal columns are spared (see Fig. 11-7).

Blood Supply to Peripheral Structures
All neural structures must receive adequate arterial blood supply in order to sustain life and maintain their integrity. The axons traveling to the periphery are gathered together into bundles or fascicles which have a connective tissue covering. Within this covering, along the entire course of the nerve, is a rich and highly anastomotic plexus of small arterioles that are derived from the branches of the major extremity vessels (Fig. 11-10). This dense anastomosis renders the peripheral nerve relatively immune to ischemic vascular disease. Such abnormality, when noted in

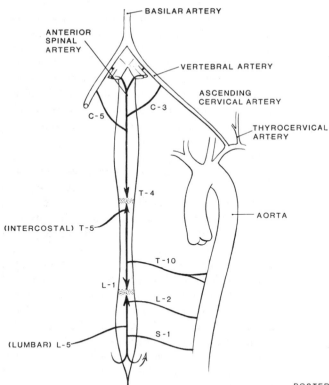

Fig. 11-8. Anterior spinal artery. Radicular arteries
are variable in location but are shown here at C-3, C-
5, T-4, T-10, L-2, L-1, and S-1. Stippled areas indicate
zones of marginal blood supply. (Redrawn from B.
Pansky and E. L. House. Review of Gross Anatomy
[3rd ed.]. New York: Macmillan, 1975.)

peripheral neural structures, is usually associated
with either direct compression of nerve or with
multiple segmental vascular lesions from small-
vessel arterial disease.

Venous Drainage of the Central Nervous System
The venous drainage of the brain is divided into
superficial and deep systems. The cortex and
outer half of the white matter drains into the
superficial system of veins located over the convexity of the brain in the subarachnoid space.
The superficial veins of the superior half of the
brain drain into the *superior sagittal sinus;* those
from the inferior half drain into the *lateral sinuses.* The deep white matter and deep nuclei of
the brain drain into the deep venous system,
which includes the *great cerebral vein of Galen,
inferior sagittal sinus,* and *straight sinus.* From

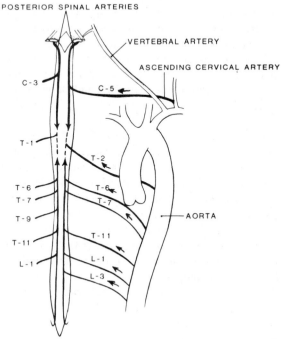

Fig. 11-9. Posterior spinal arteries supply blood to the
posterior aspect of spinal cord. They receive blood
from radicular arteries at multiple levels. (Redrawn
from B. Pansky and E. L. House. Review of Gross
Anatomy [3rd ed.]. New York: Macmillan, 1975.)

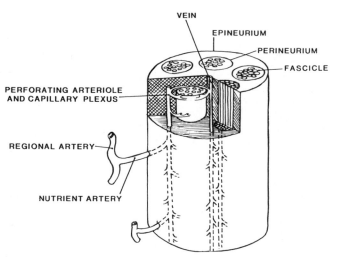

VEIN
EPINEURIUM
PERINEURIUM
FASCICLE
PERFORATING ARTERIOLE
AND CAPILLARY PLEXUS
REGIONAL ARTERY
NUTRIENT ARTERY

Fig. 11-10. Blood supply to peripheral nerve. Multiple anastomotic channels are derived from regional arteries.

these venous channels, blood empties into the transverse sinuses, the sigmoid sinuses, and ultimately the jugular veins (Fig. 11-11). Veins on the inferior surfaces of the cerebrum terminate directly or indirectly in the *cavernous sinus,* an important dural structure located on either side of the pituitary fossa containing the carotid artery; cranial nerves III, IV, and VI; and branches of cranial nerve V.

The spinal cord is drained by an anastomotic venous plexus surrounding the dural sac. Veins drain outward along both the dorsal and ventral roots into this plexus, which has numerous connections with the veins of the thoracic, abdominal, and pelvic cavities.

Physiology of the Vascular System

Cerebral Metabolism

A constant supply of energy is necessary for the support of neuronal and neurologic functions. These vital energy-dependent processes include the establishment of membrane potentials, maintenance of transmembrane ionic gradients, membrane transport, and the synthesis of cellular constituents such as proteins, nucleic acids, lipids, and neurotransmitters. The energy needed is supplied in the form of high-energy phosphate bonds from adenosine triphosphate (ATP), which is synthesized in the brain, as in other organ systems, through the glycolytic pathway, the Krebs (citric acid) cycle, and the respiratory

(electron-transport) chain (Table 11-2).

Under aerobic conditions, glucose is effectively metabolized through the glycolytic pathway, citric acid cycle, and respiratory chain to yield 38 moles of ATP per mole of glucose. Under anaerobic conditions, the Krebs (citric acid) cycle and respiratory chain cannot be activated (because of lack of oxygen), and therefore the pyruvate derived from glycolysis will be metabolized to lactate and will yield only 2 moles of ATP per mole of glucose. Another additional source of high-energy phosphate bonds is *creatine phosphate.* This compound, which is present in the brain in even greater abundance than ATP, is utilized to regenerate ATP from adenosine diphosphate (ADP) and is thus important for maintaining the level of tissue ATP. Although glycogen is present, and the brain is capable of its rapid synthesis and breakdown, the role of glycogen in brain metabolism is not completely understood and the extent of its participation in the production of high-energy phosphate bonds through glycogenolysis in the brain is not known. However, regardless of the existence of glycogen and the possible participation of amino acids in the processes of oxidative phosphorylation, *glucose is the basic substrate for brain metabolism.*

PATHOPHYSIOLOGY. Reversible alteration in cell function due to the lack of oxygen results in ischemia; irreversible alteration results in infarction. Under ischemic conditions, there is deprivation of oxygen and a depletion of glucose, which results in the decreased production of high-energy

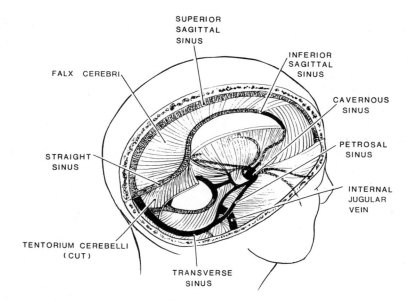

Fig. 11-11. Dura mater and its major sinuses. Dorso-lateral view illustrating falx cerebri, tentorium cere-belli, and dura lining base of skull. The dural venous sinuses are stippled or black.

Table 11-2. Glucose Metabolism

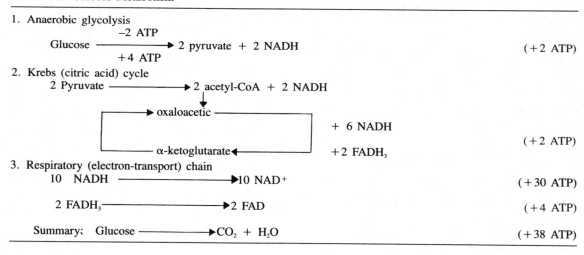

phosphate bonds. With ischemia, glucose metabolism ceases at the end of glycolysis and the end product is lactate. Because this anaerobic system is an inefficient means of producing ATP, glycolysis is more accelerated than under aerobic conditions, thus precipitating depletion of glucose. The tissue level of glucose decreases rapidly to near zero within 1 minute after total ischemia and is variable if some perfusion is retained. Because glycogenesis is also suppressed, the glycogen content in the brain promptly decreases, and glycogen cannot make a significant contribution to cerebral metabolism under anaerobic conditions. Because of this rapid depletion of substrates and inefficient ATP generation, the ATP level also decreases very rapidly. Contributing to this catastrophic situation is the extreme sensitivity of creatine phosphate to oxygen deprivation; the decline of tissue creatine phosphate under ischemic conditions is even more precipitous than that of ATP. Thus, ATP cannot be effectively regenerated from ADP and creatine phosphate, and the brain is almost totally deprived of two major sources of high-energy phosphate bonds 1 minute after ischemia (anoxic). Therefore, within seconds, a loss of blood supply produces an alteration in cellular function. Potassium rapidly leaks out of the cell (particularly at small cortical dendrites and synapses), and as the concentration of extracellular potassium increases, membrane potential is lost and cellular function ceases.

At this early stage, if the period of ischemia is short and the supply of high-energy phosphate bonds can be reestablished, neuronal function can resume. The local accumulation of carbon dioxide, the production of lactic acid, and the decrease in available oxygen all serve to produce local vasodilation in an attempt to restore an adequate blood supply. However, if the cell continues to be deprived of its nourishment, catabolic and morphologic changes occur in the neuron. Initially, the cell begins to swell (acute cell change); if its metabolic needs are then not met, the cell becomes irreversibly damaged. This is referred to as infarction, the morphologic correlate of which is *ischemic cell change* (described in Chap. 4). If the area of infarction is large, other cellular elements and the blood-brain barrier will be affected. In the region of maximal change, there is death and destruction of cells. With the catabolic changes and breakdown in the blood-brain bar-

rier, the water content of the tissue increases. The associated *brain edema* may further impair the function of cells in the regions surrounding the infarction. After reparative attempts are made and the cellular debris is removed, a cystic cavity remains.

In conditions of partial ischemia, the decline of high-energy phosphate bonds is less precipitous, and the irreversible damage occurs only after a more prolonged period of ischemia. Thus, in *cerebral hypoxia,* because there is an abundant supply of glucose, the metabolic changes are similar to those of anoxia, but lesser in extent. However, if the hypoxia is prolonged, the accumulation of lactate due to accelerated glycolysis becomes significant, and ischemia and infarction may result.

In *hypoglycemia,* the brain is supplied with adequate oxygen but lacks glucose as a substrate. Hypoglycemia produces a different metabolic pattern than that seen in cerebral ischemia. In hypoglycemia, the brain can maintain high-energy phosphate bonds through the utilization of creatine phosphate and other substances. Although function is temporarily altered, if the glucose deficiency is not present for a prolonged period, then catabolic changes are not produced and recovery can occur upon reversal of the hypoglycemic state.

The Regulation of Cerebral Blood Flow

For normal neural function, adequate blood flow and oxygenation must be maintained. The normal blood flow through the brain is approximately 750 ml per minute, or about 50 to 55 ml/100 g brain tissue per minute. Although the brain constitutes only 2 percent of the body weight, it receives 15 percent of the cardiac output and utilizes 20 percent of the oxygen consumed in the basal state. The total oxygen consumption of the brain is approximately 50 ml per minute or 3.7 ml/100 g brain tissue per minute. As has been shown, any decrease in the amount of available oxygen provided to the brain reduces neural activity. Under normal conditions, the total oxygen consumption and blood flow to the brain are nearly constant. Cortical gray matter with its increased metabolic demand has about six times the blood flow of white matter. Local changes in blood flow may occur with the changing demands of varying neural activity.

In any hemodynamic system, blood flow is directly proportional to the perfusion pressures and inversely proportional to the total resistance of the system. For the brain, this can be expressed by the following equation:

$$\text{Cerebral blood flow} \approx \frac{\text{mean arterial pressure} - \text{central venous pressure}}{\text{cerebrovascular resistance}}$$

A number of factors can modify cerebral blood flow by altering different elements in the equation above. These have been arbitrarily divided into two groups: (1) extrinsic or extracranial factors and (2) intrinsic or intracranial factors (Table 11-3).

EXTRINSIC FACTORS. Factors outside the cranial cavity that modify or regulate the cerebral blood flow are primarily related to the cardiovascular system and include the systemic blood pressure, the efficiency of cardiac function, and the viscosity of the blood. The principal force in maintaining the cerebral circulation is the pressure difference between the arteries and the veins. Since under normal circumstances, cerebral venous pressure is low (approximately 5 mm Hg),

the arterial blood pressure becomes the most important single factor in maintaining cerebral blood flow. Variations in systemic arterial blood pressure do not, however, ordinarily produce changes in cerebral blood flow in healthy persons if the intrinsic regulatory mechanisms are intact, unless the mean arterial pressure decreases to less than 50 to 70 mm Hg. The systemic arterial blood pressure is dependent on the efficiency of cardiac function (cardiac output) and the peripheral vasomotor tone or resistance. These are governed principally by autonomic control from the vasomotor center in the medulla. Alterations in cardiac rhythm and myocardial function, or the presence of cardiac disease, may result in changes in cardiac output that may secondarily influence cerebral blood flow. Baroreceptors in the carotid sinus and aortic arch participate in reflexes that mediate cardiovascular tone and help to maintain a constant blood pressure. Advancing age, the presence of atherosclerosis, and certain drugs may alter these reflex mechanisms, and a simple physiologic act such as assuming an upright posture may result in severe orthostatic hypotension and pronounced reduction in cerebral blood flow (causing fainting or syncope). In addition, the viscosity of the blood may alter cerebral

Table 11-3. Factors Regulating Cerebral Blood Flow (CBF)

Factors	Increased CBF	Decreased CBF
Extrinsic		
Systemic blood pressure		Mean arterial pressure <50 to 70 mm Hg
Cardiovascular function		Cardiac arrhythmias; orthostatic hypotension; loss of carotid sinus and aortic arch reflexes
Blood viscosity	Anemia	Polycythemia
Intrinsic		
State of the cerebral vasculature	Arteriovenous malformation	Atherosclerosis
Intracranial CSF pressure		Increased intracranial pressure
Cerebral autoregulatory mechanisms		
Myogenic factors	Decreased intraluminal pressure (vasodilation)	Increased intraluminal pressure (vasoconstriction)
Neurogenic factors	Parasympathetic stimulation (vasodilation)	Sympathetic stimulation (vasoconstriction)
Biochemical-metabolic factors	Increased carbon dioxide (vasodilation)	Decreased carbon dioxide (vasoconstriction)
	Decreased oxygen (vasodilation)	Increased oxygen (vasoconstriction)
	Decreased pH (acidosis) (vasodilation)	Increased pH (alkalosis) (vasoconstriction)
	Lactic acid (vasodilation)	

blood flow; severe anemia may increase flow as much as 30 percent, while polycythemia may decrease flow by more than 50 percent.

INTRINSIC FACTORS. The state of the cerebral vasculature also can influence cerebral blood flow. Widespread intracranial arterial disease increases cerebrovascular resistance and can result in a reduction in cerebral blood flow, while pathologic processes that are associated with a rapid shunting of blood from arteries to veins (such as occurs with an arteriovenous malformation) may produce both an increase in total cerebral blood flow and a local reduction in tissue perfusion.

Any increase in intracranial pressure is transmitted directly to the low-pressure venous system and increases cerebral venous pressure, thus decreasing cerebral blood flow. In pathologic states that are frequently accompanied by an increase in intracranial pressure (see Chap. 6), this reduction in blood flow may further accentuate the signs and symptoms produced by the primary lesion.

The normal brain has the ability to regulate its own blood supply (autoregulation) in response to changes in the arterial blood pressure and metabolic demand. *Autoregulation* is defined as the ability of an organ (for example, the brain) to maintain its blood flow constant for all but the widest extremes in perfusion pressure. Autoregulation of the cerebral blood flow occurs when the mean arterial blood pressure is between 60 and 150 mm Hg; below 60 mm Hg, blood flow decreases, and above 150 mm Hg, blood flow increases.

The brain can accomplish autoregulation by using myogenic, neurogenic, and chemical-metabolic mechanisms. Cerebral vessels, like other hollow organs that contain smooth muscle, can alter their diameter in response to intraluminal pressure. This effect (known as the Bayliss effect) results in vasoconstriction with increased intraluminal pressure and in vasodilation with a decrease in pressure. Autoregulation therefore is primarily a pressure-controlled myogenic mechanism that operates independently but synergistically with other neurogenic and chemical-metabolic factors.

Although neurogenic factors do not seem to have as great a role in regulating cerebral blood flow as do chemical-metabolic ones, the extracranial and intracranial cerebral arteries are richly supplied by a neural network, and autonomic function exerts some influence in mediating cerebral vasomotor tone. Postganglionic fibers from the cervical sympathetic chain innervate the carotid and vertebral arteries, as well as their major intracranial branches; and stimulation of the cervical sympathetic vessels produces vasoconstriction and a decrease in cerebral blood flow. Parasympathetic fibers from the geniculate ganglion traveling via the facial and superficial petrosal nerves innervate cerebral vessels of large and small diameter. Stimulation of the facial nerve produces vasodilation in pial vessels and an increase in blood flow.

Chemical-metabolic factors exert a strong influence on cerebral blood flow. *Carbon dioxide,* a substance that rapidly diffuses across the blood-brain barrier and an end product of cerebral metabolism, is also the most potent physiologic and pharmacologic agent that influences cerebral blood flow. Cerebral blood vessels react rapidly to any change in local carbon dioxide tension ($PaCO_2$). Any increase in $PaCO_2$ will produce vasodilation and increased cerebral blood flow, whereas a decrease in $PaCO_2$ will have the opposite effect. The cerebral circulation reacts to *oxygen* in the reverse manner; a reduction in PaO_2 produces vasodilation and increased cerebral blood flow, and an increase in PaO_2 produces vasoconstriction and a decrease in cerebral blood flow. The exact mechanism by which these agents exert their effects on cerebral blood vessels is unknown. They may act directly on the smooth muscle of the vessel wall, indirectly via neurogenic chemoreceptors, or they may act by producing alterations in brain hydrogen ion concentration (pH). A reduction in brain pH (acidosis) from any cause will produce vasodilation and increased cerebral blood flow, whereas an increase in brain pH (alkalosis) is associated with vasoconstriction and decreased cerebral blood flow. *Lactic acid,* which is produced by the shift to anaerobic metabolism in regions of ischemia, is therefore a potent vasodilator.

PATHOPHYSIOLOGY. Autoregulation is thus a major homeostatic and protective mechanism. In normal persons, autoregulation prevents alteration in cerebral blood flow despite variations in systemic blood pressure or regional increases in metabolic demand on the brain. In the situation of regional increase in metabolism, a corresponding increase in carbon dioxide results, to produce local vasodilation and increased blood flow, thus accommodating the increased metabolic demand. In certain disease states associated with vascular occlusion, an area of regional ischemia develops because of the reduction in available blood supply; intraluminal pressure decreases, oxygen is no longer available, $PaCO_2$ increases, lactate is produced, and the tissue becomes acidotic. These factors all produce vasodilation of nearby vessels and may provide an increase in blood flow to an area of ischemia. In certain situations, this will be sufficient to increase regional cerebral blood flow and prevent infarction; in other situations, it may reduce the size of the resultant infarct. In a region of cerebral infarction, these protective mechanisms have reduced cerebrovascular resistance to a very low value. Since there is little acute change in the central venous pressure, the major determinant of blood flow in the region of ischemic tissue becomes the mean arterial blood pressure. The proper maintenance of systemic blood pressure, therefore, may be of prime importance in the treatment of ischemic infarcts, and any pronounced reduction in systemic pressure, or the presence of cerebral edema (which will secondarily increase venous pressure), may further alter cellular function.

Pathology of the Vascular System

The symptoms and signs produced by vascular disease are a reflection of altered neuronal function in focal or diffuse areas of the nervous system. The location and nature of the underlying neural-parenchymal lesion are directly related to the abnormalities found in the blood vessels or circulatory system. Therefore, this discussion of the pathology of the vascular system will consider (1) the major derangements involving blood vessels and (2) the neural-parenchymal lesions produced by these vascular abnormalities.

Vascular Pathology

NORMAL ARTERIAL HISTOLOGY.   The normal arterial wall contains three distinct layers (Fig. 11-12): (1) the *intima,* a layer of endothelial cells surrounding the vessel lumen with a small amount of extracellular connective tissue, the internal elastic lamina; (2) the *media,* a layer of

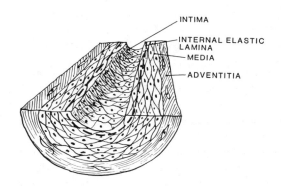

Fig. 11-12. *Cross section of normal arterial wall; note intima, internal elastic lamina, media, and adventitia.*

diagonally oriented smooth muscle cells surrounded by collagen and mucopolysaccharides; and (3) the *adventitia,* the outermost layer, containing fibroblasts and smooth muscle cells intermixed with bundles of collagen and mucopolysaccharides. An external elastic lamina is generally not found in cerebral arteries.

INTRACRANIAL ARTERIAL ANEURYSMS.   An *aneurysm* is an abnormal, localized dilation of the arterial lumen. The most commonly encountered type is a round or oval-shaped, berry-like structure that arises at the bifurcation of cerebral vessels (Fig. 11-13). The majority of cerebral aneurysms are located in the anterior half of the circle of Willis, with the most favored sites being the internal carotid-posterior communicating ar-

Fig. 11-13. *Angiographic study showing aneurysm* (arrow) *that arose from internal carotid-posterior communicating artery junction.*

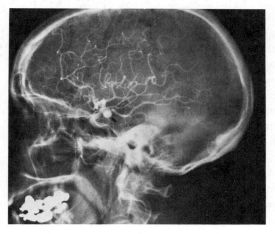

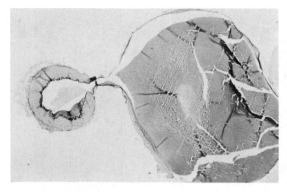

Fig. 11-14. Aneurysm (right) *of internal carotid artery* (left). *Note abrupt termination of media and internal elastic lamina of carotid artery at neck of aneurysm. (Elastic stain; ×4.)*

tery junction, the anterior cerebral-anterior communicating artery junction, and the middle cerebral artery bifurcation. Perhaps secondary to a developmental anomaly, a ballooning of the intima is seen associated with a defect in the media

Fig. 11-15. Coronal section of hemispheres showing large ruptured aneurysm of the left internal carotid artery associated with subarachnoid and intraventricular hemorrhage.

and internal elastic lamina (Fig. 11-14). Varying in size from 1 to more than 10 mm, these lesions occasionally produce symptoms by exerting pressure on adjacent structures, but more often present with rupture and bleeding into the subarachnoid space or brain (Fig. 11-15). Occasionally, aneurysms arise secondary to destruction of the arterial wall by atherosclerosis (atherosclerotic aneurysm) or to infected emboli arising from the heart (septic or mycotic aneurysm).

ARTERIOVENOUS MALFORMATIONS. Often encountered in young adults, these developmental abnormalities result from defective communication between arteries, capillaries, and veins, with dilation of one or more of the vascular elements, thus forming a variable-sized meshwork of tortuous blood vessels (Fig. 11-16). The walls of these abnormal vessels may be thin (and predisposed to rupture) or they may be hypertrophic (Fig. 11-17). Rapid shunting of blood generally occurs and may produce a chronic ischemic state in the neighboring brain. Depending on the location and structure of the malformation, there may be associated seizures and focal neurologic deficit, infarction, or bleeding into the subarachnoid space or brain.

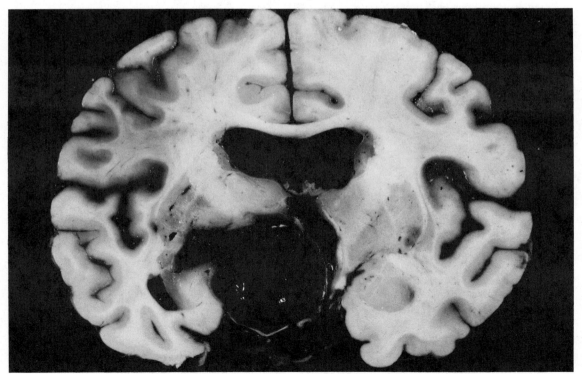

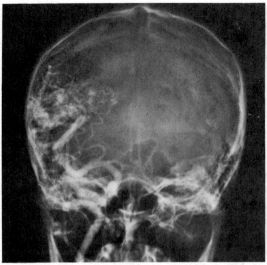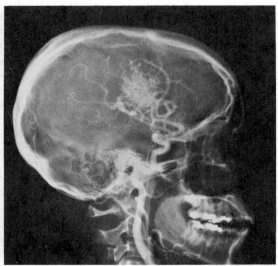

Fig. 11-16. Angiograms showing large arteriovenous malformation. Left, anteroposterior view. Right, lateral view.

Fig. 11-17. Arteriovenous malformation of left parietal lobe. Note tangled mass of dilated vessels in roughly wedge-shaped area pointing toward ventricle, with degeneration of cerebral tissue between vessels. Celloidin section. (Luxol fast-blue stain; ×1.)

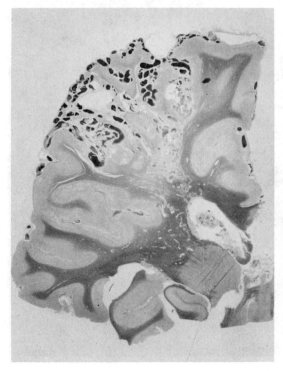

ATHEROSCLEROSIS. A generalized vascular derangement of unknown but probably multifarious etiology, atherosclerosis is the most important pathologic lesion responsible for cerebral infarction. The basic pathologic lesion is the atherosclerotic plaque. Although secondary changes may occur in other layers of the vessel wall, the intima is the layer that is principally involved in atherogenesis. Injury to the arterial wall causes focal desquamation of endothelial cells and exposes subendothelial connective tissue to circulating platelets. Stimulated by the denuded surface, platelets aggregate and adhere to the arterial wall. The process of platelet aggregation releases substances which, in association with certain lipids, induce smooth muscle and endothelial proliferation to form an elevated fibrous plaque that protrudes slightly into the arterial lumen. Although these early atherogenic lesions may regress, with further arterial injury the process is repeated, and the plaque becomes altered by ulceration, increased lipid content, hemorrhage, cell necrosis, mural thrombosis, and calcification to form the typical atherosclerotic plaque with narrowing (stenosis) or occlusion of the arterial lumen (Fig. 11-18). Clinically, many of the so-called risk factors for atherogenesis are also factors that have been shown experimentally to be capable of producing chronic injury to the arterial wall: increased shear stress hypertension, hyperlipidemia, and diabetes.

The basic processes of platelet aggregation and release and secondary plaque formation can be inhibited by certain drugs. Platelet-vessel wall in-

and dilates blood vessels. These observations suggest that pharmacologic agents that selectively inhibit thromboxane synthase or facilitate the biosynthesis of prostacyclin might be beneficial in preventing the thromboembolic complications of atherosclerosis. Although the optimal pharmacologic agent is not yet available, drugs such as acetylsalicylic acid, dipyridamole, and sulfinpyrazone are currently being used in clinical practice.

Atherosclerosis tends to chiefly affect large-caliber blood vessels; in the cerebral circulation, both the intracranial and the extracranial arteries may be involved (Fig. 11-19). Although minimal patchy involvement of the carotid and vertebral arteries is seen, significant stenosis or occlusion commonly occurs at selected sites. The carotid arteries, in their extracranial portion, tend to develop atherosclerotic plaques at the carotid bifurcations and the proximal portions of the internal carotid arteries, while the vertebral arteries are especially likely to develop lesions at their sites of origin from the subclavian arteries. Atherosclerosis of the intracranial arteries is usually limited to the larger arteries related to the circle of Willis and is found most frequently in the internal carotid, proximal middle cerebral, vertebral, and basilar arteries. The smaller distal branches of the major cerebral arteries are seldom involved by gross atheromatous plaques.

The relative importance of the intracranial compared with the extracranial arteries in the pathogenesis of cerebral ischemia is not known. Localized atheromatous plaques may occur in either site, produce focal thrombosis, and reduce blood flow distal to the lesion. This mechanism may be responsible for producing some types of cerebral infarction.

An additional danger is the development of local intraarterial thrombosis, with subsequent *embolization* to distal vessels (Fig. 11-20). These changes are frequently noted when there are lesions at the carotid bifurcation and other extracranial sites. Therefore, although it was formerly assumed that thrombosis of an intracranial artery was the most common cause of cerebral infarction, it has now become evident that atherosclerotic involvement of extracranial vessels with distal embolization is probably of equal significance; in fact this may represent the major pathogenetic mechanism for the production of transient

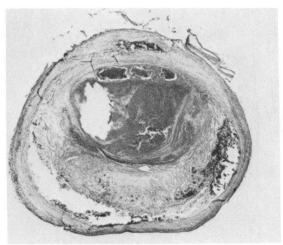

Fig. 11-18. Cross section of atherosclerotic plaque in carotid artery. Arterial wall necrosis with mural thrombosis and stenosis of lumen is seen. (H & E; ×3½.)

teraction is influenced by the selective oxygenation of arachidonic acid in both the platelet and the vascular endothelium. In the platelet, thromboxane synthase converts prostaglandin H_2 to thromboxane A_2, which is a potent aggregator of platelets as well as a constrictor of arterial conductance vessels. Vascular endothelium, however, metabolizes prostaglandin H_2 to prostacyclin, a compound that antagonizes platelet aggregation

Fig. 11-19. Location and severity of atherosclerotic lesions in major extracranial and intracranial vessels. (Redrawn from R. Escourolle and J. Poirier. Manual of Basic Neuropathology. Translated by L. J. Rubinstein, Philadelphia: Saunders, 1973.)

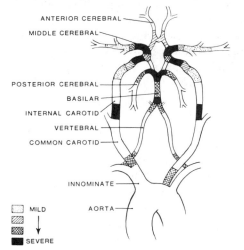

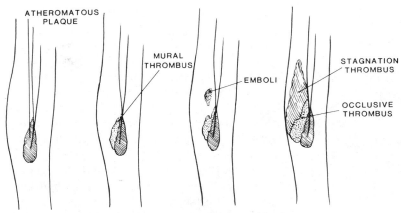

Fig. 11-20. Mechanism of thromboembolism secondary to atherosclerosis. (Redrawn from R. Escourolle and J. Poirier. Manual of Basic Neuropathology. *Translated by L. J. Rubinstein, Philadelphia: Saunders, 1973.)*

ischemic attacks. Atherosclerotic narrowing of extracranial or cerebral vessels may lead to cerebral ischemia and infarction, with or without actual thrombosis, if there is a sudden hemodynamic reduction in cerebral blood flow in an area of the brain where the blood supply is already marginal.

FIBRINOID NECROSIS. A segmental, nonatherosclerotic arteriopathy, fibrinoid necrosis (also referred to as lipohyalinosis and arteriolar sclerosis), involves primarily smaller intraparenchymal blood vessels and is found almost exclusively in the brains of hypertensive patients. The lesion is characterized by the presence of a fibrinoid material and lipid-laden macrophages in the subintimal

Fig. 11-21. Hypertensive fibrinoid necrosis. Note irregular degeneration and dilatation of wall associated with infiltration by fibrinoid material and lymphocytes. (H & E; ×100.)

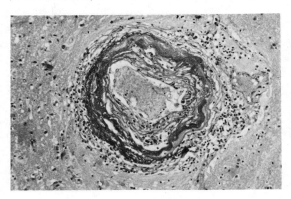

layer of cerebral vessels (Fig. 11-21). It is postulated that sustained elevations in blood pressure result in further arterial disorganization. Some of these lesions show progressive luminal obliteration and eventually result in small areas of infarction called *lacunae*, while others produce progressive weakening of the vessel wall and microaneurysm formation and eventually rupture and produce an intracerebral hemorrhage.

OTHER TYPES OF BLOOD VESSEL LESIONS. Other pathologic processes may result in disease of intracranial arteries and veins and can produce local thrombosis and resultant infarction or hemorrhage. Common examples include (1) inflammatory involvement of cerebral blood vessels, *arteritis,* which may occur secondary to infectious processes (syphilis, pyogenic meningitis) or may accompany certain systemic disorders (lupus erythematosus, periarteritis nodosa); (2) certain hematologic disorders (polycythemia, sickle cell disease); and (3) emboli of various types arising from distant sources (usually the heart).

Neural-Parenchymal Pathology
The neural-parenchymal lesions produced by the vascular lesions just discussed are of two major types: (1) hemorrhage and (2) infarction. Lesions of both types are common at the supratentorial and posterior fossa levels but less frequent at the spinal level. Symptomatic vascular disease involving the peripheral level is distinctly rare and generally occurs with lesions involving smaller

arteries and arterioles which secondarily alter the blood supply to peripheral nerves.

HEMORRHAGIC LESIONS.   Pathologic examination reveals that nontraumatic intracranial hemorrhagic disease may be defined by its anatomic location. It is usually found within the subarachnoid space as *subarachnoid hemorrhage* (refer to Fig. 6-13), within the parenchyma of the brain as *intracerebral hemorrhage* (Fig. 11-22), or as a combination of the two. Hemorrhage in either of these locations may be produced by various pathophysiologic mechanisms, the most common being (1) rupture of an intracranial aneurysm, usually producing subarachnoid hemorrhage (occasionally with an associated intracerebral hemorrhage); (2) rupture of an intraparenchymal vessel, usually producing a variably sized, blood-filled mass lesion (intracerebral hemorrhage), which often has some extension of bleeding into the ventricles; and (3) bleeding from an arteriovenous malformation, commonly producing either a sub-

arachnoid hemorrhage or an intracerebral hemorrhage, alone or in combination.

INFARCTION.   With prolonged tissue ischemia, permanent pathologic change occurs in neuronal function and structure. In the presence of diffuse oxygen deprivation, wide areas of cerebral cortex (which is more sensitive to metabolic alteration than other cerebral structures) have evidence of necrosis and cell loss, *anoxic encephalopathy* (Fig. 11-23). More commonly, the area of infarction is localized to the distribution of a diseased blood vessel (Fig. 11-24). In that region, softening and necrosis with *ischemic cell change* (see Chap. 4) are observed. The size of the infarct varies; smaller lesions (0.5 to 10 mm) are often referred to as *lacunar infarctions* and are common in the brains of hypertensive patients (Fig. 11-25). On occasion, especially with large infarctions, the original nonmass lesion may become edematous and assume the characteristics of a mass lesion. With the passage of time, the necrotic tissue in an infarcted area is removed by phagocytes and replaced by a cavity containing cystic fluid surrounded by an area of glial tissue (Fig. 11-26).

Fig. 11-22. Massive left intracerebral hemorrhage with intraventricular rupture in hypertensive patient.

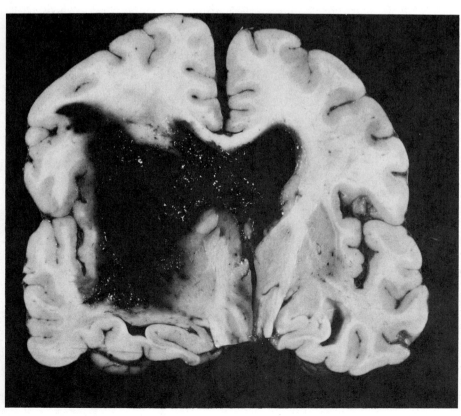

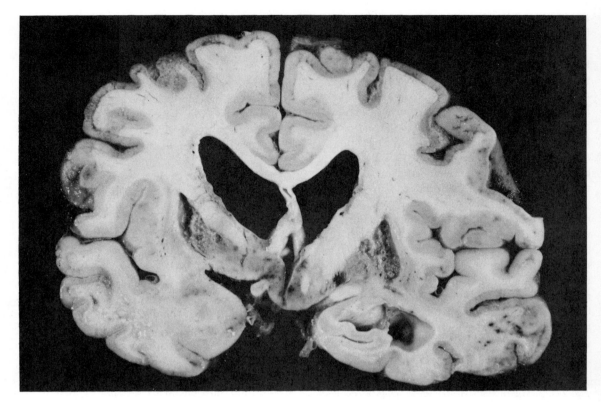

Fig. 11-23. Diffuse hypoxic brain damage in patient who survived 7 months in coma after cardiac arrest. Note infarction of cerebral cortex and basal ganglia. Cortical infarction is maximal in arterial border zones and depths of sulci.

Clinical Correlations

Risk Factors for Stroke

The goal of medical therapy in cerebrovascular disease is prevention. Epidemiologic studies have identified numerous factors, including hyperlipidemia, obesity, diabetes, and excessive smoking, that appear to be associated with atherosclerosis. Because atherosclerosis is a major cause of stroke, many of these same factors are present in the stroke-prone profile. There are, in addition, three highly specific factors that have been shown to be associated with a greatly increased risk of stroke but more importantly to result in a significant decrease in stroke incidence when promptly recognized and treated. These factors include (1) transient focal ischemic attacks, (2) hypertension, and (3) certain cardiac disorders.

TRANSIENT FOCAL ISCHEMIC ATTACKS. These spells are defined as brief (less than 24 hours, usually 5 to 30 minutes) episodes of focal neurologic dysfunction of abrupt onset, which clear without permanent neurologic deficit. These episodes may occur in the distribution of either the carotid or the vertebrobasilar arterial system. There are many theories as to the cause of these ischemic events, but current evidence suggests that the majority are caused by emboli that arise from a proximal ulcerated atherosclerotic plaque. Lesions in the region of the carotid bifurcation are a common source of transient ischemic attack. *Amaurosis fugax* (fleeting blindness) is a related episode consisting of transient monocular blindness which often arises from temporary alteration of the retinal blood supply caused by ipsilateral carotid artery disease. These events must be recognized because between 20 and 35 percent of patients experiencing these transient episodes will subsequently suffer permanent cerebral infarction.

HYPERTENSION.   Sustained elevation in systemic blood pressure increases the risk of subsequent stroke by at least four times when compared with normotension. Hypertension of even modest degree exerts its effect on the cerebral vasculature

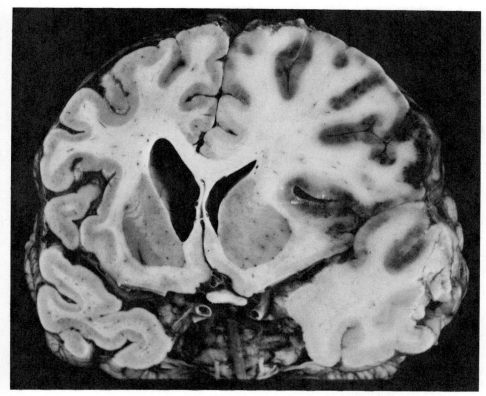

Fig. 11-24. Acute infarction in middle cerebral artery distribution. Note swelling and cortical discoloration and petechial hemorrhages in infarcted territory, with marked shift of midline structures.

by two distinct mechanisms: (1) acceleration of atherosclerosis—hypertensive patients of any age have a greater amount of atherosclerotic disease than do nonhypertensive persons, and hence are at a higher risk for the forms of atherothrombotic disease previously described, and (2) initiation of pathologic change in small arterioles (fibrinoid necrosis). This type of arterial degeneration is found almost exclusively in hypertensive patients and seems to be the vascular lesion that predisposes to both lacunar infarction and intracerebral hemorrhage. (Intracerebral hemorrhage in the absence of an arteriovenous malformation is seldom found in normal, nonhypertensive patients.)

CERTAIN FORMS OF CARDIAC DISEASE. Valvular heart disease of various types, endocarditis, and various cardiac arrhythmias (primarily atrial fibrillation) are associated with intracardiac thrombus formation. Because a large proportion of the cardiac output supplies the cerebrum, the nervous system remains a major target organ for all forms of cardiac emboli.

Generalized Cerebral Ischemia—Syncope
Under normal circumstances, cerebral blood flow remains relatively constant in spite of minor fluctuations in blood pressure. When systemic blood pressure decreases to extremely low levels and the cerebral autoregulatory mechanisms are no longer effective, a state of generalized cerebral ischemia develops. The momentary giddiness and light-headedness occasionally experienced when a person abruptly assumes an upright posture is an example of this. If cerebral perfusion remains inadequate, syncope results and consciousness is lost. States of decreased cardiac output, hypotension from many causes, vagal hyperactivity, and impairment of sympathetic vasomotor reflex activity are common causes of syncope, which should not be confused with a transient ischemic attack as previously defined. Transient ischemic attack is a *focal* ischemic event; syncope is a *generalized* ischemic event that occurs as a result of vastly different pathogenetic mechanisms and has a different prognosis. In the presence of severe focal intracranial vascular disease, syncope

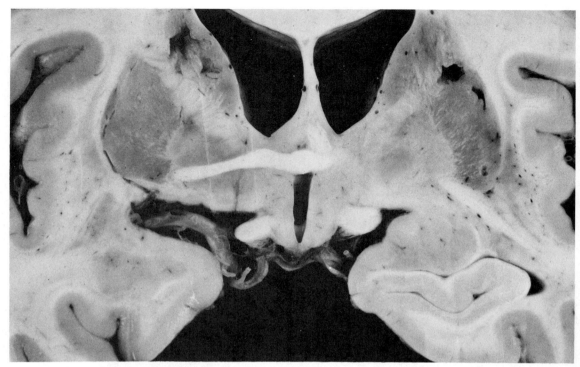

Fig. 11-25. Small, old cystic infarcts (lacunae) in basal ganglia bilaterally in hypertensive patient.

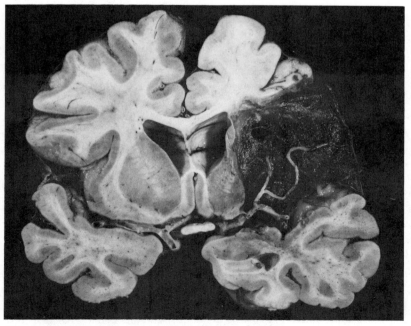

Fig. 11-26. Old infarct (20 years) in middle cerebral artery territory. Damaged brain tissue has been completely absorbed, leaving cystic area traversed by glial-vascular membranes. Note relatively intact middle cerebral artery within the area of infarction.

may infrequently be associated with focal neurologic signs and symptoms.

Radiographic Anatomy—Angiography

In the living patient, we do not have an opportunity to examine the cerebral blood vessels directly but rely on a procedure called *angiography*. High-resolution images of the cerebrovascular anatomy are obtained by cannulation of an extracranial artery and injection of a radiopaque material. As the contrast medium is carried through

the cerebral circulation, serial radiographs are obtained in both the lateral and anteroposterior projections. The contrast medium outlines the interior of the blood vessels, and the arterial, capillary, and venous phases of the circulation can be assessed.

The normal vascular anatomy as seen in a conventional cerebral angiogram is illustrated in Figure 11-27. Deviations from the normal vascular pattern may be indicative of disease and should be correlated with the clinical history and examination. Images of lower resolution, primarily displaying the extracranial arterial vessels, can be produced by electronic enhancement of the radiographs obtained after the intravenous injection of contrast medium (digital subtraction angiography). This technique, which alleviates the potential risks of an arterial puncture, is, at times, a

Fig. 11-27. Arteriographic anatomy. A, B. Lateral views. C, D. Anteroposterior views. (1) Internal carotid artery, (2) vertebral artery, (3) basilar artery, (4) branches of anterior cerebral artery, (5) branches of middle cerebral artery, (6) branches of posterior cerebral artery, (7) posterior communicating artery, (8) anterior communicating artery.

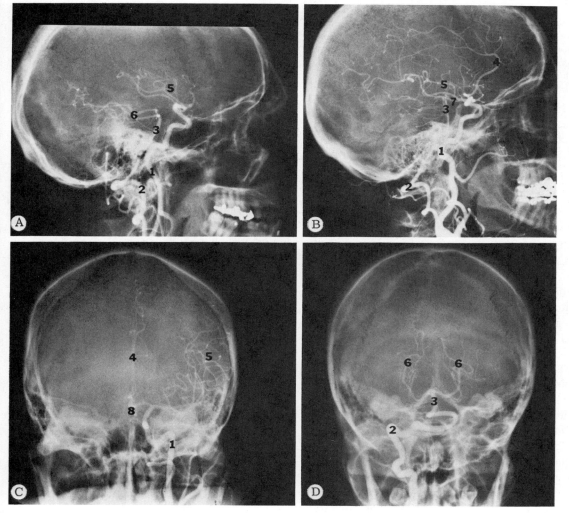

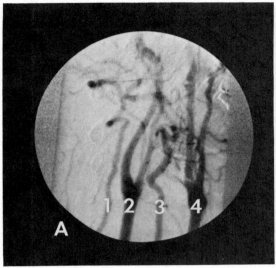
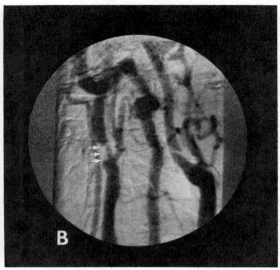
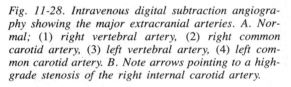

Fig. 11-28. Intravenous digital subtraction angiography showing the major extracranial arteries. A. Normal; (1) right vertebral artery, (2) right common carotid artery, (3) left vertebral artery, (4) left common carotid artery. B. Note arrows pointing to a high-grade stenosis of the right internal carotid artery.

useful alternative to conventional angiography in selected patients (Fig. 11-28). Three major types of change may be seen on the angiogram: structural abnormalities of vessels, alterations in position of vessels, and alterations in flow patterns.

STRUCTURAL ABNORMALITIES OF VESSELS. Stenosis (narrowing) of the dye column or occlusion (nonfilling) of a vessel may be seen. Vascular malformations and aneurysms are examples of this type of change. Collections of abnormal vessels may be demonstrated within neoplasms, in particular gliomas, meningiomas, and metastatic lesions, and these collections may be responsible for a so-called tumor blush or stain seen as an area of increased dye concentration.

ALTERATIONS IN POSITION OF VESSELS. Mass lesions commonly produce displacement of vessels. Such displacement may be local and result in delineation of the mass or be distant and indirect; examples of the latter include shift of the anterior cerebral artery with anteriorly placed lesions or of the internal cerebral vein with more posteriorly placed lesions. At times, such a shift or displacement of vessels is associated with a stain or blush; in other instances, as with subdural hema-

toma, only the shift is recognized, the lesion itself being represented by an avascular area. In hydrocephalus, the vessels may be stretched out over the dilated ventricular system.

ALTERATIONS IN FLOW PATTERNS. Changes in the circulatory pattern may be evident as an expression of abnormal vascular shunts, as with arteriovenous malformations or in some tumors. Collateral flow patterns may be identified in instances of thrombosis of major arteries as, for example, through the ophthalmic artery in instances of carotid artery occlusion; diminution or absence of flow is found distal to the site of vascular occlusion itself. A general slowing of the circulation may be noted when the intracranial pressure is elevated.

Measurement of Ocular Arterial Pressure

Vessel stenosis must be greater than 60 or 70 percent before flow is reduced and distal arterial pressure is lowered. An inference can be made about the presence of such a lesion by demonstrating a reduction in blood pressure along a distal segment of that artery. Thus, severe stenosis of the subclavian artery lowers the brachial blood pressure. Similarly, severe stenosis of the internal carotid artery lowers the ipsilateral ophthalmic or retinal artery pressure. A variety of simple and safe *noninvasive techniques* (ophthalmodynamometry, oculoplethysmography) are now available. Unilateral reduction in ocular arterial pressure is a reliable indicator of the presence

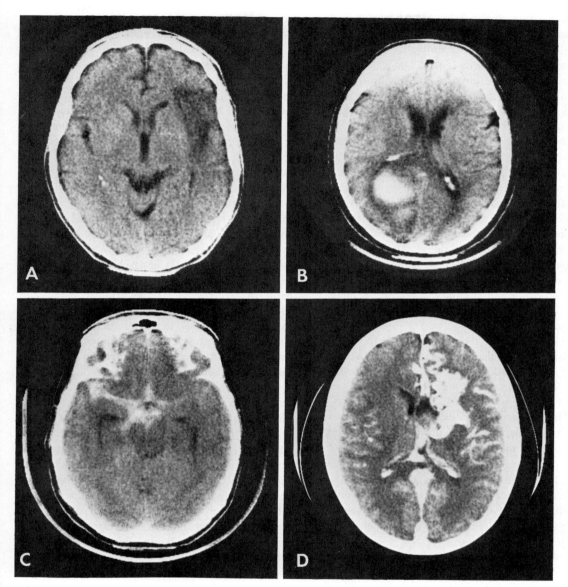

Fig. 11-29. Computed tomography. A. Infarction in left middle cerebral artery distribution. B. Area of hemorrhage in right occipital lobe. C. Blood in the basilar cisterns. D. Large predominantly left frontal arteriovenous malformation on a contrast-enhanced scan.

of a highly stenotic or occlusive lesion in the ipsilateral carotid system and may be of value in the assessment of patients with suspected carotid arterial disease.

Computed Tomography

Computed tomography is a radiographic technique capable of visualizing intracranial anatomy and pathology and has proved to be helpful in the assessment of patients with cerebrovascular disease. As shown in Figure 11-29, areas of infarction (A) often appear as regions of reduced attenuation, whereas regions of hemorrhage (B) show increased attenuation. At times, after subarachnoid hemorrhage, there is sufficient blood in the subarachnoid spaces to be identified by this technique (C). Enhancement of the vascular structures of the brain can be achieved by the injection of intravenous contrast material and can be utilized to identify large vascular anomalies, such as the arteriovenous malformation shown in D.

Examination of the Vascular System

Since "vascular" refers to both an anatomic system and an etiologic category, its evaluation requires both historical data and information obtained from the physical examination. Patients with cerebrovascular disease may present with a wide range of symptoms of diverse etiology. The evaluation of such patients should be designed to enable the clinician to determine (1) the nature of the presenting symptoms and signs; (2) the type, location, and extent of the pathologic process in the neural parenchyma; (3) the type, location, and extent of the pathologic process in the vasculature; and (4) the pathophysiologic mechanism responsible for the observed symptoms and signs. Usually this evaluation can be accomplished with reasonable accuracy through detailed history and physical examination, aided by the judicious selection of certain ancillary diagnostic studies.

Historical Aspects

From the history, it is possible to determine if a problem is vascular and if the primary pathologic process is hemorrhage or infarction and to define the likely pathophysiologic mechanism responsible for the problem.

The judgment as to whether a problem is vascular is made almost exclusively from the *temporal profile:* the onset, evaluation, and course of the presenting symptoms. An acute onset with rapid evolution (minutes to hours) to maximal deficit implies a vascular cause. In the absence of a history of a clearly defined acute onset, the diagnosis of nontraumatic cerebrovascular disease must remain uncertain.

Patients with symptoms of acute onset may be seen at any stage in the development of their symptoms. Some patients have symptoms that have resolved completely by the time they present for evaluation. They may describe the focal symptoms of transient ischemic attacks, but such events must be distinguished from seizures, labyrinthine disturbances, migraine, and generalized ischemic disorders (syncope).

Patients with symptoms of acute onset may progress and display increasing deficit while undergoing evaluation (a progressing stroke); but with these patients, careful historical inquiry must be undertaken to uncover the possibility of an underlying neoplasm, other mass lesions (that is, subdural hematoma), or superimposed metabolic or inflammatory encephalopathy.

Finally, the condition of some patients with symptoms of acute onset may have stabilized with residual deficit or may show some improvement at the time of evaluation. Most of these patients will have a *completed stroke*. Again, historical inquiry must be directed toward uncovering the pathophysiologic mechanism responsible for the deficit and must take into account other intracranial processes that could account for the symptoms.

The distinction between hemorrhage and infarction, although of major clinical importance and readily made in most cases, may be difficult in certain instances. The onset of symptoms in association with severe headache, though not invariably associated with hemorrhage, favors a hemorrhagic process. If the primary pathologic lesion is located at the supratentorial level (rather than posterior fossa), the presence of alteration in consciousness, stupor, or coma coincident with or shortly after the onset of symptoms favors the diagnosis of hemorrhagic disease.

When hemorrhage is suspected, a clinical determination of the location of the hemorrhage is often possible. The early absence of focal neurologic symptoms favors a subarachnoid hemorrhage and, in the absence of trauma, suggests the possibility of a ruptured intracranial aneurysm. The presence of focal neurologic symptoms suggests an intracerebral hemorrhage. In patients with suspected intracerebral hemorrhage, a history of significant, untreated hypertension renders the diagnosis more likely. In its absence, one must consider either the possibility of a ruptured aneurysm with associated intracerebral hemorrhage or a parenchymal hemorrhage secondary to an arteriovenous malformation (which also can present as a subarachnoid hemorrhage). The history of preexistent focal seizures, localized headache, or previous intracranial bleeding supports the diagnosis of an arteriovenous malformation.

When an ischemic process is suspected, it is necessary first to distinguish between carotid and vertebrobasilar arterial system disease. Although in most patients ischemic lesions are related to atherosclerosis, the patient's entire medical and neurologic history should be used to determine whether the symptoms are a result of (1) intracranial pathologic processes involving large-caliber or small-caliber arteries and arterioles, (2) thromboembolic disease in the major extracranial vessels, (3) emboli arising from distant sources (most often the heart), or (4) other systemic disorders.

The Neurovascular Examination

The physical evaluation of patients with suspected cerebrovascular disease must include, in addition to a general physical examination and more detailed study of neurologic function, an assessment of the neurovascular system. Cerebrovascular disease seldom occurs in isolation; the basic pathologic process often exerts its effect on multiple target organs, and therapeutic intervention can be planned only after consideration of the general well-being of the patient. A careful cardiac, pulmonary, and peripheral vascular examination (including recording of pulse rate and rhythm and measurement of the brachial blood pressures bilaterally and in the lying and standing positions) is particularly essential. In addition, the degree to which underlying disorders such as hypertension, diabetes, hyperlipidemia, and hematologic abnormalities may be contributing to the production of cerebrovascular symptoms must be determined.

The neurovascular examination includes examination of neck flexion for evidence of nuchal rigidity in patients with suspected hemorrhagic disease and three additional procedures designed to provide evidence of disease in the cerebrovascular system: auscultation of the head and neck, palpation of the cephalic vessels, and neuroophthalmologic examination.

AUSCULTATION OF THE HEAD AND NECK. The examiner should gently apply the stethoscope over the great vessels arising from the aortic arch, the carotid bifurcations, the orbits, and the skull, listening for evidence of bruits. A *bruit* is an abnormal pulsatile sound indicating turbulent blood flow through a vessel. It is usually, but not always, associated with stenosis of that vessel. A bruit may be audible over an area of abnormal arteriovenous communication, and may at times be heard over an anatomically normal vessel if there is turbulent flow.

PALPATION OF THE CEPHALIC VESSELS. Gentle palpation of the carotid arteries in the neck and of the superficial temporal arteries anterior to the ear should be performed. Altered pulsation, especially if unilateral, is usually indicative of proximal obstructive vascular disease. Although palpation of the peripheral pulses is an important part of the assessment of the general vascular system, palpation of the carotid pulses is less reliable and carries with it the potential danger of dislodging material from an atheromatous plaque. If pulsation of a carotid artery cannot be felt on gentle palpation, vigorous compression will add little diagnostic information.

NEUROOPHTHALMOLOGIC EXAMINATION. The optic fundus should be examined in all patients, as this provides valuable information about intracranial vascular disease. Atherosclerosis, hypertension, diabetes, and other systemic disorders produce recognizable retinal and vascular changes. Subhyaloid (preretinal) hemorrhages may be seen in patients with subarachnoid hemorrhage. Evidence of retinal embolic events in the form of retinal infarcts and of cholesterol (Fig. 11-30), platelet-fibrin, or calcific emboli may be seen in patients with carotid occlusive disease. These intraarterial fragments are presumed to result from an ulcerated atheromatous lesion in the circulation proximal to the ophthalmic arteries, and their presence correlates well with demonstrable lesions in the ipsilateral internal carotid artery.

Fig. 11-30. Small cholesterol embolus seen in distal arteriole of optic fundus of patient with atherosclerosis of proximal internal carotid artery.

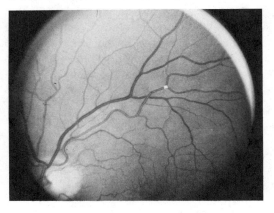

Objectives
1. Define ischemia, infarction, intracerebral hemorrhage, subarachnoid hemorrhage, aneurysm, arteriovenous malformation, embolus, transient ischemic attack, syncope, angiogram, and bruit.
2. Describe the methods of formation and the role of ATP in brain metabolism.
3. Define autoregulation, and list or discuss the factors that can alter cerebral blood flow.
4. Identify the following major vessels, and list the symptoms that *might* develop in a patient with a lesion of the affected artery:
   a. Vertebral arteries
   b. Posterior communicating artery
   c. Common and internal carotid arteries
   d. Anterior cerebral arteries
   e. Middle cerebral arteries
   f. Basilar artery
   g. Posterior cerebral artery
5. Given a patient protocol:
   a. Recognize when the problem suggests cerebrovascular disease, and list those aspects of the protocol that led to this conclusion.
   b. Localize the area of abnormality to a specific area of the neuraxis, and identify whether that area of abnormality falls within the distribution of the internal carotid, vertebrobasilar, or spinal arterial systems.
   c. Decide if the basic pathologic mechanism is hemorrhage or infarction, and state the reasons for your choice.

Clinical Problems
1. A 16-year-old boy with endocarditis noted the sudden onset of complete visual loss; within minutes, this partially cleared, and he noted only a loss of vision in the left half of the visual field of each eye. He had improved slightly when he reached the hospital, but examination still revealed a left homonymous hemianopia.
   a. What is the anatomic-pathologic nature of the lesion?
   b. What is the location of the lesion with respect to its vascular supply? Why did you make this choice?
   c. What is the pathologic term that describes the parenchymal lesion?

   d. What is the pathophysiologic mechanism responsible for the symptoms?
   e. What biochemical changes have taken place in the region of the lesion?
2. A 65-year-old woman suddenly experienced the onset of severe weakness on her left side, loss of feeling on her left side, and an inability to see in the left half of her visual fields. Examination revealed weakness of face, arm, and leg, increased reflexes with a Babinski's sign on the left, sensory loss on the left side, and a left homonymous hemianopia. A right carotid bruit was noted.
   a. What is the anatomic-pathologic nature of the lesion?
   b. What is the location of the lesion with respect to its vascular supply?
   c. What is the pathologic term that describes the parenchymal lesion?
   d. What is the pathophysiologic mechanism responsible for the symptoms?
   e. In the region immediately surrounding the lesion, the blood vessels are maximally dilated: true or false?
3. A 55-year-old hypertensive man noted the sudden onset of severe headache on the left side, loss of speech, and right hemiparesis. Within minutes, he became somnolent. Examination in the emergency room 30 minutes later revealed a comatose patient with a blood pressure of 220/120 mm Hg, a dense right hemiparesis with increased reflexes on the right, and bilateral Babinski's signs. A roentgenogram of the skull showed a 7-mm shift of the pineal gland from left to right.
   a. What is the anatomic-pathologic nature of the lesion?
   b. What is the pathologic term that describes the parenchymal lesion?
   c. What are three common causes of this type of parenchymal lesion?
   d. What clinical signs suggest the pathologic diagnosis?
   e. What other noninvasive diagnostic test would be useful in defining the pathologic lesion?
4. A 50-year-old man experienced the sudden onset of vertigo. Examination revealed dysarthria, difficulty in swallowing, a left Horner's syndrome, left palatal weakness, and loss of pain sensibility over the left face and the

right limbs and trunk. He had coarse ataxia and incoordination of his left arm.

  a. What is the anatomic-pathologic nature of the lesion?

  b. What is the location of the lesion in respect to its vascular supply?

  c. What is the pathologic term that describes the parenchymal lesion?

  d. What is the pathophysiologic mechanism responsible for the symptoms?

  e. List the tract or nucleus responsible for each of the symptoms in this patient.

5. A 62-year-old man suffered frequent, highly stereotyped episodes. He suddenly felt giddy and light-headed, lost consciousness, and fell to the ground. A physician observed one of his spells and noted that during the episode there was no peripheral pulse, and the blood pressure was too low to be detected. Both blood pressure and peripheral pulse returned to normal coincident with the patient's regaining consciousness.

  a. What is the anatomic-pathologic nature of the lesion?

  b. What is the pathophysiologic mechanism responsible for the symptoms?

  c. Define autoregulation.

  d. Under normal physiologic conditions, which of the following could be expected to produce cerebral vasodilation: inhalation of oxygen; 20 percent decrease in arterial blood pressure; 20 percent increase in arterial blood pressure; inhalation of carbon dioxide?

  e. How do these spells differ from transient ischemic attacks?

6. A 38-year-old man suddenly experienced a severe headache associated with nausea, vomiting, and neck stiffness. When examined 2 hours later, he was somnolent but easily aroused. He had no focal neurologic findings but had marked nuchal rigidity. A lumbar puncture revealed grossly bloody cerebrospinal fluid.

  a. What is the anatomic-pathologic nature of the lesion?

  b. What is the pathophysiologic mechanism responsible for the symptoms?

  c. How would you determine whether or not the bloody cerebrospinal fluid was due to a traumatic puncture?

Suggested Reading

Adams, R. D., and Victor, M. *Principles of Neurology* (2nd ed.). New York: McGraw-Hill, 1981. Pp. 529–593.

Kety, S. S., and Schmidt, C. F. The nitrous oxide method for the quantitative determination of cerebral blood flow in man: Theory, procedure and normal values. *J. Clin. Invest.* 27:476, 1948.

Lassen, N. A. Control of cerebral circulation in health and disease. *Circ. Res.* 34:749, 1974.

Raichle, M. E. The pathophysiology of brain ischemia. *Ann. Neurol.* 13:2, 1983.

Russell, R. W. R. (ed.). *Vascular Disease of the Central Nervous System* (2nd ed.). New York: Churchill Livingstone, 1983.

Siesjö, B. K. Cerebral circulation and metabolism. *J Neurosurg.* 60:883, 1984.

Horizontal
Levels

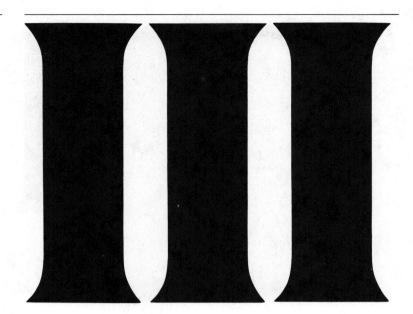

The Peripheral Level

12

Precise anatomic localization is one of the major goals of neurologic diagnosis. The study of the major longitudinal systems and the manifestations of diseases within each system permits localization of a lesion in one or more systems. In the remaining chapters, the patterns of disease at each of the four major levels will be presented. The combination of signs and symptoms as they affect each major level often allows highly specific localization of the underlying disorder.

The *peripheral* level includes all neuromuscular structures outside the skull and spinal column, including peripheral nerves, sensory receptors, muscles, and the portions of cranial nerves lying outside the cranium. The anatomy, physiology, pathophysiology, and clinical disorders of these structures, which have many common characteristics, will be considered in this chapter.

Overview

The peripheral level contains four of the longitudinal systems: motor, sensory, visceral, and vascular systems. The peripheral axon of the lower motor neuron, the neuromuscular junction, and the muscle fibers of the motor system are found at the peripheral level. The distal axon of the primary sensory neuron and the sensory receptors are peripheral. The distal axon of the visceral preganglionic and postganglionic efferent neurons and the visceral afferent axons are peripheral. Only the distal portions of the neurons of these systems are found in the periphery. The somatic cell bodies and the central processes are located in the spinal canal. The systems travel together in the periphery, and peripheral lesions typically produce combinations of symptoms and signs from all three of the neural systems. Blood vessels of the vascular system supply all these structures.

Diseases in the periphery, as in the systems, may be focal (for example, involving a single nerve) or diffuse (involving all peripheral nerves). A focal lesion may be a mass or a non-mass lesion. Diffuse lesions often involve only one type of structure in the periphery, as in primary disease of muscle. The temporal profile of peripheral diseases may be transient or may be that of one of the major disease types—inflammatory, neoplastic, degenerative-metabolic, vascular, or traumatic.

On the basis of gross anatomic features the periphery can be subdivided into nerves and end organs. Diseases of these subdivisions will have different clinical manifestations.

Nerves

PERIPHERAL AND CRANIAL NERVES. These are the gross structures carrying motor, sensory, and visceral axons to the end organs. (Some nerves contain only visceral fibers, for example, the vagus nerve.)

PLEXUS. A plexus is a complex network of axons traveling peripherally and centrally from the spinal nerves at the spinal level to the peripheral nerves.

End Organs

SENSORY RECEPTORS. The somatic receptors for the sensations of pain, touch, position, vibration, and muscle proprioception have been considered in detail in the chapters on sensory and motor systems and will not be discussed further. Primary disease of these receptors is not of clinical significance. The special sensory receptors of the cranial nerves will be considered in Chapters 14 and 15.

SOMATIC MOTOR EFFECTORS. Movement is produced by muscle. Within the muscles are the neuromuscular junctions, the muscle fibers, and the contractile elements. Tendons, bones, and joints play an integral part in movement, but are not considered further in this text.

VISCERAL RECEPTORS AND EFFECTORS. The widespread and diverse group of visceral structures was considered in Chapter 9. Although diseases of these structures are common in general medical practice, they will not be discussed further since they are more properly studied with other organ systems.

Nerve

The major peripheral structures are nerves and muscles. Nerves are a collection of nerve fibers called *axons*, which are bound together by connective tissue. At the peripheral level, nerves form the plexuses and peripheral nerves; at the spinal level, they form the nerve roots entering or leaving the spinal cord and the spinal nerves leaving the spinal column. Nerves, whether peripheral or spinal, are made up of the axons traveling between the central nervous system and the peripheral end organ. They are similar in their microscopic features, their physiology, and their pathophysiologic alterations with disease. The general features that are common to all types of nerves will be considered first, and the differences considered subsequently.

Histology

A nerve is composed of thousands of nerve fibers ranging in size from less than 1 to 20 μm in diameter. In each nerve trunk, individual fibers are surrounded by a connective tissue sheath, the *endoneurium*. Each of these is grouped with many other axons into bundles or fascicles by the *perineurium*. Groups of fascicles are bound together by an outer covering of connective tissue, the *epineurium* (Fig. 12-1). Nerves have their own blood supply. The nutrient arteries enter at

intervals along their length and form anastomotic channels within the connective tissue framework of the nerve. These anastomoses make nerves relatively resistant to vascular disease.

Nerves are made up of motor, sensory, and visceral fibers. The axons can be differentiated histologically on the basis of their size and the presence or absence of myelin. The unmyelinated fibers are small and include visceral fibers and fibers carrying pain and temperature. Proprioceptive and somatic motor fibers are large (Table 12-1). These generalizations, however, do not permit the identification of the function of an individual axon, since the afferent (carrying information centrally) axons and the efferent (carrying information peripherally) axons have a similar microscopic appearance.

Each nerve fiber consists of an axon embedded within a series of Schwann cells arranged longitudinally along the axon. Each Schwann cell covers 0.5 to 1.0 mm of axon. The junctions between Schwann cells along the axon are seen as constrictions of the nerve fiber and are called the *nodes of Ranvier* (Figs. 12-1, 12-2). A single

Table 12-1. Nerve Fiber Types

Type	Diameter (μm)	Conduction velocity (m/sec)	Function
Muscle nerve afferents			
Ia	12–20	70–120	Afferents from muscle spindle (primary endings—annulospiral)
Ib	12–20	70–120	Afferents from Golgi tendon organs
II	6–12	30–70	Afferents from muscle spindle (secondary endings—flower spray)
III	2–6	4–30	Pressure–pain afferents
IV	<2	0.5–2.0	Pain afferents
Cutaneous nerve afferents			
Aα	12–20	70–120	Joint receptor afferents
Aα	6–12	30–70	Paccinian corpuscle and touch receptor afferents
Aδ	2–6	4–30	Touch, temperature, and pain afferents
C	<2	0.5–2.0	Pain, temperature, and some mechanoreceptors
Visceral nerve afferents			
A	2–12	4–70	Variety of visceral receptors
C	<2	0.2–2.0	Visceral receptors
Efferents			
Alpha	12–20	70–120	Extrafusal skeletal muscle innervation from alpha motor neurons
Gamma	2–8	10–50	Intrafusal muscle spindle innervation from gamma motor neurons
B	<3	3–30	Preganglionic autonomic efferents
C	<1	0.5–2.0	Postganglionic autonomic efferents

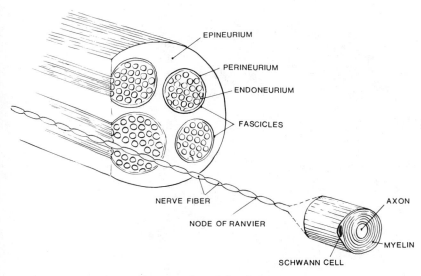

Fig. 12-1. Histologic features of peripheral nerve. Nerve is subdivided into fascicles by perineurium, with multiple motor and sensory nerve fibers intermingled in each fascicle.

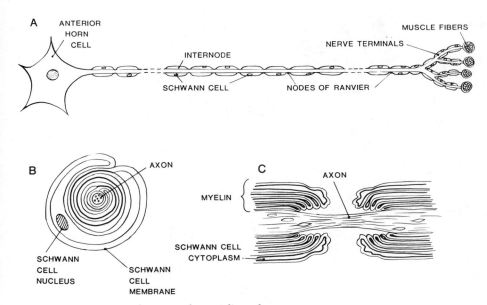

Fig. 12-2. Histologic features of a myelinated motor nerve fiber. A. Single myelinated axon extends from anterior horn cell to nerve terminals on muscle fibers. B. Cross section of nerve fiber through internode with layers of myelin formed by Schwann cell cytoplasm wrapped around it. C. Longitudinal section of node of Ranvier with Schwann cell and myelin terminations abutting around continuous central axon.

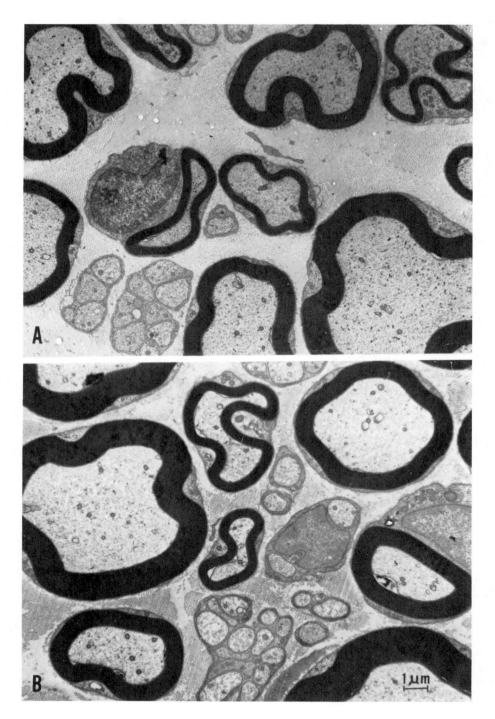

Fig. 12-3. Transverse section of a nerve fiber that contains axons of various sizes surrounded by myelin (dark areas). (A and B, ×8,500.) (From K. Sugimura, et al. Interstitial hyperosmolarity may cause axis cylin-der shrinkage in streptozotocin diabetic nerve. J. Neuropathol. Exp. Neurol. 39:710, 1980. By permission of The American Association of Neuropathologists, Inc.)

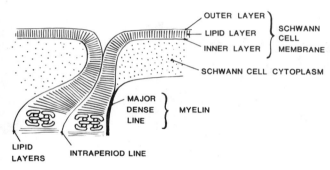

OUTER LAYER ⎱
LIPID LAYER ⎰ SCHWANN CELL MEMBRANE
INNER LAYER

SCHWANN CELL CYTOPLASM

MAJOR DENSE LINE ⎱ MYELIN

LIPID LAYERS
INTRAPERIOD LINE

Fig. 12-4. Formation of myelin from layers of Schwann cell membrane. Major dense lines are formed from protein layers of membrane and are separated by the lipid layer, which contains cholesterol, cerebroside, sphingomyelin, and phosphatidylserine.

Schwann cell surrounds either a number of unmyelinated axons or one myelinated axon. During development, either many unmyelinated axons become embedded in the Schwann cell or the Schwann cell wraps around one axon in concentric circles to form the myelin of the myelinated nerve fiber (Fig. 12-3). Although the fibers in a nerve are adjacent to one another, the electrical activity in each nerve fiber is independent of the activity in all the other fibers in the nerve. The action potentials are isolated from each other by the endoneurium and the myelin.

As the Schwann cell encircles an axon, layers of plasma membrane fuse to form myelin (Fig. 12-4). *Myelin* is thus a series of concentric layers of lipids and proteins. The lipids include cerebrosides, sulfatides, proteolipids, sphingomyelin, inositol phosphatides, glycolipids, glycoproteins, and cholesterol. There are three proteins in myelin, a glycoprotein and two basic proteins. The basic proteins in nerve have similarities to the basic myelin protein in the central nervous system, but are different proteins.

Although myelin is relatively inert metabolically, it has a significant turnover and responds to various disease states. For instance, myelin may be lost (demyelination) in certain immunologic disorders. When myelin is lost along a peripheral nerve, it is usually lost in the region of a single Schwann cell, which extends from one node of Ranvier to another. This loss is called *segmental demyelination* and alters the function of a nerve fiber. Myelin also may be formed abnormally or may accumulate myelin metabolites in abnormal quantities. This condition occurs in genetic disorders due to enzyme defects, such as *metachromatic leukodystrophy* in which a deficit of arylsulfatase A results in the accumulation of metachromatic sulfatides in nerve fibers and loss of function in myelinated axons.

The axons of all nerve fibers consist of the axon membrane, or *axolemma*, and the axoplasm. The axoplasm contains mitochondria, microtubules, microfilaments, and neurofilaments. The *mitochondria* mediate the generation of energy needed to establish the concentration gradients across the axolemma. The *microtubules* participate in the transport of proteins, enzymes, and other materials down the axon from the cell body to the periphery. The function of the neurofilaments and microfilaments is unknown but may be related to axoplasmic transport or axon growth.

Axonal Transport
Two transport mechanisms, a slow and a fast, distribute proteins, neurotransmitters, synaptic vessels, mitochondria, and other cellular elements that are formed in the cell body to the distal axons. The slow axoplasmic flow, moving 1 to 3 mm per day, conveys three types of filamentous proteins—neurofilaments, microtubules (formed from two types of tubulin subunits), and microfilaments (which contain neural actin and myosin)—down the axon to the nerve terminal. These filamentous proteins account for 80 percent of the substances transported by axoplasmic flow. The remainder are enzymes and neurotransmitters. The slow transport system furnishes new axoplasm to developing or regenerating neurons and continuously renews the axoplasms of mature neurons.

The fast axonal transport, traveling 400 mm per day, carries particulate matter such as new membrane materials, synaptic vesicles, and precursors of receptor structures from the cell body, where they are synthesized down the axon to the

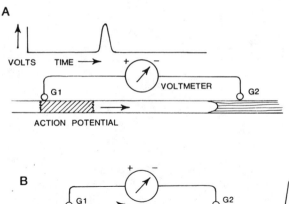

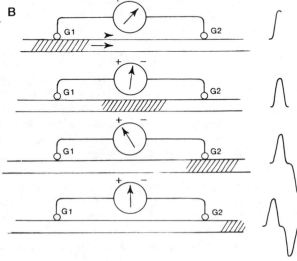

Fig. 12-5. Recording action potentials from nerve trunk with electrodes (G1 and G2). A. With G2 over damaged nerve and G1 over active nerve, a monophasic action potential is recorded as depolarization passes under G1. B. If both electrodes are over active nerve fibers, potentials of opposite polarity are recorded as depolarization passes under G1 and G2, a biphasic action potential. When G1 and G2 are close together, the two potentials fuse to form a smooth biphasic response.

nerve terminal. Some of this material is deposited along the axon to maintain and replace the axolemma; the rest goes to the nerve terminals to form the synaptic vesicles and receptor structures at the nerve endings. Fast axonal transport moves materials not only away from the cell body but also back from the nerve terminal to the cell body, where they are restored or degraded. The intracellular membranes that are degraded within neuronal lysosomes constitute the major component of the retrograde transport back to the cell body. Retrograde transport is also the mechanism by which neurotropic viruses, such as herpes sim-

plex, rabies, and polio, ascend up the peripheral nerves to reach the central nervous system.

Physiology

The resting potential and action potentials in single axons have been described in detail in Chapter 5. In this chapter, we will focus on the physiology of whole nerve trunks. The function of the axons is to carry information in the form of electrical activity from one area to another. A measure of the ability of a nerve to perform this function would be of major clinical value in the identification of disease involving a nerve. However, during normal function, the electrical activities of the fibers in a nerve are asynchronous and cancel each other out. Therefore, physiologic electrical activity from an active nerve trunk cannot be recorded with surface electrodes.

The action potential of a single axon can be recorded experimentally with an intracellular microelectrode that records it as a monophasic wave

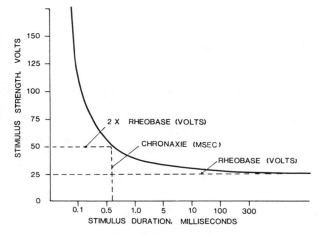

Fig. 12-6. Strength-duration curve. Threshold voltage for each duration is plotted. Rheobase is 25 V, and chronaxie is 0.6 msec.

of depolarization. The electrical activity in a single nerve fiber also can be monitored by placing electrodes in the extracellular fluid very close to the nerve fiber. This method does not detect transmembrane potential changes; rather, it senses potential changes in the extracellular fluid which result from longitudinal current flow between the depolarized and nondepolarized regions of an axon. The extracellular recording is improved (a bigger voltage change is measured) if the extracellular resistance is artificially increased by recording from the nerve experimentally in air or in oil.

Extracellular recording from single axons is difficult because of their small size; however, it is possible to record from groups of axons or from whole nerve trunks, if all axons discharge synchronously. This recording is obtained experimentally and from patients by applying an electrical shock that activates all axons simultaneously. The potential recorded from a nerve activated in this way is the *compound action potential.* The voltage signal obtained from an extracellular recording of the nerve impulse depends on the electrode arrangement. A monophasic potential change is observed from nerve fibers conducting an impulse if only one of the electrodes is placed over an active nerve. A biphasic potential is recorded if both electrodes are placed over the active nerve (Fig. 12-5).

As in the stimulation of a single axon, the whole nerve trunk is activated by passing a current between the cathode (negative pole) and the anode (positive pole). The cathode depolarizes the underlying axons, and the anode hyperpolarizes them. Depolarization requires current flow in the axons. Because large axons have lower internal resistance, the threshold for activation is lowest for the larger fibers. The *threshold stimulus* for a nerve trunk is that which just excites the large fibers. Supramaximal stimuli activate all fibers, including the small fibers, and require greater current flow. Excitability, therefore, depends on axon size.

The *excitability* of a nerve can be defined in terms of the two parameters of a stimulus: voltage and duration. If the strength of the current (or voltage) is plotted against the duration of a stimulus needed to produce excitation of a nerve, a curve is obtained which is called a *strength-duration curve.* A shift in the strength-duration curve indicates a change in excitability and is seen in nerve diseases. The strength-duration curve is often characterized in terms of two points. The *rheobase* is the minimal voltage needed to produce excitation with an infinitely long stimulus duration (usually 300 msec) and the *chronaxie* is the time required to excite a nerve by a stimulus with a voltage twice as large as the rheobase (Fig. 12-6).

The compound action potential recorded from a nerve trunk after supramaximal stimulation is the summation of action potentials from many axons. Its amplitude can be graded by varying the strength of the stimulus. A threshold stimulation evokes only a small potential resulting from activity in a few large fibers. As the stimulus strength is increased, more fibers are excited, and their activity is added to the compound action potential as each additionally activated fiber produces a small increment in the recorded voltage. When all the fibers are excited, the amplitude of the compound action potential is maximum; it will not increase in amplitude with further increases in the stimulus strength (supramaximal). The compound action potential thus can be graded in amplitude, while action potentials in single axons are not graded but fire in an all-or-nothing fashion.

Variation in axon diameter in a nerve trunk results in different conduction velocities as well as different thresholds for activation. The rate at which an axon conducts is a function of the amount of longitudinal current flow and will be greater with larger axons. The *conduction velocity* is calculated by dividing the distance a potential travels by the time it takes to travel that distance. It is approximately five times the axon's diameter in microns; for example, 5 to 100 meters per second for axons of 1 to 20 µm in diameter. If a nerve trunk is stimulated at a distance from the recording electrodes, the compound action potential exhibits several components (Fig. 12-7) because of the dispersion of the potentials from fibers of different diameters. The impulses in the large fibers reach the recording site first. The components of the compound action potential thus distinguish activity in groups of fibers whose diameters are within certain size ranges. The af-

Table 12-2. Fiber Types in a Mixed Nerve

Diameter (µm)	Conduction velocity (m/sec)	Type
12–20	70–120	Ia, Ib, A_a, alpha efferent
6–12	30–70	II, A_a, gamma efferent, visceral afferent
2–6	4–30	III, Aδ, gamma efferent, visceral afferent
<2	0.5–2.0	IV, B, C

ferent fibers in cutaneous nerves (to joints and skin) are subdivided into groups named by letters (Aα, Aδ, and C). The afferent fibers in muscle nerves (nerves to muscle) are subdivided into groups designated by Roman numerals (I, II, III, IV). These are listed in Table 12-1.

Nerves that innervate muscle contain both sensory and motor fibers. The motor fibers arise from the alpha and gamma motor neurons and innervate the extrafusal and intrafusal muscle fibers. The sensory fibers are the group Ia and II fibers from muscle spindles and the group Ib fibers from Golgi tendon organs. Cutaneous nerves innervate joints and skin and are commonly considered sensory nerves, although both they and the muscle nerves contain efferent and afferent fibers of the visceral system, the "C" or group IV fibers. Table 12-2 lists by size the components of a mixed nerve.

In addition to transmitting action potentials, axons move proteins along their length. This process is known as *axoplasmic transport* and is important for the production of neurotransmitter in the nerve terminal, for maintaining the integrity of the distal parts of the axon, and for the release of trophic factors from the nerve terminal. The *trophic factors* are undefined substances, released from nerve terminals, which are necessary for the normal function of the postsynaptic cell. Loss of these trophic factors occurs in some nerve diseases and results in physiologic and histologic abnormalities of the postsynaptic cell.

Pathophysiology
A nerve may be altered in a number of ways by disease processes. These can be classified as diseases of the axolemma, the axoplasm, or the myelin sheath.

Fig. 12-7. Compound action potential of cutaneous nerve in vitro, showing peaks generated by different fiber types.

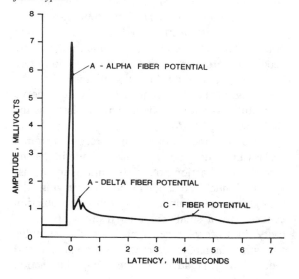

AXOLEMMAL DISORDERS. The axon membrane may undergo physicochemical alterations that block conduction without destruction or histologic alteration of the axon. Such alterations may occur by electrical, pharmacologic, thermal, or mechanical means. The alterations are usually transient and reversible and include the familiar phenomenon of a leg "going to sleep."

Electrical conduction blocks do not occur clinically but can be obtained by the application of steady depolarizing (cathodal block) or hyperpolarizing (anodal block) currents to a nerve fiber or nerve trunk. A depolarizing current may initially evoke an action potential and then block impulse transmission. An anodal block results from a hyperpolarization of the axon membrane, which moves the membrane potential away from threshold.

A clinically useful method of producing conduction block is the application of pharmacologic agents (local anesthetics) to a nerve. These include compounds such as procaine hydrochloride (Novocain), benzocaine, cocaine, and other esters of benzoic acid. Local anesthetics interfere with nerve conduction by preventing the membrane permeability changes that occur with depolarization (Table 12-3). The membrane is said to be "stabilized" by local anesthetics. Small, unmyelinated nerve fibers, such as those mediating pain, are more sensitive to local anesthetics than are the larger myelinated fibers and are blocked at low concentrations of the drug which do not appreciably affect large fibers (see Table 12-1).

A transient, reversible conduction block can be

Table 12-3. Sequence of Events of Local Anesthetic Block

Displacement of calcium ions from nerve receptor site
↓
Binding of local anesthetic to receptor site
↓
Blockade of sodium channel
↓
Decrease in sodium conductance
↓
Decreased depolarization of nerve membrane
↓
Failure to achieve threshold potential level
↓
Lack of development of propagated action potential
↓
Conduction blockade

obtained by lowering the temperature of nerve fibers. This method of blocking nerve impulse transmission is accomplished by the local application of ice or an ethyl chloride spray and is used clinically to produce superficial anesthesia. Mechanical conduction blocks occur with distortion of a nerve and may be due to alteration of the blood supply or to changes in the configuration of the membrane, with secondary changes in its ionic permeability.

AXOPLASMIC DISORDERS. Axons may be affected by acute or chronic disorders of the axoplasm. An acute lesion is one in which the axon is disrupted. This may occur with complete division of the nerve in a laceration or with a severe local crush, traction, or ischemia. In laceration, the connective tissue framework is destroyed; in the other lesions, it remains intact. But in each instance, the continuity of the axons is lost, the distal axon is deprived of axoplasmic flow from the neuron, and it undergoes dissolution in a process called *wallerian degeneration*. Central chromatolysis and peripheral muscle atrophy accompany wallerian degeneration (Fig. 12-8). In most lesions other than laceration, not all axons are destroyed and some function may remain. The smaller fibers are more resistant to such injuries and are more likely to be spared. After acute axonal disruption, recovery occurs only through the growth of new axons.

If a nerve is completely severed, reinnervation is poor because the axonal sprouts have no pathway to follow. Axonal sprouts may grow in the wrong direction and produce spirals or large bulbous tips. These sprouts, with their Schwann cells and connective tissue, may form a *neuroma*. The neuroma may not only prevent proper regrowth of the nerve but may also be painful.

The activity of Schwann cells in the distal nerve stump provides an aid to reinnervation across a gap, as they divide, elongate, and migrate toward the proximal nerve stump. If axonal sprouts manage to reach this Schwann cell outgrowth, they may eventually reinnervate the denervated organs. However, the amount of functional recovery is always less than that seen in a crush injury. One reason for this is that most axonal sprouts will not find their way along the pathway followed originally by their parent fibers and will reinnervate an inappropriate organ. A

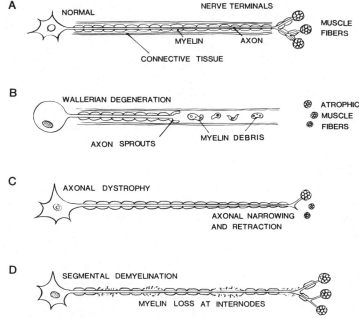

Fig. 12-8. Pathologic changes in peripheral nerve fibers. A. Normal. B. Wallerian degeneration occurs distal to local destruction of an axon and is associated with central chromatolysis and muscle fiber atrophy. Regeneration occurs along connective tissue path. C. Axonal dystrophy results in distal narrowing and "dying back" of nerve terminals due to either intrinsic axon or motor neuron disease. D. Segmental demyelination destroys myelin at scattered internodes along axon without axonal damage.

motor axon that establishes a connection with a sensory receptor organ will not function, and a motor axon that reinnervates a different muscle from the one that it originally supplied cannot take part in the same reflex actions. *Synkinesis* is the result of such aberrant reinnervation, in which attempts to activate one group of muscles produce concomitant contraction in other muscles innervated by that nerve. The patient can no longer selectively activate a muscle. In injuries to long nerves, the end organs may atrophy before reinnervation can occur, thus preventing normal recovery.

The rate of nerve regeneration varies with the type of injury. Recovery is quicker with crush injuries than with nerve severance. The delay in recovery depends on axonal growth, reversal of atrophy of the end organ, reinnervation of the end organ, and remyelinization and maturation of the axon. In humans, the overall rate of functional

recovery under optimal conditions is about 1 to 3 mm per day. The recovery rate in a limb may be quicker proximally than distally.

Axoplasmic disorders may be chronic or slow in evolution and present with different findings than do acute lesions. When the process is complete, the axons degenerate just as they do in acute lesions; however, there are intermediate stages in which the axons first lose their integrity distally, a so-called dying back. This occurs first in the longest axons and results in loss of function in the most distal parts of the body. The axons also may atrophy or become narrowed in chronic disorders, referred to as axonal *atrophies* or axonal *dystrophies* (Fig. 12-8). In either situation, there are abnormalities of the axon prior to changes in the myelin. Therefore, unless major narrowing of an axon is present, the conduction of the axons is slowed very little. Chronic axonal disorders occur with many diseases, including genetic, toxic, metabolic, and deficiency states.

The narrow axons seen in some axoplasmic disorders also occur with local compression of a nerve and in regenerating fibers. Moderate narrowing of an axon results in slowing of conduction velocity, but by itself it usually causes little functional impairment. A nerve with slowed conduction velocity can still transmit impulses, though not at as high rates as normal. High-frequency impulses, such as rapid vibrations, the output from muscle spindles, and motor activity in strong muscle contraction, are poorly transmitted so that vibratory sensation and reflexes are lost.

MYELIN DISORDERS.   Genetic, immunologic, and toxic disorders can produce primary damage to myelin. In these disorders, myelin is usually lost at internodes, with normal myelin remaining at other internodes. This scattered loss of myelin is segmental demyelination (Fig. 12-8). The loss of myelin results in slowing of conduction velocity, with mild impairment of vibratory sensation, loss of reflexes, some loss of proprioceptive sensation, and loss of strong muscle contractions. However, with moderate demyelination, the action potential is blocked, producing more severe deficits. Genetic disorders can be associated with a lack of myelin (hypomyelination) or abnormal myelin and can result in functional disturbances similar to those seen with segmental demyelination.

In each of these disorders, there may be varied severity of damage and selective involvement of one or another fiber type. In localized lesions, there is loss of function in the areas supplied by the nerve. In generalized nerve disease, the axons are affected randomly throughout the cross section of a nerve and randomly along the length of the nerve, so that the most likely areas to lose function are the distal regions supplied by the longest nerves. This produces a characteristic distribution of *abnormalities in the distal portions* of the extremities. This distal deficit also occurs in primary neuronal disease in which the neuron is unable to provide sufficient nutrients to the most distal portion of the nerve, with a resultant dying back of the distal portions of the long nerves.

SUMMARY.   Because the function of peripheral nerves is to conduct action potentials from one area to another, three general kinds of functional abnormality occur:

1. The excitability of axons may be increased with spontaneous or excessive firing of an axon. This occurs in many disorders, but especially in ischemic or metabolic diseases.
2. The axon may be unable to conduct an action potential, either because of transient metabolic changes or because of structural damage to the axon. If an axon is severed, the distal portion will undergo wallerian degeneration but will be able to conduct an impulse in the distal part of the nerve for 3 to 5 days. The proximal portion of the axon will continue to function normally.
3. The axon may conduct an impulse slowly or at low rates of firing. This may occur from loss of myelin or be due to narrowing and deformation of the axon. The latter may be seen in the area of compression or in regenerating fibers. Slow conduction results in mild clinical symptoms or signs except for the ability to carry high-frequency information such as vibration, which is severely impaired.

The physiologic alterations seen with diseases of the nerves are associated with two clinically important manifestations. The threshold for activation of some portion of lower motor neurons may be low, and they may discharge spontaneously. If this occurs, all the muscle fibers in the motor unit will contract simultaneously. Such a single, spontaneous contraction of a motor unit is visible as a small twitch under the skin called a *fasciculation*. It is evidence of irritability of the motor unit and occurs in many disorders. Similar irritability in sensory fibers is perceived as paresthesia (tingling) in large fibers, or as pain in small fibers.

Table 12-4. Examples of Denervation Hypersensitivity

Site	Clinical finding	Due to destruction of	Hypersensitivity to
Striated muscle	Fibrillation	Alpha efferents	Acetylcholine
Anterior horn cell	Spasticity, clonus, hyperreflexia	Descending pathway	Local sensory input
Pupil	Miosis	Postganglionic sympathetic	Epinephrine analogs
Pupil	Mydriasis	Postganglionic parasympathetic	Acetylcholine analogs

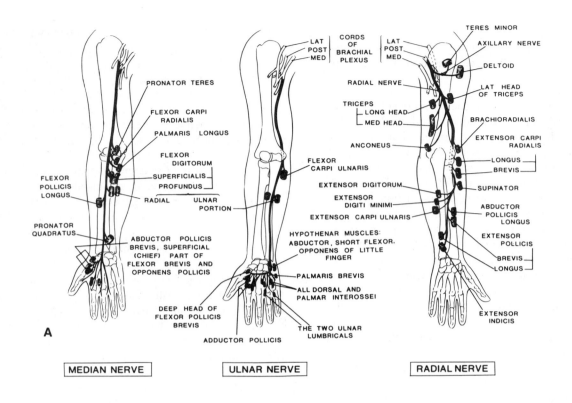

MEDIAN NERVE   ULNAR NERVE   RADIAL NERVE

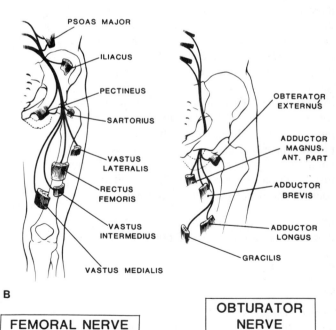

FEMORAL NERVE   OBTURATOR NERVE

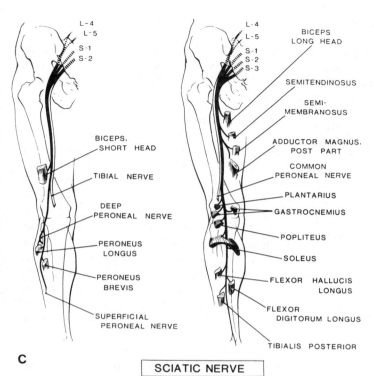

C

SCIATIC NERVE

COMMON PERONEAL
NERVE DIVISION (In black)

TIBIAL NERVE
DIVISION (In black)

Fig. 12-9. Major nerves in upper and lower extremities, showing their location and muscles that they innervate. A. Arm and hand. B. Hip and thigh. C. Leg. D. Lower leg and foot. (From W. H. Hollingshead. Textbook of Anatomy [3rd ed.]. New York: Harper & Row, 1974. Pp. 158-160, 357-360. By permission.)

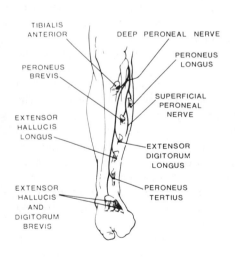

D

COMMON PERONEAL
NERVE

MEDIAL and LATERAL PLANTAR NERVES
(Plantar view of the foot)

A second important manifestation is the result of the loss of trophic factors of the nerve acting on muscle. A denervated muscle will atrophy and undergo changes in its membrane. These changes include a hypersensitivity to acetylcholine. Normally, most of the acetylcholine receptors are confined to the area immediately adjacent to the end plate. After denervation, the sensitivity spreads along the surface, until the entire fiber responds to the drug. This is one form of denervation hypersensitivity (Table 12-4). Muscle fibers undergo denervation hypersensitivity and begin to discharge and twitch approximately 2 weeks after losing their innervation. Such spontaneous, regular twitching of single muscle fibers is called *fibrillation*.

Peripheral Nerves

Anatomy
The peripheral nerves are the major nerve trunks in the extremities and are derived from the plexuses. They have the histologic and physiologic features described in the previous section. Each nerve has a well-defined anatomic course in an

Table 12-5. Peripheral Nerve Distributions

Nerve	General innervation	
Median	Sensory:	Palmar surface of thumb and first three fingers
	Motor:	Finger and wrist flexion
Ulnar	Sensory:	Fourth and fifth fingers
	Motor:	Intrinsic hand muscles
Radial	Sensory:	Dorsum of the hand
	Motor:	Forearm, wrist, and hand extension
Femoral	Sensory:	Anterior aspect of thigh and medial part of leg
	Motor:	Hip flexion and knee extension
Sciatic	Sensory:	Posterior aspect of thigh and portion of leg below the knee
	Motor:	Knee flexion and all ankle and foot motion
Peroneal	Sensory:	Lateral aspect of leg and dorsum of foot
	Motor:	Foot and toe dorsiflexion
Tibial	Sensory:	Posterior part of leg and sole of foot
	Motor:	Foot and toe plantar flexion

extremity, supplies a specific area of skin, and provides innervation for specific muscles (Fig. 12-9). The major peripheral nerves and their important areas of innervation are described in Table 12-5. More detailed distributions are shown in Figure 12-10.

Clinical Correlations
The proximity of some nerves to bony structures makes them particularly vulnerable to lesions at those sites. The *median nerve* passes through a tunnel at the wrist (the carpal tunnel) where it is easily and often compressed, producing arm pain, sensory loss of the first three digits, and weakness of the thenar muscles—the carpal tunnel syndrome. The *ulnar nerve* is commonly compressed at the elbow, where it passes around the medial epicondyle in an exposed position (the "funny bone"). Lesions here produce sensory loss in the ring and fifth fingers, with flaccid weakness and atrophy of the intrinsic muscles of the hand. The *radial nerve* is particularly susceptible to injury as it curves around the humerus in the spiral groove in the mid-upper arm. Lesions at this site produce a wrist drop and weakness of finger extension. The *peroneal nerve* is in an exposed position over a bony prominence where it curves around the head of the fibula at the knee. Damage at this site produces footdrop and sensory loss of the dorsum of the foot. The deep, protected locations of the sciatic, tibial, and femoral nerves result in fewer injuries. These and all other lesions of the peripheral nerves can be recognized by an analysis of the distribution of the motor, sensory, and reflex changes. The type of lesion may be any of those previously described—with total, irreversible destruction due to wallerian degeneration or with mild, reversible changes due to membrane or myelin alterations. The use of nerve conduction studies to determine the location of slowing or block of conduction is of particular value in identifying the location and severity of such lesions.

Peripheral nerves also may be involved in *diffuse disease* of the myelin or axons. In either instance, the clinical features are similar. There is distal loss of sensation in the upper and lower extremities (more severe in the lower extremities), usually for all modalities, although in some disorders there may be selective involvement of certain fiber types and therefore of certain modalities of sensation. There may be paresthesia, dys-

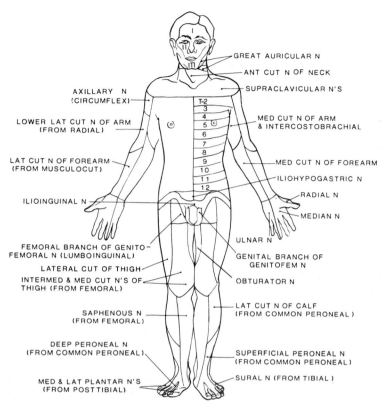

GREAT AURICULAR N

ANT CUT N OF NECK

SUPRACLAVICULAR N'S

AXILLARY N
(CIRCUMFLEX)

T-2
3
4
5
6
7
8
9
10
11
12

LOWER LAT CUT N OF ARM
(FROM RADIAL)

MED CUT N OF ARM
& INTERCOSTOBRACHIAL

LAT CUT N OF FOREARM
(FROM MUSCULOCUT)

MED CUT N OF FOREARM

ILIOHYPOGASTRIC N

RADIAL N

ILIOINGUINAL N

MEDIAN N

ULNAR N

FEMORAL BRANCH OF GENITO-
FEMORAL N (LUMBOINGUINAL)

GENITAL BRANCH OF
GENITOFEM N

LATERAL CUT OF THIGH

INTERMED & MED CUT N'S OF
THIGH (FROM FEMORAL)

OBTURATOR N

LAT CUT N OF CALF
(FROM COMMON PERONEAL)

SAPHENOUS N
(FROM FEMORAL)

DEEP PERONEAL N
(FROM COMMON PERONEAL)

SUPERFICIAL PERONEAL N
(FROM COMMON PERONEAL)

MED & LAT PLANTAR N'S
(FROM POST TIBIAL)

SURAL N (FROM TIBIAL)

Fig. 12-10. Cutaneous distribution of peripheral nerves. (Redrawn from W. Haymaker and B. Woodhall. Peripheral Nerve Injuries: Principles of Diagnosis [2nd ed.]. Philadelphia: Saunders, 1953.)

esthesia, or hyperalgesia, usually in the same distribution. Reflexes are generally lost. Distal muscles are weak and flaccid and eventually atrophy. Atrophy of distal muscles produces deformities, for example, pes cavus and hammer toes (high arches with cocked-up toes) with loss of intrinsic foot muscles.

Although many peripheral nerve diseases affect both axon and myelin, if the disease process primarily affects the axon, there is more severe atrophy, with loss of innervation and prominent fibrillation in distal muscles. Disorders primarily producing myelin damage are associated with less atrophy, are more readily reversible, and have little or no fibrillation.

Plexus

Anatomy
A *plexus* is a complex recombination of axons as they rearrange themselves in passing from one

area to another. There are three major somatic plexuses: the brachial, the lumbar, and the sacral (lumbosacral) plexuses. The *brachial plexus* is derived from spinal nerves C-5 through T-1 and gives rise to the major nerves of the upper extremity. The axons of the spinal nerves are rearranged into trunks, divisions, and cords of the plexus just beneath and behind the clavicle (Fig. 12-11).

The *lumbar plexus*, derived from L-2 through L-4 spinal nerves, and the *sacral plexus*, derived from L-4 through S-3 spinal nerves, give rise to the major nerves of the lower extremity. The femoral and obturator nerves arise from the lumbar, and the sciatic nerve arises from the sacral plexus. The rearrangements of the axons in the lumbosacral plexus occur in the pelvis, posteriorly, deep to the psoas major muscle (Fig. 12-11).

Clinical Correlations
Each of these plexuses may undergo the same physiologic or histologic alterations described previously. They are most commonly involved in trauma, tumor, or hemorrhage. The diagnosis of disease in these regions depends on the presence

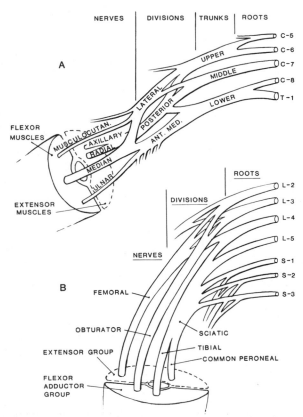

Fig. 12-11. Major components of plexuses. A. Brachial plexus showing origin of the three trunks, three cords, and peripheral nerves. B. Lumbosacral plexus divisions forming nerves of lower extremity.

of involvement of proximal muscles innervated by multiple roots, multiple dermatomal involvement, and sparing of the paraspinal muscles. The changes involve motor and sensory fibers and, when severe, result in autonomic disturbances such as loss of sweating, thinning of the skin, and trophic changes in the skin. Reflex changes are also seen.

A number of major plexuses are purely visceral and are a part of the visceral nervous system. While these plexuses may be involved in localized disease processes, this involvement is uncommon and not of clinical significance. The spinal nerves and nerve roots are within the spinal canal and will be discussed in the next chapter.

The Neuromuscular Junction

The *neuromuscular junction* is the site at which the motor nerve terminal meets a muscle fiber

and where the efferent nerve terminals evoke a contraction of the muscle. This contraction is accomplished through the production of an excitatory synaptic potential called an *end-plate potential*. In the normal skeletal muscle fiber, the end-plate potential always reaches threshold for the production of an action potential, which then propagates along the muscle fiber. The action potential in turn triggers a contraction.

Histology

Each junction consists of a presynaptic portion derived from the nerve terminal and a postsynaptic portion derived from the muscle fiber. As an axon enters a muscle, it branches into many nerve terminals, each of which innervates one muscle fiber. As the terminal approaches the muscle fiber, the axon loses its myelin sheath and comes to lie in a depression in the muscle fiber. The nerve terminal is covered by a Schwann cell, but the inferior portion of the axolemma is directly apposed to the sarcolemma of the muscle fiber, with a synaptic cleft of 500 Å intervening. The postsynaptic portion of the junction consists of complex folds of sarcolemma immediately be-

A

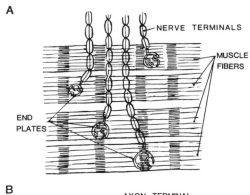

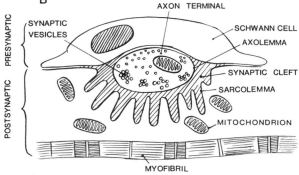

Fig. 12-12. Neuromuscular junction. A. End plates where single nerve terminals innervate single muscle fibers. B. Cross section of an end plate. Axon terminal lies in depression on muscle surface covered by Schwann cell. Postsynaptic, sarcolemmal folds contain acetylcholine receptors. Acetylcholine is stored in synaptic vesicles in nerve terminal.

neath the nerve terminal. This region can be demonstrated with histochemical techniques that stain acetylcholinesterase (Fig. 12-12). The sarcolemma, with its folds, forms the subneural apparatus. The cytoplasm of the nerve terminal contains a concentration of mitochondria and many synaptic vesicles. Often, the synaptic vesicles seem to be clustered near a region of density of the presynaptic membrane. These specialized areas are located opposite the postsynaptic folds. Acetylcholine is bound to the vesicles in the nerve terminal.

Physiology

Small electrical potentials can be recorded from the region of the neuromuscular junction of skeletal muscle fibers, even in the absence of nerve impulses in the motor fibers. These potentials have all the electrical and pharmacologic properties of end-plate potentials, except that they are small and occur in a random fashion without the need of nerve activity. These have been called *miniature end-plate potentials.*

The miniature end-plate potentials are due to leakage of the neurotransmitter acetylcholine from the presynaptic terminals. The leakage occurs in "quanta" of transmitter; that is, the miniature end-plate potentials are produced by thousands of molecules of acetylcholine released together. The end-plate potential in contrast is produced by the near synchronous release of many quanta triggered by the nerve impulse. The *synaptic vesicles* are the storage sites of quanta of acetylcholine.

When the resting potential of the motor axon terminal at a neuromuscular junction is reduced, the frequency of release of miniature end-plate potentials is increased. The relationship is not a linear one, however. There is a tenfold increase in frequency for every 15 mV of depolarization. The depolarization associated with an action potential in the motor axon terminal speeds up the frequency of the miniature end-plate potentials sufficiently to result in the release of a burst of several hundred acetylcholine quanta, thus accounting for the end-plate potential. The number (M) of quanta (Q) released by a presynaptic

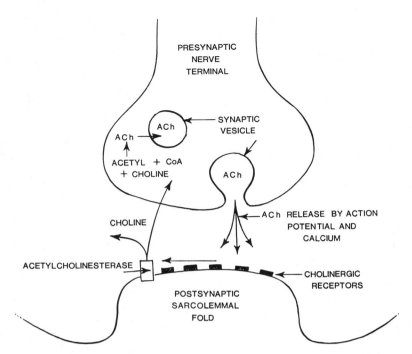

Fig. 12-13. Neurotransmitter action at neuromuscular junction. Acetylcholine (ACh) is formed and stored in nerve terminal. It is released by nerve terminal depolarization in the presence of calcium and binds with receptors on postsynaptic membrane. After producing an ionic conductance charge, it is hydrolyzed by acetylcholinesterase.

action potential can be calculated by dividing the average end-plate potential amplitude (EPP) by the average miniature end-plate potential amplitude (MEPP):

$$M = \frac{EPP}{MEPP}$$

Acetylcholine increases the permeability of the postsynaptic membrane to both sodium and potassium ions. The membrane potential is thus only partially depolarized; the synaptic currents do not flow long enough for the membrane to be depolarized to zero. The end-plate potential is therefore considerably smaller than the action potential; nevertheless, it is well above the threshold for generating a muscle fiber action potential. When the end-plate potential reaches threshold, it triggers the action potential of the muscle. The acetylcholine is rapidly broken down by the enzyme acetylcholinesterase after binding with the postsynaptic membrane and producing the end-plate potential.

Acetylcholine is synthesized by *choline acetylase* from acetyl-CoA and choline in the nerve terminal. It is stored in or on the vesicles and released by the action potential through calcium binding in the membrane. The acetylcholine diffuses across the synapse and binds with the cholinergic receptor until it is broken down by acetylcholinesterase for partial reuptake into the terminal. A summary of the events occurring at the neuromuscular junction is shown in Figure 12-13.

Pharmacology

A number of important drugs affect neuromuscular transmission. For instance, curare, the poison used by some South American Indians on the tips of their blowgun arrows, prevents acetylcholine from reacting with the receptor sites of the muscle membrane by competitively binding with the sites and causes paralysis. In contrast to the effect of the acetylcholine, the reaction between the curare molecule and the acetylcholine receptor molecule does not change conductance in the membrane. Curare thus blocks neuromuscular transmission.

Another substance that blocks neuromuscular transmission is botulin, the agent that causes botulism in food contaminated by *Clostridium botulinum*. Botulin blocks the release of acetylcholine from the motor nerve terminals, causes a loss of end-plate potentials, and results in paralysis.

Neuromuscular transmission is enhanced by drugs that block the action of acetylcholinesterase. In the absence of this enzyme, the acetylcholine released by nerve impulses has a greater and more prolonged action. However, if too much acetylcholine accumulates, it may cause a depolarizing block of the muscle membrane. Excess acetylcholine may also desensitize the acetylcholine receptor molecules and reduce the response to acetylcholine. Normally this interaction occurs but is only transient, because the acetylcholine is removed by the esterase. An example of an anticholinesterase used to treat patients clinically is *physostigmine.* Some insecticides and nerve gases are also anticholinesterases. Several drugs can mimic the action of acetylcholine at the neuromuscular junction. One of these is *nicotine.* In low doses, nicotine has an excitatory effect on skeletal muscle, while in high doses, it blocks neuromuscular transmission.

Clinical Correlations

Disorders of neuromuscular transmission theoretically can involve a number of mechanisms, including the synthesis of acetylcholine, packaging of acetylcholine in the vesicles, release of vesicles from the nerve terminal, diffusion of acetylcholine across the synaptic cleft, binding of the acetylcholine with the receptor, response of the receptor to the transmitter, and breakdown of the acetylcholine by acetylcholinesterase. Two of these disorders are well known clinically. Both are manifested as weakness without sensory loss. One of these is *myasthenia gravis,* in which there is partial receptor blockade resulting in weakness that increases after exercise. In the other disorder, the *myasthenic syndrome,* there is an impairment of release of acetylcholine from the nerve terminal. This also results in weakness; however, it can be partially overcome by continued activity because, with continued activation, changes in the nerve terminal membrane facilitate release. Thus, patients with this syndrome show increasing strength with a brief period of exercise. In myasthenia gravis, both the end-plate potentials and the miniature end-plate potentials are small. In the myasthenic syndrome, a disorder often associated with carcinoma, the miniature end-plate potentials are normal, but the end-plate potentials

are small because of a reduction in the number of quanta released.

Muscle

All body movements are produced by muscles. Through their activity, all the behavior of the organism is affected. The function of muscle is to produce force, to obtain motion, or to stabilize a part. Striated muscles act through their attachment to tendons and bones, but they depend foremost on their contractile elements. They vary in size and structure, from the very tiny stapedius muscle of the ear to the large, powerful gastrocnemius muscle of the leg. Each is designed to perform specific functions, whether they be finely controlled, rapid, skilled movements, powerful, sudden contractions, or slow, continuous, steady exertion of force. Muscles' size and shape (fusiform, unipennate, bipennate, and multipennate) vary with their function, as does their microscopic anatomy. Muscles requiring sudden, strong, or phasic contractions are made up predominantly of type II, white, or fast-twitch muscle fibers that can function anaerobically; while those requiring steady, continuous contractions are made up primarily of type I, red, slow-twitch muscle fibers that depend on aerobic metabolism. The size of motor units, the innervation ratios, and the number of motor units in a muscle also are designed to efficiently perform the appropriate activity. The extraocular muscles, for example, which must perform rapid, quick, very finely controlled movements, have large numbers of motor units—more than a thousand per muscle. Each motor unit has a low innervation ratio, controlling only 5 to 10 muscle fibers. In contrast, the gastrocnemius muscle is a much larger muscle with approximately the same number of motor units. However, the innervation ratio is much higher, each lower motor neuron controlling as many as 2,000 muscle fibers.

Muscles have long been classed as "red" or "white" on the basis of their color. More recently, other biochemical and histochemical differences, such as the content of glycogen, mitochondria, and particular enzymes, have been used to identify different types of muscle fiber (Fig. 12-14). Red fibers contain large amounts of oxidative enzymes (lactic dehydrogenase, succinic dehydrogenase, and cytochrome oxidase), while white fibers contain little of these enzymes

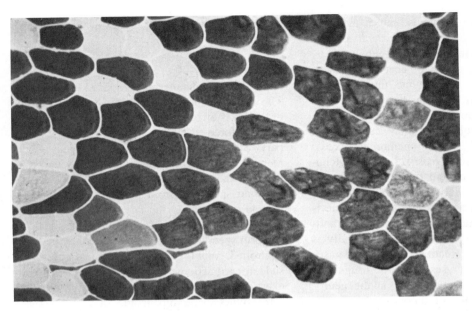

Fig. 12-14. Transverse section of muscle fiber, treated with an ATPase stain, showing normal random checkerboard pattern of the two types of muscle fibers. Type I fibers are stained lightly, while type II fibers are stained darkly. (ATPase stain; ×200.) (Courtesy of Dr. Andrew G. Engel.)

Table 12-6. Characteristics of Motor Units

Tonic	Phasic
Motor neuron (type I)	Motor neuron (type II)
Small alpha motor neuron	Large alpha motor neuron
Small axon	Large axon
Low firing frequency	High firing frequency
Slow-twitch fibers	Fast-twitch fibers
Muscle fibers (red)	Muscle fibers (white)
Aerobic oxidative enzymes	Anaerobic glycolytic enzymes
Small quantities of glycogen	Large quantities of glycogen
Rich in myoglobin	Poor in myoglobin
Lower threshold to stretch	Higher threshold to stretch
Longer contraction time	Shorter contraction time
More mitochondria	Fewer mitochondria
Lower muscle tension	Higher muscle tension
Lower metabolism	Higher metabolism
Lower oxygen consumption	Greater oxygen consumption
Constant good blood flow	Rapidly insufficient blood flow
Low fatigability	Pronounced fatigability

but relatively large amounts of phosphorylase and glycolytic enzymes. The fibers in any one motor unit are *uniform;* that is, all muscle fibers innervated by a single anterior horn cell are identical in their histochemical and physiologic properties. These properties are determined by the anterior horn cell; and reinnervation of muscle fibers by other anterior horn cells after denervation changes the muscle fiber type in addition to the size of the muscle fiber. Some of the differences in type I and type II motor units are shown in Table 12-6.

Structure

Each muscle is made up of large numbers of muscle fibers arranged in parallel along the longitudinal axis of the muscle. The fibers range from 2 to 15 cm in length and from 30 to 60 μm in diameter. Each is attached to the tendon of the muscle via connective tissue attachments. Individual muscle fibers are multinucleated cells containing *myofibrils,* the contractile elements, as well as mitochondria, nuclei, and other cellular constituents. Each muscle fiber has a single end plate located approximately halfway along its length.

The myofibrils of the muscle are banded and give the muscle fiber a banded appearance. Each muscle contains bundles of myofibrils arranged with their bands in register (Fig. 12-15). The bands are due to the overlapping of the component fibrillar protein of the myofibrils. Each myofibril is approximately 1 μm in diameter and

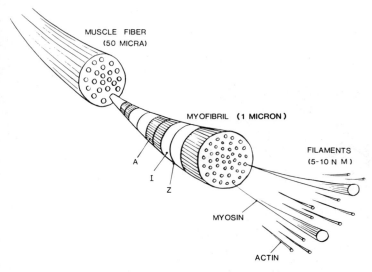

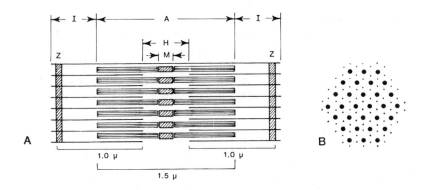

Fig. 12-15. Ultrastructure of muscle fiber. Each fiber is made up of many myofibrils containing filaments of actin and myosin organized in bands A, I, and Z. (NM = nanometers.)

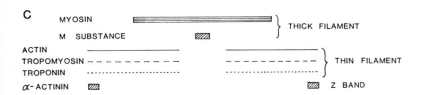

Fig. 12-16. Organization of protein filament in a myofibril. A. Longitudinal section through one sarcomere (Z disk to Z disk) showing overlap of actin and myosin. B. Cross section through A band, where the thin actin filaments interdigitate with the thick myosin filaments in a hexagonal formation. C. Location of specific proteins in sarcomere.

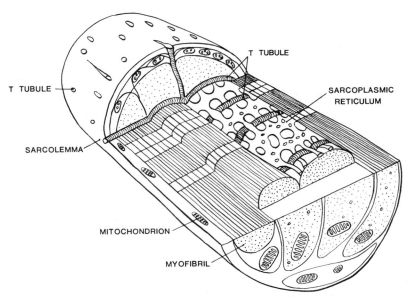

Fig. 12-17. Structure of single muscle fiber cut both horizontally and longitudinally. Individual myofibrils are surrounded and separated by sarcoplasmic reticulum. T tubules are continuous with extracellular fluid and interdigitate with sarcoplasmic reticulum.

contains two types of filaments: thin filaments and thick filaments. The thick filament contains *myosin,* a large protein material of approximately 100 Å in diameter, with lateral projections of meromyosin. *Actin,* the thin filament, is 50 Å in diameter. Actin has two proteins, *troponin* and *tropomyosin,* associated with it; these can prevent the interaction of actin and myosin. The actin and myosin filaments are arranged in a hexagonal formation where they overlap (Fig. 12-16). The area of overlap is darker and is called the *A band.* The area which includes only thin actin filaments is lighter and is called the *I band.* The thin actin filaments are attached to a crystalline structure, which is also dark and is called the *Z disk.* The region including only myosin filaments is the *H band.* The myosin filaments are bound together at an area of darkness centrally called the *M line* within the H band.

A muscle fiber can be divided longitudinally into areas called *sarcomeres,* which extend from one Z disk to the next. The sarcomere is approximately 2 μm long and consists (in order) of I band, A band, H zone, A band, and I band between two Z disks. Running throughout the muscle and intertwined with the myofibrils is

sarcoplasmic reticulum, which forms a longitudinal, anastomotic network of irregular tubular spaces surrounding the myofibrils (Fig. 12-17). At specific locations along the length of the myofibrils, usually at the junction of the A and the I bands, there are transverse tubular structures, the *T tubules,* which are near the sarcoplasmic reticulum. The T tubules are hollow structures, continuous with the surface membrane (or sarcolemma), and therefore are open to the extracellular fluid. They run perpendicularly from the surface membrane into the muscle fiber, encircling the myofibrils.

Physiology

The contraction of a muscle is initiated by the action potential. When the end-plate potential reaches threshold, an action potential is initiated in the end-plate region, which propagates in both directions down the length of the muscle fiber. As the action potential sweeps down the fiber, the current flow generated by the potential passes internally into the depths of the fiber via the T-tubule system. These currents cause the release of calcium from the sarcoplasmic reticulum. The calcium binds with troponin, a protein attached to the surface of the actin filaments, and breaks the troponin-tropomyosin linkage. This linkage, which exists at rest, prevents the interaction of the thin and the thick filaments. When calcium eliminates this inhibition, the filaments interact, attach briefly, and move relative to each other, to result in shortening of the sarcomere. The attachments are brief, rapidly broken, and remade with elements further along the filaments as they slide past one another. Thus, contraction is initiated by the inhibition of an inhibition and is accomplished by the sliding of the filaments. The energy required to break the attachments between the actin and myosin is provided by adenosine triphosphate (ATP) acting with magnesium. If a muscle runs out of energy sources, the binding between actin and myosin can no longer be broken, and the muscle becomes rigid (as in rigor mortis). In normal muscle, the reuptake of calcium by the sarcoplasmic reticulum terminates each contraction.

The generation of tension depends on overlap of actin and myosin filaments. If a muscle is stretched too far, there will be only minimal overlap and little opportunity for interaction. The muscle, therefore, has optimal lengths for contraction, as shown on a length-tension diagram (Fig. 12-18).

The rate at which tension develops varies with

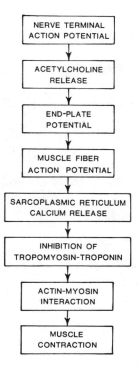

Fig. 12-19. Sequence of events leading to muscle contraction.

Fig. 12-18. Length-tension diagram of muscle fiber in relation to its sarcomere length. A. Tension generated at different sarcomere lengths. B. Extent of overlap of actin and myosin filaments at different sarcomere lengths.

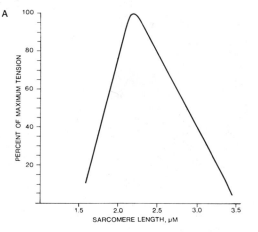

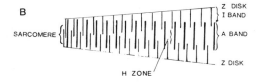

muscle fiber type. In a slow-twitch muscle in which the twitch lasts 100 msec, repetitive stimulation at 10 per second results in a steady contraction. The same rate of activation in a fast-twitch fiber with a twitch time of 25 msec results in a series of brief distinct twitches with each impulse. The sequence of events leading to the contraction of a muscle is illustrated schematically in Figure 12-19.

Clinical Correlations

A disease may damage a muscle directly, as in a *myopathy,* or indirectly by damaging nerves to cause *neurogenic atrophy.* In either instance, there is weakness and atrophy of the muscle. However, myopathy and neurogenic atrophy are histologically and physiologically distinct. If a muscle loses its innervation because of disease of the lower motor neuron, the muscle fibers fibrillate and atrophy. In disorders with incomplete denervation, scattered muscle fibers atrophy. If the process is chronic, viable axons in the muscle reinnervate the denervated fibers, resulting in motor units with a higher innervation ratio and large motor unit potentials. If the large units are lost,

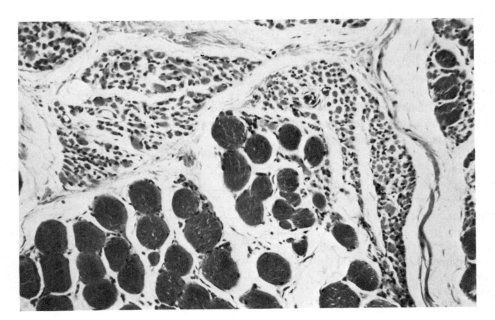

Fig. 12-20. Histologic changes in neurogenic atrophy. Transverse section of muscle fibers showing groups of atrophic fibers and increased connective tissue where many axons have degenerated, (H & E; ×200.) (Courtesy of Dr. Andrew G. Engel.)

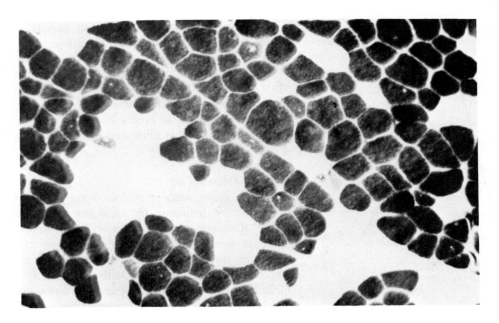

Fig. 12-21. Transverse section of reinnervated muscle fiber. Type I fibers are stained lightly and type II darkly. Note the loss of the normal checkerboard pattern; instead there is a grouping of the same type of fibers. (ATPase stain; ×200.) (Courtesy of Dr. Andrew G. Engel.)

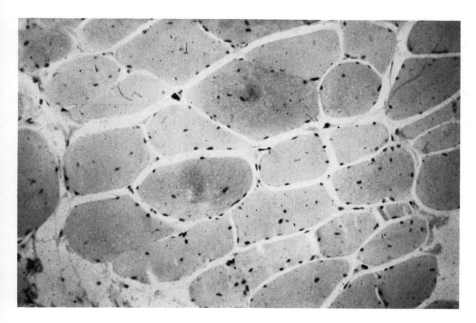

Fig. 12-22. Transverse section of muscle showing general histologic features of myopathy. There is random variation in fiber diameter, with both large and small fibers. Many fibers have internal migration of nuclei; some are splitting or degenerating; and there is an increase in connective tissue. (H & E; ×200.) (Courtesy of Dr. Andrew G. Engel.)

the atrophy subsequently appears in large groups of fibers to produce the typical histologic pattern of neurogenic atrophy (Figs. 12-20, 12-21).

In many myopathies, entire muscle fibers degenerate in a random process, affecting muscle fibers of many motor units, with a loss of fibers from all motor units. With this loss, a smaller force is generated when the motor units are activated. In addition to weakness, the loss of muscle fibers results in smaller motor unit potentials, a feature that can be recognized by needle electromyography. Whereas many primary muscle diseases or myopathies have specific histologic changes, some features are common to all myopathies: random variation in fiber size, internal migration of nuclei, increased connective tissue, and degenerative changes in the muscle fibers (Fig. 12-22).

Although these abnormalities may affect all muscles in the body, most primary muscle diseases affect the proximal muscles to a greater extent than the distal muscles. Proximal muscle weakness is therefore characteristic of myopathy. It is associated with normal sensation and normal

reflexes as long as there is muscle left to contract. The weakness is not associated with an alteration of tone.

Destruction of muscle fibers in their entirety or segmentally along their length is the most common manner for disease processes to affect a muscle. However, two other specific pathophysiologic alterations can occur:

1. Disorder of the sarcolemma, preventing it from generating normal action potentials.
2. Disorder of the excitation-contraction coupling mechanism within the muscle fiber.

DISORDERS OF THE SARCOLEMMA. These result in two types of abnormalities: (1) inability to generate action potentials, as in periodic paralysis in which altered ionic conductance in the membrane results in altered resting potential and loss of action potentials and electrical activity, leaving the muscle contraction weak, and (2) other membrane disorders, such as myotonias, which produce excessive firing or irritability of the membrane, excess muscle contraction, prolonged contraction, or inability to stop contraction.

DISORDERS OF THE CONTRACTILE MECHANISM. In these disorders, muscle fibers generate normal electrical activity but do not generate normal force. In the genetic disorder of phosphorylase deficiency, there is inability to generate sufficient energy. As the muscle runs out of energy, it cramps without electrical activation. Other metabolic and toxic disorders interfere with the excitation-contraction coupling and produce weakness similar in distribution and character to that described with muscle fiber degeneration.

Clinical Findings with Lesions in the Periphery

Muscle Disease

Patients with primary myopathy have weakness often accompanied by a significant atrophy. Voluntary movement is otherwise normal, with no involuntary movements or spasticity. The common types of myopathy, such as muscular dystrophy and polymyositis, involve proximal muscles. There is relative preservation of reflexes because the neural apparatus is intact. Fasciculations (twitching of the muscles), which are indicative of disease of the lower motor neuron, are not present. Patients with disease of muscle show no evidence of damage to the longitudinal systems of the central nervous system. They do not have involvement of mental function, and they do not have sensory symptoms or signs.

Muscular dystrophy is a disease primarily affecting muscle. It is of genetic origin but unknown pathophysiology. There are a number of forms of muscular dystrophy with different clinical patterns. The three major types are Duchenne, fascioscapulohumeral, and limb-girdle. Each of these shows the histologic alterations typical of a myopathy, with random, patchy degeneration of muscle fibers, central nuclei, and connective tissue proliferation. *Polymyositis,* a connective tissue disease, is an immunologic disorder. It shows pathologic changes similar to those of a dystrophy but with inflammatory cell infiltrates, particularly in and around blood vessels. These changes are more prominent in the peripheral areas of the muscle. Muscular dystrophies have the characteristic temporal profile of degenerative disorders; that is, they are diffuse, chronic, and progressive. Polymyositis, however, has the histologic features of an inflammatory disorder and can be expected to show a subacute temporal profile.

Neuromuscular Junction Disease

The major symptom in patients with defects of neuromuscular transmission is weakness, usually in proximal or cranial muscles. There is no atrophy, and tone is normal. The major features differentiating neuromuscular junction disease from muscle disease are fluctuation of weakness with exertion and the response to drugs acting at the neuromuscular junction, which do not occur in myopathies.

Myasthenia gravis, a disorder affecting the neuromuscular junction, is an autoimmune disease in which antibodies are formed against acetylcholine receptors in the postsynaptic membrane at the motor end plate. The reduction in the number of receptor sites at the motor end plate results in a decrease in the response of the muscle fiber to the neurotransmitter acetylcholine. Clinically, myasthenia gravis is characterized by a fatigable weakness that is induced or increased by exercise and improved by rest or anticholinergic agents.

Peripheral Nerve Disease

Diseases involving the peripheral nerves have a combination of motor, sensory, and visceral symptoms and signs. There is flaccid weakness and atrophy and sensory loss involving all modalities of sensation in the same distribution as the motor findings. Deep tendon reflexes and superficial reflexes are absent in the distribution of the involved peripheral nerves. Damage to the sympathetic fibers, traversing the peripheral nerves, may result in alterations in sweating and skin temperature. Other visceral disturbances such as hypotension and impotence also may occur.

Diseases of the peripheral nerves are of two types: (1) symmetric polyneuropathies, usually distal and due to a disturbance involving many nerves, and (2) localized mononeuropathies involving a single peripheral nerve, often due to trauma, neoplasm, or compression. In mononeuropathy, or plexus disease, the weakness, pain, sensory deficit, and reflex loss are within the distribution of a specific peripheral nerve, for example, sciatic, radial, median, and ulnar.

Peripheral neuropathy in which there is death or destruction of a portion of the axon results in degeneration of the distal part of the axon in a process called *axonal degeneration* in diffuse disorders and *wallerian degeneration* with focal lesions (see Chap. 4). Axonal degeneration occurs in generalized disorders of peripheral nerve, such as toxic neuropathies, diabetic neuropathies, and

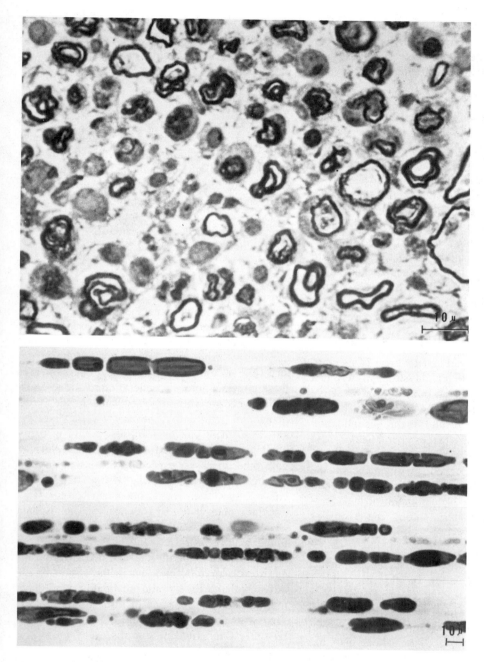

Fig. 12-23. Phase microscopy of a damaged nerve fiber secondary to a crush injury. The upper segment is a transverse section of the nerve showing dilatation, fragmentation, and collapse of the myelin sheaths and an increase in the number of nuclei. The lower segment is a longitudinal section of the nerve showing rows of myelin ovoids indicating a disintegration of the myelin. (From P. J. Dyck. Ultrastructural Alterations in Myelinated Fibers. In J. E. Desmedt [ed.], New Developments in Electromyography and Clinical Neurophysiology, Vol. 2. Basel: Karger, 1973. By permission.)

neuropathies due to nutritional deficiencies. In these disorders, the peripheral nerves show loss of axons, fragmentation of axis cylinders, and breakdown of myelin into fragments or myelin ovoids (Fig. 12-23).

Other peripheral neuropathies are characterized primarily by *segmental demyelination*. In the Guillain-Barré syndrome (postinfectious allergic neuritis), there is edema and swelling of myelin and Schwann cell cytoplasm, with cellular infiltration and segmental loss of myelin. If severe, this may be associated with axonal destruction and wallerian degeneration. In the genetic hypertrophic neuropathies, such as Charcot-Marie-Tooth disease, there is repeated demyelination and remyelination of nerve fibers. Each episode leaves a layer of connective tissue forming concentric layers around the axon. Such nerves become very large and firm, and the axons may finally be lost, leaving only the connective tissue stroma.

Peripheral neuropathy may be only one manifestation of a widespread genetic error of metabolism. In metachromatic leukodystrophy, there is a deficit of *arylsulfatase,* an enzyme that is active in the breakdown of myelin products. The absence of the enzyme results in the accumulation of abnormal sulfatides in peripheral nerves and produces the clinical pattern of peripheral neuropathy. There is associated involvement of the white matter of the central nervous system. Pathologically, there is the accumulation of metachromatically staining material along the axons as well as the breakdown of myelin.

Refsum's disease is another genetically determined disease in which the metabolic defect results in an accumulation of phytanic acid, a fatty acid. The disease is characterized by a chronic, sensorimotor polyneuropathy associated with hypertrophic changes and onion-bulb formation of peripheral nerves. The patient also has ichthyosis (dry, rough, scaly skin), retinitis pigmentosa, and deafness. In the past, this was considered an untreatable degenerative neurologic disorder; however, it has now been shown that a diet low in phytanic acid is helpful in treating this condition.

Laboratory Studies in the Identification of Lesions in the Periphery

In addition to the clinical features previously listed, a number of laboratory tests are helpful in differentiating diseases involving the peripheral structures. These include biochemical, electrophysiologic, and histologic studies.

General Medical Tests

Peripheral neuromuscular disorders are often found with, or secondary to, systemic disease processes. For example, neuropathies occur with diabetes, nutritional deficiencies, kidney diseases, carcinoma, and poisonings. Myopathies occur with endocrine diseases, connective tissue diseases, metabolic disorders, and neoplasm. Therefore, a general medical assessment is important in the evaluation of peripheral disease.

Muscle Enzymes

Muscle contains a number of enzymes that are important in their metabolism, such as aldolase, serum glutamic-oxaloacetic transaminase (SGOT), and lactic dehydrogenase (LDH). Muscle damage from any disease that results in destruction or degeneration of muscle fibers releases these enzymes into the general circulation. Thus, their levels are commonly elevated in the blood of patients with active primary muscle diseases. However, these enzymes are also found in many other tissues, and their levels can be elevated with other diseases, especially those that damage the heart or liver. *Creatine kinase* (CK) is an enzyme that transfers a phosphate group from creatine phosphate to adenosine diphosphate (ADP) to form creatine and ATP. This enzyme is found mainly in muscle and is therefore a more specific indicator of muscle disease. Creatine kinase levels may be elevated in the serum in patients with early or mild myopathy who have minimal clinical evidence of disease, and in persons who are carriers of the abnormal gene in recessively inherited muscle disease.

Nerve Conduction Studies

Often, it is not possible to be certain on the basis of clinical findings whether a patient has a peripheral disorder. To help in this differentiation, the function of peripheral nerves can be evaluated by nerve conduction studies that quantitatively measure their responses to stimulation. Nerve conduction studies are of particular value in localizing disease in peripheral nerves, in assessing

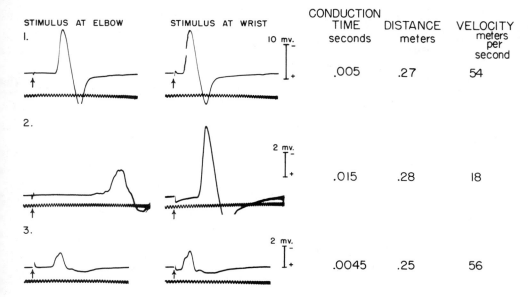

		CONDUCTION TIME seconds	DISTANCE meters	VELOCITY meters per second
		.005	.27	54
		.015	.28	18
		.0045	.25	56

Fig. 12-24. Measurement of conduction velocity. 1. Normal. 2. Neuropathy: conduction velocity is slowed along entire nerve, and amplitude is reduced with proximal stimulation because of dispersion of the response. 3. Myopathy: conduction velocity is normal, but amplitude is reduced because of muscle atrophy. (From Department of Neurology and Department of Physiology and Biophysics, Mayo Clinic and Mayo Foundation. Clinical Examinations in Neurology [3rd ed.]. Philadelphia: Saunders, 1971. By permission.)

the severity of the disease, and in characterizing nerve disease.

The natural activity in individual axons of a peripheral nerve is random and cannot be readily recorded; however, with the application of an electrical stimulus, all the large myelinated fibers can be discharged simultaneously, and the resulting compound action potential can be recorded and measured. If an electrical stimulus (20 to 100 V for 0.1 msec) is applied to a mixed peripheral nerve, action potentials will be initiated that travel in both directions along the nerve. Action potentials traveling centrally will be perceived by the patient as a shock in the distribution of the nerve stimulated. Those traveling peripherally will invade each of the terminal branches of the nerve, where they can be recorded either from cutaneous sensory branches or from muscles innervated by motor branches. Thus, either the motor or the sensory components of the peripheral nerves can be selectively studied.

These two types of potentials, the sensory nerve action potential and the compound muscle

action potential, are measured on an oscilloscope. The *amplitude* of the potential is a function of the number of axons that can carry activity from the point of stimulation to the recording site. The *latency* is a function of the rate at which the largest fibers in the nerve propagate action potentials down the axon. By measuring the distance traveled and dividing this value by the time, the *conduction velocity* can be determined (Fig. 12-24). Conduction velocity depends on the diameter of the axon and the extent of myelination of the axons. If a nerve is stimulated repetitively at rates of 2 to 40 per second, a normal muscle can respond with the same number of fibers, and the compound action potential with each stimulus will be identical.

The presence of peripheral nerve disease is reflected in the nerve conduction studies. In an axolemmal disorder, the action potential is blocked in the region of the abnormality. Stimulation distal to this point results in normal responses, but proximal stimulation produces either no response or only a reduced amplitude response. Axoplasmic disorders with axonal narrowing result in slowing of conduction, while those with axonal degeneration result in a reduced amplitude or absent response to stimulation. In myelin disorders, there is slowing of conduction, with progressive loss of amplitude on more proximal stimulation.

Localized lesions of a peripheral nerve produce a local block or a slowing of conduction in the

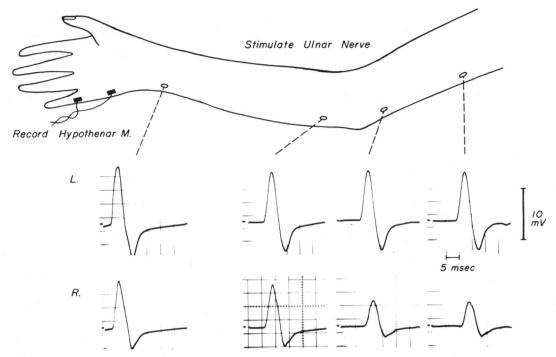

Fig. 12-25. Nerve conduction studies in patient with ulnar neuropathy at the elbow. Normal responses from left arm (L); abnormal on right (R). There is a localized partial block of conduction (decreased amplitude above the elbow) and localized slowing of conduction velocity at the elbow. (Courtesy of E. H. Lambert, Mayo Clinic.)

region of the damage. The block results in a smaller evoked response with proximal rather than with distal stimulation (Fig. 12-25). In generalized disorders of peripheral nerves, there may be a generalized slowing of conduction in segmental demyelinating disorders (Fig. 12-26), a loss of amplitude of responses, especially distally in axonal dystrophies, or a combination of both.

Disorders of neuromuscular transmission are characterized by progressive loss of amplitude of an evoked motor response with repetitive stimulation, especially at rates of 2 to 5 per second. The evoked responses in primary muscle disease with atrophy are of low amplitude but are without other changes in nerve conduction. In upper motor neuron lesions, results of nerve conduction studies are normal.

Nerve conduction studies are usually performed in conjunction with electromyography because they utilize similar techniques and complement each other in arriving at diagnoses of peripheral nerve and muscle disease.

Electromyography

Muscle function can be evaluated by measuring the electrical activity by electromyography (EMG or needle examination) (Fig. 12-27). Electromyography provides information about the presence and type of disease involving muscle. Since nerve disorders produce secondary changes in muscle, EMG is valuable not only in diagnosing primary muscle diseases but also in differentiating neurogenic disorders, diseases of neuromuscular transmission, and diseases of the central nervous system.

In EMG, a needle electrode is inserted into a muscle, and the electrical activity is recorded on an oscilloscope and a loudspeaker. The recorded potentials are characterized by their amplitude, duration, and firing patterns (Fig. 12-28). Recordings are made in multiple muscles in three states: at rest, with needle movement, and with voluntary activity.

At rest, there is electrical silence in a normal muscle, except in the region of motor end plates where end-plate potentials or other small potentials may be recorded (Fig. 12-28). If the needle is moved in the muscle, the mechanical stimula-

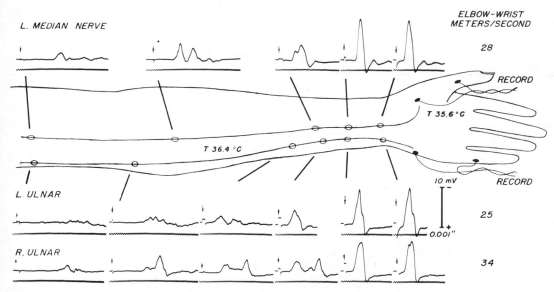

Fig. 12-26. Nerve conduction studies in generalized demyelinating neuropathy. The evoked muscle action potentials with nerve stimulation are shown. Conduction velocity is listed at right. All nerves are affected, with slowing of conduction and dispersion of potentials along their entire length. (Courtesy of E. H. Lambert, Mayo Clinic.)

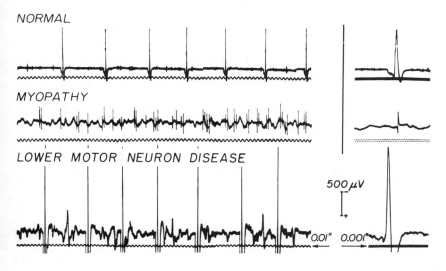

Fig. 12-27. Potentials recorded in electromyography. Motor unit potentials during voluntary contraction in a normal person, muscular dystrophy (myopathy), and amyotrophic lateral sclerosis (lower motor neuron disease). Potentials on left are displayed with a slow time base; on right, with a fast time base.

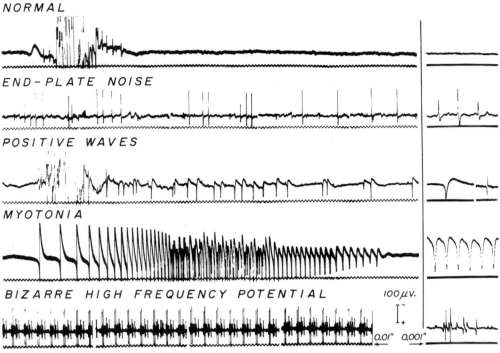

NORMAL

END-PLATE NOISE

POSITIVE WAVES

MYOTONIA

BIZARRE HIGH FREQUENCY POTENTIAL

100μv.

0.01"   0.001"

Fig. 12-28. Examples of EMG activity in response to insertion of the needle into the muscle. The top segment shows a normal discharge; the second segment shows biphasic spikes arising in the end-plate region; the third segment shows abnormal positive waves (downward deflections) from denervated muscle; the fourth segment shows a rapid burst of potentials that is characteristic of myotonia; the bottom segment shows a complex repetitive discharge in a chronic neurogenic atrophy.

tion produces a discharge of the muscle fibers in a characteristic brief burst called *insertional activity* (Fig. 12-28). With voluntary contraction of the muscle, the motor units fire repetitively, in an orderly fashion, with a frequency and number proportional to the effort exerted. The motor unit potentials are measured to determine their amplitude, duration, and firing rate.

If there is a primary myopathy with random degeneration of muscle fibers, each motor unit will have a reduced innervation ratio and the motor unit potential will be of short duration and low amplitude (Fig. 12-29). Because of the reduction in power of each motor unit, many more will fire for any given strength than in a normal muscle. If there is partial destruction of some muscle fibers, the still viable portions may fire spontaneously (fibrillate). In sarcolemmal disor-

ders, there will be an overall reduction in activity, with small motor unit potentials. In disorders of excitation-contraction coupling, there will be no abnormality recorded on EMG.

In contrast to the changes in myopathy, a neurogenic disorder results primarily in a loss of number of motor unit potentials and will be seen as poor recruitment with increasing effort and a small number of units firing rapidly with maximal effort. In addition, if there has been a chronic denervation with opportunity for reinnervation and resultant increase in innervation ratio, the motor unit potentials will be of long duration and high amplitude. Any muscle fibers that are denervated because of axonal degeneration will fibrillate. If a motor unit is irritable, single brief twitches or fasciculation of the motor units will occur (see Fig. 12-27).

Diseases of neuromuscular transmission are characterized by variable conduction blocks across individual neuromuscular junctions and result in variations in the amplitude of the motor unit potentials with voluntary contraction. In upper motor neuron disease, the motor units appear normal and recruit normally but fire slowly (poor activation).

By combining the findings from EMG and nerve conduction studies, it is often possible to

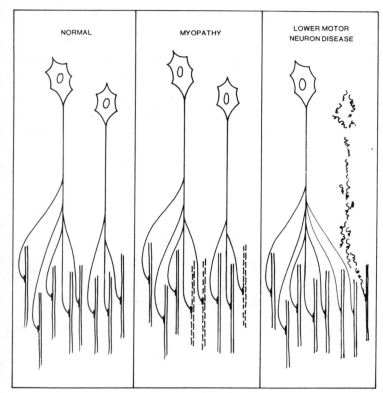

Fig. 12-29. Alteration in innervation patterns in peripheral disease. Myopathy shows random loss of muscle fibers from all motor units. Neurogenic atrophy shows loss of innervation of all fibers in motor unit, with partial reinnervation by surviving axons.

localize the disease in the periphery and at times to specific sites, to characterize the general type of disorder, and to assist in determining the severity or prognosis in the disorder.

Nerve Biopsy

In some peripheral nerve diseases, the clinical, biochemical, and electrophysiologic studies do not reveal the nature of the abnormality. For these patients, a nerve biopsy specimen, usually of a fascicle of the sural nerve, is studied. Nerve biopsy specimens are best studied in three ways: by light microscopy of nerve bundles, teased fiber studies, and cross-sectional fiber counts. For ordinary light microscopy, a piece of nerve is fixed and stained with standard histologic stains and special stains for specific diseases. For instance, in leprosy, the *Mycobacterium leprae* can be stained with acid-fast stains; and in metachromatic leukodystrophy or amyloid, other specific stains demonstrate the accumulation of the abnormal materials.

If another portion of the nerve is fixed and stained for myelin, it can be teased or pulled apart into single fibers. These single fibers then can be examined for the presence of segmental demyelination, paranodal loss of myelin, or other characteristic changes, such as the presence of linear rows of myelin ovoids after axonal degeneration. In addition, the diameter and the length of the internodes can be measured. Plots of the internodal length compared with the axon diameter can give quantitative estimates of the presence of myelin disorders.

Cross sections of a portion of the nerve also can be stained with myelin stains, and the diameters of the fibers can be measured and plotted as density of fibers. The presence of selective loss of certain fiber types then can be quantitatively determined.

Muscle Biopsy

Although at times the clinical history or pattern of muscle impairment in a patient can permit the diagnosis of a myopathy, often neither the clinical nor the electrophysiologic findings can provide a specific diagnosis. In these situations, muscle biopsy is of clinical diagnostic value. It, like the EMG and nerve conduction studies, can differentiate muscle abnormalities secondary to neurogenic disorders (neurogenic atrophy) from those due to primary myopathy. In the latter case, they can often provide an even more specific diagnosis.

Muscle biopsy specimens are taken from a muscle that shows moderate (but not severe) weakness. In severe weakness, there may be so much replacement of muscle by fat or connective tissue that a diagnosis cannot be made. The specimen is stained with routine stains such as hematoxylin and eosin or trichrome and with various histochemical stains that permit the identification of different fiber types. It is also stained for specific abnormalities, such as glycogen in glycogen-storage diseases or lipid in lipid-storage diseases. Fiber type grouping provides evidence of neurogenic disease, while the presence of specific materials may allow the diagnosis of a specific myopathy.

Objectives

1. Name the four major systems represented at the peripheral level and describe the location, histologic features, and function of each.
2. Name the four subdivisions of the peripheral level at which lesions occur, and describe their gross anatomic location and histologic features.
3. List the neurologic deficits that would be associated with damage in each of these subdivisions of the peripheral level and explain their mechanism of occurrence.
4. Describe the mechanism of muscle contraction.
5. Name the location of, function of, and deficit (motor, sensory, and reflex) resulting from a lesion of each of the following: spinal nerves C-5, C-6, C-7, C-8, L-4, L-5, and S-1; brachial and lumbosacral plexuses; radial, ulnar, median, sciatic, femoral, peroneal, and tibial peripheral nerves.
6. Describe the application of the EMG and nerve conduction studies to neurologic diseases.

Clinical Problems

1. A 47-year-old bank manager has had diabetes for 14 years. The diabetes is controlled by insulin. He is seen with a complaint of impotence of 6 months' duration. He has had 2 to 3 years of gradually progressive burning and numbness, first of his feet and recently of his hands. He has occasional dizzy spells on arising. On examination his blood pressure is 115/75 mm Hg supine but decreases to 80/40 mm Hg, with no change in pulse when he arises. He has mild weakness of his toe and foot dorsiflexors but no other weakness. His ankle reflexes are absent. Other reflexes are hypoactive. He has moderate loss of all modalities of sensation in a glove-and-stocking distribution. There is an absence of hair on his legs, and his skin is very dry. On nerve conduction studies, no sensory potentials could be obtained, and motor responses were of low amplitude, with a mild slowing of conduction velocity. The EMG showed fibrillation in distal muscles bilaterally.

   a. What is the localization and type of disease?
   b. What is this disorder called?
   c. What is the significance of low-amplitude evoked potentials?
   d. What is the significance of fibrillation?
   e. How is fibrillation differentiated from fasciculation?

2. A 57-year-old man has been in good health except for a chronic "smoker's cough." During the past 6 months, he has noted gradually increased difficulty in climbing steps and more recently has had trouble in arising from chairs. He has had some dryness of his mouth. Examination revealed no abnormalities other than weakness of proximal muscles and very hypoactive reflexes. Both the strength and the reflexes appear to improve somewhat with exercise. Results of laboratory studies are unremarkable other than for changes in the EMG suggesting the presence of a defect of neuromuscular transmission. On the roentgenogram of the chest, there is a mass in the right hilum of the lung. An intercostal muscle biopsy was performed, and electrophysiologic recordings

were made from the muscle. The following data were obtained:

	Patient	Normal
Average resting potential (mV)	75.6	74.7
Average MEPP amplitude (mV)	0.3 ± 0.3	0.3 ± 0.4
Average EPP amplitude (mV)	3.2 ± 0.9	15 +
Average single fiber action potential amplitude (mV)	97 ± 3	98 ± 3
Threshold (mV)	60	60

a. What two factors determine the size of the end-plate potential (EPP)?
b. Which of these is abnormal in this patient?
c. What is the quantum content in this patient?
d. How could this produce weakness?
e. What is this disorder?

3. A 55-year-old woman developed proximal symmetric weakness during a 2-week period, with mild muscle soreness. On examination, reflexes, sensation, and mentation were normal. All proximal muscles were moderately weak, distal muscles mildly so. There was no fatigue with exercise.

a. What specific disease is this likely to be?
b. What is the location and cause of this disorder?

Results of motor and sensory nerve conduction studies on this patient were normal, except for a borderline low-amplitude compound muscle action potential. A needle electrode (EMG) was inserted in a weak muscle and recordings were made of the motor unit potentials. Two abnormalities were noted: The potentials were small and they fired rapidly with minimal contraction.

c. With disease of the motor unit, if neuromuscular transmission is normal, weakness is due to either of two losses. What are they?
d. What are the two mechanisms used to increase force of contraction?
e. In what way will scattered loss of some muscle fibers alter the firing pattern and size of motor unit potentials?
f. What pattern of histologic change would you expect in this patient?
g. Would muscle fibers innervated by a single anterior horn cell be grouped together?
h. In what general situation does fiber type grouping occur?
i. How could a person with moderately severe motor neuron disease have no weakness?
j. What do the T tubules, sarcoplasmic reticulum, and calcium have in common?
k. This patient had an elevation of serum creatine kinase. Why did this occur?

Suggested Reading

Brooke, M. H. *A Clinician's View of Neuromuscular Diseases.* Baltimore: Williams & Wilkins, 1977.

Dyck, P. J., et al. *Peripheral Neuropathology* (2nd ed.). Philadelphia: Saunders, 1984.

Engel, A. G., and Banker, B. Q. *Myology.* New York: McGraw-Hill, 1985.

Hubbard, J. I. *The Peripheral Nervous System.* New York: Plenum, 1974.

Schwartz, J. H. Axonal transport: Components, mechanisms, and specificity. *Annu. Rev. Neurosci.* 2:467, 1979.

Swash, M., and Schwartz, M.S. *Neuromuscular Diseases: A Practical Approach to Diagnosis and Management.* New York: Springer-Verlag, 1981.

Waxman, S. G. *Physiology and Pathobiology of Axons.* New York: Raven, 1978.

The Spinal Level

13

The spinal level includes the vertebral column and its contents. The spinal canal within the vertebral column is the passage formed by the vertebrae, extending from the foramen magnum of the skull through the sacrum of the spinal column. It contains the spinal cord, nerve roots, spinal nerves, meninges, and the vascular supply of the spinal cord. Five of the major systems are represented in the spinal canal: sensory, motor, visceral, vascular, and cerebrospinal fluid systems. Diseases in the spinal canal therefore will involve one or more of these systems to produce patterns of disease distinctive to this level. The anatomic and physiologic characteristics of the spinal cord and spinal nerves that permit identification and localization of diseases in the spinal canal are presented in this chapter.

Overview

Two distinct patterns of abnormality occur with disease of the nervous system: segmental and longitudinal. Damage to segmental structures, as already noted for peripheral lesions, produces signs localized in a single segment of the body. These signs include flaccid weakness, atrophy, loss of reflexes, and loss of all modalities of sensation in a focal distribution. Lesions in the spinal cord usually damage longitudinal systems in addition to segmental structures. Damage to a longitudinal system produces deficit in that system for all functions below the level of the lesion. It is the combination of these patterns of involvement that permits a precise definition of the location of a disease process.

Localized lesions at the spinal level may produce only segmental signs by damage to the spinal nerves and roots within the spinal column. Segmental signs can occur with spinal level lesions because of the origin and termination of primary sensory neurons and lower motor neurons in the spinal cord. The primary sensory endings in the cord distribute information widely within the cord, but in an organized fashion. For example, muscle spindle afferents send excitatory fibers to motor neurons of synergistic muscles and inhibitory fibers to antagonistic muscles. Such connections result in complex reflexes mediated at the spinal cord level. The motor neurons of the somatic and visceral efferent pathways, located in the ventral and intermediolateral gray matter of the spinal cord, are the origin of the peripheral motor axons. These motor neurons integrate information from multiple sources in determining the activity of the peripheral muscles and glands.

Lesions at the spinal level can damage these central components of the primary sensory neurons or lower motor neurons and result in disorders of the peripheral structures manifested as:

1. Atrophy, fasciculation, and weakness, occurring with death or damage of the motor neurons in the ventral horns.
2. Preganglionic sympathetic disturbances occurring with damage to the neurons in the intermediolateral cell column.
3. Loss of sensation with destruction of the central processes of the primary sensory neurons.

These segmental signs permit the localization of disease along the length of the spinal cord. They are recognized as originating at the spinal level by the associated involvement of ascending or descending tracts which produces intersegmental signs. The location of a lesion within the spinal canal often can be defined further by the pattern of involvement among the structures in the cross section of the cord. The spinal cord, therefore, is subdivided both along its length and cross section to aid in the recognition of disease.

Spinal Cord Subdivisions

The segments along the length of the spinal cord are named to correspond to the vertebrae through which the spinal nerves pass.

1. Cervical. The cephalad portion of the spinal cord from which eight pairs of ventral and seven pairs of dorsal roots arise to form the cervical spinal nerves.
2. Thoracic. The middle portion of the spinal cord from which 12 pairs of nerve roots arise to form the thoracic spinal nerves.
3. Lumbar. The upper caudal portion of the spinal cord from which five lumbar nerve roots arise to form the lumbar spinal nerves.
4. Sacral. The caudal end of the cord from which five pairs of sacral nerve roots arise. The conus medullaris is the termination of the cord from which sacral nerve roots arise.

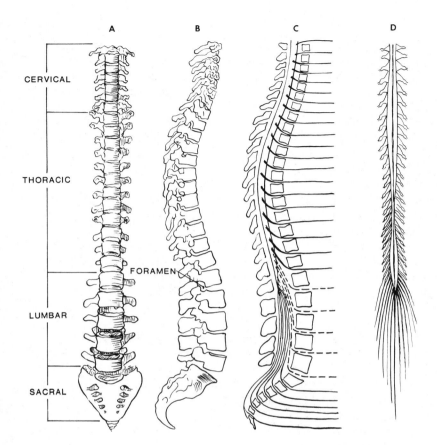

CERVICAL

THORACIC

FORAMEN

LUMBAR

SACRAL

A   B   C   D

Fig. 13-1. Spinal column and cord showing relationships to each other. A. Anterior view of spine. B. Lateral view of spine. C. Lateral view of spinal cord and roots in spine. D. Dorsal view of spinal cord.

The cross section of the spinal canal is subdivided into major structures from the center to the periphery.

1. Central canal. The central remnant of the ependymal lining of the neural tube.
2. Gray matter. Accumulations of neurons in columns and clusters surrounding the central canal.
3. White matter. Longitudinal fiber tracts in the periphery of the spinal cord.
4. Blood vessels. Vascular supply of the spinal cord located on its external surface.
5. Nerve roots and spinal nerves. The segmental axons of motor and sensory fibers leaving or entering the cord bilaterally along its entire length.
6. Meninges and subarachnoid space. The connective tissue coverings of the spinal cord in the spinal canal and the space they surround.

Anatomy of the Spinal Cord

External Morphology

The spinal cord lies within the vertebral canal and, in the adult, extends from the foramen magnum to the lower border of the first lumbar vertebra (L-1). The spinal cord is roughly cylindrical with a slight anteroposterior flattening. It has two wider areas, the *cervical* and *lumbar enlargements,* from which the innervation of the upper and lower extremities arises. The caudal end of the spinal cord tapers to form the *conus medullaris* (Fig. 13-1).

Nerve fibers enter and exit from the spinal cord via the *spinal nerve roots.* These roots form from the union of smaller rootlets and leave the cord dorsolaterally and ventrolaterally. The dorsal and ventral roots join laterally at the intervertebral foramina to form the spinal nerves. Thirty-one pairs of spinal nerves are thus formed and divide the cord into 8 cervical, 12 thoracic, 5 lumbar, and 5 sacral segments and 1 coccygeal segment. Each spinal segment except the first and last has a dorsal (afferent) root and a ventral (efferent) root,

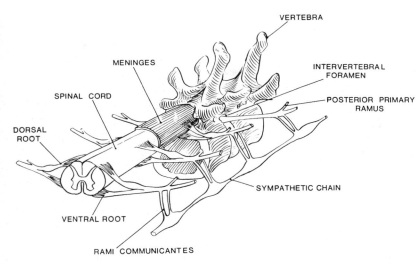

Fig. 13-2. Formation of a spinal nerve as it leaves spinal canal through intervertebral foramen.

which emerge on each side of a spinal segment and become ensheathed by dura as they unite to form the spinal nerve. The dorsal root ganglion, which contains the cell bodies of the nerve fibers in the dorsal root, is an enlargement of the dorsal root at the intervertebral foramen. In the intervertebral foramen, the dura merges with the perineurium of the peripheral nerve.

There are thus four nerve roots arising from each spinal cord segment, a dorsal and ventral root on each side. They are contained entirely within the spinal canal and are bathed in cerebrospinal fluid. They follow a lateral or, in the lower portions of the spinal canal, a descending course to the intervertebral foramen, where the dorsal and ventral roots join to form the spinal nerve (Fig. 13-1). The ventral roots carry the myelinated axons of the alpha and gamma motor neurons to the somatic musculature and the myelinated axons of the preganglionic neurons of the sympathetic (parasympathetic in the sacral region) nerves to viscera. The dorsal roots carry the sensory input from cutaneous, somatic, muscular, and visceral receptors in myelinated and unmyelinated axons. The cell bodies of these axons are in the dorsal root ganglia.

The spinal nerves are very short nerves in which the motor, sensory, and autonomic components of a single cord segment are united in a single structure as they exit from the spinal canal through the intervertebral foramen (Fig. 13-2). The *foramen* is the bony canal formed by two

adjacent vertebrae. Because the nerve is surrounded by this bony structure, it is particularly vulnerable to local compression by a tumor, a herniated nucleus pulposus, or arthritic changes in the bones. Each of the spinal nerves is derived from a segment of the spinal cord, and the names of the nerves correspond to the names of the segments. Since there are only seven cervical vertebrae, the C-1 through C-7 spinal nerves exit *above* the pedicle of the vertebra of the same number, while the C-8 spinal nerves emerge *between* the C-7 and T-1 vertebrae. Caudal to T-1, the spinal nerves all exit below the vertebrae of the same number.

Each spinal nerve is distributed to a well-defined area of skin called a *dermatome* (Fig. 13-3). Dermatomes of adjacent spinal nerves overlap. This overlap accounts for the variation in sensory loss seen in patients with spinal nerve lesions. The spinal nerves are also distributed to specific groups of muscles called *myotomes* (Table 13-1).

The nerve roots are anchored in the intervertebral foramina at the point where their dural sleeves terminate. Flexion of the spinal cord or traction on a peripheral nerve (such as with a disk herniation or local tumor) can stretch and irritate a spinal nerve and cause pain.

Early in development, the spinal cord segments are at the same level as the corresponding vertebrae. With growth, the vertebral column elongates more than the spinal cord does, and the spinal roots are displaced caudally. The roots of rostral cord segments are displaced less than those of caudal segments. The lumbar and sacral nerves, therefore, have long spinal roots that de-

Table 13-1. Myotomes Listed
by Spinal Nerve and Muscle

Spinal nerve	Muscles
C-5	Biceps, deltoid, infraspinatus
C-6	Biceps, deltoid, infraspinatus, wrist flexors, wrist extensors, forearm pronators
C-7	Wrist extensors, wrist flexors, finger flexors, finger extensors, triceps
C-8	Intrinsic hand muscles
L-4	Iliopsoas, quadriceps, anterior tibial
L-5	Anterior tibial, toe dorsiflexors, hamstrings, posterior tibial
S-1	Gluteus maximus, hamstring, gastrocnemius, intrinsic foot muscles

Muscles	Spinal nerves*
Neck flexors	C-1 to C-6
Neck extensors	C-1 to C-6
Shoulder external rotator	C-5, C-6
Deltoid	C-5, C-6
Biceps brachii	C-5, C-6
Triceps	C-6, <u>C-7</u>, C-8
Wrist extensors	C-6, C-7, C-8
Wrist flexors	C-6, C-7, C-8, T-1
Digit extensors	<u>C-7</u>, C-8
Digit flexors	C-7, C-8, T-1
Thenar	C-8, T-1
Hypothenar	C-8, T-1
Interossei	C-8, T-1
Abdomen	T-6 to L-1
Rectal sphincter	S-3, S-4
Iliopsoas	<u>L-3</u>, L-4
Thigh adductor	L-2, L-3, L-4
Quadriceps	L-2, L-3, L-4
Thigh abductor	L-4, <u>L-5</u>, S-1
Gluteus maximus	<u>S-1</u>, S-2
Hamstrings	L-4, <u>L-5</u>, <u>S-1</u>
Anterior tibial	L-4, L-5
Toe extensors	L-4, <u>L-5</u>, S-1
Peronei	<u>L-5</u>, S-1
Posterior tibial	<u>L-5</u>, S-1
Toe flexors	L-5, S-1
Gastrocnemius	L-5, <u>S-1</u>, S-2

* Spinal nerves underlined provide the major innervation for that muscle.

scend within the dural sac to reach their appropriate vertebral level of exit. These roots are called the *cauda equina* because they have an appearance similar to a horse's tail. Because of the difference in length between the vertebral column and the spinal cord, care must be taken to specify vertebral level or spinal segment level in indicating the location of a lesion. Generally in a neurologic problem, the affected spinal segment is defined first, and then an attempt is made to correlate that with the appropriate vertebral level. However, in cases of vertebral lesions, the level of the vertebral involvement is often seen on the roentgenogram and then the level of a possible spinal injury is determined.

The general guidelines for locating the level of a spinal cord injury with respect to the vertebrae are:

1. Between T-1 and T-10, add two to the number of the vertebral spine to determine the spinal cord segment at the same location.
2. The lumbar segments of the cord are approximately at the level of the spinous processes of T-11 and T-12.
3. Sacral and coccygeal segments are at the level of the L-1 spinous process.
4. There are eight cervical segments and only seven cervical vertebrae, so that the cervical enlargement at C-7 cord segment is centered at the C-7 vertebral level.

The surface of the spinal cord shows several longitudinal furrows. The anterior (ventral) surface is indented by the deep anterior median fissure. The posterior surface contains a shallow posterior median sulcus. The dorsal spinal roots enter each side of the spinal cord along the posterolateral sulci. Posterior intermediate sulci extend from the rostral cervical to the midthoracic spinal cord, between the dorsal root entry zone and the midline.

Meninges
The spinal cord is ensheathed by three membranous coverings, the *meninges*. The outer membrane is a tough, relatively inelastic connective tissue sheath called the *dura mater*. The inner two membranes, or *leptomeninges,* are the *arachnoid* and the *pia mater*. These membranes are much thinner than the dura mater and consist of deli-

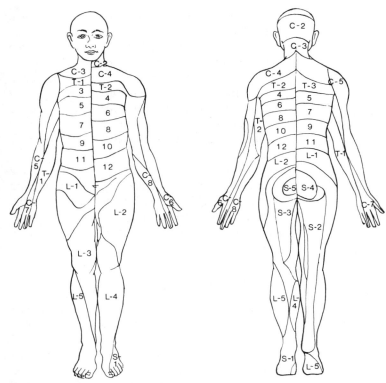

Fig. 13-3. *Cutaneous distribution of spinal nerves (dermatomes). (Redrawn from F. R. Ford. Diseases of the Nervous System: In Infancy, Childhood and Adolescence [6th ed.]. Springfield, Ill.: Thomas, 1973.)*

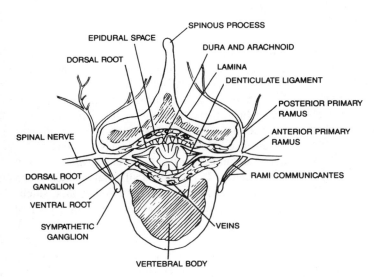

Fig. 13-4. *Cross section of spinal canal showing spinal cord, its meningeal coverings, and manner of exit of spinal nerves.*

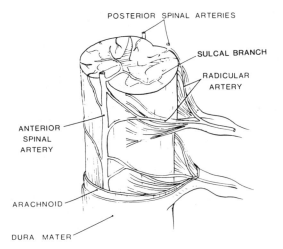

POSTERIOR SPINAL ARTERIES

SULCAL BRANCH

RADICULAR ARTERY

ANTERIOR SPINAL ARTERY

ARACHNOID

DURA MATER

Fig. 13-5. The arterial supply of a spinal cord segment enters via the radicular arteries.

cate, interlacing collagen fibers. The arachnoid is a nonvascular membrane separated from the pia mater by the *subarachnoid space* containing cerebrospinal fluid. The pia mater is a vascular membrane that adheres to the spinal cord and is invaginated into the cord to form the outer wall of the perivascular space surrounding blood vessels entering and exiting from the spinal cord (Fig. 13-4).

The spinal cord is anchored to the inner surface of the dura mater by a series of lateral collagenous bands called *denticulate ligaments,* derived from the pia mater. From 18 to 24 of these ligaments firmly attach the pia mater midway between the dorsal and ventral roots to the arachnoid and the dura mater on each side of the spinal cord. The dural sheath terminates at the level of the second sacral vertebra. A pial extension, the *filum terminale,* arises from the caudal tip of the conus medullaris and pierces the end of the dural sac. It continues as connective tissue, the *coccygeal ligament,* to attach to the periosteum of the coccyx.

Blood Supply

One anterior and two posterolateral arteries run the length of the spinal cord and form an irregular plexus around the spinal cord. The *spinal arteries* receive their supply from the *vertebral arteries* and from the intercostal, lumbar, and sacral arteries through six to eight *radicular arteries* (see Fig. 11-8), the largest usually entering at

the lower thoracic or upper lumbar region of the cord (Fig. 13-5). The spinal arteries are interconnected by anastomoses circling the surface of the cord and sending short branches inside the cord. *Sulcal* branches from the anterior spinal artery in the anterior median fissure go alternately right and left. The *posterior spinal arteries* provide the blood supply for the posterior columns. The remainder of the cord is supplied by the *anterior spinal artery.*

The venous plexus is irregular and there may be six or seven longitudinal veins at the surface of the cord. This plexus communicates with the occipital and marginal sinuses and with the basal plexus of veins above the level of the foramen magnum.

Internal Morphology

A cross section of the spinal cord reveals a central H-shaped gray area surrounded by white matter (Fig. 13-6). The gray matter consists of a longitudinally continuous matrix of neuronal cell bodies, dendrites, myelinated and unmyelinated axons, and glial cells. The gray matter is divided into *dorsal horns, intermediate gray,* and *ventral horns.* The interconnecting gray in the midline is separated into a *posterior gray commissure* and an *anterior gray commissure* by the central canal. A lateral projection of the intermediate gray, the *lateral horn,* is present in the first thoracic (T-1) through the second lumbar (L-2) spinal cord segments.

WHITE MATTER.   The white matter is composed of longitudinally arranged myelinated and unmyelinated nerve fibers, with an abundance of myelin that gives it a glistening white appearance. The white matter is divided into columns. The large bundle of fibers between the dorsal gray horns is divided into two posterior funiculi, or dorsal columns, by the *posterior median septum.* This septum is composed of glial elements and pia and extends from the posterior median sulcus to the posterior gray commissure. From the first cervical spinal segment (C-1) to about the sixth thoracic segment (T-6), each dorsal white column or posterior funiculus is divided into a laterally located fasciculus cuneatus and a medially located fasciculus gracilis by the posterior intermediate septum. The remainder of the white matter constitutes the anterior and lateral funiculi. The

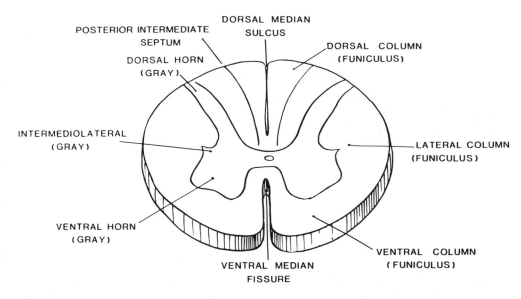

Fig. 13-6. *Major horizontal subdivisions of the spinal cord.*

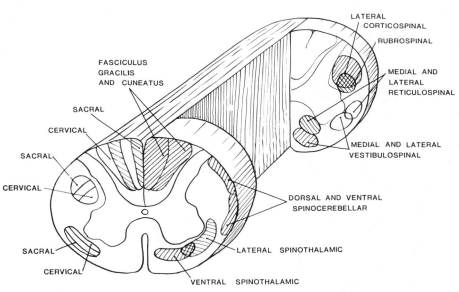

Fig. 13-7. *Principal tracts of the spinal cord. Lamination in the posterior columns and corticospinal and spinothalamic tracts is shown in the left half of the diagram. The location of the sensory pathways is shown at the same level on the right and the location of the motor pathways is shown at another level on the far right.*

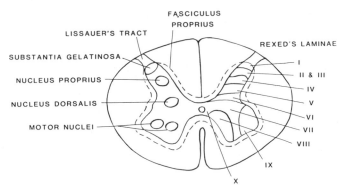

Fig. 13-8. Groups of nuclei in the spinal cord (left) *and laminae of the spinal cord* (right).

anterior white commissure consists of a band of transversely oriented nerve fibers located between the anterior gray commissure and the anterior median fissure. The locations and functions of the major ascending and descending fiber tracts in the white matter have been presented with the longitudinal systems. Their location in the spinal cord and lamination are illustrated in Figure 13-7.

GRAY MATTER.   There are three types of neurons present in the spinal gray matter. One sends axonal projections out of the central nervous system via the ventral spinal roots. These efferent fibers arise from neurons located in the ventral and intermediate horns. A second type of neuron, the *tract cell,* sends ascending axonal projections to supraspinal centers. The location of the cell bodies of tract cells is known only in some cases (for example, Clarke's column). The third type of neuron has axonal projections that remain in the spinal cord. These cells are called *internuncial cells* or *interneurons,* and they constitute the bulk of spinal neurons.

Many interneurons have axonal terminations within the cord segment where they originate. Others have axonal projections that course in a rostral or caudal direction for several spinal segments before terminating. Intersegmental axonal projections may course along several segments in the surrounding white matter before reentering the gray matter to terminate. These are termed *propriospinal* fibers and form the *fasciculi proprii,* which surround the spinal gray matter. The dorsolateral fasciculus (Lissauer's tract) is located at the apex of the dorsal horn (see Fig. 13-6) and contains many propriospinal fibers. The axons

may remain on the same side of the cord (ipsilateral) or cross the midline to terminate in the contralateral gray matter. Interneurons that send projections across the midline are termed *commissural neurons.* Such cells are found in abundance in the medial portion of the ventral horn. An interneuron is not restricted to a single pattern of axonal projection; instead, it may have several branches with different areas of termination. For example, a commissural neuron also may have an axonal branch that terminates ipsilaterally. Thus, spinal cord interneurons integrate segmental and intersegmental activity, both ipsilaterally and contralaterally.

The distribution of neurons in the spinal gray matter is not random. Scattered throughout the gray matter are clusters of neurons that extend longitudinally for varied distances along the spinal cord as cell columns (Fig. 13-8). Conspicuous groups of cells are found in the ventral horns. The axons of these cells emerge from the spinal cord to innervate skeletal muscle fibers. These cells are called *alpha motor neurons,* and the cell columns in which they reside are *somatic motor (efferent) nuclei.* Alpha motor neurons innervate the extrafusal muscle fibers, while the small *gamma motor neurons,* scattered nearby, innervate the intrafusal muscle fibers of muscle spindles. Alpha motor neurons are up to 80 μm in diameter and are among the largest neurons in the nervous system.

Another class of efferent fibers, exiting from the cord via the ventral root, arise from a distinct column of cells located in the lateral aspect of the intermediate gray matter (lateral horn). These cells form the *intermediolateral cell column,* which extends from the first thoracic spinal segment (T-1) to the second lumbar spinal segment (L-2). The axons of these neurons synapse with

Table 13-2. Projections to and from Rexed's Lamina

Projections	Lamina
To lamina	
Nociceptors	1, 2, 5
Mechanoreceptors	3–6
Group Ia (primary endings in muscle spindles)	6, 7, 9
Group II (secondary endings in muscle spindles)	4–6, 7, 9
Group Ib (Golgi tendon organs)	5–7
Nonmyelinated C fibers	2
Corticospinal tract	3–6, 7
Reticulospinal tract	1, 2, 5, 6, 7, 8
Propriospinal fibers	1, 2
From lamina	
Ventrospinocerebellar	5, 6, 7
Spinothalamic	4, 5, 6
Postsynaptic dorsal column neurons	3, 4, 5

ganglion cells of the sympathetic (thoracolumbar) division of the visceral nervous system. Therefore, the intermediolateral cell column is termed a *visceral efferent nucleus*. The parasympathetic motor (efferent) neurons are in the sacral cord. However, they do not form a well-defined cell group but are located throughout the ventral horn of S-2 to S-4. The reflex center for micturition is in this area of the cord.

The *nucleus dorsalis (Clarke's column)* is a distinct group of cells located in the medial portion of the base of the dorsal horn. This nucleus is distinguishable from the eighth cervical (C-8) to the second lumbar (L-2) spinal segment. The cells of the nucleus dorsalis are tract cells that send axons to the cerebellum via the dorsal spinocerebellar tracts.

The *substantia gelatinosa* forms the prominent caplike portion of the dorsal horn. It consists of small cells (6 to 20 μm) with axonal projections that remain within the substantia gelatinosa. This column of cells processes sensory information entering via dorsal root fibers (see Fig. 13-6).

The cell bodies of primary afferent fibers are located in the dorsal root ganglia. These cells have a distal axon segment that terminates in a sensory receptor and a central axon segment that enters the spinal cord via the dorsal root. The central or proximal axon segment may take several courses on entering the spinal cord. It may turn rostrally and join the dorsal columns to ascend to supraspinal centers, or it may divide into

ascending and descending branches which course over several segments in the white matter while sending collateral branches into the gray matter. The collateral branches of the different types of receptors in turn synapse with cells in specific areas of the gray matter of the spinal cord, predominantly in the dorsal horn. Descending pathways from the brain also send projections to localized areas of the spinal cord. Output pathways likewise arise from cells in particular areas of the spinal gray matter (Table 13-2).

The spinal gray matter is subdivided histologically by cell characteristics into lamina (Rexed's lamina) (Fig. 13-8), as follows:

Lamina 1, the most dorsal layer, receives input from propriospinal and nociceptors. It contains marginal cells, important cells of the dorsal horn that project to the other segments of the spinal cord, the cervical area, the nuclei of the dorsal columns, the reticular formation, the thalamus (forming part of the spinothalamic tracts), and the cerebellum (forming part of the spinocerebellar pathways).

Lamina 2 is the substantia gelatinosa and contains interneurons and substance P, considered to be a neurotransmitter of small axons. It receives input from nonmyelinated C fibers and nociceptors.

Lamina 3 represents the dorsal part of the nucleus proprius and receives input from mechanoreceptors.

Lamina 4 represents the ventral part of the nucleus proprius. It contains a number of types of sensory cells. It receives input from mechanoreceptors and group II fibers from muscle spindles and gives rise to spinothalamic tract fibers.

Lamina 5 forms the base of the dorsal horn, is continuous with the reticular formation, and receives input from the reticulospinal tract, lamina 4, mechanoreceptors, group II fibers, and group Ib fibers from Golgi tendon organs.

Lamina 6 contains exteroceptive and proprioceptive sensory cells with a large receptive field.

Lamina 7 contains Clarke's column. The lateral horn is a lateral extension of this lamina. It receives input from the corticospinal tract, the reticulospinal tract, and afferents from muscle spindles and Golgi tendon organs.

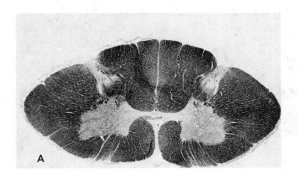

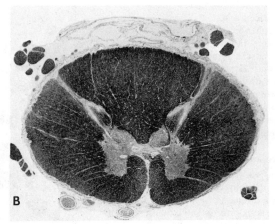

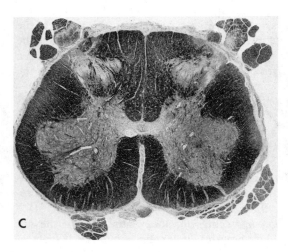

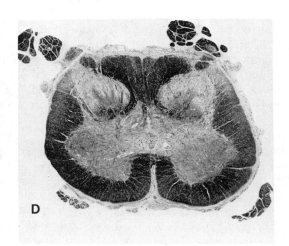

Fig. 13-9. Cross sections of spinal cord with myelin stain showing proportions of white matter (dark areas) and gray matter (light areas) at various levels. A. Cervical; B. thoracic; C. lumbar; D. sacral.

Lamina 8 contains cells with projections mainly to the contralateral ventral horn and the ventral funiculus.

Lamina 9 is a collection of motor neurons.

The gray matter thus consists of multiple interacting cell groups that process inputs from the periphery, the spinal cord, and descending pathways from the brain; mediate reflexes; and give rise to ascending spinal tracts.

The variations in the configuration of the gray and white matter at different segments of the spinal cord help in identifying the level of a section of the cord (Fig. 13-9 and Table 13-3). The nerve roots and spinal nerves are made up of myelinated and unmyelinated axons with the same histologic and physiologic characteristics as the peripheral axons described in Chapter 12. The pathophysiologic alterations of nerve roots are, therefore, also the same.

Spinal Cord Physiology

The major functions of the spinal cord are the transmission of activity via the longitudinal pathways and the mediation of local reflexes. The reflex activity of the spinal cord depends on the

Table 13-3. Configurational Characteristics
of the Spinal Cord

Shape of cord	Oval at cervical segments, nearly circular at lumbar segments, and almost quadrangular at sacral segments
Proportion of white to gray matter	Progressively increasing from below up
Size of anterior horn	Enlargement at cervical and lumbar segments
Posterior intermediate sulcus	Present in cervical and upper thoracic segments
Lateral horn	Well marked at thoracic segments
Nerve roots	Many present around cord at lumbar and sacral segments

neuronal activity of the cells in the gray matter of the cord.

Neuronal Activity

A transmitter substance released from an axonal terminal at spinal cord neurons acts on specialized areas of the subsynaptic membrane (the area of the postsynaptic membrane lying under the presynaptic terminal bouton or knob) called *receptor sites,* causing a selective increase in the permeability of the subsynaptic membrane to certain ions. The ionic currents arising from these permeability changes result in changes in the potential difference across the subsynaptic membrane. Such a potential change electrotonically propagates to an adjacent membrane by current flow in the intracellular and extracellular fluids. Electrotonic propagation is a passive process, and a potential change propagated in this manner decrements with distance. Therefore, the largest potential change occurs at the subsynaptic membrane, while the potential change across an area of membrane at a distance from the synaptic junction is reduced in proportion to the distance from the synapse and in proportion to the geometry of the cell.

Each neuron receives synaptic inputs from many sources. Synaptic activity occurring concurrently at several of these sites results in *spatial summation,* membrane potential changes that summate over the surface of the neuron. Synaptic transmission occurring consecutively at one or more sites on the neuron produces *temporal summation,* potential changes that summate if the time interval between successive synaptic activity is less than the time course of the potential change produced by such activity.

The potential changes occurring across the postsynaptic membrane during synaptic activity, *postsynaptic potentials,* can be monitored with a microelectrode, as depolarizing postsynaptic potentials, the excitatory postsynaptic potential, and as hyperpolarizing potentials, the inhibitory postsynaptic potential. The amplitude and time course of postsynaptic potentials vary with the number, distribution, and functional capability of synapses engaged in transmission, as well as with the duration of action of the transmitter substance. The membrane potential at the axon hillock is the sum of the potentials over the entire cell, and is a *graded response,* in contrast to the action potential that occurs in an all-or-none fashion.

The excitatory postsynaptic potential is a transient depolarization of the neuronal membrane resulting from the action of a transmitter substance released from depolarized axon terminals. The transmitter substance combines with receptor sites in the subsynaptic membrane, causing a selective increase in its permeability to Na^+ and K^+, with an influx of Na^+ and an efflux of K^+. The net effect of these ionic currents is to drive the membrane potential in a depolarizing direction to a level between the equilibrium potentials for Na^+ and K^+.

If, during the course of the excitatory postsynaptic potential, the neuronal membrane is depolarized to threshold (10 mV above the resting potential), an action potential is generated at the axon hillock and conducted throughout the neuron. If the excitatory postsynaptic potential is of insufficient amplitude to trigger an action potential, the excitability of the neuronal membrane is increased during the subthreshold depolarization, but no action potential is generated. On termination of the action of the excitatory transmitter substance by enzymatic degradation, diffusion, reuptake by axonal terminals, or a combination of these mechanisms, the excitatory postsynaptic potential decays exponentially.

The inhibitory postsynaptic potential is a transient hyperpolarization of the neuronal membrane, resulting from the action of a neurotransmitter released from presynaptic endings.

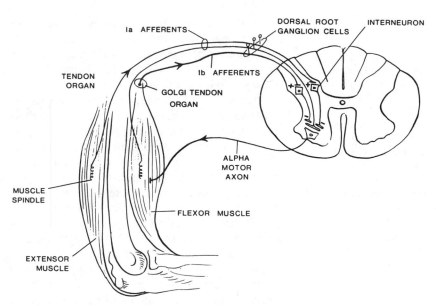

Fig. 13-10. Mechanism of presynaptic inhibition. Type Ia afferents from flexors are inhibited by Golgi tendon organ and antagonistic spindle afferents.

The transmitter reacts with receptor sites in the subsynaptic membrane, selectively increasing its permeability to K^+ and Cl^- and producing a hyperpolarization. The inhibitory postsynaptic potential decreases the excitability of a neuron in two ways: (1) the membrane potential is displaced away from threshold and (2) the increased permeability of the subsynaptic membrane tends to buffer or shunt local depolarizing currents. Like the excitatory postsynaptic potential, the inhibitory postsynaptic potential is a graded response that summates spatially and temporally.

A neuron does not merely relay information; rather it processes information by the integration of its total synaptic input. The soma and dendrites of a neuron are covered with presynaptic terminals. In a given time interval, excitatory and inhibitory synaptic transmission may be occurring at any number of these synaptic junctions. The neuronal membrane integrates the potential changes by spatial and temporal summation. The excitability of a neuron, therefore, is changing from moment to moment, depending on the relative effectiveness of the excitatory and inhibitory input in altering the state of polarization of the postsynaptic membrane. However, once the membrane is depolarized to threshold, the neuron responds in an all-or-none fashion, with the generation of an action potential.

The amount of transmitter released from a presynaptic ending when an action potential is conducted into the nerve terminal is dependent on the absolute potential change produced across the nerve terminal membrane. A subthreshold depolarization of the terminal membrane reduces the amplitude of an impulse being conducted into the terminal; hence, the amount of transmitter substance released is reduced. Such a subthreshold depolarization is produced in presynaptic endings by activity in axo-axonal synapses. In *axo-axonal synapses,* an axon terminal ends on another axonal ending, which is presynaptic to the dendrite of a neuron. Depolarization of the presynaptic ending by axo-axonic synaptic transmission reduces the amplitude of the excitatory postsynaptic potential. The reduction in the effectiveness of synaptic transmission produced by this mechanism is termed *presynaptic inhibition* (Fig. 13-10). Presynaptic inhibition that occurs on afferent nerve fibers is termed *primary afferent depolarization.* Primary afferent depolarization reduces the input of sensory information to the central nervous system.

The motor neurons in the autonomic and somatic efferent pathways of the spinal cord have similar physiologic characteristics. Both act as integrators of information, summating the excitatory postsynaptic potentials (EPSPs) and inhibitory postsynaptic potentials (IPSPs) from multiple sources and firing only when the membrane potential reaches threshold. The firing pattern in

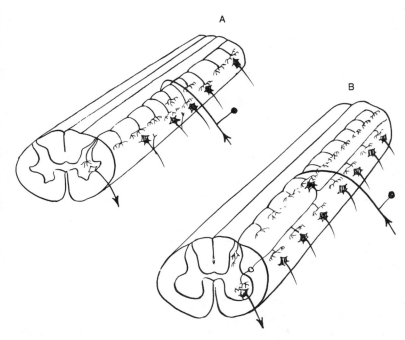

Fig. 13-11. Reflex connections of primary afferents. A. Monosynaptic (no interneurons). B. Polysynaptic (one or more interneurons). Note longitudinal spread of connections in both types of reflex.

both is similar. These neurons do not normally produce single discharges but fire repetitively at a rate that is a function of the level of depolarization of the cell. Firing is initiated at low frequencies of four to eight per second and gradually increases in frequency as more and more excitation occurs. The neurons innervating the same muscle lie together in groups, are influenced by similar inputs, and therefore tend to fire at the same time. However, differences in size of neurons result in differences in threshold of firing and different firing rates. The number of cells firing in a given motor neuron pool, therefore, is a function of the amount of inhibitory and excitatory input coming to the entire pool of neurons.

Disorders of motor neurons can alter response to input so that the neurons fire spontaneously or with minimal input, as occurs in tetanus or in strychnine poisoning. Disorders may also result in single, spontaneous discharges, such as fasciculations, or in reduced response to input, as in the weakness seen in motor neuron disease. If the neuron degenerates, it no longer provides the neurotrophic factors needed for normal function of the end organ, which then atrophies. A dener-

vated end organ also undergoes denervation hypersensitivity, becoming more sensitive to the transmitter.

Spinal Reflexes

The simplest level of motor control is a reflex, in which a specific sensory input induces a specific motor response. Such reflex responses can either promote movements (phasic muscle contractions promote reposition of limbs) or maintain posture (tonic muscle contractions counteract gravity and maintain the body in an upright position). The segmental circuits mediating movement reflexes primarily involve excitation of the flexor motor neurons, while those mediating posture involve excitation of extensor and axial motor neurons. Spinal reflex patterns are subjected to increasing amounts of control from supraspinal levels during the course of development. The magnitude of this reflex subordination in the adult is indicated by the complete areflexia and flaccidity that follow spinal cord transsection.

A reflex arc consists of the receptor, an effector, and the interconnecting neural elements. The simplest reflex, the *monosynaptic reflex,* involves only two neural elements, an afferent neuron and a motor neuron in synaptic contact with each other. *Polysynaptic reflexes* involve one or more interneurons interposed between the afferent and efferent neurons (Fig. 13-11).

Table 13-4. Summary of Spinal Reflexes

Reflex	Receptor	Afferent fiber	Responses
Phasic stretch reflex	Muscle spindle (primary endings)	Group Ia (large, myelinated)	Brisk, transient contraction of muscle from which the Ia activity arises
Tonic stretch reflex	Muscle spindle (secondary endings)	Group II (intermediate, myelinated)	Sustained contraction of muscle from which the II activity arises
Clasp-knife response	Muscle spindle (secondary endings)	Group II (intermediate, myelinated)	Relaxation of muscle from which Ib activity arises
Flexion reflex (withdrawal from noxious stimulus)	Nociceptors (free nerve endings)	Small myelinated and unmyelinated cutaneous afferents (A-delta, C) and muscle afferents (group III, C)	Withdrawal of stimulated limb and extension of contralateral limb (crossed extension)
Tension feedback	Golgi tendon organs	Group Ib (large, myelinated)	Adjusts contraction in response to tension changes

These reflexes are effected through the alpha motor neurons whose axons exit from the spinal cord via the ventral roots to innervate the extrafusal muscle fibers that make up the bulk of the muscle mass. Alpha motor neurons are somatotopically arranged in the ventral horn. Alpha motor neurons supplying axial musculature are located medial to those that innervate the muscles of the extremities. Alpha motor neurons that innervate extensor muscles are called *extensor motor neurons,* while those that innervate flexor muscles are *flexor motor neurons.* Muscles that functionally aid one another are called *synergists,* and those that act in functional opposition are *antagonists.* For example, both the gastrocnemius and the soleus muscles are responsible for plantar flexion of the foot; therefore, they are synergists. The anterior tibial muscle is responsible for dorsiflexion of the foot and so is an antagonist of the gastrocnemius and soleus muscles.

There are many types of reflex activity controlled at the spinal cord level. These will be illustrated by the stretch reflex, flexion reflex, clasp-knife response, recurrent inhibition, and bladder control (Table 13-4).

STRETCH REFLEX.   The response initiated by an afferent discharge from the muscle spindles is a *stretch reflex.* This reflex continuously activates extensor and axial muscles and results in stabilization of the trunk and limbs to counteract the downward force of gravity and maintain upright posture. This reflex is not clearly functional in humans until approximately the seventeenth week of gestation. Subsequently, it becomes integrated with other postural influences that descend from pontomedullary levels. The stretch reflex is of two types: phasic and tonic.

The *phasic stretch reflex* is elicited by muscle stretch sufficient to discharge the primary spindle afferents (group Ia). These large, myelinated, primary afferent fibers enter the dorsomedial portion of the spinal cord dorsal horn and project directly onto homonymous motor neurons (neurons innervating the muscle from which the spindle discharge originated) to produce contraction of the homonymous muscle; concurrent monosynaptic reflex activation of the synergistic muscles results in stabilization of the joint across which the synergists attach. Even though the motor neurons supplying synergistic muscles receive excitatory input, they are normally not depolarized to threshold. They are said to be in the *subliminal fringe.*

In addition to making monosynaptic contact with alpha motor neurons, group Ia afferents send collateral branches into the medial aspect of the base of the dorsal horn. Here they form excitatory synapses with inhibitory interneurons. These interneurons send axonal projections to alpha motor neurons innervating muscles antagonistic to muscles from which the group Ia afferent activity arises. When a muscle is stretched, the alpha motor neurons innervating that muscle and its synergists are excited, while those innervating antagonistic muscles are inhibited. This pattern of

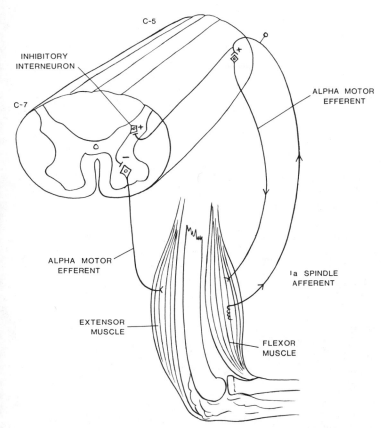

Labels on figure:
C-5
INHIBITORY
INTERNEURON
C-7
ALPHA MOTOR
EFFERENT
ALPHA MOTOR
EFFERENT
Ia SPINDLE
AFFERENT
EXTENSOR
MUSCLE
FLEXOR
MUSCLE

Fig. 13-12. Pathways for monosynaptic reflex and reciprocal innervation. A flexor Ia afferent is shown making monosynaptic contact with a flexor motor neuron and an inhibitory interneuron. Interneuron sends axonal projections to extensor motor neuron, providing the pathway for reciprocal inhibition.

excitation of one group of muscles and simultaneous inhibition of antagonistic muscles is termed *reciprocal innervation* (Fig. 13-12).

This form of stretch reflex elicits a dynamic, or *phasic*, response, initiated by a rapid rate of change in the length of a muscle and producing a burst of excitatory synaptic input to alpha motor neurons supplying the muscle and its synergists. If the change in length of the muscle is sufficiently sudden, then a brisk contraction of the muscle occurs.

A second type of response to muscle stretch is the *static*, or *tonic*, response, initiated by a change in the length of the muscle. It provides a continuous background of excitatory input to alpha motor neurons via group II afferents. This activity is responsible for clinical muscle tone and is described as the *tonic stretch reflex*.

During a voluntary contraction, the muscle shortens and the muscle spindles tend to go slack. As a result, the intrafusal fibers are stretched less and the spindle afferent discharge decreases. If the muscle is passively stretched, the intrafusal fibers are also stretched, and the spindle sensory discharge increases. The excitation of motor units within a muscle in response to muscle stretching provides a normal level of resistance to passive movement of a joint, which is called *muscle tone*. In the absence of muscle tone, there is no resistance to passive movement and the muscle is *flaccid*. Dorsal rhizotomy (section of the dorsal roots) interrupts the afferent limb of the tonic stretch reflex and results in a dramatic reduction in muscle tone. Obviously, such a procedure also would abolish the phasic stretch reflex.

Clinically, the monosynaptic reflex is elicited by tapping on a tendon to produce a sudden stretch of a muscle. A commonly observed monosynaptic reflex is that involving the contraction of the quadriceps muscle (knee-jerk), elicited by tapping on the patellar tendon. A number of such

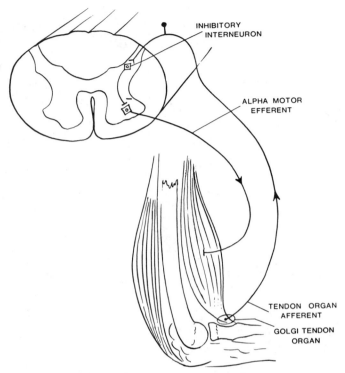

Fig. 13-13. Clasp-knife pathway. Potentially injurious tension development in flexor muscle produces activity in group Ib afferents innervating Golgi tendon organs of that muscle. This results in inhibition of alpha motor neurons supplying the muscle and a relaxation of muscle.

monosynaptic reflexes are routinely tested in the neurologic examination of a patient. The monosynaptic reflex has been given many names (*myotatic reflex,* stretch reflex, tendon-jerk reflex, and deep tendon reflex). The last term, *deep tendon reflex,* is used extensively and may be misleading. It implies that the receptors for the reflex reside in the tendon, which they do not. The tap on the tendon stretches the muscle and produces a phasic, synchronous discharge of primary spindle afferents, which triggers the monosynaptic stretch reflex. Hyperactive tendon jerks (hyperactive stretch reflexes) on one side of the body are indicative of upper motor neuron damage. The increased resistance to passive movement caused by increased tonic stretch reflexes is termed *spasticity.* In a patient with spasticity, if a constant stretch is applied to the muscle and a tendon tap or sudden additional stretch is superimposed, not one but a series of tendon-jerk reflexes results. This repetitive jerking is called *clonus* and

reflects the highly sensitive state of the alpha motor neurons to synchronous afferent volleys.

Patients with lesions of the internal capsule and other upper motor neuron lesions typically have spasticity with increased resistance to passive stretch of the muscle. However, if a spastic muscle is stretched beyond a given length, there is an abrupt decrease in the resistance to stretching, which is known as the *clasp-knife reflex.* A clasp knife has an initial resistance to being closed, and then at a certain point, the knife suddenly snaps shut. In the clasp-knife reflex, an initial resistance (increased tone) at the beginning of the stretch of a flexor or extensor muscle persists up to a certain point, and is then followed by sudden loss of muscle tone. The clasp-knife reflex is due to the activation of group II spindle afferents, which produces a length-dependent inhibition of the stretch reflex.

The Golgi tendon organs appear to act as a sensitive feedback to individual motor units on the tension they are generating. *Tendon organs are receptors located within the fascia of muscle tendons. These receptors are phasically discharged by stretch of the muscle tendon. Because*

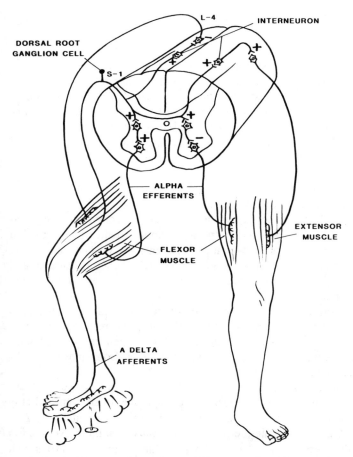

Fig. 13-14. Flexion reflex pathway. Afferent supply and interneuronal connections for flexion reflex in lower extremity are illustrated in spinal cord section. Noxious stimulus applied to lower extremity results in ipsilateral flexion (withdrawal) and, provided that stimulus strength is sufficiently high, extension of contralateral limb (crossed extension reflex).

the tendon organs are in series with the muscle fibers, muscle contraction with resultant phasic stretch of the tendon results in tendon-organ discharge. The tendon-organ afferents first project centrally through fibers (group Ib) only slightly smaller in diameter than the spindle primary fibers and then enter the dorsomedial portion of the dorsal horn. A disynaptic relay is made to the homonymous motor neurons (Fig. 13-13). Tendon-organ discharge inhibits the homonymous motor neurons and their synergists and excites the antagonist motor neurons. Opposite effects occur in neurons in the contralateral gray matter.

FLEXION REFLEX. The term *flexion reflex* is a general one encompassing various polysynaptic reflexes. These can range from the reflex withdrawal of a portion of the body from a noxious stimulus to flexion of the lower extremities during walking. The receptors involved in flexion reflexes may be nociceptors, touch and pressure receptors, and some joint receptors.

The flexion reflex response is thus known by a number of terms, including withdrawal reflex, nociceptive reflex, and cutaneous reflex. This reflex results in limb movement mediated by flexor muscle contraction away from the source of stimulation. Both ontogenetically and phylogenetically, the flexion reflex is one of the most primitive reflexes of the central nervous system. It is found in all the vertebrates, and in humans it is present by the seventh to eighth week of gestation. In the adult, the circuit underlying this reflex is incorporated into the more complex volitional movements of cortical initiation.

Stimuli that evoke the flexion reflex cause a

discharge of cutaneous receptors, which in turn triggers action potential discharges along unmyelinated and finely myelinated fibers that enter the dorsolateral portion of the dorsal horn of the spinal cord. This input is then transmitted through short, multisynaptic relays to the ventral motor neuronal pool (Fig. 13-14).

During flexor reflex activation, there is ipsilateral flexor motor neuron excitation and extensor inhibition (reciprocal innervation). Contralateral to the side of stimulation there is flexor motor neuron inhibition and extensor excitation (double reciprocal innervation). This *crossed extension reflex* stabilizes the body as the ipsilateral limb is flexed.

Because the flexion reflex is polysynaptic, there is afterdischarge in the interneuronal relays, and the motor response outlasts the stimulus. Activation of the flexor motor neurons is typically widespread so that flexor muscles at the ankle, knee, and hip contract to withdraw the whole limb.

Most cutaneous reflex responses activate underlying muscles (local sign), so that, for example, cutaneous stimulation over an extensor muscle results in extensor contraction to move the muscle away. However, painful cutaneous stimulation in the distal portions of the limb induces reflex withdrawal, or flexion, and thus represents the common usage of the term flexion reflex for cutaneous reflex activation.

A number of cutaneous, or superficial, reflexes are included in neurologic examinations. In general, these reflexes are mediated by polysynaptic segmental circuits similar to those of the cutaneous flexion reflex. Abnormalities in specific superficial reflexes can be diagnostic of central nervous system lesions. For example, in the normal person, plantar flexion of the toes occurs with noxious stimulation of the sole of the foot. In the presence of corticospinal tract disease, however, these local cord reflexes are altered and a more primitive form of flexion reflex occurs— *Babinski's sign*. The great toe responds to plantar stimulation with dorsiflexion. The abdominal contractions normally induced by cutaneous stimulation of the abdomen and the cremasteric contractions normally induced by cutaneous stimulation along the inner side of the thigh (both forms of flexion reflex) are no longer elicitable after a corticospinal tract (direct activation pathway) lesion.

LONG-LATENCY REFLEXES.   Reflex responses to disturbance of voluntary movement or to electrical stimulation have been found in the human arm at approximately 60 msec. These long-latency (long loop) reflexes involve supraspinal pathways and areas and reflect higher levels of control of motor function.

Gamma Loop

The gamma motor neurons receive the same inputs as do the alpha motor neurons, except that primary spindle afferents do not project to the gamma motor neurons. In general, gamma and alpha neurons innervating the same muscle are activated in the same way by an incoming stimulus. However, compared with alpha motor neurons, gamma motor neurons respond at lower thresholds to segmental influences and descending activity, especially that from indirect pathways.

Contraction of the whole muscle would cause the length of muscle spindles to shorten and stop firing, unless a mechanism were available to regulate the length of the muscle spindle. Regulation is achieved by the gamma motor neurons that innervate the muscle spindles. The muscle spindle consists of sensory receptors on the center of specialized muscle fibers, the *intrafusal fibers*. Gamma motor neurons activate the intrafusal fibers, with contraction and shortening of the intrafusal fibers on either side of the central noncontractile region. Contraction of the ends of the intrafusal fibers stretches the central region and activates the sensory receptors and the afferent nerve terminals. Thus, an afferent spindle discharge may occur as a direct effect of gamma motor neuron excitation of the intrafusal fibers. When the gamma motor neurons are active during muscle contraction, the resultant intrafusal fiber contractions are sufficient to overcome the slack in the spindle that would result from the whole muscle contraction. This allows the spindle to maintain a high degree of sensitivity over a wide range of different lengths during voluntary and reflex movements. The spindle discharge due to gamma motor neuron activation of the intrafu-

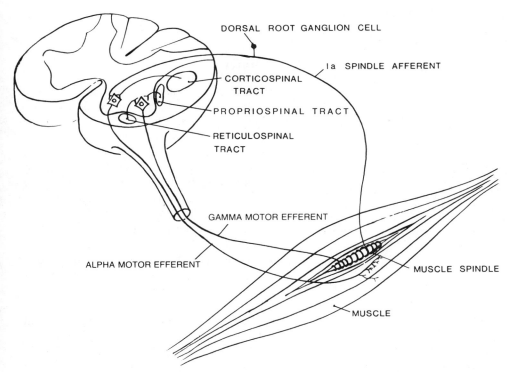

DORSAL ROOT GANGLION CELL

Ia SPINDLE AFFERENT

CORTICOSPINAL
TRACT

PROPRIOSPINAL TRACT

RETICULOSPINAL
TRACT

GAMMA MOTOR EFFERENT

ALPHA MOTOR EFFERENT

MUSCLE SPINDLE

MUSCLE

Fig. 13-15. Pathways for monosynaptic reflex and gamma loop. Group Ia afferent fiber from muscle spindle makes monosynaptic contact with alpha motor neuron supplying that muscle. Gamma motor neuron sends efferent fiber, via ventral root, to innervate intrafusal muscle fibers of muscle spindle. Loop is completed by group Ia afferent fiber terminating on alpha motor neuron. Input to gamma motor neuron is from both segmental and supraspinal sources (corticospinal, reticulospinal, propriospinal tracts).

sal fibers is called the *gamma bias* of the spindle (Fig. 13-15).

If a muscle is being continuously contracted, an additional phasic contraction of the muscle—such as that induced by a tendon-jerk reflex—produces a transient (approximately 100 msec) reduction of activity of the motor units. This "silent period" after phasic muscle contraction reflects the action of several important reflex mechanisms: (1) the decrease or cessation of muscle spindle discharge, (2) the inhibitory discharge of the tendon organs, (3) recurrent inhibition of the alpha motor neurons, and (4) the refractory period of the alpha motor neurons. In hypertonia or hypotonia, there is absence or prolongation of the silent period due to an abnormally high or low gamma bias.

Direct excitation of alpha motor neurons alone can produce a contraction of the extrafusal muscle fibers and a reduction in the length of the muscle spindles. This "unloading effect" reduces the activity in group Ia afferents and, therefore, the excitability of alpha motor neurons supplying that muscle. Reduced motor neuron firing results in a lack of smoothness in the muscle contraction. To counteract this force fluctuation, movements are normally initiated by coactivation of both gamma and alpha motor neurons.

Renshaw Cell System

As axons of alpha motor neurons exit from the gray matter of the ventral horn, they give off collateral branches that terminate on interneurons located in Rexed's lamina VII in the ventral horn. These cells, called *Renshaw cells,* send axonal projections to terminate on alpha motor neurons. Excitation of Renshaw cells causes inhibition of alpha motor neurons. Thus, excitation of alpha motor neurons causes the excitation of Renshaw cells which, in turn, inhibits motor neurons. This mechanism is termed *recurrent inhibition* and is an example of negative feedback (Fig. 13-16).

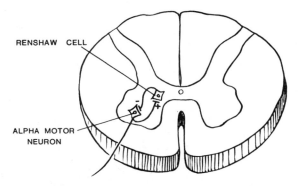

RENSHAW CELL

ALPHA MOTOR
NEURON

Fig. 13-16. Pathways for recurrent inhibition. Recurrent collateral of the axon of an alpha motor neuron making excitatory synaptic contact with a Renshaw cell. Excitation of Renshaw cell produces inhibition of alpha motor neuron.

Interneurons

The coordination of activity in the neuronal populations of the spinal cord is achieved by interneurons, neurons that are interposed between incoming (afferent) and outgoing (efferent) fibers in the spinal cord. Interneurons receive input from the periphery, local spinal segments, and descending pathways from higher centers; they form multisynaptic, divergent or convergent connections with motor neurons, afferent neurons, and other neuronal groups within the spinal cord. This convergence of input and divergence of output allow individual neurons to influence the activity of multiple neurons and allow individual neurons to receive input from multiple sources. The interneurons thus serve as a link among the peripheral nervous system, the descending pathways from the brain, local neuronal groups, and the motor neurons. The interneurons (1) regulate voluntary and reflex motor acts, (2) coordinate the activity in muscle groups with the appropriate degree of contraction and relaxation of agonists and antagonists, (3) transmit information from the periphery and higher centers to motor neurons, (4) modulate afferent impulses by allowing or preventing transmission of afferent impulses from the periphery and local spinal circuits, and (5) provide a background of spontaneous activity and readiness to respond.

The interneurons at the spinal level thus serve as the basis for regulating voluntary movements, local control of motor behavior, automatic movements, and other integrated activities.

Micturition

As the bladder fills with urine, a constant low intravesical pressure is maintained as a result of the inherent tone of the smooth muscle. Urine is held within the bladder by the configuration of the internal urethral sphincter and contraction of the external urethral sphincter. With increased stretching of the smooth muscle, proprioceptive sensations, which give rise to feelings of bladder fullness and of a desire to void, are carried to the *reflex micturition center* in the spinal cord by sensory fibers in the pelvic nerves. The sensation of the desire to urinate is then transmitted to higher centers in the brain by way of the fasciculus gracilis. If the time and place for voiding are appropriate, the brain sets in motion a reflex voiding contraction by means of impulses transmitted through the descending pathways to the neurons in the micturition center.

Motor impulses arising in the neurons of the micturition center travel over the parasympathetic efferent fibers of the pelvic nerve, ganglionic synapses, and neuromuscular endings to stimulate contraction of the detrusor muscle of the bladder and of the internal vesical sphincter. The contraction of the detrusor muscle results in increased intravesical pressure, and the longitudinal contraction of the smooth muscle of the internal vesical sphincter pulls open the vesical neck, widens and shortens the urethra, and thereby decreases urethral resistance; as a result of these changes urine passes into the urethra. The presence of urine in the urethra initiates a reflex that results in relaxation of the external urethral sphincter and permits the passage of urine through the entire urethra. The afferent limb of this reflex arc is in the pelvic nerve, whereas the efferent limb is in the pudendal nerve. Voluntary cessation of micturition occurs by contraction of the external urethral sphincter.

Clinical Correlations

Diseases at the spinal level, like those at other levels, can be classified as focal or diffuse. *Focal disease* at the spinal level may be *segmental* with symptoms and signs at only one level, as in lesions of the spinal nerve in the intervertebral foramen. Or focal disease at the spinal level may present with a combination of *segmental* and *longitudinal* symptoms and signs, if there is involvement of the ascending or descending pathways in the spinal cord along with the segmental structures.

Diffuse disease in the spinal level may involve only a *single system* such as the motor system in motor neuron disease, or the ventriculosubarachnoid system in meningitis. Or it may involve *multiple systems,* as in some degenerative and inflammatory disorders.

Focal Disorders at the Spinal Level

Focal lesions at the spinal level are characterized by segmental signs or symptoms specific for a particular level of the spinal canal. These may be due to damage to a spinal nerve, a dorsal or ventral nerve root, a single vertebra, or a spinal cord function found only at a single level.

SEGMENTAL LOCALIZATION. Lesions of the spinal nerves are often due to (or related to) disease of the vertebral column and are at the spinal level. However, many of their clinical features are similar to those of peripheral nerve lesions. Lesions of the spinal nerves are recognized by their pattern of distribution. They are associated with motor, sensory, autonomic, and reflex changes.

1. *Motor Involvement.* These are the findings of lower motor neuron damage, that is, lesions affecting the final common pathway (Table 13-5). There is flaccid weakness in a myotomal distribution. When present for sufficient duration, there is associated atrophy. There also may be fasciculation and fibrillation in muscles in the appropriate myotome. Because the lesion is proximal to the origin of the posterior primary ramus of the spinal nerve, the paraspinal muscles will be involved as well as other proximal muscles (see Table 13-1). This involvement is in contrast to lesions that involve the peripheral nerve.

2. *Sensory Involvement.* There is sensory loss in a dermatomal distribution, a loss usually best recognized in regard to pain, temperature, or touch. There may be paresthesia from spontaneous firing of the larger axons or dysesthesia from abnormal firing of large and small axons. Spontaneous pain in a dermatomal distribution is common and is probably due to local swelling, edema, and ionic changes in the spinal nerve, with spontaneous firing of small pain fibers. The pain is often perceived beyond the distribution of the spinal nerve because of intraspinal spread of electrical activity (referred pain). Irritable spinal nerves are more sensitive to stretch, and pain is produced when the extremities are put in certain positions, as for example, when a leg is put through a straight leg raising test.

3. *Autonomic Involvement.* Autonomic fibers also are involved, but because of their more extensive overlapping, autonomic disturbances do not occur with lesions of single spinal nerves. Bilateral sacral spinal nerve or cauda equina damage, however, may result in abnormalities of bladder function.

4. *Reflex Involvement.* Peripheral reflexes may be lost if either the motor or the sensory component of the reflex arc is damaged. They are, therefore, an important sign of spinal nerve disease (Table 13-6).

The term *radiculopathy* refers specifically to disease of the nerve root that is located within the

Table 13-5. Summary of Findings in Upper and Lower Motor Neuron Lesions

Finding	Upper motor neuron[a]	Lower motor neuron[b]
Strength	Decreased	Decreased
Tone	Increased	Decreased
Deep tendon reflexes	Increased	Decreased
Superficial reflexes	Decreased	Decreased
Babinski's sign	Present	Absent
Clonus	Present	Absent
Fasciculations	Absent	Present
Atrophy	Absent	Present

[a] Involves direct and indirect activation pathways.
[b] Involves final common pathway.

Table 13-6. Deep Tendon Reflexes

Reflex	Spinal nerves*	Plexus	Peripheral nerves
Biceps jerk	C-5, C-6	Brachial	Musculocutaneous
Triceps jerk	C-7, C-8	Brachial	Radial
Knee jerk	L-3, L-4	Lumbar	Femoral
Ankle jerk	L-5, S-1	Sacral	Sciatic, tibial

*Spinal nerves underlined provide the major innervation.

vertebral column and spinal canal. Localized nerve root disease produces purely motor or purely sensory deficits, depending on whether the ventral or dorsal root is affected. However, the nerve roots have the same segmental derivation as the spinal nerves, and it is common usage to refer to disease of the spinal nerve (in which the dorsal and ventral roots have joined) as radiculopathy.

Localization to a specific spinal level may be on the basis of:

1. Local anterior root or anterior horn signs such as segmental atrophy, flaccid weakness, hypotonia, or some combination of these.
2. Local sensory abnormalities such as segmental (radicular) loss of all modalities of sensation.
3. Local segmental loss or depression of deep tendon reflexes due to interruption of the stretch reflex arc. This may occur because of damage to efferent or afferent limbs of the reflex arc.
4. Segmental signs of vertebral column involvement. Occasionally, this may be seen as localized pain and tenderness of a vertebra, but more commonly it depends on roentgenographic visualization of a structural abnormality at one level.
5. Segmental signs of bladder involvement, such as evidence of a nuclear lesion in the conus of the spinal cord, or an infranuclear lesion in the cauda equina with an autonomous (nonreflex) bladder, loss of voluntary control, loss of anal reflex, and large residual urine.

In the absence of specific signs of spinal cord involvement, it may be difficult to distinguish a purely segmental lesion at the spinal level from a more peripheral disorder. However, if the lesion is in the distribution of a single spinal nerve, it can be assumed to be at the spinal level or within the vertebral column (see Chap. 12). Other clues to a lesion at this level are the presence of bilateral abnormalities, the presence of proximal involvement such as in the paraspinal muscles, and signs of meningeal or subarachnoid involvement such as Brudzinski's sign (in which neck flexion with leg extension produces pain).

INTERSEGMENTAL LOCALIZATION. The most convincing evidence of a focal lesion at the spinal level is the combined presence of segmental signs of the type previously described in association with *intersegmental signs* due to involvement of the long ascending or descending pathways of the spinal cord. There are three major types of intersegmental signs that appear with focal diseases in the spinal canal:

1. A long tract motor level. These findings are those of an upper motor neuron lesion that involves the direct and indirect pathways (see Table 13-5). They are spastic paralysis, increased deep tendon reflexes, and Babinski's sign below the level of the lesion. Other abnormal reflexes due to damage of the direct and indirect activation pathways also may be seen, such as loss of the abdominal reflexes, flexion reflexes, and crossed extension reflexes.
2. A long tract sensory level. This level is indicated by posterior column or lateral spinothalamic tract deficits on the appropriate side below the level of the lesion.
3. Autonomic disturbances below the level of the lesion. The most striking is supranuclear (reflex or automatic) neurogenic bladder dysfunction, with incontinence due to contractions of a spastic bladder. There also may be other evidence of autonomic disturbances, such as loss of blood pressure control, abnormalities of sweating, and loss of rectal control.

Combinations of segmental and long tract signs permit the identification of the site of cord disease with some accuracy. Some characteristic patterns of abnormality are:

1. Upper cervical. This pattern includes long tract signs in the upper and lower extremities for motor and sensory modalities and a supranuclear bladder dysfunction.
2. Middle and lower cervical. Segmental signs of motor and sensory dysfunction appear in the upper extremities, along with long tract signs in the lower extremities and supranuclear bladder dysfunction.
3. Thoracic. Long tract signs in the lower extremities appear with a segmental sensory finding (level of sensation) in the trunk and a supranuclear bladder dysfunction.
4. Lumbar and upper sacral. This pattern includes segmental motor and sensory signs in

the lower extremities with a supranuclear bladder dysfunction.

5. Conus medullaris. Segmental signs appear in the lower extremities with an infranuclear bladder disturbance.

6. Cauda equina. There is pain and asymmetric motor and sensory involvement of multiple roots with or without infranuclear bladder.

SPINAL SHOCK. Focal lesions may be acute, subacute, or chronic. An acute lesion of the spinal cord may be accompanied by *spinal shock,* which may mask some of the signs previously outlined. When the spinal cord is suddenly severely damaged, essentially all cord functions immediately become depressed. The normal activity of spinal cord neurons depends to a great extent on continual tonic discharges from higher centers, particularly discharges transmitted through the vestibulospinal tract and the excitatory portion of the reticulospinal tracts. The acute loss of this input results in loss of neuronal activity.

After a few days to a few weeks, the spinal neurons gradually regain their excitability. This is characteristic of neurons in the nervous system— that is, after loss of facilitatory impulses, they increase in excitability. In most nonprimates, the excitability of the cord centers returns to normal within a few hours to a few weeks, but in humans, the return often may be delayed for several months and occasionally is never complete. However, in some patients, the recovery of excitability is excessive, with hyperexcitability of reflexes.

Some major functions are affected by spinal shock. The arterial blood pressure rapidly decreases, sometimes to as low as 40 mm Hg, with loss of sympathetic activity. The pressure ordinarily returns to normal within a few days. All muscle reflexes are blocked during the initial stages of shock. Some reflexes eventually become hyperexcitable, particularly if a few facilitatory pathways remain intact between the brain and the cord. The sacral reflexes for control of bladder and colon evacuation are suppressed in humans for the first few weeks after cord transection, but eventually they return.

The first reflexes to reappear are flexion reflexes, especially in response to stimulation of the plantar surface of the foot (Babinski's reflex). After 3 to 4 weeks, flexion reflexes can be triggered from a broader area and are more generalized. After several months, hyperexcitability has developed to the point that plantar stimulation may induce flexion responses on both sides of the body as well as profuse autonomic discharge (for example, sweating, contractions of bladder and rectum). Such mass reflexes may occur even with no obvious source of stimulation. Even after flexion reflexes reappear, the limbs remain flaccid in

Table 13-7. Effects of Lesions at Spinal Cord Segments

Segment	Deficit	Independence	Aids required
C-4, C-5	Tetraplegia Impaired respiration Reflex bladder	None	Wheelchair Constant care
C-6, C-7	Tetraplegia	Minimal	Wheelchair Hand splints
C-8, T-1	Impaired respiration Reflex bladder Paraplegia Hand weakness	Personal care Drives car	Wheelchair Special braces
T-2, T-3	Impaired respiration Reflex bladder Paraplegia	Complete	Wheelchair Leg braces
T-12, L-1	Paraplegia Reflex bladder	Complete	Wheelchair Leg braces
L-4, L-5	Paraplegia Reflex bladder	Complete	Foot braces
S-2, S-3	Nonreflex bladder	Complete	Catheter

the absence of tonic stretch reflex activation. After several months, a return of muscle tone and the tendon reflexes may occur.

After recovery from spinal shock, a patient who has suffered a major spinal cord injury will be left with major deficits that are a function of the level of the lesion. The primary task of the physician, after localizing a lesion and minimizing the damage, is to enable the patient to achieve maximal use of whatever residual function remains. Some of the effects of spinal cord lesions are listed in Table 13-7.

Transverse lesions of the spinal cord can be further localized in cord cross section. In chronic or subacute lesions, it is often necessary to localize a lesion in this manner in order to identify the most likely type of lesion. It is of particular importance to determine if a lesion is *extrinsic* (extramedullary) or *intrinsic* (intramedullary). Extrinsic lesions arise outside the substance of the spinal cord and compress it. These are more common than intrinsic lesions and often can be removed surgically, with recovery of some or all functions.

Extrinsic lesions commonly damage the dorsal or ventral roots and are therefore usually associated with radicular pain. Because the dorsal root ganglion contains the cell bodies that maintain the axons traveling both peripherally and centrally in the sensory system, the destruction of it can result in wallerian degeneration in both the peripheral nerves and the central pathways. In contrast, a lesion that destroys the dorsal root proximal to the ganglion produces sensory loss and reflex loss, with degeneration in the central processes but not in the peripheral nerve. Destruction of the root distal to the ganglion produces the same clinical symptoms and signs but is associated with peripheral but not central wallerian degeneration. The presence or absence of peripheral wallerian degeneration often can be determined by electrical studies of patients. Ventral root damage produces degeneration of the peripheral nerves, with associated reflex loss, atrophy, and weakness.

Intrinsic lesions arise within the substance of the spinal cord and often spare the more peripheral pathways of the spinal cord. Although sensory symptoms are prominent, they are often painless. A review of Figure 13-7 shows that the pathways of the lumbar and sacral segments in the spinothalamic and corticospinal tracts are localized more superficially. Intrinsic lesions preferentially damage the pathways from higher levels and may manifest sacral sparing, in which the long tract signs spare the most caudal segments, because they are more laterally placed in the cord. A syrinx or tumor in the cervical cord gray matter may produce sacral sparing.

Localization is aided by knowledge of the decussations of the pathways. Because the spinothalamic pathways cross to the opposite side within two or three segments of their entry, a lesion of one side of the spinal cord produces dissociation of the sensations of pain and temperature (lost contralaterally below the lesion), from position and vibration (lost ipsilaterally below the lesion). Similarly, a lesion in the region of the central canal destroys the spinothalamic fibers decussating in the anterior commissure and gives segmental loss of pain and temperature, with segmental signs of motor neuron destruction if the lesion extends into the ventral horns, but sparing of other modalities of sensation.

Focal disorders of the spinal cord may be either mass or nonmass in type. The same criteria applied at other levels can be used to differentiate a mass from a nonmass. In the clinical history, progression favors a mass, as does the presence of distortion, destruction of tissue, or obstruction of the subarachnoid spaces on special studies (myelography). The pathologic changes can be identified by the temporal profile and may include vascular lesions (infarct of the cord, arteriovenous malformations, hematomas), neoplastic diseases (tumors of the nerve roots, intramedullary or extramedullary cord tumors), inflammatory disease (poliomyelitis, abscess, arachnoiditis), and traumatic lesions (cord transection, ruptured intervertebral disks). Focal lesions are typically single. However, in multiple sclerosis, there are multifocal lesions, which can produce complex findings.

MULTIPLE SCLEROSIS. This is a disorder associated with localized areas of demyelination in the white matter of the central nervous system (Fig. 13-17). Although spinal cord involvement is common, the lesions also may appear in the white matter of the brain stem, cerebellum, and cerebrum. The focal lesions develop over a few days, and the symptoms may resolve over a few

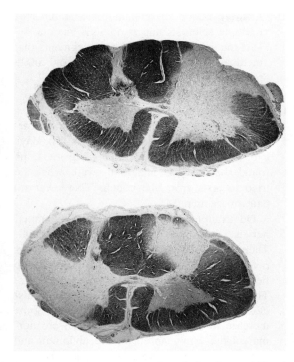

Fig. 13-17. Sections of spinal cord showing multifocal areas of demyelination in a patient with multiple sclerosis.

days to weeks or leave a persistent deficit. They occur in scattered areas to produce a *multifocal* disorder. The disease is of unknown cause, but its subacute course, some of the histologic features, and laboratory findings suggest that it may be an autoimmune disorder with inflammatory features. The areas of demyelination vary in size from a few millimeters to several centimeters in diameter and show myelin breakdown, with preservation of the axis cylinders (see Fig. 4-21). In the acute lesions, there may be perivascular infiltrations of lymphocytes. Later during the course of a lesion, there are predominantly macrophages phagocytosing the myelin products. As the lesion resolves, it becomes gliotic. Severe lesions may be associated with axonal destruction, and the disorder may clinically appear to be degenerative late in the course as remissions no longer occur. The clinical history of multiple sclerosis is one of recurrent episodes of deficit in widespread areas, corresponding to the intermittent occurrence of such lesions in disseminated areas. Any single such lesion in the spinal cord could be associated with segmental signs at the level of the lesion, or with longitudinal tract deficits below the level, or with both.

Diffuse Disorders at the Spinal Level

Diffuse disorders of the spinal canal are generally chronic and progressive, thus suggesting a degenerative cause. These may involve a single system or multiple systems. Motor neuron diseases (amyotrophic lateral sclerosis or progressive muscular atrophy) are examples of diffuse single system disorders in the spinal cord. In motor neuron disease, there is a progressive destruction of the motor neurons in the anterior horn of the spinal cord, with or without degeneration of neurons in the direct and indirect activation pathways (see Chap. 9).

However, not all diffuse, progressive system diseases of the spinal level (or elsewhere) are degenerative. *Combined system disease* is a motor and sensory system degeneration affecting the posterior and lateral columns which is due to vitamin B_{12} deficiency (Fig. 13-18). The major pathologic change is that of demyelination of these regions. If the metabolic defect persists, the process becomes more severe, with axonal destruction and necrosis but little gliosis initially. In patients with long-duration, progressive disease who are not treated, gliosis also develops. There is often peripheral nerve and cerebral involvement as well. These lesions result in the clinical pattern of a slowly progressive sensory ataxia, with upper motor neuron signs, some lower motor neuron signs (depressed ankle reflexes), paresthesia, and occasionally dementia. The disorder is also often associated with macrocytic anemia

Fig. 13-18. Section of thoracic spinal cord showing demyelination of posterior columns secondary to pernicious anemia.

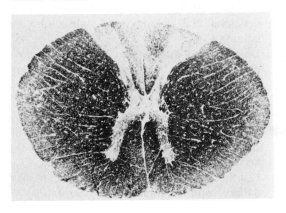

(pernicious anemia) that is also due to vitamin B_{12} deficiency. The reclassification of this degenerative disease as a metabolic disorder due to a nutritional deficiency was a major medical advance. It can be hoped that other degenerative disorders seen in a neurologic practice will soon have their causes determined in the same way, to permit appropriate treatment.

Spinal nerve lesions as described thus far have been lesions of single spinal nerves. There also may be diffuse involvement of spinal nerves in *polyradiculopathy*. Although polyradiculopathy may be difficult to recognize clinically, demonstrating the involvement of paraspinal muscles at multiple levels by EMG is strong evidence of it. Proximal weakness, which is more commonly seen in muscle disease, may also occur in polyradiculopathy, but usually there are additional abnormalities such as reflex and sensory loss. One form of polyradiculopathy is the Guillain-Barré syndrome, a subacute, inflammatory disorder that produces segmental demyelination predominantly in nerve roots.

Objectives

1. Name and identify the four major longitudinal subdivisions and the six major horizontal subdivisions at the spinal level.
2. Describe the differences in the horizontal components at the four longitudinal subdivisions.
3. Describe the relationship of cord segment to spinal nerve and vertebrae.
4. Name the longitudinal systems found at the spinal level, and describe the location of each.
5. Describe the functions of the alpha and gamma motor neurons, interneurons, the Renshaw cell, Clarke's nucleus, intermediolateral cell column, and substantia gelatinosa.
6. Describe and differentiate EPSP, IPSP, temporal and spatial summation, presynaptic inhibition, and spinal shock.
7. Describe with examples the stretch reflexes and flexion reflexes.
8. List the symptoms and signs associated with lesions of the spinal cord at C-6, T-6, L-5, and S-2.
9. List the features that differentiate an extramedullary from an intramedullary lesion.
10. List the major clinicopathologic features of multiple sclerosis and pernicious anemia.
11. List the spinal nerves and cord segments that mediate the biceps, triceps, knee, and ankle reflexes.

Clinical Problems

1. A 55-year-old man underwent surgery for carcinoma of the prostate 1 year ago. Six days ago, while watching TV after a big meal, he found that he was unable to walk when he tried to arise from the couch. There was no pain or trauma.

   On examination, the mental status, cranial nerves, and upper extremities were normal. There was a severe flaccid paralysis, with hypotonia of the lower abdominal muscles, hip flexors, hip adductors, and knee extensors. There was a moderate weakness of other muscles of the lower extremities but with some increase in tone (spastic). Reflexes were normal in the arms, absent at the abdomen and knees, and hyperactive at the ankles. He had bilateral Babinski's reflexes and loss of sensation for pain and temperature over both lower extremities. Position, vibration, and two-point discrimination were normal. All findings were symmetric.
   a. What is the level, side, and type of lesion?
   b. What is the longitudinal and horizontal location of the lesion?
   c. Is the conus medullaris involved in the lesion?
   d. What type of bladder dysfunction would occur with lesions of the lumbar cord and sacral cord?
   e. What is the most likely cause?
2. A 60-year-old woman first noted numbness of all fingers of the right hand 2½ years ago. Clumsiness of the right hand developed shortly thereafter. Defective appreciation of temperature with the right hand had been noted 1½ years ago; and 7 months prior to her admission, a similar numbness of all fingers of the left hand developed. At the same time, a stiffness of both lower extremities was noted, accompanied by an unsteadiness on rapid turning.

   On neurologic examination, the mental status and cranial nerves were intact. Fasciculations and a minor degree of atrophy were present in muscles of both shoulders. Fasciculations were not present in the lower extremities. Strength was decreased bilaterally as follows: moderate weakness in shoulder abductors and elbow flexors and extensors. There was a marked weakness of intrinsic hand muscles. The lower extremities had minimal weakness. Spasticity was noted on passive motion in the lower extremities and her gait was spastic. The triceps, quadriceps, and Achilles reflexes were increased bilaterally. Plantar responses were extensor bilaterally. Abdominal reflexes were absent. Pain and temperature were decreased at the C-4 to T-1 segments bilaterally, with total loss in her right hand and lower arm. In these segments, touch sensation was intact.

a. What is the level and type of lesion?
b. Which systems and which subdivisions of each are involved?
c. Which cord segments are involved and in what horizontal location?
d. What is the most likely cause?

3. A 52-year-old woman is hospitalized because of ataxia and mental symptoms. She is unable to give a history, but her husband relates that for the past 3 years she has complained of a "pins and needles" sensation in her feet and hands that gradually spread to her knees and elbows. For the past 18 months, she has had a progressive gait ataxia and weakness of the legs. For about the same length of time, she has had mental symptoms. At first, she was irritable and uncooperative. At present, she has impaired memory, thinks her husband is trying to poison her, and is confused at night. She is also incontinent of urine and stool.

On examination, she is demented and is ataxic when she walks. The Romberg sign is positive. Both legs are moderately and symmetrically weak. Tendon reflexes are normal in the arms and absent in the legs. There are bilateral Babinski's signs. Position sense is impaired in her toes. Vibration sense is absent in her legs. Touch, pain, and temperature sensations are not significantly impaired. She has a bladder catheter in place.

a. What is the location and type of lesion?
b. Which sensory pathways are involved?
c. Why are tendon reflexes absent and Babinski's reflex present?

d. What is one identifiable cause for certain neurologic disorders previously classified as "degenerative" diseases?

4. A 30-year-old man had an acute onset of severe back and right leg pain after falling while carrying a sack of bagels. His symptoms have worsened over the 4 weeks since onset. On examination, there is a slight hypalgesia on the lateral aspect of his leg. Reflexes are normal. There is mild weakness of hip abductors, hamstrings, ankle dorsiflexors, and toe extensors on the right. He experiences severe pain when he coughs or when his leg is elevated.

a. What is the site and type of lesion?
b. What neural structure is involved?
c. In a patient with footdrop, at what sites could the lesion be located?
d. What produces pain on straight leg raising?

Suggested Reading

Adams, R. D., and Victor, M. (eds.). *Principles of Neurology* (2nd ed.). New York: McGraw-Hill, 1981. Pp. 867–1007.

Brookhart, J. M., et al. (eds.). *Handbook of Physiology,* Section 1, Vol. II, Part 1. Bethesda, Md.: American Physiological Society, 1981.

Burke, R. E., and Rudomin, P. (eds.). Spinal Neurons and Synapses. In *Handbook of Physiology,* Section 1, Vol. I, Part 2. Bethesda, Md.: American Physiological Society, 1977. Pp. 877–944.

Crago, P. E., Houk, J. C., and Hasan, Z. Regulatory actions of human stretch reflex. *J. Neurophysiol.* 39:925, 1976.

DeMyer, W. Anatomy and Clinical Neurology of the Spinal Cord. In A. B. Baker and L. H. Baker (eds.), *Clinical Neurology,* Vol. 3. Philadelphia: Harper & Row, 1971. Pp. 1–32.

Homma, S. (ed.). *Understanding the Stretch Reflex.* New York: Elsevier, 1976.

Kuyper, H. G. J. M. The Anatomical Organization of the Descending Pathways and Their Contributions to Motor Control Especially in Primates. In J. E. Desmedt (ed.), *New Developments in Electromyography and Clinical Neurophysiology,* Vol. 3. New York: Karger, 1973. Pp. 38–68.

Lundberg, A. Convergence of excitatory and inhibitory action on interneurones in the spinal cord. *UCLA Forum in Medical Science,* 11:231, 1969.

Lundberg, A. Control of Spinal Mechanisms from the Brain. In D. B. Tower (ed.), *The Nervous System,* Vol. 1. New York: Raven, 1975. Pp. 253–265.

Matthews, P. B. C. Muscle spindles and their motor control. *Physiol. Rev.* 44:219, 1964.

Merton, P. A. How we control the contraction of our muscles. *Sci. Am.* 226:30, May 1972.

The Posterior Fossa Level

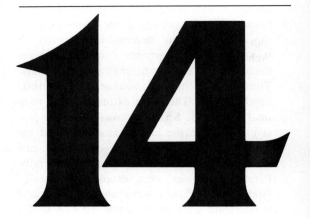

The posterior fossa level contains all the structures located within the skull below the tentorium cerebelli and above the foramen magnum (Fig. 14-1). These structures are derivatives of the primitive mesencephalon, metencephalon, and myelencephalon and include portions of all the systems discussed earlier. The major structures of this level are the brain stem (medulla, pons, and midbrain), the cerebellum, and segments of cranial nerves III through XII, prior to their emergence from the skull. The brain stem, the central core of the posterior fossa level, is a specialized rostral extension of the embryonic neural tube that preserves, even in the mature state, many of the longitudinal or intersegmental features found in the spinal cord and also provides for the segmental functions of the head.

This chapter describes the general features of each major longitudinal system as they relate to the posterior fossa level and discusses in further detail the cranial nerves and internal anatomy of the medulla, pons, midbrain, and cerebellum. Three additional systems (oculomotor, auditory, and vestibular), which are located primarily at this level, are introduced and described.

Overview

The brain stem contains ascending and descending pathways traveling to the thalamus, hypothalamus, cortex, cerebellum, cranial nerve nuclei, and spinal cord. The main sensory pathways include those that originate in the spinal cord (the spinothalamic tracts, medial lemniscus, and the spinocerebellar pathways), as well as those that arise from the cranial nerve nuclei (the descending tract of the trigeminal nerve, the trigeminal-thalamic tract, and the lateral lemniscus). The main motor pathways include the direct activation pathways (the corticospinal and corticobulbar pathways) and the indirect activation pathways (reticulospinal, rubrospinal, and vestibulospinal pathways). Additional important intersegmental pathways found at this level include the medial longitudinal fasciculus, the ascending and descending fibers of the consciousness and visceral systems, and many of the structures of the oculomotor, auditory, and vestibular systems.

It is traditional to subdivide the brain stem into three parts: the medulla (derived from myelencephalon), which contains the motor neurons for swallowing, tongue movement, talking, and cer-

tain visceral-motor functions; the pons (derived from metencephalon), which contains the nuclei associated with motor, sensory, and parasympathetic innervation of the face and abduction of the eye; and the midbrain (derived from mesencephalon), which contains the nuclei of the ascending reticular activating system, the nuclei that govern eye movements (except abduction), and the fibers involved in pupillary constriction and accommodation.

The brain stem has 10 pairs of cranial nerves (Fig. 14-2), which perform segmental functions comparable to the functions of the spinal nerves. The portions of these nerves contained within the bones of the cranium are considered part of the posterior fossa level; the segments of these nerves distal to the bones of the skull are considered part of the peripheral level. The location and general function of the cranial nerves at the posterior fossa level are summarized in Table 14-1.

The *cerebellum* (a derivative of metencephalon) lies dorsal to the pons and medulla and consists of a midline vermis and two lateral hemispheres. The cerebellum is functionally and anatomically divided into three lobes: the flocculonodular lobe, responsible for equilibration and balance; the anterior lobe, responsible for gait and posture; and the large posterior lobe, responsible for coordinated movements of the extremities.

The cerebrospinal fluid system is represented at the posterior fossa level by the aqueduct of Sylvius, the fourth ventricle, the meninges, the extraventricular subarachnoid cisterns, and the cerebrospinal fluid itself. The entire blood supply to the posterior fossa level is derived from the vertebrobasilar arterial system supplying paramedian, short, and long circumferential arteries to the brain stem and cerebellum. The major long circumferential arteries are the posterior inferior cerebellar arteries at the medullary level, the anterior inferior cerebellar arteries at the pontine level, and the superior cerebellar artery at the level of the midbrain.

The major components of three additional systems are also found at this level. The oculomotor system is represented by: cranial nerve nuclei III, IV, and VI; their axons traveling toward the extraocular muscles; the medial longitudinal fasciculus; and the fibers for supranuclear control of eye movement descending from the cortex. The

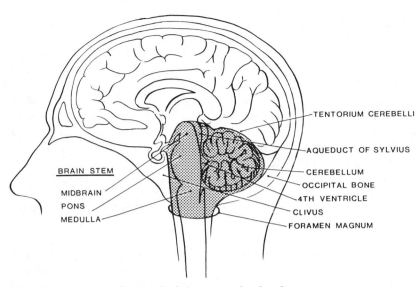

Fig. 14-1. Posterior fossa (stippled area) *is bordered by foramen magnum, tentorium cerebelli, clivus, and occipital bones.*

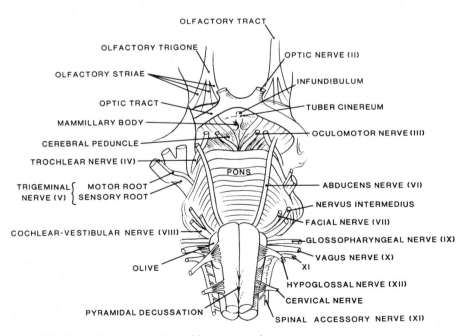

Fig. 14-2. Ventral (anterior) view of brain stem showing the cranial nerves. (Only cranial nerves III through XII are in the posterior fossa level.)

Table 14-1. The Location and General Function of Cranial Nerves at the Posterior Fossa Level

Level	Cranial nerve	General function
Medulla	XII Hypoglossal	Motor to muscles of tongue
	XI Spinal accessory	Motor to sternocleidomastoid and trapezius muscles
	X Vagus	Motor to muscles of soft palate, pharynx, and larynx; parasympathetic fibers to thoracic and abdominal viscera; sensory fibers from pharynx and external auditory meatus; visceral sensory fibers from chest and abdominal cavity
	IX Glossopharyngeal	Motor to stylopharyngeus muscle; sensory from pharynx and tongue; taste from posterior tongue
Pons	VIII Cochlear-vestibular	Hearing and equilibration
	VII Facial	Motor to muscles of facial expression; parasympathetic to salivary glands; taste sensation from anterior tongue
	VI Abducens	Motor to lateral rectus muscle of eye
	V Trigeminal	Sensory from face; motor to muscles of mastication
Midbrain	IV Trochlear	Motor to superior oblique muscle of eye
	III Oculomotor	Motor to medial, superior, and inferior recti, and inferior oblique muscles of eye, and levator palpabrae of eyelid; parasympathetic to constrictors of pupil

auditory system is represented by the auditory nerves, cochlear nuclei, trapezoid bodies, and multiple, bilateral pathways that ascend to the inferior colliculi en route to the thalamus and temporal cortex. The vestibular system is represented by the vestibular nerves, vestibular nuclei, and their multiple connections with the cerebellum, spinal cord, medial longitudinal fasciculus, and structures at the supratentorial level.

Lesions can be precisely localized at the posterior fossa level, when there is a combination of intersegmental and segmental involvement. Lesions at the posterior fossa level are unique in that unilateral brain-stem lesions may produce involvement of the ipsilateral side of the face and the contralateral side of the body. Other types of neurologic dysfunction that help localize a lesion at the posterior fossa level are disturbances of cerebellar function or involvement of the intracranial portions of cranial nerves III through XII.

General Anatomy of the Posterior Fossa Level

Posterior Cranial Fossa and Tentorium

The posterior cranial fossa is formed by the occipital bones at the base of the skull and the temporal bones anteriorly and laterally (Fig. 14-3). The inferior limit of the posterior fossa is the foramen magnum, where the cervical cord merges with the medulla. The rostral limit of the posterior fossa is the tentorium cerebelli, which lies between the cerebellum and the occipital lobe. The tentorium is attached posteriorly and posterolaterally to the transverse sinus and anterolaterally to the petrous ridge. The anterior border is not attached to bone but forms the tentorial notch through which the midbrain passes to merge with the diencephalon.

Systems Contained in the Posterior Fossa Level

The neural structures of the posterior fossa level consist of cranial nerves III through XII, the midbrain, pons, medulla, and cerebellum. Each of the previously studied neural systems is represented at the posterior fossa level.

THE CEREBROSPINAL FLUID SYSTEM. Cerebrospinal fluid flows into the posterior fossa in the *aqueduct of Sylvius,* a narrow canal in the midbrain between the third and fourth ventricles. The fourth ventricle is located at the level of the medulla and pons, which form its floor. The roof of the fourth ventricle is the ventral midline portion of the cerebellum. Cerebrospinal fluid leaves the fourth ventricle through the foramen of Magendie (at the caudal end of the ventricle) and through the two foramina of Luschka (at each lateral an-

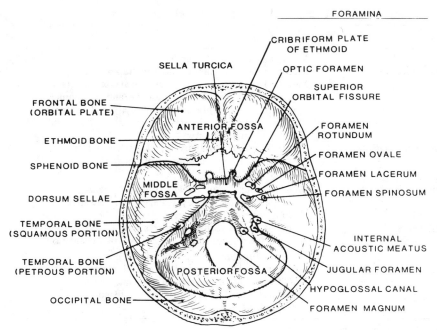

FORAMINA

CRIBRIFORM PLATE
OF ETHMOID

SELLA TURCICA

OPTIC FORAMEN

SUPERIOR
ORBITAL FISSURE

FRONTAL BONE
(ORBITAL PLATE)

ANTERIOR FOSSA

FORAMEN
ROTUNDUM

ETHMOID BONE

FORAMEN OVALE

SPHENOID BONE

FORAMEN LACERUM

FORAMEN SPINOSUM

MIDDLE
FOSSA

DORSUM SELLAE

TEMPORAL BONE
(SQUAMOUS PORTION)

INTERNAL
ACOUSTIC MEATUS

TEMPORAL BONE
(PETROUS PORTION)

POSTERIOR FOSSA

JUGULAR FORAMEN

HYPOGLOSSAL CANAL

OCCIPITAL BONE

FORAMEN MAGNUM

Fig. 14-3. Base of skull with major bones and foramina.

gle of the ventricle) to enter the subarachnoid space, where it circulates through the cisterna magna, cerebellopontine, prepontine, interpeduncular, and ambient cisterns.

THE SENSORY SYSTEM. The brain stem contains ascending pathways mediating (1) pain and temperature (lateral spinothalamic); (2) conscious proprioception and discriminative sensation (dorsal column–medial lemniscal); (3) unconscious proprioception (anterior and posterior spinocerebellar); and (4) touch (anterior spinothalamic and dorsal column–medial lemniscal). In addition, sensory input from the face and head enters at this level.

THE CONSCIOUSNESS SYSTEM. The central core of the brain stem contains the reticular formation and its ascending projectional pathways. The brain stem, along with other areas of the nervous system, thus serves the important function of mediating consciousness, attention, and sleeping and waking cycles.

THE MOTOR SYSTEM. All subdivisions of the motor system are represented at the posterior fossa level. The lower motor neurons of several

of the cranial nerves contain the final common pathway to muscles of the head and neck. The direct activation pathways are represented by the corticospinal tracts, which descend through the brain stem and decussate in the lower medulla en route to the spinal cord, and the corticobulbar pathways, which provide supranuclear innervation to brain-stem motor nuclei. The indirect activation pathways in the brain stem consist of short multineuronal descending pathways of the reticulospinal, rubrospinal, and vestibulospinal tracts arising in the brain stem. Much of the cerebellar control circuit is located at this level, and portions of the basal ganglia control circuit (substantia nigra and red nucleus) are present in the midbrain.

THE VISCERAL SYSTEM. The posterior fossa not only contains the reticular formation and the ascending and descending pathways that mediate visceral function but also is the location of preganglionic parasympathetic fibers traveling with cranial nerves III, VII, IX, and X and of the visceral vasomotor, respiratory, and vomiting regulatory centers.

THE VASCULAR SYSTEM. The structures in the posterior fossa receive their blood supply from the vertebrobasilar arterial system (Fig. 14-4). The vertebral arteries enter the cranial cavity

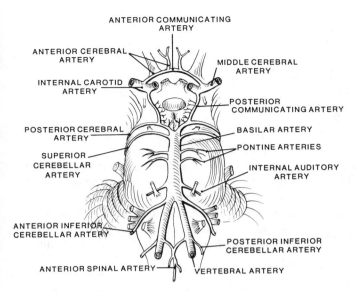

ANTERIOR COMMUNICATING
ARTERY

ANTERIOR CEREBRAL
ARTERY

MIDDLE CEREBRAL
ARTERY

INTERNAL CAROTID
ARTERY

POSTERIOR
COMMUNICATING ARTERY

POSTERIOR CEREBRAL
ARTERY

BASILAR ARTERY

SUPERIOR
CEREBELLAR
ARTERY

PONTINE ARTERIES

INTERNAL AUDITORY
ARTERY

ANTERIOR INFERIOR
CEREBELLAR ARTERY

POSTERIOR INFERIOR
CEREBELLAR ARTERY

ANTERIOR SPINAL ARTERY

VERTEBRAL ARTERY

Fig. 14-4. Blood supply of posterior fossa structures is from the vertebral and basilar arteries.

through the foramen magnum and then course rostrally along the ventral-lateral surface of the medulla where they give off branches to form the anterior spinal artery, which descends on the anterior aspect of the lower medulla to the cervical spinal cord. At the level of the pons, the two vertebral arteries merge to form the basilar artery, which continues rostrally to the upper midbrain level, where it branches to form the posterior cerebral arteries.

Branches of the vertebral and basilar arteries are subdivided into three groups which supply each level of the brain stem and the cerebellum. The paramedian zone on either side of the mid-

Fig. 14-5. Blood supply of the medulla. Lateral zone is from the posterior inferior cerebellar artery, paramedian zone from the anterior spinal artery, and intermediate zone from the vertebral artery.

line is supplied by paramedian branches; the intermediate zone is supplied by short circumferential branches; and the lateral zone is supplied by long circumferential branches (Fig. 14-5). The *paramedian* and *lateral zones* are often involved by vascular lesions, with significant clinical deficit. The paramedian area of the medulla is supplied by paramedian branches of the anterior spinal artery, while the intermediate zone is supplied by the vertebral arteries. The paramedian areas of the pons and midbrain are supplied by the paramedian branches of the basilar artery. The lateral areas of the brain stem are supplied by three pairs of long circumferential arteries: the *posterior inferior cerebellar artery* arising from the vertebral arteries and supplying the lateral area of the medulla and posterior inferior aspect of the cerebellum; the *anterior inferior cerebellar artery,* a branch of the basilar artery that supplies the lateral area of the pons and the anterior inferior aspect of the cerebellum; and the *superior*

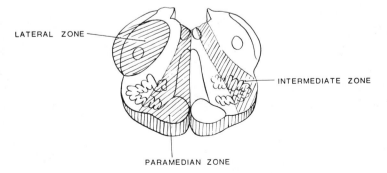

LATERAL ZONE

INTERMEDIATE ZONE

PARAMEDIAN ZONE

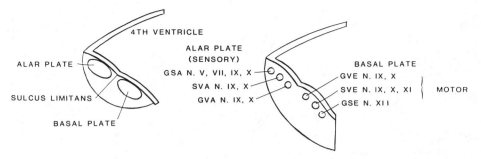

Fig. 14-6. Alar and basal plates of brain stem at the level of the medulla in (left) *5-week and* (right) *10-week embryo (see Table 14-2).*

cerebellar artery, a branch of the basilar artery that supplies the lateral area of the midbrain and superior surface of the cerebellum.

Three additional special systems are found primarily at the posterior fossa level: (1) the oculomotor system, which mediates eye movement; (2) the auditory system, which mediates hearing; and (3) the vestibular system, which mediates balance and equilibrium.

Embryologic Organization of the Brain Stem

The primitive neural tube displays an anatomic organization similar to that of the spinal cord,

Fig. 14-7. Location of cell columns within brain stem. Sensory nuclei are shown on left and motor nuclei on right.

with functional areas for sensation (alar plate) and motor activity (basal plate) separated by the sulcus limitans. Within these sensory and motor areas, further segregation occurs in the brain stem into somatic and visceral regions (Fig. 14-6). This separation persists into the adult, with minor variations.

These functional divisions exist as rostrocaudal cell columns from which the cranial nerve nuclei are derived. Some cranial nerves contain components from more than one of these columns. The appearance of new structures in the brain stem and the enlargement of the embryonic central canal into the fourth ventricle displace some of these nuclear columns from their embryonic position. The location of the cell columns in the adult brain stem and the cranial nerves arising from each is shown in Figure 14-7. These functionally oriented cell columns provide an important framework for learning the intrinsic anatomy of

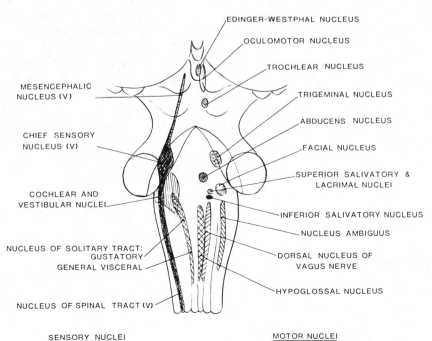

Table 14-2. Components of the Cranial Nerves

Component	Function	Cranial nerve
Efferent	Motor	
General somatic efferent (GSE)	Somatic striated muscles	III, IV, VI, XII
General visceral efferent (GVE)	Parasympathetic glands and smooth muscles	III, VII, IX, X
Special visceral efferent (SVE)	Branchial arch muscles	V, VII, IX, X, XI
Afferent	Sensory	
General somatic afferent (GSA)	Somesthetic senses	V, IX, X
Special somatic afferent (SSA)	Hearing and balance, vision	II, VIII
General visceral afferent (GVA)	Pharynx and viscera	IX, X
Special visceral afferent (SVA)	Smell, taste	I, VII, IX, X

each of the major subdivisions of the posterior fossa. The components of each of these cell columns, found in each of the cranial nerves, are shown in Table 14-2.

The Medulla

The medulla oblongata is that portion of the brain stem extending from the level of the foramen magnum to the caudal border of the base of the pons. Many of the features of the medulla are similar to those of the spinal cord (Fig. 14-8). The major ascending and descending pathways present in the spinal cord are also present in this area; however, there are several important changes that occur in this region, including (1) the location of the corticospinal tracts in the medial-ventral portion of the medulla (the medullary pyramids), (2) the termination of the fasciculus gracilis and cuneatus on their respective nuclei and the subsequent course of the second-order neurons in the *medial lemniscus*, (3) the replacement of the zone of Lissauer by the *de-*

scending tract of the trigeminal nerve, (4) the replacement of the central gray portion of the spinal cord by the reticular formation, (5) the entrance of the dorsal spinocerebellar tracts into the inferior cerebellar peduncle, and (6) the replacement of the central canal of the spinal cord by the fourth ventricle.

Further important anatomic features of the medulla include the following.

DECUSSATION OF THE PYRAMIDS.   At the lower end of the medulla, most of the fibers in the descending corticospinal pathways cross to the opposite side of the brain stem before descending in the spinal cord as the lateral corticospinal tracts (Fig. 14-8).

DECUSSATION OF THE MEDIAL LEMNISCUS.   In the caudal medulla rostral to the pyramidal decussation, second-order axons originating from the nucleus gracilis and cuneatus sweep ventromedially around the central gray matter as the *internal arcuate fibers*. These fibers then cross the midline to the opposite side and continue rostrally as the medial lemnisci (Fig. 14-9).

Fig. 14-8. Cross section of low medulla at the decussation of pyramids. Myelin-stained section on right.

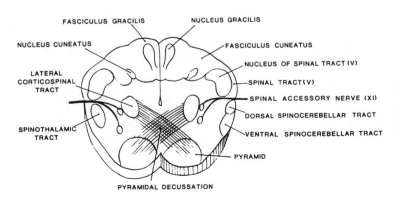

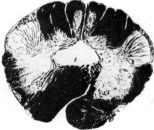

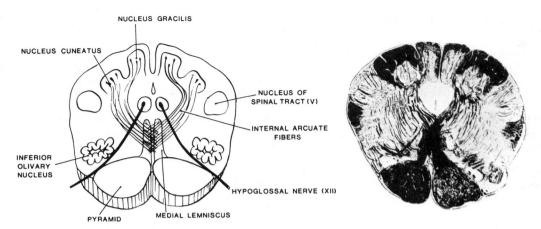

Fig. 14-9. Cross section of low medulla at the decussation of medial lemnisci. Myelin-stained section on right.

INFERIOR OLIVARY NUCLEI. The convoluted bands of cells located in the ventrolateral portion of the medulla are the inferior olivary nuclei which receive fibers from the dentate nucleus of the cerebellum, red nuclei, basal ganglia, and cerebral cortex. The olivary nuclei relay fibers to the opposite cerebellar hemisphere to form the olivocerebellar pathway via the inferior cerebellar peduncle. The inferior olive is a major relay station in the cerebellar pathways. It provides tonic cerebellar support for reflex movements and triggers phasic motor programs in the cerebellum.

MEDIAL LONGITUDINAL FASCICULUS. This fiber tract is located in the paramedian regions of the brain stem dorsal to the medial lemniscus (Fig. 14-10). The medial longitudinal fasciculus extends rostrally from the cervical cord to the upper

Fig. 14-10. Midportion of medulla at origin of hypoglossal and vagus nerves. Myelin-stained section on right.

midbrain level and transmits information for the coordination of head and eye movements.

INFERIOR CEREBELLAR PEDUNCLE (RESTIFORM BODY). One of the three major connections between the cerebellum and brain stem, this pathway is located in the dorsolateral portion of the medulla and contains dorsal spinocerebellar, olivocerebellar, vestibulocerebellar, and reticulocerebellar fibers traveling to the cerebellum, as well as cerebellovestibular fibers traveling from the cerebellum to the brain stem (Fig. 14-10).

Hypoglossal Nerve (Cranial Nerve XII)

FUNCTION. The hypoglossal nerve supplies motor innervation to the intrinsic muscles of the tongue. It is a motor nerve whose nuclei arise from the general somatic efferent (GSE) group of cranial nerve nuclei.

ANATOMY. The hypoglossal nucleus is located in the paramedian area of the caudal medulla in the floor of the fourth ventricle (Figs. 14-9, 14-10).

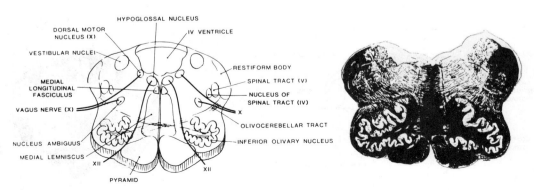

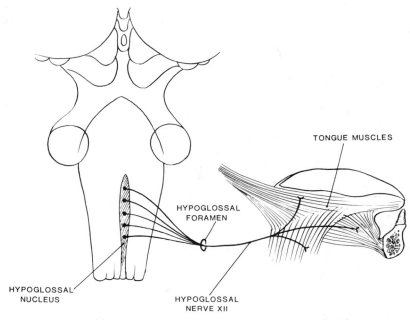

Fig. 14-11. Origin, course, and distribution of hypoglossal nerve fibers.

The fibers course ventrally and exit from the ventral aspect of the medulla between the medullary pyramids and the olive. After exit from the brain stem, these fibers pass through the hypoglossal foramen and innervate the striated musculature of the tongue (Fig. 14-11).

PATHOPHYSIOLOGY. Diseases involving the hypoglossal nucleus or cranial nerve XII are associated with atrophy, paresis, and fasciculations of tongue muscles. Unilateral weakness causes the tongue to deviate toward the side of the weakness on protrusion of the tongue. Involvement of upper motor neuron pathways innervating the hypoglossal nuclei produces slowing of alternating movements of the tongue and weakness, without atrophy. The structure and function of the hypoglossal nerve are summarized in Table 14-3.

Spinal Accessory Nerve (Cranial Nerve XI)

FUNCTION. The spinal accessory nerve is a motor nerve that supplies motor innervation to the sternocleidomastoid and trapezius muscles. It is a special visceral efferent (SVE) nerve innervating striated muscles that are derivatives of the branchial arches.

ANATOMY (FIG. 14-12). Cranial nerve XI arises from cell bodies in the ventral gray horn of the upper five cervical cord segments. The nerve ascends in the spinal canal lateral to the spinal cord, enters the skull through the foramen magnum, and leaves the cranial cavity via the jugular foramen to innervate the sternocleidomastoid and trapezius muscles.

PATHOPHYSIOLOGY. The spinal accessory nerve may be compressed by lesions in the region of the foramen magnum (where the nerve enters the skull) or in the region of the jugular foramen as it

Table 14-3. Structure and Function of the Hypoglossal Nerve

Component	Function	Nucleus of origin or termination	Ganglion	Foramen	Signs of dysfunction
GSE	Motor innervation of the tongue	Hypoglossal		Hypoglossal	Weakness of tongue movement

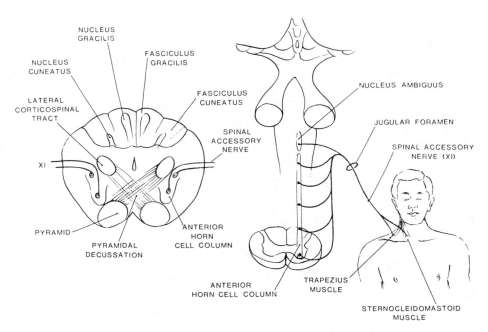

Fig. 14-12. Spinal accessory nerve. Origin of axons in the upper cervical cord and their course to trapezius and sternocleidomastoid muscles are shown on right. Nuclei of origin in the medulla are shown in the cross section on the left.

exits from the skull. Signs of dysfunction of cranial nerve XI include weakness of head rotation (sternocleidomastoid muscle) and inability to elevate or shrug the shoulder (trapezius muscle) on the side of the lesion. The sternocleidomastoid muscle rotates the face to the opposite side so that damage to the spinal accessory nerve results in weakness in turning the head toward the side contralateral to the lesion. The structure and function of the spinal accessory nerve are summarized in Table 14-4.

Vagus Nerve (Cranial Nerve X)

FUNCTION. The vagus nerve is a mixed nerve with special visceral efferent (SVE), general visceral efferent (GVE), general somatic afferent (GSA), general visceral afferent (GVA), and special visceral afferent (SVA) functions. The functions of cranial nerve X are innervation of the striated muscles of the soft palate, pharynx, and larynx derived from branchial arches (SVE); parasympathetic innervation to the thoracic and abdominal viscera (GVE); sensory innervation of the external auditory meatus (GSA); sensory innervation of the pharynx, larynx, and thoracic and abdominal viscera (GVA); and innervation of taste receptors on the posterior pharynx (SVA).

ANATOMY (FIG. 14-13). The SVE fibers of the vagus nerve innervating the striated muscles of the soft palate, pharynx, and larynx arise from the *nucleus ambiguus,* a structure located in the lateral medullary region dorsal to the inferior olive. The GVE components of the vagus nerve contain preganglionic parasympathetic fibers arising in the *dorsal motor nucleus* to supply the thoracic and abdominal viscera. These preganglionic fibers synapse with postganglionic neurons in the

Table 14-4. Structure and Function of the Spinal Accessory Nerve

Component	Function	Nucleus of origin or termination	Ganglion	Foramen	Signs of dysfunction
SVE	Motor to sterno-cleidomastoid and trapezius muscles	Anterior horn cells of cervical cord		Jugular	Weakness of head rotation and shoulder elevation

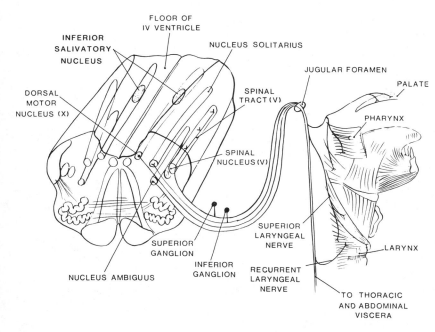

Fig. 14-13. *Motor and sensory nuclei of the vagus nerve in the medulla and the course and distribution of some of its SVE fibers.*

cardiac, pulmonary, esophageal, or celiac plexuses or within the visceral organs themselves.

The afferent fibers carried in the vagus nerve arise from three different sources: (1) GSA fibers carrying general sensation from the external auditory meatus have their cell bodies in the *superior (jugular) ganglion,* and central processes from this ganglion enter the medulla with the vagus and terminate in the spinal nucleus of the trigeminal nerve; (2) GVA fibers carrying information from abdominal and thoracic viscera have their cell bodies in the *inferior (nodose) ganglion,* and the central processes terminate in the *nucleus of the tractus solitarius;* and (3) SVA fibers in the vagus nerve carrying taste from the posterior pharynx also have their cell bodies located in the *inferior (nodose) ganglion,* and central processes terminate in the nucleus of the tractus solitarius.

The vagus nerve emerges from the lateral aspect of the medulla, dorsal to the olives, and leaves the skull through the jugular foramen. The superior and inferior ganglia of the vagus nerve are located in (or just below) the jugular foramen. The vagus nerve then passes down the neck near the carotid artery and the jugular vein. At the base of the neck, the vagus nerve passes in front of the subclavian artery. At this point on the right side, the right vagus nerve gives off the *right*

recurrent laryngeal nerve, which loops below and behind the subclavian artery and runs upward to the larynx to innervate most of the laryngeal muscles on the right side. On the left side, the vagus nerve descends in front of the arch of the aorta and gives off the *left recurrent laryngeal nerve,* which loops under the arch of the aorta and then runs upward to the larynx to provide innervation of most of the laryngeal muscles on the left side. The vagus nerve, after giving off the recurrent laryngeal nerves, descends into the thorax and abdominal cavities to supply the esophagus, heart, lungs, and abdominal viscera.

PATHOPHYSIOLOGY. Because of the dual innervation of many viscera and their independence of innervation, unilateral disease processes that involve this nerve do not produce symptoms involving the viscera. Instead, the neurologic signs usually consist of weakness of the striated muscles of the larynx and pharynx and difficulty in swallowing and speaking. Injury to the recurrent laryngeal nerves results in vocal cord paresis and a hoarse voice. The structure and function of cranial nerve X are summarized in Table 14-5.

Glossopharyngeal Nerve (Cranial Nerve IX)

FUNCTION. The glossopharyngeal nerve is also a mixed nerve with SVE, GVE, GSA, GVA, and SVA components. The functions of cranial nerve IX are innervation of the stylopharyngeus muscle

Table 14-5. Structure and Function of the Vagus Nerve

Component	Function	Nucleus of origin or termination	Ganglion	Foramen	Signs of dysfunction
SVE	Motor to muscles of soft palate, pharynx, and larynx	Nucleus ambiguus		Jugular	Hoarseness, dysphagia, decreased gag reflex
GVE	Parasympathetic to thoracic and abdominal viscera	Dorsal motor nucleus of nerve X		Jugular	Visceral disturbance, tachycardia
GSA	Sensation: external auditory meatus	Spinal nucleus of nerve V	Superior (jugular)	Jugular	Decreased sensation: external auditory meatus
GVA	Sensation: pharynx, larynx, and thoracic and abdominal viscera	Nucleus of tractus solitarius	Inferior (nodose)	Jugular	Decreased sensation: pharynx
SVA	Taste: posterior pharynx	Nucleus of tractus solitarius	Inferior (nodose)	Jugular	Not clinically significant

of the pharynx (SVE); parasympathetic innervation to the parotid gland (GVE); sensory innervation to the back of the ear (GSA); sensory innervation to the pharynx, tongue, eustachian tube, carotid body, and carotid sinus (GVA); and innervation of taste receptors from the posterior one-third of the tongue (SVA).

Fig. 14-14. Motor and sensory nuclei of the glossopharyngeal nerve in the medulla and the course and distribution of SVE fibers to the stylopharyngeus muscle and GVE fibers to the parotid gland.

ANATOMY (FIG. 14-14).   The SVE fibers to the stylopharyngeus muscle originate in the nucleus ambiguus. The GVE components of the glossopharyngeal nerve carry preganglionic parasympathetic fibers that arise in the inferior salivatory nucleus and terminate in the otic ganglion. Postganglionic fibers from this ganglion supply the parotid salivary glands; stimulation will increase salivary flow.

The afferent fibers carried in the glossopharyngeal nerve arise from three sources: (1) GSA fibers, carrying general sensation from behind the

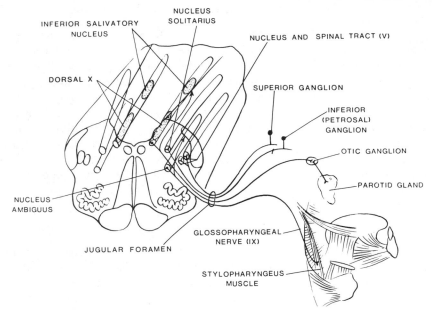

Table 14-6. Structure and Function of the Glossopharyngeal Nerve

Component	Function	Nucleus of origin or termination	Ganglion	Foramen	Signs of dysfunction
SVE	Motor to stylopharyngeus muscle	Nucleus ambiguus		Jugular	Not clinically significant
GVE	Parasympathetic to parotid gland	Inferior salivatory nucleus	Otic	Jugular	Decreased salivation
GSA	Sensation: back of ear	Spinal nucleus of nerve V	Superior	Jugular	Decreased sensation: back of ear
GVA	Sensation: pharynx, tongue, carotid receptors	Nucleus of tractus solitarius	Inferior (petrosal)	Jugular	Decreased gag reflex
SVA	Taste: posterior one-third of tongue	Nucleus of tractus solitarius	Inferior (petrosal)	Jugular	Decreased taste posterior

ear, have their cell bodies in the superior ganglion and their central connections terminate in the spinal nucleus of the trigeminal nerve; (2) GVA fibers carrying sensation from the pharynx; and (3) SVA fibers carrying taste sensation from the posterior tongue. The latter two arise from cell bodies contained in the inferior (petrosal) ganglion and have central connections that terminate in the nucleus of the tractus solitarius. Within the medulla there are segmental reflex connections between the pharyngeal sensory fibers and the motor neurons supplying the muscles of the pharynx to mediate the gag reflex.

The glossopharyngeal nerve emerges from the medulla, dorsal to the inferior olivary nuclei, and passes through the jugular foramen (which is also the location of its ganglia) to innervate peripheral structures. The components and structure of the glossopharyngeal nerve are thus similar to those of the vagus (Table 14-6).

PATHOPHYSIOLOGY. Isolated lesions of the glossopharyngeal nerve are rare but, with or without vagus damage, result in loss of pharyngeal sensation and of the gag reflex. Occasionally, lesions give rise to a paroxysmal pain syndrome of unknown cause (glossopharyngeal neuralgia). In this disorder, the patient experiences brief attacks of severe pain which usually begin in the throat and radiate down the side of the neck in front of the ear and to the back of the lower jaw. On occasion, the pain may begin deep in the ear. Attacks of discomfort may be precipitated by swallowing or protrusion of the tongue.

Clinical Correlations—Medulla and Lower Cranial Nerves

JUGULAR FORAMEN SYNDROME. Cranial nerves IX, X, and XI leave the skull along with the jugular vein through the jugular foramen (Fig. 14-15). A lesion (usually a mass) within or adjacent to the jugular foramen may affect all three cranial nerves and result in ipsilateral weakness of the pharyngeal and laryngeal muscles (nerve X), decreased sensation of the ipsilateral pharynx (nerve IX), and weakness of the ipsilateral trapezius and sternocleidomastoid muscles (nerve XI). One lesion that causes this syndrome is a glomus tumor or chemodectoma arising in chemoreceptors found along the jugular vein.

BULBAR AND PSEUDOBULBAR PALSY. Dysfunction of the motor components of the cranial nerves of the lower portion of the brain stem (particularly the medulla or "bulb") occurs with lower or upper motor neuron lesions. Lesions affecting the final common pathway result in bulbar palsy, which is manifest as flaccid weakness of the muscles associated with talking, chewing, swallowing, and movement of the tongue and lips. Supranuclear lesions involving the cerebral cortex or direct and indirect activation pathways result in upper motor neuron dysfunction of bulbar musculature, manifest as slow movements and a harsh, strained, spastic speech dysarthria. Because there is bilateral cortical innervation of most bulbar motor nuclei, a unilateral supranuclear lesion does not usually produce significant bulbar dysfunction; however, bilateral supranu-

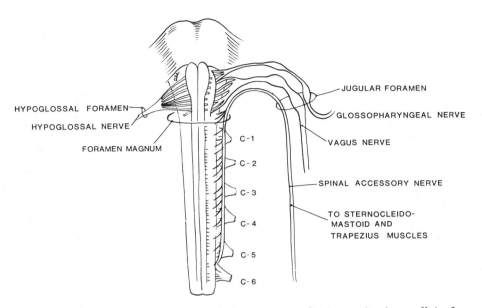

HYPOGLOSSAL FORAMEN

HYPOGLOSSAL NERVE

FORAMEN MAGNUM

JUGULAR FORAMEN

GLOSSOPHARYNGEAL NERVE

VAGUS NERVE

SPINAL ACCESSORY NERVE

TO STERNOCLEIDO-MASTOID AND TRAPEZIUS MUSCLES

C-1
C-2
C-3
C-4
C-5
C-6

Fig. 14-15. Ventral view of medulla and cranial nerves IX, X, and XI exiting together through the jugular foramen. Dorsal roots of C-1 through C-6 in the upper cervical spinal cord are also shown.

clear lesions result in severe paresis of bulbar muscles, characterized by spastic weakness with dysarthria, dysphagia, and reduced mouth and tongue movements. This involvement of bulbar function by bilateral supranuclear lesions is called *pseudobulbar palsy.*

The Pons

The pons is that portion of the brain stem located between the rostral and caudal borders of the basis pontis. Dorsoventrally, it is divided into the

Fig. 14-16. Cross section of lower pons at level of cranial nerves VI and VII.

basis pontis (ventrally), formed by the crossing fibers of the middle cerebellar peduncle, and the *tegmentum* (dorsally), which is the area between the fourth ventricle and the base. The basis pontis, which dominates the anatomy of the pons, contains the corticospinal, corticobulbar, and corticopontine fibers, as well as the pontine nuclei, which relay information to the cerebellum via the numerous transverse fibers forming the middle cerebellar peduncle. Within the tegmentum are the lateral spinothalamic tracts, medial lemnisci, medial longitudinal fasciculus, reticular formation, and the pathways of the consciousness and visceral systems. In addition, the tegmentum of the pons contains structures relating to the following cranial nerves: acoustic and vestibular divisions of nerve VIII, facial (nerve VII), abducens (nerve VI), and trigeminal (nerve V). The locations of these structures are shown in

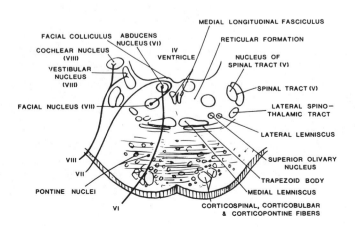

FACIAL COLLICULUS ABDUCENS NUCLEUS (VI)

COCHLEAR NUCLEUS (VIII)

VESTIBULAR NUCLEUS (VIII)

FACIAL NUCLEUS (VII)

IV VENTRICLE

MEDIAL LONGITUDINAL FASCICULUS

RETICULAR FORMATION

NUCLEUS OF SPINAL TRACT (V)

SPINAL TRACT (V)

LATERAL SPINO-THALAMIC TRACT

LATERAL LEMNISCUS

SUPERIOR OLIVARY NUCLEUS

TRAPEZOID BODY

MEDIAL LEMNISCUS

VIII
VII
PONTINE NUCLEI
VI

CORTICOSPINAL, CORTICOBULBAR & CORTICOPONTINE FIBERS

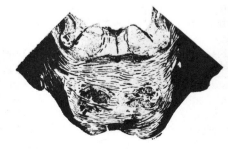

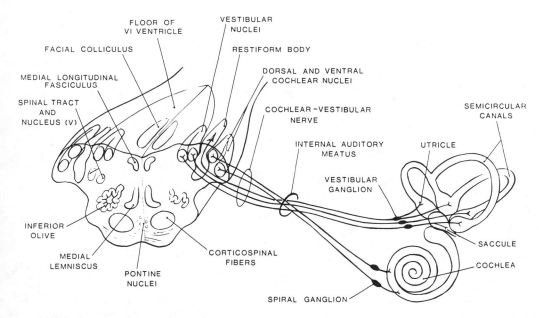

Fig. 14-17. Cochlear-vestibular nerve. The cell bodies are located in ganglia near the cochlea and semicircular canals with primary afferent terminations in the lateral pons.

Figure 14-16. Dorsal to the tegmentum is the fourth ventricle.

Cranial nerve VIII (auditory, vestibulocochlear, "statoacoustic") is made up of two divisions, one mediating hearing and the other conducting vestibular sensations. Since by gross inspection it is often difficult to denote any separation between these divisions as they travel together in an identical course from the brain stem to the internal auditory meatus, they have traditionally been grouped together (Fig. 14-17). However, because they have different nuclei of origin, innervate different receptors, have different central connections, and mediate different functions, they will be discussed separately. In addition, these divisions are part of two important subsystems found primarily at the posterior fossa level (the auditory and vestibular systems), which will be discussed in later sections of this chapter.

Acoustic Division of Cranial Nerve VIII

FUNCTION. The acoustic division of cranial nerve VIII is an afferent nerve conducting impulses for hearing from the ear. Audition is a special somatic afferent (SSA) function.

ANATOMY. Fibers that are carried in this division of cranial nerve VIII arise from cell bodies in the spiral ganglion located in the cochlea of the ear. Axons of these primary sensory neurons pass centrally through the internal auditory meatus and enter the dorsolateral area of the medulla at the pontomedullary junction. In its course to this point, cranial nerve VIII passes through the subarachnoid space at the caudal-lateral pontine border known as the *cerebellopontine angle,* and the fibers synapse in the dorsal and ventral cochlear nuclei (Fig. 14-17). Pathways arise from the cochlear nuclei that relay auditory potentials to the medial geniculate bodies of the thalamus and the auditory cortex of the temporal lobes bilaterally (see The Auditory System).

Table 14-7. Structure and Function of the Acoustic Division of Cranial Nerve VIII

Component	Function	Nucleus of origin or termination	Ganglion	Foramen	Signs of dysfunction
SSA	Hearing	Dorsal and ventral cochlear nuclei	Spiral	Internal auditory meatus	Decreased hearing

PATHOPHYSIOLOGY. Lesions of the acoustic division of cranial nerve VIII produce a unilateral loss of hearing. The physiology and pathophysiology of hearing will be discussed with the auditory system. The structure and function of the acoustic division of cranial nerve VIII are summarized in Table 14-7.

Vestibular Division of Cranial Nerve VIII

FUNCTION. The vestibular division of cranial nerve VIII is an afferent nerve conducting gravitational and rotational information from the ear. This information is necessary to maintain proper balance and equilibrium, which are special somatic afferent (SSA) functions.

ANATOMY. Fibers that are carried in this division of cranial nerve VIII arise from bipolar cells in the vestibular (Scarpa's) ganglion located within the internal auditory meatus (Fig. 14-17). They innervate the organs of balance (utricle, saccule, and semicircular canals) in the ear. Axons of these primary sensory neurons travel toward the brain stem, along with the acoustic division of nerve VIII, and make synaptic contact with the four vestibular nuclei (superior, medial, lateral, and inferior) located beneath the floor of the fourth ventricle in the upper medulla and pons (Fig. 14-17). Pathways arise from the vestibular nuclei, which conduct information to the cerebellum, spinal cord, reticular formation, and nuclei of cranial nerves III, IV, and VI via the medial longitudinal fasciculus (see The Vestibular System).

PATHOPHYSIOLOGY. Lesions of the vestibular division of cranial nerve VIII result in the sensations of vertigo (hallucination of rotatory movement) or disequilibrium. The physiology and pathophysiology of equilibrium will be discussed with the vestibular system. The structure and function of the vestibular division of cranial nerve VIII are summarized in Table 14-8.

Facial Nerve (Cranial Nerve VII)

FUNCTION. The facial nerve provides innervation to the muscles of facial expression derived from branchial arches. It is a mixed nerve with special visceral efferent (SVE), general visceral efferent (GVE), and special visceral afferent (SVA) functions. In addition to supplying the muscles of the face (SVE), it also provides parasympathetic innervation to the submandibular, sublingual, and lacrimal glands (GVE) and innervation of taste receptors on the anterior two-thirds of the tongue (SVA).

ANATOMY. The SVE fibers of the facial nerve innervating the striated muscles of the face arise in the facial nucleus located in the lateral tegmentum of the pons. Fibers arising from the facial nucleus pass medially and arch dorsally, forming a loop or genu around the abducens nucleus before proceeding to the lateral surface of the pons and emerging as the facial nerve (Figs. 14-16, 14-18). This looping of facial nerve fibers around each nucleus of cranial nerve VI creates a slight bulge in the floor of the fourth ventricle. These paired structures (which can be seen on gross inspection) are called the *facial colliculi*.

The parasympathetic (GVE) fibers of the facial nerve supplying the salivary and lacrimal glands arise from the superior salivatory nucleus and join the SVE fibers as they emerge from the pons (Fig. 14-19).

The SVA components of the facial nerve that mediate taste from the anterior two-thirds of the tongue arise from cell bodies located in the geniculate ganglion (situated at the bend of cranial nerve VII as it runs in the facial canal of the temporal bone). The central process from this ganglion enters the pons with GVE fibers as part of a smaller subdivision of the facial nerve (the nervus intermedius). In the pons, these fibers turn caudally to synapse, along with other taste fibers, in the nucleus of the tractus solitarius.

Table 14-8. Structure and Function of the Vestibular Division of Cranial Nerve VIII

Component	Function	Nucleus of origin or termination	Ganglion	Foramen	Signs of dysfunction
SSA	Balance and equilibrium	Vestibular nuclei	Vestibular	Internal auditory meatus	Disequilibrium, vertigo

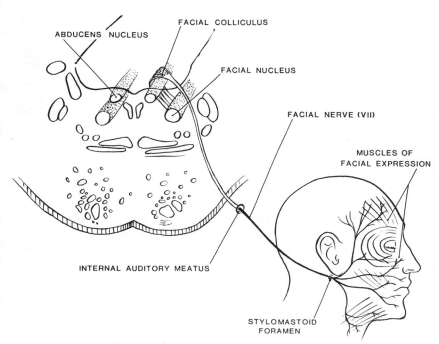

Fig. 14-18. Facial nerve nucleus in pons and course and distribution of motor axons. The loop of the facial nerve over the abducens nucleus forms the facial colliculus in the floor of the fourth ventricle.

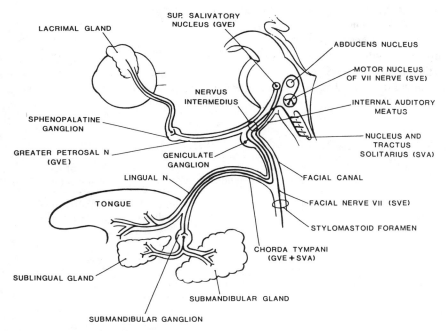

Fig. 14-19. Course of visceral efferent and afferent divisions of the facial nerve. (Redrawn from R. C. Truex and M. B. Carpenter. Strong and Elwyn's Human Neuroanatomy [5th ed.]. Baltimore: Williams & Wilkins, 1964.)

The facial nerve, as it leaves the pons, thus contains two divisions: a large SVE division supplying voluntary motor fibers to the face and the smaller nervus intermedius containing GVE and SVA fibers (Fig. 14-19). Both divisions leave the cranial cavity through the internal auditory meatus and enter the facial canal. The SVE fibers to the face continue through the canal, exiting at the stylomastoid foramen below the ear (Fig. 14-19). In addition to innervating the facial muscles, the SVE fibers provide innervation to the stapedius, a small muscle of the inner ear, the platysma, and other submental muscles. The nervus intermedius does not traverse the entire facial canal but splits into two branches that leave the canal in the region of the geniculate ganglion: the greater superficial petrosal nerve (containing the GVE fibers for lacrimation) and the chorda tympani nerve (carrying fibers for salivation and taste).

Preganglionic parasympathetic fibers in the greater superficial petrosal nerve synapse in the sphenopalatine ganglia; postganglionic fibers then proceed toward the lacrimal gland. After the chorda tympani nerve leaves the facial canal, it enters the middle ear cavity, arches over the tympanic membrane, and emerges from the petrous bone to join the lingual nerve of cranial nerve V on its way to the tongue and salivary glands (Fig. 14-19). The preganglionic parasympathetic fibers synapse in the submandibular ganglion, where postganglionic parasympathetic fibers arise to supply the submandibular and sublingual salivary glands in the mouth.

PATHOPHYSIOLOGY. Disorders of the facial nerve result in paresis of the muscles of facial expression and loss of taste on the anterior two-thirds of the tongue. Facial weakness, however, also results from a lesion involving the direct activation pathways descending from the cortex to innervate the facial nuclei. It is of clinical importance to distinguish between upper motor neuron (central) facial weakness involving the lower part of the face and lower motor neuron (peripheral) facial weakness involving both the upper and lower portions of the face (see Fig. 9-16).

Bell's palsy is a relatively common disorder usually of unknown (but perhaps inflammatory) cause which produces a peripheral weakness of nerve VII. Patients with this condition have weakness of both upper and lower facial muscles, with inability to completely close the eye on the side of the lesion. In addition (depending on the site of involvement of the facial nerve in the facial canal), such patients can have decreased lacrimation, salivation, and taste and hyperacusis (due to involvement of the nerve innervating the stapedius muscle).

The structure and function of the facial nerve are summarized in Table 14-9.

Abducens Nerve (Cranial Nerve VI)

FUNCTION. The abducens nerve is a general somatic efferent (GSE) nerve that provides innervation to the lateral rectus muscle of the eye.

Table 14-9. Structure and Function of the Facial Nerve

Component	Function	Nucleus of origin or termination	Ganglion	Foramen	Signs of dysfunction
SVE	Motor to muscles of facial expression	Facial nucleus		Internal auditory meatus: stylo- mastoid	Facial weakness, hyperacusis
GVE	Parasympathetic: lacrimal gland	Superior salivatory nucleus	Spheno- palatine	Internal auditory meatus	Decreased tearing
	salivary glands		Subman- dibular		Decreased salivation
SVA	Taste: anterior two- thirds of tongue	Nucleus of tractus solitarius	Geniculate	Internal auditory meatus	Decreased taste

Table 14-10. Structure and Function of the Abducens Nerve

Component	Function	Nucleus of origin or termination	Ganglion	Foramen	Signs of dysfunction
GSE	Motor to lateral rectus muscle	Abducens		Superior orbital fissure	Diplopia, medial deviation of eye

Contraction of the lateral rectus produces lateral movement (abduction) of the eyeball.

ANATOMY. The abducens nuclei are located in the GSE cell column near the midline, beneath the floor of the fourth ventricle (see Fig. 14-16). Efferent fibers pass through the tegmentum and basis pontis to emerge on the ventral surface near the pontomedullary junction. They ascend ventral to the base of the pons, traverse the cavernous sinus (along with cranial nerves III, IV, and branches of V), and leave the cranial cavity through the superior orbital fissure to supply the lateral rectus muscles of the eye (Fig. 14-20).

PATHOPHYSIOLOGY. Lesions affecting the abducens nerve result in weakness of the lateral rectus muscle, with medial deviation of the eye and diplopia (see The Oculomotor System). The intracranial course of cranial nerve VI is unusually long, and, as a result, the nerve may be affected by multiple pathologic processes involving the pons, base of the skull, cavernous sinus, superior

Fig. 14-20. The abducens nerve arises from nucleus in pons and has a long intracranial course to the lateral rectus muscle via cavernous sinus and superior orbital fissure.

orbital fissure, and orbit. The structure and function of the abducens nerve are summarized in Table 14-10.

Trigeminal Nerve (Cranial Nerve V)

FUNCTION. The trigeminal nerve is the sensory nerve to the face. It is a mixed nerve with general somatic afferent (GSA) and special visceral efferent (SVE) components. In addition to carrying touch, pain, temperature, and proprioceptive information (GSA) from the face, cranial nerve V provides motor innervation to the muscles of mastication, which are derived from branchial arches (SVE).

ANATOMY. The GSA fibers mediating touch, pain, temperature, and proprioception from the face have a slightly divergent course (Fig. 14-21). Fibers mediating touch, pain, and temperature arise from cell bodies in the trigeminal (semilunar or gasserian) ganglion. Axons travel proximally from the ganglion to enter the lateral aspect of the pons. Touch fibers synapse directly in the main (or chief) sensory nucleus of nerve V located in the dorsolateral pons. Second-order fibers ascend via crossed and uncrossed pathways in the trigeminothalamic tracts to synapse in the

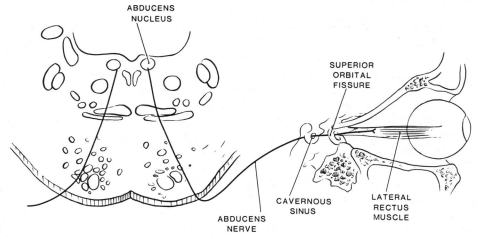

ABDUCENS NUCLEUS

SUPERIOR ORBITAL FISSURE

CAVERNOUS SINUS

LATERAL RECTUS MUSCLE

ABDUCENS NERVE

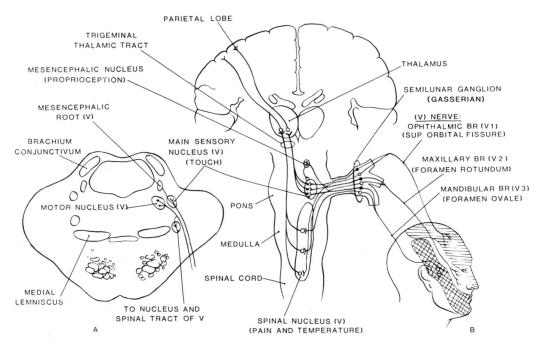

Fig. 14-21. Trigeminal nerve. A. Midpontine cross section. B. Horizontal section with course and distribution of sensory axons.

ventral posteromedial nucleus of the thalamus.

Pain and temperature fibers do not synapse in the main sensory nucleus but turn caudally to descend the length of the medulla into the upper three or four segments of the cervical spinal cord. This group of fibers is called the *descending tract of the trigeminal nerve* (Fig. 14-21). Axons from this tract synapse with cell bodies of second-order neurons that are in the nucleus of the spinal (or descending) tract of the trigeminal nerve (located medial to the tract). Along its course, the small GSA components of nerves IX and X (from the skin of the external ear) are added to the spinal tract of nerve V. There is a topographic relationship imposed on these descending paths, such that fibers from the upper-outer aspects of the face descend further into the cervical cord than do fibers from the lower-central facial regions. Second-order fibers for pain and temperature from the nucleus of the spinal tract thus cross at various levels to the opposite side and ascend to the thalamus in the trigeminothalamic tract running very near the medial lemniscus. These fibers synapse in the ventral posteromedial nucleus of the thalamus, where third-order neurons arise to terminate in the parietal lobe.

Proprioceptive fibers carried in the nerve, in contrast to all other first-order afferent neurons studied thus far, arise from cell bodies located inside the central nervous system in the mesencephalic nucleus of nerve V, which lies along the lateral border of the rostral fourth ventricle and aqueduct of Sylvius (Fig. 14-21). The distal axons of these first-order neurons arising from receptors in the muscles of mastication (and perhaps others) travel without synapse through the gasserian (semilunar) ganglion. Axons from the mesencephalic nucleus connect directly with the motor nucleus of nerve V to mediate a monosynaptic jaw reflex.

The SVE fibers providing voluntary motor innervation to the muscles of mastication arise from cell bodies in the motor nucleus of nerve V located medial to the main sensory nucleus (Fig. 14-22). Axons course anterolaterally and exit from the lateral surface of the pons and run near the gasserian ganglion. They join with the mandibular division to exit the skull through the foramen ovale and innervate the temporalis, masseter, medial and lateral pterygoid, and tensor tympani muscles. The temporalis and masseter muscles cause closure of the jaws, the pterygoids facilitate lateral jaw movement, and the tensor tympani is a small muscle of the inner ear.

From the gasserian ganglion, fibers of nerve V course peripherally via three major divisions: the ophthalmic nerve (V_1) exits in the superior orbital

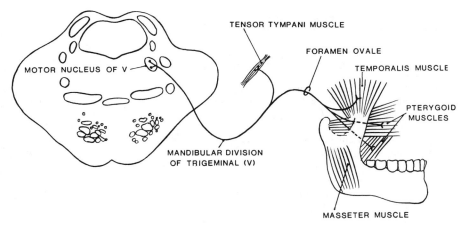

Fig. 14-22. Motor division of trigeminal nerve with nucleus in pons and course of axons to muscles of mastication.

fissure to innervate the upper face; the maxillary nerve (V_2) exits in the foramen rotundum to innervate the midface; and the mandibular nerve (V_3)—carrying both motor and sensory fibers—exits via the foramen ovale to innervate the lower face and muscles of mastication.

PATHOPHYSIOLOGY. Lesions involving cranial nerve V produce loss of facial sensation and (if motor fibers are involved) weakness of the masticatory muscles, resulting in deviation of the jaw to the side of the weakened muscles when the jaw is opened.

Trigeminal neuralgia (tic douloureux) is a disorder characterized by transient, brief, repetitive paroxysms of pain occurring in the distribution of one or more branches of cranial nerve V. The pain is very severe and disabling and occurs either spontaneously or is triggered by relatively minor sensory stimulation of the face. Although pathologic changes have been noted in the region of the gasserian ganglion, the precise cause of this syndrome is unknown.

Two reflexes tested as part of the neurologic examination involve cranial nerve V. The *jaw jerk* is the only muscle-stretch reflex that can be elicited in the head. It is mediated entirely by the mandibular branch of nerve V. Tapping the jaw places the muscles of mastication on a brief stretch. Proprioceptive impulses travel centrally and synapse with the motor nucleus of nerve V and result in reflex contraction of the jaw. Although a decrease in the jaw jerk occurs with

lesions in the reflex arc, the reflex is often difficult to elicit in healthy persons and is therefore usually regarded as abnormal only when it is hyperactive. This generally occurs with bilateral upper motor neuron lesions affecting the direct and indirect activation pathways to the motor nuclei of nerve V.

The *corneal reflex* is elicited by stroking the cornea of one eye with a piece of cotton. The afferent limb of this reflex is the ophthalmic division of nerve V. The nature of the central pathways is not entirely clear, but connection is made with both facial nuclei. Impulses traveling via the facial nerves bilaterally cause contraction of both orbicularis oculi muscles, resulting in a blink. Unilateral lesions of nerve V, the tegmentum of the pons, or the facial nerve alter this reflex. The structure and function of the trigeminal nerve are summarized in Table 14-11.

The Midbrain

The midbrain is that portion of the brain stem located between the rostral border of the pons and the upper border of the superior colliculus. The rostral limit of the midbrain gradually merges with structures of the diencephalon. Although the gross appearance of this mesencephalic derivative resembles the primitive neural tube, the presence of certain structures unique to the midbrain modifies the primitive embryonic arrangement. The midbrain is divided dorsoventrally into three main regions: the tectum (dorsal), tegmentum, and base (ventral) (Fig. 14-23).

The *tectum* or roof is the dorsal surface of the midbrain and lies above the transverse plane of the aqueduct of Sylvius. The tectum contains two paired structures, the inferior and superior collic-

Table 14-11. Structure and Function of the Trigeminal Nerve

Division of trigeminal nerve V	Component	Function	Nucleus of origin or termination	Ganglion	Foramen	Signs of dysfunction
Ophthalmic (V$_1$)	GSA	Sensation: forehead pain	Spinal nucleus of nerve V	Gasserian (semilunar)	Superior orbital fissure	Decreased forehead pain Decreased corneal reflex
		Touch: forehead	Main sensory nucleus of nerve V	Gasserian (semilunar)	Superior orbital fissure	Decreased forehead touch Decreased corneal reflex
Maxillary (V$_2$)	GSA	Sensation: cheek pain	Spinal nucleus of nerve V	Gasserian (semilunar)	Rotundum	Decreased cheek pain
		Touch: cheek	Main sensory nucleus of nerve V	Gasserian (semilunar)	Rotundum	Decreased cheek touch
Mandibular (V$_3$)	GSA	Sensation: jaw pain	Spinal nucleus of nerve V	Gasserian (semilunar)	Ovale	Decreased jaw pain
		Touch: jaw	Main sensory nucleus of nerve V	Gasserian (semilunar)	Ovale	Decreased jaw touch
		Proprioception	Mesencephalic nucleus		Ovale	Decreased jaw jerk
	SVE	Motor to muscles of mastication	Motor nucleus of nerve V		Ovale	Weakness of muscles of mastication, decreased jaw jerk

uli (the corpora quadrigemina). The inferior colliculi in the caudal midbrain act as a relay station for auditory fibers that pass to the thalamus via the brachium of the inferior colliculi. The superior colliculi located in the rostral midbrain are part of the oculomotor system and are associated with ocular control. The central canal persists as a narrow conduit (the aqueduct) surrounded by a zone of periaqueductal gray matter.

The *tegmentum* is that region lying ventral to the aqueduct and dorsal to the substantia nigra. In addition to the major longitudinal pathways (medial lemniscus, lateral lemniscus, lateral spinothalamic tracts, medial longitudinal fasciculus, indirect activating pathways, autonomic fibers, and projectional pathways of the reticular formation), it contains fibers and nuclei of cranial nerves III and IV, the red nucleus, and the decussation of the superior cerebellar peduncles (Fig. 14-23A).

THE SUPERIOR CEREBELLAR PEDUNCLE (BRACHIUM CONJUNCTIVUM). Efferent fibers from the cere-

bellum travel rostrally and ventrally into the tegmentum of the midbrain. In the caudal midbrain they cross to the opposite side, forming the decussation of the brachium conjunctivum (Fig. 14-24A). The fibers then pass to the red nucleus and thalamus.

THE RED NUCLEUS. The red nucleus is a large, round mass of gray matter that occupies the central portion of the tegmentum on each side of the upper midbrain (Fig. 14-23B). It is visible to the naked eye, with a slightly red color that is due to dense capillaries and high iron content. The red nuclei receive fibers from the cerebellum and the cerebral cortex and give rise to (1) descending fibers that synapse in the ipsilateral inferior olivary nuclei and then terminate in the contralateral cerebellum and (2) the rubrospinal tract, which decussates caudal to the red nucleus in the ventral tegmental decussation and then descends through the opposite side of the brain stem to the spinal cord.

The *base of the midbrain,* also known as the

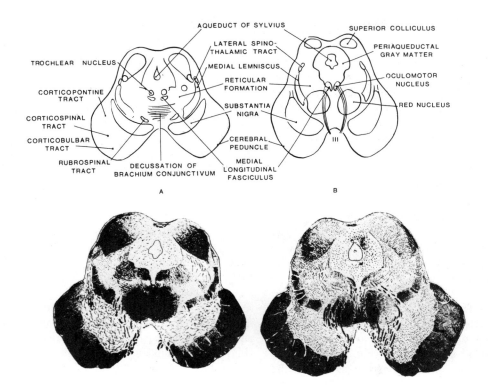

Fig. 14-23. Cross section of midbrain. A. Lower mid-brain at level of inferior colliculus. B. Upper midbrain at level of superior colliculus. Myelin-stained sections are shown below.

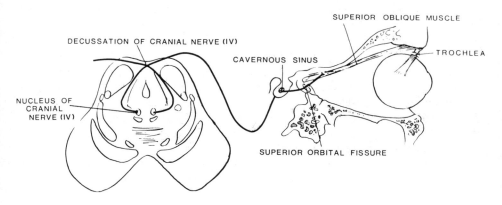

Fig. 14-24. Trochlear nerve. Cross section of lower midbrain showing nucleus and course and distribution of axons to the superior oblique muscle of the opposite eye.

basis pedunculi, consists of the cerebral peduncles (the corticospinal, corticobulbar, and corticopontine fibers descending from the internal capsule) and the substantia nigra lying dorsal to each peduncle (Fig. 14-23A). The substantia nigra contains melanin-containing neurons (hence its dark appearance), which are functionally related to the basal ganglia and motor system.

Trochlear Nerve (Cranial Nerve IV)

FUNCTION. The trochlear nerve is a general somatic efferent (GSE) nerve that supplies motor innervation to the superior oblique muscle of the eye. Contraction of the superior oblique muscle causes a downward deviation of the eye in the adducted position.

ANATOMY. The fibers contained in each trochlear nerve arise from the trochlear nucleus on the opposite side of the brain stem, just ventral to the periaqueductal gray matter (Fig. 14-24). The fibers course dorsolaterally and cross behind the tectum to emerge from the opposite side of the midbrain on its dorsal aspect. Thus, it is the only crossed cranial nerve in the brain stem and the only one not emerging from the ventral or lateral surfaces of the brain stem (Fig. 14-24). The nerve then passes around the cerebral peduncles to enter the cavernous sinus. It enters the orbit via the superior orbital fissure to innervate the superior oblique muscle.

PATHOPHYSIOLOGY. Lesions of the trochlear nerve cause weakness of the superior oblique muscle and result in diplopia on downward and inward gaze. The patient may, at times, compensate for this by tilting the head slightly to the opposite side. Isolated lesions of cranial nerve IV are uncommon (except after head trauma), and the nerve is most often involved along with nerves III, V, and VI by lesions in the cavernous sinus, superior orbital fissure, or orbit. The structure and function of the trochlear nerve are summarized in Table 14-12.

Oculomotor Nerve (Cranial Nerve III)

FUNCTION. The oculomotor nerve is a mixed motor nerve providing general somatic efferent (GSE) innervation to the following muscles of the eye: superior rectus, inferior rectus, medial rectus, inferior oblique, and the voluntary elevator of the eyelid (the levator palpebrae superioris). In addition, cranial nerve III supplies general visceral efferent (GVE)—parasympathetic—innervation to the pupil and ciliary muscle controlling the lens of the eye.

ANATOMY. The GSE fibers of cranial nerve III arise from the oculomotor nucleus, ventral to the aqueduct at the level of the superior colliculus (Fig. 14-25). Fibers pass ventrally through the tegmentum and base of the midbrain and emerge in the interpeduncular fossa.

The GVE fibers providing preganglionic parasympathetic innervation to the pupil arise in the Edinger-Westphal nuclei (a small group of neurons located at the rostral end of each oculomotor nucleus). Preganglionic fibers join with GSE fibers and, after emerging from the brain stem, pass through the cavernous sinus and superior orbital fissure to enter the orbit (Fig. 14-25). GSE fibers continue directly to innervate the muscles of the eye, while GVE fibers synapse in the ciliary ganglion, where postganglionic parasympathetic fibers arise and proceed to the pupilloconstrictor muscle of the iris and to the ciliary body.

PATHOPHYSIOLOGY. Lesions involving the GSE component of cranial nerve III produce weakness

Table 14-12. Structure and Function of the Trochlear Nerve

Component	Function	Nucleus of origin or termination	Ganglion	Foramen	Signs of dysfunction
GSE	Motor to superior oblique muscle	Trochlear nucleus on opposite side		Superior orbital fissure	Diplopia

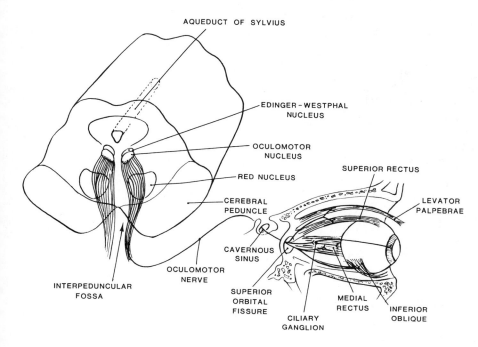

AQUEDUCT OF SYLVIUS

EDINGER-WESTPHAL NUCLEUS

OCULOMOTOR NUCLEUS

RED NUCLEUS

SUPERIOR RECTUS

LEVATOR PALPEBRAE

CEREBRAL PEDUNCLE

CAVERNOUS SINUS

OCULOMOTOR NERVE

INTERPEDUNCULAR FOSSA

SUPERIOR ORBITAL FISSURE

CILIARY GANGLION

MEDIAL RECTUS

INFERIOR OBLIQUE

Fig. 14-25. Oculomotor nerve. Cross section of upper midbrain with nucleus and course and distribution of axons to the eye.

of all voluntary eye muscles except the lateral rectus and superior oblique. Diplopia and ptosis (due to weakness of the levator palpebrae) are often present, and the eye is deviated downward and outward. Ptosis due to levator palpebrae weakness must be distinguished from ptosis due to lesions affecting the sympathetic innervation of the eye. The latter causes mild drooping of the lid from loss of innervation to the smooth muscle in the upper eyelid (Müller's muscle) and is associated with a small pupil. Diseases affecting the neuromuscular junction or muscle fibers of the levator palpebrae (for example, in myasthenia gravis and in ocular myopathy) also cause ptosis, but the pupil is normal.

Lesions involving the GVE component result in loss of parasympathetic innervation to the eye and produce mydriasis (pupillary dilation).

Observation of pupillary inequality (anisocoria) and testing of the pupillary light reflex are an integral part of the neurologic examination. The size of the pupil is influenced by many factors, primarily the intensity of light falling on the ret-

ina. The afferent pathway for the pupillary light reflex is conducted by cranial nerve II (optic) via the optic chiasm, optic tracts, and brachium of the superior colliculus to the pretectal region (Fig. 14-26). After synapse with the Edinger-Westphal nuclei, the pathway continues in cranial nerve III (oculomotor).

The normal pupil constricts briskly when light is focused on the ipsilateral retina (providing the reflex pathway is intact) and produces the direct light reflex. As a result of the semidecussation of fibers in the optic chiasm and in the pretectal region, the contralateral pupil also constricts (consensual light reflex). Unilateral lesions of the optic nerve generally do not produce anisocoria but alter both the direct and the consensual light reflexes when the involved eye is tested; these responses will be normal on testing the opposite eye.

Lesions that involve the parasympathetic innervation of the pupil result in ipsilateral mydriasis, a loss of the direct pupillary reflex, and the presence of a consensual reflex upon testing the involved eye. Shining a light in the opposite eye results in normal direct response but loss of the consensual reflex. Anisocoria occurs with lesions involving the sympathetic innervation of the pupil

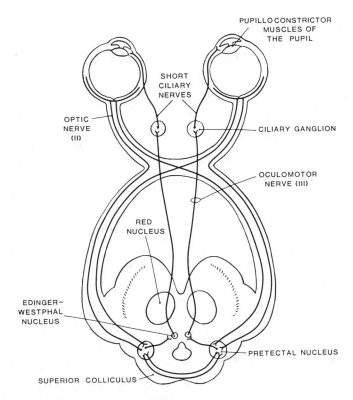

Fig. 14-26. Pathways for the pupillary light reflex with the afferent arc in the optic nerve and efferent arc in the oculomotor nerve.

(as in Horner's syndrome) and results in ipsilateral miosis with normal pupillary reflexes. The structure and function of the oculomotor nerve are summarized in Table 14-13.

The Cerebellum

The cerebellum represents the largest single structure in the posterior fossa. It is not part of the brain stem but lies dorsal to the pons and medulla and forms the roof of the fourth ventricle. Although the cerebellum is an embryonic derivative of the metencephalon (the rhombic lip and alar plate) and is an important structure for the integration of unconscious proprioception, its function is closely related to the motor system, and it forms the central structure in the cerebellar control circuit (see Chap. 9).

Gross Anatomy

The cerebellum is composed of two lateral lobes,

Table 14-13. Structure and Function of the Oculomotor Nerve

Component	Function	Nucleus of origin or termination	Ganglion	Foramen	Signs of dysfunction
GSE	Motor to medial rectus, superior rectus, inferior rectus, inferior oblique, and levator palpebrae	Oculomotor		Superior orbital fissure	Diplopia, ptosis
GVE	Parasympathetic pupilloconstrictor muscles, ciliary muscle	Edinger-Westphal	Ciliary	Superior orbital fissure	Mydriasis, loss of direct pupillary reflex, loss of lens accommodation

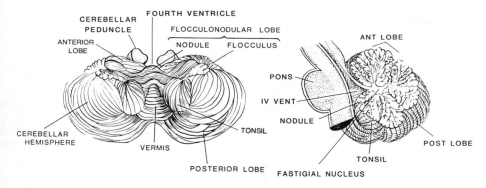

Fig. 14-27. Lobes of the cerebellum from the inferior surface.

the cerebellar hemispheres, and a midline portion called the vermis (Fig. 14-27). The cerebellum is also subdivided in the transverse plane into three lobes:

1. The flocculonodular lobe—the posterior vermis rolled into the caudal roof of the fourth ventricle is called the nodulus. The nodulus and the immediately adjacent flocculus on either side make up the flocculonodular lobe.
2. The anterior lobe—that portion of the vermis and cerebellar hemispheres located anterior to the primary fissure.
3. The posterior lobe—the remaining vermis and hemispheres.

There are also two inferomedial lobules on the posterior lobes of the hemispheres (the cerebellar tonsils), which are situated just above the foramen magnum.

Fig. 14-28. Afferent and efferent fibers in the cerebellar peduncles.

Functional Anatomy

Clinically, it is convenient to discuss the cerebellum in terms of its functional anatomy: (1) the anterior lobe and vermis receive spinocerebellar connections and are predominantly concerned with the muscle synergies involved in walking; (2) the flocculonodular lobe receives input from the vestibular system and is primarily concerned with the maintenance of equilibrium; and (3) the posterior lobes (the cerebellar hemispheres) receive the corticopontocerebellar connections and are involved with the coordination of ipsilateral voluntary limb movements.

The Cerebellar Peduncles

The cerebellum is connected to the brain stem by the three pairs of peduncles that contain afferent and efferent fibers carrying information to and from the cerebellum (Fig. 14-28).

The inferior cerebellar peduncle (restiform body) contains both afferent and efferent fibers and carries to the cerebellum most of the information that it receives from the spinal cord and medulla. The most important pathways going to

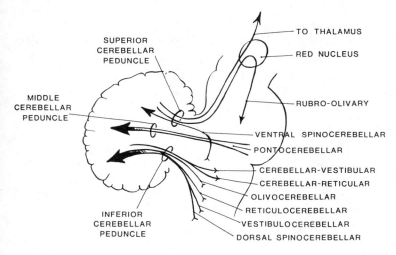

the cerebellum (afferent) via the restiform body include the dorsal spinocerebellar tract and cuneocerebellar pathway carrying unconscious proprioception, vestibulocerebellar pathways, reticulocerebellar pathways, and the olivocerebellar pathways (arising in the contralateral inferior olivary nucleus). The main efferent fibers of the restiform body include the cerebellovestibular and cerebelloreticular pathways.

The middle cerebellar peduncle (brachium pontis) contains only afferent fibers that originate in neurons in the contralateral pontine nuclei. These nuclei, in turn, receive innervation from the cerebral cortex via the corticopontine tracts. Thus, a crossed corticopontocerebellar pathway is established, whereby each cerebellar hemisphere can monitor the activity of the opposite cerebral hemisphere.

The superior cerebellar peduncle (brachium conjunctivum) contains both afferent and efferent fibers but represents the main outflow pathway of the cerebellum. Efferent fibers (originating primarily in the dentate nucleus) bound for the opposite red nucleus, thalamus, and inferior olive all leave via the superior cerebellar peduncle and cross the midline in the decussation of the brachium conjunctivum. This results in two additional loops (cortico-ponto-cerebello-dentato-rubro-thalamo-cortical pathway and the cerebello-dentato-rubro-olivo-cerebellar pathway), which allow the cerebellum to monitor activity in other areas of the nervous system. The afferent pathway of the brachium conjunctivum is the ventral spinocerebellar fibers.

Internal Anatomy

The internal structure of the cerebellum consists of a three-layered, highly convoluted cortex and an internal mass of white matter containing four

pairs of deep nuclei (dentate, emboliform, globose, and fastigial), which function as relay stations for efferent fibers originating in the cerebellar cortex (Fig. 14-29). The dentate is the largest of these nuclei and is situated in a lateral position; it receives fibers primarily from the posterior lobe. The emboliform and globose nuclei receive fibers from the anterior lobe, and the medially located fastigial nuclei receive fibers from the flocculonodular lobe.

The cortex of the cerebellum consists of the molecular, Purkinje cell, and granular cell layers (Fig. 14-30). The outermost (molecular) layer contains few cells (predominantly basket cells) and consists primarily of axons and dendrites. The middle layer consists of a single row of large goblet-shaped neurons, called *Purkinje cells*. The innermost (granular cell) layer is composed of densely packed small neurons called *granule cells*, which have scattered among them larger neurons called *Golgi cells*.

Afferent (incoming) fibers terminate either as mossy fibers or as climbing fibers. The mossy fibers, which constitute most cerebellar afferents, synapse with granule or Golgi cells. These cells, in turn, send processes into the molecular layer, where they synapse with Purkinje cell dendrites. The arborization of the Purkinje cell dendrites is at right angles to the dendrites of the Golgi cells and the parallel fibers of the granule cells in the molecular layer to provide spatial organization to cerebellar function.

Climbing fibers, which are the axons of the olivocerebellar pathway, synapse directly on Purkinje cells via an array of terminal axon branches that wind around and "climb" the Purkinje cell body and dendritic tree. The granular cell and the climbing fiber inputs to Purkinje cells are excitatory. Purkinje cells, in turn, send their axons to the deep cerebellar nuclei. The Purkinje cell–cerebellar nuclei synapses are inhibitory.

Fig. 14-29. Cerebellar nuclei in horizontal section.

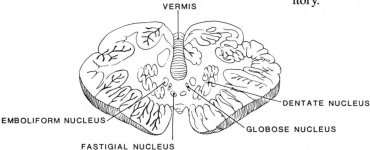

VERMIS

DENTATE NUCLEUS

EMBOLIFORM NUCLEUS

GLOBOSE NUCLEUS

FASTIGIAL NUCLEUS

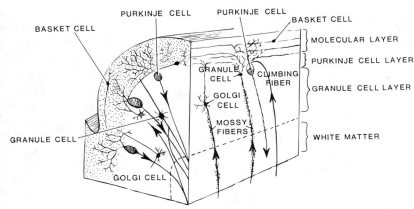

Fig. 14-30. Cell layers and connections of the cerebellar hemisphere.

Pathophysiology

As described in Chapter 9, disturbances of cerebellar function are manifest as a loss of balance and equilibrium or as a disorder in the modulation of the range, force, rate, and direction of movement. The flocculonodular lobe is primarily responsible for balance and equilibrium, and lesions involving this region of the cerebellum result in an inability to sit or stand without swaying or falling (truncal ataxia). The anterior lobe is primarily responsible for posture and coordination of gait; lesions involving this region of the cerebellum result in an unsteady and staggering gait (gait ataxia). The posterior lobe is primarily responsible for coordination of ipsilateral voluntary movements of the extremities; lesions involving this region of the cerebellum result in loss of motor coordination of the extremities, dysmetria, and, if the dentate nucleus or its outflow path, the brachium conjunctivum, is involved, intention tremor (limb ataxia).

New Systems in the Posterior Fossa Level

Besides the major longitudinal systems already discussed, three additional special systems (oculomotor, auditory, and vestibular) are found primarily at the posterior fossa level.

The Oculomotor System

The oculomotor system controls eye movements and is part of the motor system. Major components are located in the posterior fossa level, although, as with other efferent systems, the pathways for supranuclear control originate at the supratentorial level, and elements of the final common pathway are located at the peripheral level. Vision itself is exclusively a supratentorial function. The anatomy and physiology of the visual system will be discussed with that level in Chapter 15.

OVERVIEW. Movement of the eyes is accomplished by the action of cranial nuclei and nerves III, IV, and VI and the extraocular muscles. Most of the input to these nuclei is indirect, through the pontine paramedian reticular formation, which coordinates the activity of the lower motor neurons for both reflex and voluntary eye movements. Input to the pontine reticular formation for voluntary and pursuit movements comes via descending supranuclear pathways from the frontal and occipital cortex. Reflex movements are mediated by input from the vestibular nuclei via the medial longitudinal fasciculus and from the retina via the superior colliculus and pretectal region.

Lesions at the supratentorial, posterior fossa, and peripheral levels can result in oculomotor disorders: paresis of one or more extraocular muscles with diplopia, gaze paresis, nystagmus, or loss of conjugate movements.

PHYSIOLOGY. Eye movements subserve a number of different functions that utilize different neural mechanisms. *Saccadic* eye movements are rapid reflex movements that bring a visual image to the fovea. *Smooth pursuit* movements keep the fovea focused on a moving target. *Vergence* movements maintain the visual image on the fovea when objects move toward the eyes (convergence) or away (divergence). *Vestibular reflex* movements maintain a visual image on the fovea during movements of the head. Finally, *optokinetic* movements rapidly change the visual images on the fovea in a moving visual scene.

Each of these eye movements is mediated via the nuclei of cranial nerves III, IV, and VI and is coordinated through cells in the pontine paramedian reticular formation. The different pathways acting on the reticular formation to produce these movements have not been fully defined, but some anatomic differences in the control systems can be described.

ANATOMY.   The five major areas of oculomotor control are (1) the nuclei of the lower motor neurons of cranial nerves III, IV, and VI, described earlier in this chapter; (2) the pontine paramedian reticular formation; (3) the superior colliculus and pretectal region; (4) vestibular connections via the medial longitudinal fasciculus; and (5) the cortical eye fields.

The anatomy of the oculomotor, trochlear, and abducens nuclei and nerves forming the final common pathway for the oculomotor system has

Fig. 14-31. A. Attachment of eye muscles. B. Eye movement produced by each muscle. (Redrawn from A. B. Baker. Clinical Neurology [2nd ed.], Vol. 1. Hagerstown, Md.: Harper & Row, 1962.)

been described in this chapter. The eye muscles generally act in pairs, moving the eyes in the same direction simultaneously (conjugately). The six cardinal directions of gaze correspond to the direction of eye movement subserved by individual eye muscles (Fig. 14-31). Ocular movements are tested by having the patient look in the six cardinal directions (horizontally to the right and left, and up and down with the eyes looking right and left). A deficit in the function of any one muscle will impair movement of the eye in that direction. A lesion of one of the nerves will result in a deficit in each of the muscles innervated by that nerve (Table 14-14).

The *pontine paramedian reticular formation* is located between the abducens and the trochlear nuclei and receives input from all other areas concerned with eye movements, including the medial longitudinal fasciculus, the mesencephalic reticular formation, the superior colliculi, the pretectal region, and the cerebellum and the cortical eye fields. This region is made up of small groups of scattered nuclei whose cells show different patterns of firing with eye movements. Some cells fire tonically, others fire in bursts,

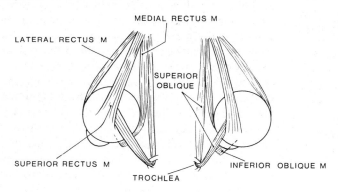

A

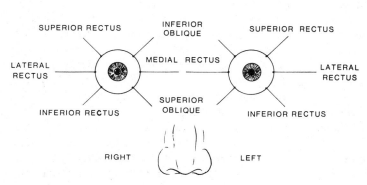

B

Table 14-14. Functions of the Ocular Nerves

Nerve	Muscles	Function (deviation of the eye)	Signs of dysfunction
III	Medial rectus	Medially	Eye is deviated down
	Superior rectus	Up and out	and out with complete
	Inferior rectus	Down and out	paralysis of nerve III
	Inferior oblique	Up and in	(usually associated with ptosis and mydriasis)
IV	Superior oblique	Down and in	Limitation of downward gaze when eye is looking medially, extorsion of eye
VI	Lateral rectus	Laterally	Eye is deviated medially

some pause, and others show complex patterns of firing. This area coordinates the input from multiple regions to produce the varied types of eye movements already outlined. It controls primarily horizontal movement, although vertical movements are also partially mediated there.

While eye movements usually need to be conjugate to maintain a visual image on the fovea of both eyes, if the object moves closer to the observer, the eyes need to converge (move together) to maintain the image on the fovea. *Convergence* is mediated by Perlia's nucleus, a small midline nucleus between the oculomotor nuclei which sends impulses to the neurons of both medial rectus muscles to produce simultaneous contraction and convergence. Two other reflexes normally accompany convergence: accommodation and miosis. Impulses from the nucleus of Perlia also travel to the Edinger-Westphal nuclei immediately medial to the oculomotor nuclei, which give rise to parasympathetic fibers traveling in nerve III to the ciliary ganglion. These fibers contract the ciliary muscle, which relaxes the tension on the lens and focuses the image closer. The parasympathetic activity also shortens the pupillary muscle fibers to constrict the pupil at the same time the convergence occurs.

The superior colliculus and immediately rostral pretectal region receive major input directly from the retina, with additional input from the cortical eye fields. Fibers from these regions connect with the mesencephalic and the pontine reticular formation, mediating eye movements. The superior colliculi mediate rapid fixation of the fovea to a target; the tectal region appears to be involved in control of vertical eye movements.

The vestibular nuclei provide major input to the oculomotor system to correct eye position and maintain a visual image on the fovea during head movement, the vestibuloocular reflex. Fibers from the superior and medial vestibular nuclei pass via the ipsilateral and contralateral medial longitudinal fasciculus, respectively, to the pontine reticular formation and the oculomotor nuclei (Fig. 14-32). The *medial longitudinal fasciculus* is a major component of the oculomotor system, coordinating the individual eye movements, vestibular input, and head position. It is located close to the midline just beneath the aqueduct of Sylvius and fourth ventricle and extends bilaterally from the upper end of the cervical spinal cord to the midbrain.

Activation of the vestibular nuclei results in compensatory eye movements, called *nystagmus*, which are asymmetric, with a slow movement in one direction and a faster corrective movement returning the eye to its original position. Vestibular nystagmus is mediated via the medial longitudinal fasciculus and may be horizontal, vertical, or rotatory.

There are two *cortical eye fields*, frontal and occipitoparietal (Fig. 14-33). The frontal eye field is located in the posterior portion of each middle frontal gyrus, Brodmann's area 8, and is responsible for the voluntary control of conjugate gaze. Fibers from this region project to the pontine reticular formation and the superior colliculus. Stimulation of the frontal eye field results in conjugate deviation of the eyes to the opposite side, and acute destruction results in conjugate deviation of the eyes toward the side of the lesion.

The occipitoparietal eye fields are located at the parietooccipital junction of each hemisphere, Brodmann's area 19, and are responsible for involuntary smooth pursuit, in which the eyes are fixed on an object and maintain visual fixation as

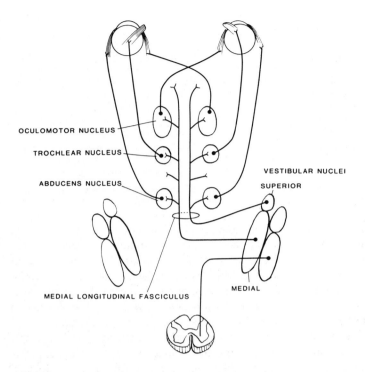

OCULOMOTOR NUCLEUS

TROCHLEAR NUCLEUS

ABDUCENS NUCLEUS

VESTIBULAR NUCLEI

SUPERIOR

MEDIAL

MEDIAL LONGITUDINAL FASCICULUS

Fig. 14-32. Medial longitudinal fasciculus and its connections with vestibular and ocular nuclei.

the object moves. Fibers from area 19 project to nuclei in the pretectal region and to the superior colliculus and from there to the reticular formation. The voluntary fixation on a visual target is broken when the target reaches the limit of the visual field. The eyes then make a quick conjugate movement in the opposite direction to fix on a new target. This movement is called *optokinetic nystagmus* and depends on an intact occipitoparietal eye field.

Fig. 14-33. Cortical eye fields. Areas 17 and 18 are primary visual cortex. Cortical gaze centers are in areas 8 and 19.

PATHOPHYSIOLOGY. Disturbances of ocular movement are important localizing signs in neurologic diagnosis. Lesions affecting the final common pathway occur at either the posterior fossa level (nucleus or nerve) or the peripheral level (nerve or muscle) and produce diplopia. The final common pathway can be damaged by lesions at the nucleus, nerve, neuromuscular junction, or extraocular muscle.

Diplopia, or double vision, occurs when the conjugate movement of the eyes is altered and the images no longer fall on corresponding areas of the two retinas. The brain interprets this as seeing two images instead of one (Fig. 14-34). Usually, the diplopia occurs secondary to a lesion affecting one (or more) of the ocular nerves or the

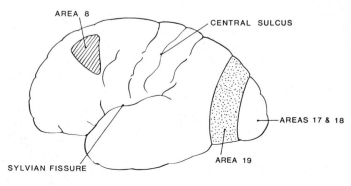

AREA 8

CENTRAL SULCUS

AREAS 17 & 18

AREA 19

SYLVIAN FISSURE

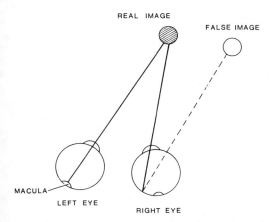

Fig. 14-34. Diplopia occurs when the images of one object fall on different parts of the two retinas. The brain interprets this as seeing two images. In this example, the right lateral rectus muscle is paretic, and the patient cannot rotate the right eye to the right. The image of the object falls on the nasal aspect of the retina of the right eye, and the brain interprets this as a second image (false image) to the right of the real image.

ocular muscles; the affected eye shows restricted movement in the field of the paralyzed muscle.

If diplopia is present when gaze is tested in the six cardinal directions, the two images will be seen maximally separated in the direction of gaze of the paretic muscle. In the position of maximal image separation, the image falling on the paretic eye will always be the more peripheral image. In a cooperative patient, the weak muscle can be determined by covering one eye and noting which image disappears, or by placing a colored lens in front of one eye and having the patient note the color of the peripheral image.

Lesions of the pontine reticular formation can cause paresis of conjugate gaze of both eyes to the side of the lesion or cause deviation of both eyes to the opposite side. Lesions of the pretectal region cause paresis of conjugate upward gaze (Parinaud's syndrome).

A lesion of the medial longitudinal fasciculus results in a syndrome of disconjugate eye movements called internuclear ophthalmoplegia, in which lateral gaze results in contraction of the lateral rectus but not the opposite medial rectus. In this syndrome, function of the medial rectus is intact, as demonstrated by normal convergence. This syndrome typically also has associated nystagmus.

Nystagmus is a common manifestation of dis-

ease in the vestibular system and is associated with lesions involving the labyrinth, vestibular nerve, vestibular nuclei, or vestibulo-cerebellar pathways. Destruction of the labyrinth or vestibular nerve on one side results in nystagmus with the slow component toward the injured side; an irritative lesion results in nystagmus with the slow component to the opposite side. Nystagmus may occur alone or in association with vertigo, the subjective sensation of rotation.

Acute supratentorial lesions involving the frontal eye fields produce loss of voluntary conjugate gaze to the opposite side or conjugate deviation of the eyes toward the side of the lesion. Focal motor seizures are associated with tonic deviation of the eyes to the opposite side. Destructive processes involving the occipitoparietal eye fields produce asymmetric responses on testing optokinetic nystagmus.

Generalized metabolic disorders can also affect the oculomotor system. Thiamine deficiency results in small hemorrhages in the mammillary bodies and around the third and fourth ventricles, which in turn cause diplopia, nystagmus, and ataxia, often with impairment of mentation. This combination is known as Wernicke's encephalopathy and is seen most commonly in alcoholic persons.

The Auditory System

The auditory system is located at the posterior fossa and supratentorial levels. The auditory structures transform mechanical energy (sound) into action potentials and relay them to the brain stem and cerebral cortex. Auditory information is used for alerting and communication.

OVERVIEW. Sound waves are transformed into electrical signals by the structures in the middle and the inner ear. Afferent impulses pass centrally via the acoustic division of cranial nerve VIII and ascend bilaterally to the superior temporal gyrus of the temporal lobe via the trapezoid body, lateral lemniscus, inferior colliculus, and medial geniculate bodies. Although lesions central to the cochlear nuclei result in some alteration in auditory function, unilateral loss of hearing is found only with lesions of cranial nerve VIII or the peripheral receptors.

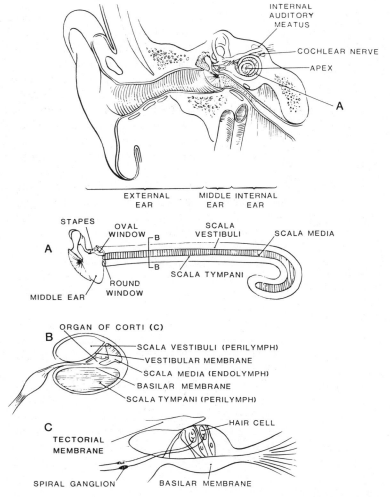

Fig. 14-35. Structures of the external, middle, and inner ear at top. A. Cochlea uncoiled and showing the three chambers. B. Cross section of cochlea (B-B in Fig. 14-35A) showing three chambers and basilar membrane. C. Close-up view of organ of Corti.

THE EAR. The receptors for the auditory and vestibular systems are found in the ear, which is subdivided into three major regions (Fig. 14-35): (1) the external ear, consisting of the pinna, which collects and directs sound waves through the external auditory meatus; (2) the middle ear or tympanic cavity, containing the tympanic membrane (eardrum) and the auditory ossicles, which convert sound waves to fluid motion; and (3) the inner ear, or labyrinth, a series of fluid-filled membranous channels in the petrous portion of the temporal bone. The membranous labyrinth duplicates the shape of the bony labyrinth and is divided into two channels: one containing endolymph and the other containing perilymph. The ionic compositions of these two fluids are different: Perilymph is similar to spinal fluid, whereas endolymph has a high potassium and low sodium content. The labyrinth is further subdivided into the cochlea, containing the receptors for sound, and the vestibule, consisting of the utricle, saccule, and three semicircular canals, with the receptors for head movement.

ANATOMY OF THE AUDITORY SYSTEM. The cochlea contains three parallel chambers coiled 2¾ turns into the shape of a helix (Fig. 14-35). The two outer chambers, the scala vestibuli and scala tympani, contain perilymph and are in continuity at the apex of the coil. The middle chamber, the

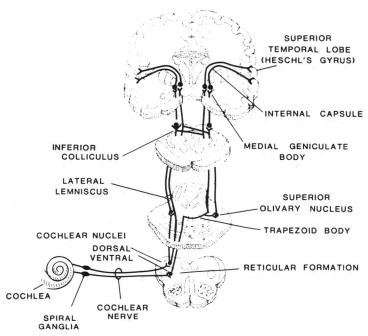

SUPERIOR
TEMPORAL LOBE
(HESCHL'S GYRUS)

INTERNAL CAPSULE

INFERIOR
COLLICULUS

MEDIAL GENICULATE
BODY

LATERAL
LEMNISCUS

SUPERIOR
OLIVARY NUCLEUS

TRAPEZOID BODY

COCHLEAR NUCLEI
DORSAL
VENTRAL

RETICULAR FORMATION

COCHLEA

COCHLEAR
NERVE

SPIRAL
GANGLIA

Fig. 14-36. Auditory pathways. Auditory impulses can ascend directly up the ipsilateral lateral lemniscus or synapse in the trapezoid body or superior olivary nucleus. They also may cross over to the opposite side and ascend in the contralateral lateral lemniscus. Fibers thus ascend bilaterally to the inferior colliculus, medial geniculate bodies, and auditory cortex.

scala media (also called the cochlear duct), contains endolymph.

The scala vestibuli and scala media are separated by the vestibular (Reissner's) membrane, and the scala tympani and scala media are separated by the basilar membrane. At the base of the cochlea, the scala vestibuli ends at the oval window, and the scala tympani ends at the round window. The organ of Corti lies on the surface of the basilar membrane and contains mechanically sensitive hair cells, the *auditory receptors*. These cells generate electrotonic potentials in response to movement of the basilar membrane produced by sound waves. The base of a hair cell is enmeshed in a network of cochlear nerve endings. These cochlear fibers emerge from the coils of the cochlea in the central axis of the coil and join the acoustic division of cranial nerve VIII. Cell bodies for these cochlear fibers are located in the spiral ganglion, the primary sensory ganglion for hearing, within the axis of the helix. Fibers pass-

ing centrally enter the brain stem and synapse in the dorsal and ventral cochlear nuclei (Fig. 14-36).

From the cochlear nuclei, second-order neurons travel via several pathways to the thalamus. Some fibers enter the reticular formation and participate in the alerting functions of the consciousness system. Some fibers ascend directly in the ipsilateral lateral lemniscus, while other fibers synapse in the nuclei of the trapezoid body or superior olivary nuclei located in the ventral tegmentum of the pons (Fig. 14-36). Many, but not all, of these fibers cross to the opposite side in the trapezoid body before they pass rostrally. Thus, there are auditory fibers conducting information from both ears in each lateral lemniscus. Some fibers synapse in the nucleus of the lateral lemniscus on their way to the inferior colliculus. At the inferior colliculus, some fibers again synapse and a few may pass to the opposite side. Fibers traveling via the brachium of the inferior colliculus terminate in the medial geniculate body of the thalamus, which gives rise to axons that pass via the sublenticular portion of the internal capsule to the auditory cortex of the superior temporal gyrus (Heschl's gyrus) (Fig. 14-36). Because of the partial decussation of auditory fibers, sound entering each ear is transmitted to both cerebral hemispheres.

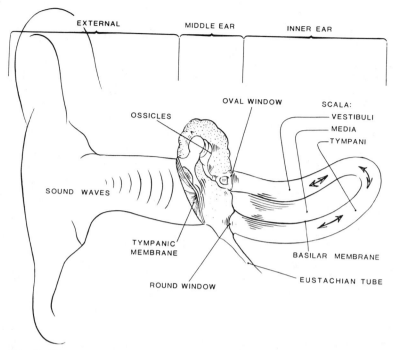

Fig. 14-37. Conversion of sound waves to movements of the basilar membrane.

PHYSIOLOGY OF AUDITION. The ear converts sound waves of the external environment into action potentials in the auditory nerves. Sound waves in the atmosphere move the tympanic membrane (Fig. 14-37). This movement is transmitted to the ossicles (malleus, incus, and stapes) of the middle ear, which amplify and transform the movements of the eardrum into smaller but more forceful motions of the footplate of the stapes resting against the oval window of the inner ear. The movement of the stapes against the oval window produces traveling waves in the perilymph of the scala vestibuli. At the apex of the cochlea, these waves pass into the scala tympani and are dissipated by movement of the round window. As the sound waves enter the perilymph of the scala vestibuli, they are also transmitted through the vestibular membrane into the endolymph of the scala media. This causes displacement of the basilar membrane, which stimulates the hair-cell receptors of the organ of Corti. The movement of the hair cells generates electrotonic potentials, which are converted into action potentials in the auditory nerve fibers.

From the stapes to the apex, the basilar membrane varies in width and tension, resulting in different portions of the membrane responding to different frequencies. The cochlea thereby mechanically separates the activation of different hair cells by different frequencies of sound.

PATHOPHYSIOLOGY. Patients with disease of the auditory division of cranial nerve VIII or its receptors complain of tinnitus (buzzing or ringing) or deafness (loss of hearing). These alterations can be important segmental signs in localizing a pathologic process in the posterior fossa level. Lesions within the central nervous system seldom produce significant alteration in hearing. Therefore, unilateral hearing loss most commonly indicates disease in the ipsilateral ear, in cranial nerve VIII or its nuclei. It is of primary importance to distinguish between the types of hearing deficit found in ear disease and in neural disease. Conduction deafness is due to disease of the external or middle ear, which prevents the sound waves from being transmitted to the cochlea. Sensorineural deafness is due to disease of the cochlea or the auditory nerve or its nuclei. This distinction can often be made with a tuning fork by performing the Weber and Rinné tests, as outlined in Table 14-15. Audiometric testing identifies the frequencies that are most impaired. Middle ear

Table 14-15. The Weber and Rinné Tests for Unilateral Deafness

Test	Method	Normal response	Conduction deafness	Sensorineural deafness
Weber	Base of vibrating tuning fork placed on vertex of skull	Heard equally in both ears (or center of the head)	Sound louder in abnormal ear	Sound louder in normal ear
Rinné	Each ear is tested separately—base of vibrating tuning fork is placed on the mastoid region until subject no longer hears sound (bone conduction), then held in air next to the ear (air conduction)	Air conduction is better than bone conduction	Bone conduction is better than air conduction in involved ear	Air conduction is better than bone conduction in involved ear

disease is associated with low-frequency loss, and nerve damage is associated with high-frequency loss.

Patients with lesions central to the cochlear nuclei do not complain of hearing loss. Although bilateral lesions of the inferior colliculi, medial geniculate bodies, or superficial temporal gyri

Fig. 14-38. Normal brain-stem auditory evoked potentials in a 26-year-old man. Top segment represents the response of the left ear; bottom segment represents the response of the right ear. (The responses represent an average of 2,048 samples.) (Cz = central vertex area; A1 = left ear; A2 = right ear.)

produce hearing loss, examples of these are so rare as to be of no practical clinical importance. Unilateral lesions in the region of the auditory receptive areas of the cerebral cortex do not cause hearing loss, but they produce a deficit in sound localization or discrimination. Focal seizures involving the cortical auditory receptive areas in the temporal lobe produce hallucinations of sound. Electrical potentials evoked by click stimuli (named brain-stem auditory evoked potentials) can be recorded on the scalp from the nuclei along the auditory pathway (Fig. 14-38). Abnormalities in these potentials can identify and localize lesions in this system.

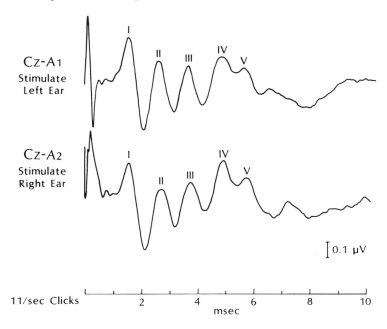

The Vestibular System

The vestibular structures provide the nervous system with information concerning gravity, rotation, and acceleration (which is necessary for the maintenance of balance and equilibrium) and are located primarily at the posterior fossa level.

OVERVIEW. Receptors adapted to detect gravitational pull, rotational movements, and acceleration are located in the utricle, saccule, and semicircular canals of the inner ear. These receptors transmit information about head movement to the central nervous system via the vestibular division of cranial nerve VIII. Numerous connections exist between the vestibular nuclei and the cerebellum, spinal cord, reticular formation, medial longitudinal fasciculus, and cerebral cortex, to allow integration of vestibular impulses with other sensory information for normal balance and equilibrium. Lesions affecting the vestibular structures result in a sense of imbalance (disequilibrium). Vertigo, a highly specific symptom of vestibular system dysfunction, is often accompanied by severe visceral disturbances: nausea, vomiting, tachycardia, and sweating. Nystagmus

Fig. 14-39. Vestibular receptors. A. Nerve supply to vestibular receptors (utricle, saccule, and semicircular canals). B. Macula of utricle and saccule. C. Ampulla of semicircular canals.

also occurs with lesions of the vestibular system or its connections.

ANATOMY AND PHYSIOLOGY. The receptors for the vestibular system are enclosed in the vestibular portion of the labyrinth in the utricle, the saccule, and the three semicircular canals (Fig. 14-39). The receptors are hair cells that respond to mechanical movement and initiate impulses that are transmitted via the vestibular division of cranial nerve VIII to the vestibular nuclei in the medulla and pons (see Fig. 14-17). The cell bodies for the primary sensory neurons are in the vestibular ganglion located within the internal auditory meatus. Movement of the hair cells produces local generator potentials that increase or decrease the frequency of action potentials in the nerve. The hair cells in the utricle and saccule respond to positional or gravitational change, while those in the semicircular canals respond to rotational or angular acceleration.

The utricle and saccule contain endolymph; in their walls are specialized areas of epithelium called *maculae* (Fig. 14-39B). The macula is a tuft of ciliated columnar epithelial cells embedded in a gelatinous matrix containing small calcified particles (otoliths). When the head is tilted from a vertical position, gravitational pull on the otoliths distorts the hair cells and initiates action potentials in the vestibular nerve. The three semi-

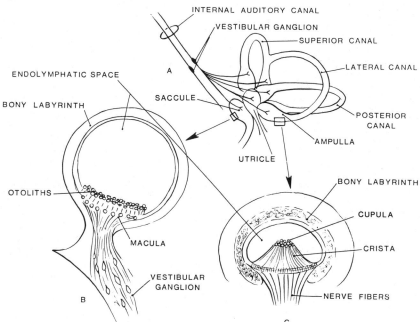

circular canals monitor acceleration in any plane. At one end of each canal, there is an enlargement, the *ampulla* (Fig. 14-39A). The ampulla contains a specialized region of epithelium (much like the maculae of the saccule and utricle) located in a transverse ridge projecting into the lumen, known as *cristae* (Fig. 14-39C). During rotational movement, the endolymph of the semicircular canals moves and distorts the cristae, thus stimulating the hair cells and initiating action potentials. Each of the three semicircular canals lies in a different plane, and each is thereby sensitive to rotation about a different axis.

Fibers of the vestibular division of cranial nerve VIII synapse in the superior, medial, lateral, and inferior vestibular nuclei located near the floor of the fourth ventricle. The vestibular nuclei have connections with several areas of the nervous system. Some fibers of the vestibular nerve pass directly to the cerebellum via the inferior cerebellar peduncle; others synapse in the inferior and medial vestibular nuclei prior to entering the cerebellum and terminating in the flocculonodular lobe. The flocculonodular lobe, in turn, sends fibers via the fastigial nucleus to the lateral vestibular nuclei, the origin of the vestibulospinal tracts, to regulate muscle tone in response to changing position. All of the vestibular nuclei send fibers to the reticular formation which can modify the activity in the visceral and consciousness systems. The medial longitudinal fasciculus receives fibers from the vestibular nuclei that coordinate head and eye movements (see Fig. 14-32). Pathways ascending to the cerebral cortex are not clearly defined; however, vestibular function is represented at the cortical level in the temporal lobes.

PATHOPHYSIOLOGY. There is continuous, balanced afferent input from the vestibular apparatus on each side. When the receptor activity is altered by motion, the afferent impulses change and a subjective sensation of motion is produced. When sensations of motion are in harmony with other sensory input, they are perceived as a correct response to a changing environment. When a lesion renders one portion of the vestibular system either hypoactive or hyperactive, the centrally integrated afferent impulses are not in accord with other sensory stimuli, and a sensation of disequilibrium is experienced. Dizziness, light-headedness, giddiness, and wooziness are common but nonspecific examples of disequilibrium and are frequently not associated with disease of the vestibular system. However, *vertigo,* the hallucination of rotatory movement, is a highly specific form of disequilibrium suggestive of disease involving the vestibular system. Vertigo is, on rare occasions, a manifestation of focal seizures involving the temporal lobe; it is, however, most often a manifestation of disease involving the peripheral receptors, vestibular nerve, or brain stem, and thus usually represents an important neurologic symptom of disease at the posterior fossa level or in the ear. The central stimulation accompanying the sensation of vertigo produces changes in other systems, with nausea, vomiting, ataxia, and nystagmus.

The function of the vestibular system is tested by using caloric stimulation and by testing the oculocephalic reflexes. In caloric testing, the outer canal of each ear is irrigated with either warm or cold water. The temperature gradient of the water causes convection currents and movement of the endolymph within the semicircular canals. This results in nystagmus if the labyrinth, vestibular nerves, medial longitudinal fasciculus, and oculomotor system in the brain stem are intact. Quantitative electrical measures of the direction and amplitude of the eye movements with nystagmus produced by caloric testing are used in electronystagmography to help define the location and severity of vestibular lesions. The oculocephalic (doll's eye) reflexes are tested by rapidly turning the head from side to side or up and down. This results in stimulation of the semicircular canals and movement of the eyes in the opposite direction. Clinical caloric testing and doll's eye movements are commonly employed to test the integrity of these brain-stem pathways in patients with altered states of consciousness and, when abnormal, are helpful in localizing the responsible lesion to the posterior fossa level.

Clinical Correlations

Lesions that involve the posterior fossa level are associated with abnormalities in cranial nerve, cerebellar, or brain-stem function. Because components of each of the major longitudinal systems are found at this level, dysfunction in any of these systems may be present. Lesions in all etiologic categories are found at this level, and the pathologic nature of these lesions can be determined, as at other levels, by applying the general principles of neurologic diagnosis outlined in Chapter 4. In this section, the clinical correlates of ischemic lesions and certain types of neoplasms, which are relatively common at this level, will be discussed, as well as the effects of expanding supratentorial mass lesions that may secondarily involve the posterior fossa level (herniations of the brain).

Ischemic Lesions of the Brain Stem

The blood supply of the brain stem is derived from the vertebrobasilar arterial system. The pattern of supply to each level is relatively constant, with the midline region being supplied by small penetrating paramedian branches of the vertebral and basilar arteries and the lateral area being supplied by larger circumferential branches: the posterior inferior cerebellar artery at the level of the medulla, the anterior inferior cerebellar artery at the level of the pons, and the superior cerebellar artery at the level of the midbrain. Ischemic le-

Fig. 14-40. A. Paramedian infarct of medulla. B. Lateral medullary infarct of medulla (Wallenberg's syndrome).

sions involving the brain stem usually occur either in the paramedian region or in the lateral region. Infarction of the paramedian region involves the descending motor pathways, medial lemniscus, and the nuclei of cranial nerves III, IV, VI, and XII. Infarction of the lateral region involves the cerebellum, cerebellar pathways, descending sympathetic pathways, the lateral spinothalamic tract, and the nuclei of cranial nerves V, VII, VIII, IX, or X.

VASCULAR LESIONS OF THE MEDULLA.   The paramedian region of the medulla is supplied by vessels from the anterior spinal and vertebral arteries. An infarction in the paramedian medulla involves the medullary pyramids, medial lemniscus, and cranial nerve XII, resulting in contralateral hemiparesis, impaired conscious proprioceptive sensation, and ipsilateral tongue weakness (Fig. 14-40).

The lateral regions of the medulla and portions of the cerebellum are supplied by the long, circumferential, posterior inferior cerebellar artery. Occlusion or thrombosis of this artery (or its parent vertebral artery) produces infarction of the lateral medulla and results in a constellation of signs and symptoms referred to as *Wallenberg's*

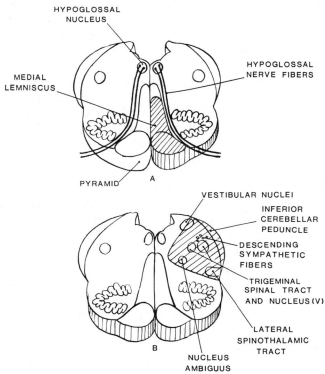

syndrome (Fig. 14-40). This syndrome includes dysarthria and dysphagia due to involvement of the nucleus ambiguus; ipsilateral impairment of pain and temperature on the face due to involvement of the descending nucleus and tract of nerve V; contralateral loss of pain and temperature in the trunk and extremities due to involvement of the spinothalamic tract; an ipsilateral Horner's syndrome due to involvement of the descending sympathetic fibers in the lateral part of the brain stem; ipsilateral limb ataxia due to involvement of the inferior cerebellar peduncle; and vertigo, which is due to involvement of the vestibular nuclei or vestibulocerebellar fibers located in the tegmentum of the medulla.

VASCULAR LESIONS OF THE PONS. An infarct of the paramedian area of the pons results in ipsilateral sixth nerve palsy due to involvement of the nucleus of nerve VI, ipsilateral facial weakness secondary to involvement of the facial nerve as it passes around the abducens nucleus, contralateral hemiparesis due to involvement of the corticospinal tracts in the basis pontis, and a contralateral impairment of conscious proprioception secondary to involvement of the medial lemniscus (Fig. 14-41).

An infarct of the lateral portion of the pons results in ipsilateral facial paralysis secondary to

involvement of the facial nucleus; impairment of touch, pain, and temperature on the same side of the face secondary to involvement of the main sensory nucleus and tract of cranial nerve V; loss of pain and temperature on the contralateral side of the body due to involvement of the lateral spinothalamic tract; ipsilateral deafness due to involvement of the nuclei of nerve VIII; ipsilateral Horner's syndrome secondary to involvement of the descending sympathetic fibers; and ipsilateral cerebellar signs secondary to involvement of the middle cerebellar peduncle.

VASCULAR LESIONS OF THE MIDBRAIN. Infarction of the lateral midbrain is uncommon; however, ischemic lesions involving the paramedian region (Fig. 14-42) are occasionally seen and produce diplopia, ptosis, and mydriasis due to involvement of cranial nerve III and a contralateral hemiparesis secondary to involvement of the cerebral peduncle. This constellation of symptoms is called *Weber's syndrome.*

Neoplasms of the Posterior Fossa

Certain tumors of the posterior fossa are more commonly encountered in children and young adults. Ependymomas and medulloblastomas frequently arise in the region of the fourth ventricle and are associated with ataxia, nausea, and vomiting. As these lesions increase in size, they obstruct the outflow of cerebrospinal fluid from the ventricular system and result in a noncommunicating hydrocephalus and signs of increased intra-

Fig. 14-41. Paramedian infarct of pons (shaded area) with involvement of VI nerve nucleus, facial nerve, medial lemniscus, and corticospinal tract.

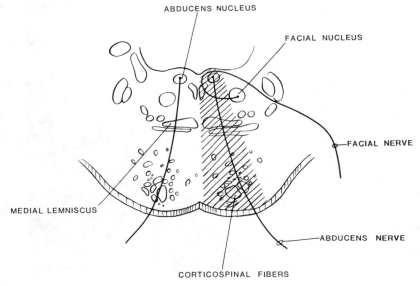

ABDUCENS NUCLEUS

FACIAL NUCLEUS

FACIAL NERVE

MEDIAL LEMNISCUS

ABDUCENS NERVE

CORTICOSPINAL FIBERS

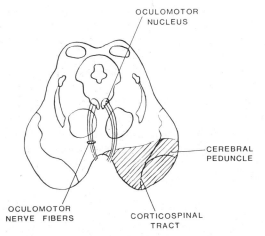

OCULOMOTOR
NUCLEUS

CEREBRAL
PEDUNCLE

OCULOMOTOR
NERVE FIBERS

CORTICOSPINAL
TRACT

Fig. 14-42. Paramedian infarct of midbrain—Weber's syndrome (shaded area). Involvement of nerve III and cerebral peduncle.

cranial pressure. Astrocytomas of the cerebellum also are common in childhood; they arise within the cerebellar hemisphere (resulting in ipsilateral limb ataxia). These tumors, which are frequently cystic in structure, display a unique biologic behavior; the early diagnosis and surgical removal of cerebellar astrocytomas, in contrast to astrocy-

Fig. 14-43. Gross specimen of brain-stem glioma. Transverse section showing diffuse asymmetric enlargement.

tomas of other locations, are associated with a good prognosis.

Astrocytomas also arise from glial cells located within the substance of the brain stem to result in a brain-stem or pontine glioma (Fig. 14-43). These tumors, which involve either the base or the tegmentum, are usually associated with progressive (often bilateral) symptoms of cranial nerve, motor, and sensory dysfunction. If the reticular formation is affected, consciousness is altered.

Certain tumors arise from outside the parenchyma of the brain stem (extraaxial tumors), often from the meninges (meningiomas) or from the supporting cells found in the cranial nerves. Extraaxial tumors initially produce alteration in cranial nerve function and secondarily affect brain-stem function by compression or direct invasion. The most common tumor of this group, an acoustic neuroma (schwannoma, cerebellopontine angle tumor), arises in the cerebellopontine angle from the Schwann cells of cranial nerve VIII (Fig. 14-44). Early signs of an acoustic neuroma are unilateral tinnitus, decreased hearing, and disequilibrium. As the tumor enlarges, there is erosion of the internal auditory meatus which can be seen on roentgenograms of the skull, ipsilateral facial paresis, loss of the corneal reflex, and ipsilateral limb ataxia. With further increase in size, signs of brain-stem compression and increased intracranial pressure are present.

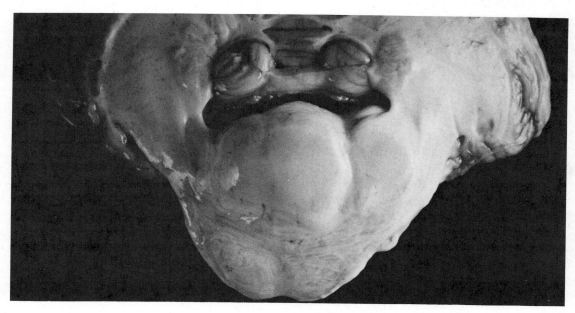

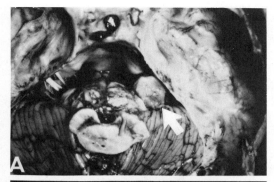

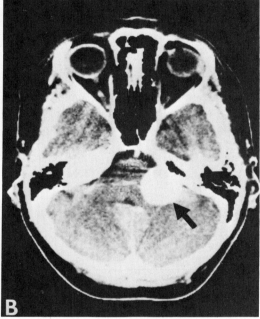

Fig. 14-44. Acoustic neuroma. A. Gross specimen with posterior fossa and contents viewed from above with tumor (arrow) of cranial nerve VIII. (Note normal cranial nerves VII and VIII on the opposite side.) B. Computed tomographic scan of posterior fossa at the level of the pons showing tumor in cerebellopontine angle compressing pons.

Herniations of the Brain

Expanding supratentorial mass lesions may secondarily affect the structures located in the posterior fossa. The cranial cavity is a closed space and cannot accommodate to changes in intracranial volume. In the presence of a supratentorial or posterior fossa mass, intracranial pressure increases, and with further expansion, the brain adjusts to the increased volume by compression and slight shifts in position. With further compression and shift, the function in areas of the nervous system remote from the expanding mass is also compromised, and further deterioration in clinical condition occurs. The changes in shape and position that occur secondary to intracranial mass lesions are called *herniations of the brain*.

UNCAL HERNIATION. Uncal herniation characteristically occurs when unilateral, expanding supratentorial lesions, especially in the middle fossa, shift the inner basal edge of the uncus of the hippocampal gyrus toward the midline and over the lateral edge of the tentorium, compressing the adjacent midbrain (Fig. 14-45A and Table 14-16). Cranial nerve III and sometimes the posterior cerebral artery on the side of the expanding temporal lobe are compressed by the overhanging swollen uncus. The clinical sign resulting from compression of cranial nerve III is an ipsilateral third-nerve paresis, usually beginning with dilatation of the pupil. Compression of the contralateral cerebral peduncle against the free edge of the tentorium can result in a hemiparesis ipsilateral to the expanding lesion. Midbrain compression also affects the ascending reticular activating system, and there is progressive loss of consciousness. If the posterior cerebral artery is compressed, infarction of the occipital lobe occurs and results in a homonymous hemianopia.

CENTRAL OR TRANSTENTORIAL HERNIATION. This type of herniation occurs as a further progression of uncal herniation and in association with parasagittal or bilateral supratentorial masses. It consists of a caudal displacement of the diencephalon, midbrain, and pons (Fig. 14-45B and Table 14-16). Caudal displacement of the basilar artery (which is attached to the circle of Willis via the posterior cerebral arteries) does not occur to the same degree, resulting in stretching and shearing of paramedian perforating vessels, with secondary infarction and hemorrhage in the brain stem. This type of herniation blocks the flow of cerebrospinal fluid through the aqueduct of Sylvius, thus further increasing the volume of the supratentorial contents. The clinical signs of central herniation are oculomotor paresis, progressive alteration of consciousness, and decerebrate rigidity.

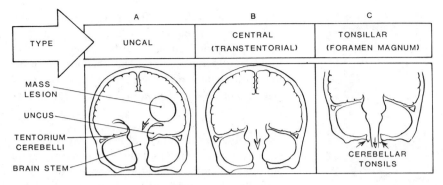

Fig. 14-45. Herniations of the brain. A. Uncal hernia-tion. B. Central (transtentorial) herniation. C. Tonsil-lar (foramen magnum) herniation. (Redrawn from F. Plum and J. B. Posner. The Diagnosis of Stupor and Coma *[2nd ed.]. Philadelphia: Davis, 1972.)*

TONSILLAR OR FORAMEN MAGNUM HERNIATION. As a result of an expanding mass in the posterior fossa, or further progression of uncal or transten-torial herniation, herniation of the cerebellar ton-sils through the foramen magnum occurs, with compression of the medulla (Fig. 14-45C and Ta-ble 14-16). Signs of tonsillar herniation include neck pain and stiffness, the result of stretching and irritation of the lower cranial nerves supply-ing the neck muscles; progressive loss of con-sciousness secondary to involvement of the ascending reticular activating system; generalized flaccidity; alteration of vital signs, with slowing of the pulse and vasomotor instability; and peri-odic or irregular respiration, the result of involve-ment of visceral centers in the medulla.

The three types of herniation of the brain are summarized in Figure 14-45 and Table 14-16.

Table 14-16. Herniations of the Brain

Type	Location	Cause	Anatomic structures involved	Clinical effects
Uncal	Tentorial notch, midbrain	Mass lesion in temporal lobe or middle fossa	Hippocampal gyrus and uncus Oculomotor nerve Cerebral peduncle Midbrain ascend-ing reticular ac-tivating system Posterior cerebral artery	Paresis of nerve III Hemiparesis Coma Homonymous hemianopia
Central (transtentorial)	Tentorial notch, midbrain	Mass lesion in frontal, parietal, or occipital lobe Progression of uncal hernia-tion	Midbrain and pons Ascending reticular activating system	Decerebrate rigid-ity Coma
Tonsillar (foramen mag-num)	Foramen magnum, medulla	Mass lesion in posterior fossa Progression of uncal or trans-tentorial herniation	Cerebellar tonsils Indirect activation pathways Ascending reticular activating system Vasomotor centers	Neck pain and stiff-ness Flaccidity Coma Alteration of pulse, respiration, blood pressure

Neurologic Examination of the Posterior Fossa Level

The integrity of the posterior fossa is examined by testing the function of each of the major longitudinal systems found at this level (see Chaps. 6 through 11) and the functions associated with the oculomotor, auditory, and vestibular systems and cranial nerves III through XII.

The Oculomotor System and Cranial Nerves III, IV, and VI

It is customary to begin by observing the eyes at rest. The presence of ptosis, conjugate deviation, or any extraocular muscle imbalance is noted. Ocular movements are tested by having the patient turn his eyes in the six cardinal directions of gaze. The medial and lateral rectus muscles are tested by having the patient first look to one side and then to the other. The patient, while looking to one side, is instructed to look up and down. In this position, the out-turning eye is elevated and depressed by the superior and inferior rectus muscles, respectively, and the in-turning eye by the inferior and superior oblique muscles, respectively. The procedure is repeated with the patient looking in the opposite direction. The presence of extraocular weakness or subjective diplopia is recorded. At this point, nystagmus also should be tested by having the patient follow the examiner's finger from one extreme of gaze to the other in both the horizontal and vertical planes, while observing for rapid to-and-fro movements of the eyes. A few low-amplitude jerks at the extremes of lateral gaze are not uncommon in normal subjects.

Pupillary size and shape are noted, and the pupillary light reflex is tested by shining a light into each eye individually, while observing the direct and consensual pupillary responses. The convergence (accommodation) reflex is tested by asking the patient to shift gaze from a distant object to the examiner's finger, held a few inches in front of the patient's nose. Convergence is normally accompanied by bilateral pupillary constriction.

Cranial Nerve V

Sensory function is examined by testing the patient's ability to perceive pinprick and light touch applied to the skin supplied by the three divisions of the trigeminal nerve. The corneal reflex (which also involves cranial nerve VII) is tested by asking the patient to look to one side while the cornea is gently touched with a wisp of cotton, brought toward the cornea from the opposite direction. The normal response is prompt, bilateral blinking.

Motor function is tested by having the patient open the jaw. In the presence of unilateral pterygoid weakness, there is deviation of the jaw to the weak side. The patient is also asked to bite firmly while the examiner palpates the masseter and temporalis muscles on each side. Jaw jerk is tested by placing the examiner's forefinger on the relaxed jaw and by striking the finger with a reflex hammer.

Cranial Nerve VII

The examination of the facial nerve begins with the initial observation of the patient. As the patient talks and smiles, facial asymmetry or reduced contraction becomes apparent. Specific muscle groups are then examined. The frontalis muscles are tested by asking the patient to wrinkle his forehead, and strength can be assessed by attempting to smooth the wrinkles on each side. The orbicularis oculi can be tested by asking the patient to close his eyes tightly and then try to open them. The lower facial muscles are tested by asking the patient to smile or show his teeth. Taste is not examined unless a peripheral facial nerve lesion is suspected. It is tested by having the patient protrude his tongue and then asking him to identify sugar, salt, or other substances applied to the side of the tongue.

The Auditory and Vestibular Systems and Cranial Nerve VIII

Audiometry provides the best means of examining hearing, but a rough estimate of the functioning of the acoustic system can be made by determining if the patient can hear the sound of a watch or the sound produced by rubbing the forefinger and thumb together in front of the ear. Auditory acuity of one side is compared with the acuity of the other. The Weber and Rinné tests should be performed (see Table 14-15).

Vestibular function is ordinarily not examined unless disease of cranial nerve VIII, sensory ataxia, or brain-stem disease is suspected. Caloric testing (irrigating the outer ear canal with cold water and observing for nystagmus, conjugate deviation of the eyes, or subjective vertigo) is a convenient means of testing vestibular function, but usually is reserved for comatose patients.

Cranial Nerves IX and X

The glossopharyngeal and vagus nerves are often tested together by listening to the patient talk and inquiring about difficulty in speaking or swallowing. A soft, breathy voice associated with nasal escape of air is suggestive of weakness in the oropharynx, while a hoarse or husky voice suggests a lesion of the nerve supply to the larynx. The patient is also asked to open his mouth and say "ah." Normally, the palate will rise in the midline; unilateral palatal weakness will cause the uvula to deviate toward the intact side. The gag reflex is examined by touching the back of the throat with a tongue blade and noting the contraction of pharyngeal muscles.

Cranial Nerve XI

The sternocleidomastoid muscle is tested by asking the patient to turn his head to the side, against resistance applied by the examiner to the patient's jaw. The contracting muscle (on the side opposite the turn of the head) can be observed and palpated. The trapezius muscle is examined by having the patient elevate his shoulders against resistance applied by the examiner.

Cranial Nerve XII

The patient is asked to protrude his tongue in the midline and then to wiggle it from side to side. With upper motor neuron lesions, there is slowing of the alternate motion rate of the tongue. With unilateral lower motor neuron weakness, there are ipsilateral atrophy and fasciculations, and the protruded tongue deviates toward the side of the lesion.

Speech

Verbal communication includes both cognitive and motor skills. The cognitive aspects of verbal communication are considered language and are described in Chapter 15. Some motor speech disorders may result from disease of the brain stem and cranial nerves (flaccid dysarthria) or cerebellum (ataxic dysarthria). Spastic, hypokinetic, and hyperkinetic dysarthrias result from disease at the supratentorial level.

Tests for disorders of speech, the dysarthrias,

are commonly administered at the same time as the testing of cranial nerve function. Speech can be evaluated by listening to spontaneous speech or by having the patient repeat the syllables *pa-pa-pa* (facial muscle and nerve function), *ta-ta-ta* (tongue and hypoglossal nerve function), and *ka-ka-ka* (pharyngeal muscle and ninth and tenth nerve function). The syllables *pa-ta-ka-pa-ta-ka* test cranial muscle coordination (cerebellar function).

Objectives

1. Name and identify the nuclei and peripheral portions of cranial nerves III through XII. Describe their functions, clinical examination, and the signs and symptoms which indicate their dysfunction.
2. Identify the major anatomic features of the medulla, pons, midbrain, and cerebellum as described in the text, and state their function.
3. Outline the physiologic and anatomic features of the auditory and vestibular systems, and identify the signs and symptoms of their dysfunction.
4. Describe the actions of the ocular muscles, the significance of diplopia, the anatomy of the pupillary light reflex, and the significance of nystagmus, the oculocephalic reflex (doll's eye phenomenon), and ptosis.
5. List the major herniations of the brain, and briefly describe their mechanisms of symptom production.

Clinical Problems

1. A 68-year-old woman, previously in good health, suddenly became extremely nauseated and dizzy—as if the room were spinning around her. She remained conscious and could describe her symptoms to a companion, who noted that her voice was hoarse. Examination in the emergency room several hours later revealed the following abnormalities: The patient could not sit or stand because of vertigo. She was anxious and perspiring, except on the left side of her face. Her left pupil was small, and her left eyelid drooped slightly. There was horizontal and rotatory nystagmus. The left palate was drooping, and the left gag reflex was absent. There was loss of pain and temperature sensation on the left side of her face. Touch

was preserved. Muscle strength and stretch reflexes were normal in the extremities. There was moderate incoordination of her left arm and leg. Sensory examination revealed loss of pain and temperature sensation in her right arm, trunk, and leg.

   a. What is the location and type of pathology?
   b. Specifically, what is the site of the lesion?
   c. What artery supplies the involved area?
   d. What anatomic structures are responsible for the loss of pain and temperature sensation on the left side of the face and on the right side of the trunk?
   e. What is the cause of the ptosis, miosis, and anhidrosis on the left?

2. A 50-year-old man was well until 6 months ago when he noted some difficulty in swallowing. Food seemed to "stick" in the right side of his throat, and liquids occasionally entered the right side of his nose. In the past 3 months, he had noted a progressive hoarseness of his voice and difficulty in reaching overhead with his right arm. Examination revealed that the soft palate sagged on the right side. When the left posterior pharynx was stimulated, the soft palate pulled upward and to the left. When the right side was similarly stimulated, nothing happened and the patient said he could barely feel the touch. Indirect laryngoscopy revealed that the right vocal cord did not move with phonation. Muscle testing revealed weakness and atrophy of the right trapezius and sternocleidomastoid muscles. Results of the remainder of the examination were normal.

   a. What is the location and type of lesion?
   b. What neural structures are involved?
   c. Through what foramen do these structures leave the skull?
   d. What other structure also passes through this foramen?
   e. Name one lesion that can produce the above syndrome.

3. A 70-year-old woman had a sudden onset of weakness of her right arm and leg and difficulty in moving her tongue. When seen in the emergency room a few hours later, she had weakness of her right arm and leg and decreased ability to perceive proprioceptive and tactile stimuli on the right. When her tongue was protruded, it deviated to the left.

   a. What is the location and type of lesion?
   b. What structures are involved?
   c. What is the pathologic nature of the lesion?

4. A 25-year-old man awoke one morning and noted that the left side of his face seemed weak. On looking into a mirror, he noted that he could not retract the left corner of his mouth as well as the right. He also noted that he could no longer close his left eye completely or smile with the left side of his face. A neurologic examination revealed no abnormality except for the following: At rest, the left side of his face drooped and the left palpebral fissure was wider than the right. The left side of his forehead did not wrinkle when he tried raising his eyebrows. He could not close his left eye completely. When he attempted to show his teeth, his mouth pulled to the right. Testing of sensations of pain, temperature, and touch of the face was normal. Taste was absent on the left side of his tongue. Strips of filter paper were placed in the conjunctival sacs; the one on the right became moist within a few minutes and the left side remained dry.

   a. What is the location and type of lesion?
   b. Why was taste involved?
   c. Why was there decreased lacrimation?
   d. What is the name of this clinical entity?

5. A 60-year-old woman had ringing (tinnitus) of her right ear for the past year, as well as intermittent episodes of feeling that the room was spinning around her. In the past 6 months, she began staggering to the right and had difficulty with coordination of her right hand. Three weeks ago, she noted that the right side of her face was weak. Examination revealed a loss of hearing and an absent caloric response on the right. She could not wrinkle her forehead or retract the right side of her face when asked to smile. She had trouble with coordination in her right hand and had an intention tremor on finger-to-nose and heel-to-shin testing of the right upper and lower extremities.

   a. What is the location and type of lesion?
   b. What specific anatomic structures are involved?
   c. What is the general anatomic term used

to describe the region of involvement?

d. Name one pathologic lesion that can produce this syndrome.

e. What diagnostic studies might be useful in defining the location of this lesion?

6. A 60-year-old woman suffered a myocardial infarction. Several days later, however, she complained to the nurse that she had an abrupt onset of seeing double whenever she looked to the left and that she was having some difficulty in using her right arm. Testing of cranial nerves revealed a paralysis of the left lateral rectus muscle. Her speech was slightly slurred, and the left nasolabial fold was flattened. Her mouth pulled to the right on smiling. Her left eye could not be closed tightly, and her left eyebrow could not be raised as high as the right. Facial sensation and taste were normal. Testing of the extremities revealed weakness of the right arm and leg, with hyperactive reflexes and Babinski's sign on the right. There was loss of joint position and vibration sense in the right arm and leg.

a. What is the location and type of lesion?

b. What anatomic structures are involved?

c. What is the pathologic nature of the lesion?

7. A 73-year-old diabetic woman entered the hospital because of the abrupt onset of double vision and left-sided weakness. Examination several hours later revealed that her right pupil was 4 mm and her left was 3 mm. The direct and consensual light response of the right pupil was less brisk than the left. There was slight ptosis of the eyelid on the right. On following a light with her eyes, she reported seeing two images when the light was moved directly to her left and to her right and upward. A red glass was placed over her right eye. When the light was moved to the left, the red image was seen to the left of the white image. When the light was moved to her right and upward, the red image was above the white image. In each instance, the separation increased as the light was moved further. The only other abnormalities on neurologic examination were slight drooping of the left corner of her mouth, slight weakness of her left arm and leg with hyperactive deep

tendon reflexes, reduced abdominal reflexes, and Babinski's sign on the left.

a. What is the location and type of lesion?

b. What anatomic structures are involved?

c. Diplopia testing indicated weakness of which muscles?

d. Why was the pupillary light reflex altered?

e. What is the pathologic nature of the lesion?

8. A 10-year-old boy was seen because of trouble with coordination of his left side. He had been well until 3 months ago, when he experienced severe headaches. Two months ago, he began to note that his left hand shook when he reached for an object. One month prior to admission, he noted increasing clumsiness of his left leg. Because of the headaches, nausea and vomiting, and increased clumsiness of the left arm and leg, he was examined. Examination showed that his optic nerve heads were swollen and that the patient took frequent missteps with his left leg and had an intention tremor on finger-to-nose and heel-to-shin testing. His tone was slightly decreased on the left, but strength and sensation were intact.

a. What is the location and type of lesion?

b. What specific area of the neuraxis seems to be involved?

c. What signs and symptoms suggest the presence of increased intracranial pressure?

d. Name the most common lesion occurring in children that can produce this syndrome.

9. A 55-year-old man had noted progressive difficulty in swallowing and talking during the past year; liquids had tended to go down his "windpipe" or out his nose, and he had felt that his trouble with speech was due to his "tongue not working right." Examination revealed fasciculations and atrophy of the tongue bilaterally. He had trouble protruding his tongue and moving it from side to side. When he was asked to say "ah," his palate showed only a minimal elevation. When asked to say "ka, ka, ka," he had nasal emission of speech. When asked to show his teeth, he was noted to have bilateral facial

weakness, left greater than right, and he could not whistle. Slight distal extremity weakness and fasciculations also were seen. Deep tendon reflexes were reduced, but bilateral Babinski's sign was present. Results of the remainder of the examination were normal.

   a. What is the location and site of the lesion?

   b. What system(s) is involved?

   c. What component(s) of the system(s) is involved?

   d. Name one disorder that can produce this syndrome.

10. A 13-year-old girl awoke one morning complaining of a left earache and a dull generalized headache. Her temperature was 102°F (38.7°C) orally. She did not improve with aspirin and bed rest, and that evening she was taken to her family physician, who diagnosed acute otitis media and gave her an injection of penicillin. For the next several days, she continued to have some ear drainage and mild left-sided ear pain and headache. During the next week, she suffered increasingly severe headaches, with nausea and vomiting. One day prior to admission, she experienced progressive weakness of the right face, arm, and leg and difficulty in speaking. She also seemed to have difficulty in thinking of what word she wanted to say, and she had difficulty in understanding what people were saying to her.

   a. At this point, what is the suspected location and type of lesion?

When seen at the local hospital, she was stuporous but could be aroused by strong stimuli. Her left pupil was dilated and reacted poorly to light. The right pupillary reflex was intact. The left eye was deviated down and out, and she had ptosis of the left eyelid. During the examination, her right hemiparesis became much worse.

   b. What is the reason for her change in level of consciousness?

   c. How do you explain the eye findings?

   d. Why was there worsening of her hemiparesis?

   e. What is the term used to describe the above process?

It was decided to send the patient to the nearest neurosurgical facilities, which were several hours away. On arrival at the second hospital, she was deeply comatose. Respirations were deep and rapid. Her temperature was 105°F (40.3°C). Her pupils were slightly dilated and did not react to light. Her jaw was tightly clenched. Her spine was extended and arched posteriorly. Her arms were stiffly extended and the fists clenched. Her legs were also stiffly extended.

   f. The findings present at this point suggest involvement at what level of the neuraxis?

   g. What term describes her body position and tone?

   h. What term describes the process producing this clinical picture?

Suggested Reading

Burde, R. M. Eye Movements. In S. Eliasson, A. L. Prensky, and W. B. Hardin, Jr. (eds.), *Neurological Pathophysiology*. New York: Oxford University Press, 1978. Pp. 237-252.

Ellenberger, C., Jr. The Visual System. In S. Eliasson, A. L. Prensky, and W. B. Hardin, Jr. (eds.), *Neurological Pathophysiology*. New York: Oxford University Press, 1978. Pp. 215-236.

Hardin, W. B., Jr., and Merson, R. M. The Higher-Order Dysfunctions: Apraxia, Agnosia, and Aphasia. In S. Eliasson, A. L. Prensky, and W. B. Hardin, Jr. (eds.), *Neurological Pathophysiology*. New York: Oxford University Press, 1978. Pp. 198-214.

Lance, J. W., and McLeod, J. G. *A Physiological Approach to Clinical Neurology* (3rd ed.). Boston: Butterworth, 1981. Pp. 219-262.

Leigh, R. J., and Zee, D. S. *The Neurology of Eye Movements*. Philadelphia: Davis, 1983.

Villiger, E. *Atlas of Cross Section Anatomy of the Brain*. (Revised by A. T. Rasmussen.) New York: Blakiston, 1951.

Zuleger, S., and Staubesand, J. *Atlas of the Central Nervous System in Sectional Planes: Selected Myelin Stained Sections of the Human Brain and Spinal Cord*. Baltimore-Munich: Urban & Schwarzenberg, 1977.

The Supratentorial Level

15

The nervous system has been presented as six major systems combined in different ways at four major levels. Each of these systems has a specific function, and each level has representations of most of these systems. The final level, the supratentorial, like the posterior fossa, has two additional minor systems, which have been discussed only briefly heretofore, located within this one level. These are the limbic system and the visual system.

This chapter discusses the important features of the two major anatomic areas at the supratentorial level—the diencephalon and the telencephalon—and the anatomy, physiology, and clinical correlates of these two systems.

Overview

The supratentorial level includes all structures located within the skull above the tentorium cerebelli. These structures have evolved from the embryonic prosencephalon and therefore include derivatives of the diencephalon and telencephalon (Fig. 15-1). The *diencephalon* is composed of those structures between the midbrain and the cerebral hemispheres that surround the third ventricle. The diencephalon has four subdivisions: thalamus, ventral thalamus, hypothalamus, and epithalamus.

The *thalamus* is the largest structure in the diencephalon and consists of nuclei that act as a relay and integrating station for ascending and descending activity in the major neural systems. The *ventral thalamus* lies between the thalamus and the midbrain and contains nuclei and pathways closely related to the motor system and the basal ganglia control circuit. The major nucleus in the ventral thalamus is the subthalamic nucleus.

The *hypothalamus* lies anterior and inferior to the thalamus and contains the hypothalamic nuclei, the tuber cinereum, and the mammillary bodies. The pituitary gland, although not part of the hypothalamus, is attached to it by the pituitary stalk at the tuber cinereum. The hypothalamus regulates visceral functions, temperature control, osmolality of blood, eating, sleeping, and endocrine functions.

The *epithalamus* is situated in the dorsal diencephalon and contains the pineal gland—a midline structure that has endocrine function and which, when calcified, can be used as roentgenographic evidence to identify its position.

The *cerebral hemispheres* are the adult derivatives of the *telencephalon* and are subdivided into three anatomic regions: basal ganglia, subcortical white matter, and cerebral cortex. The *basal ganglia* are large masses of gray matter situated deep in the cerebral hemispheres, lateral and anterior to the thalamus. The basal ganglia and their connections form one of the motor control pathways. The *subcortical white matter* is composed of dense fiber tracts connecting cortical and subcortical structures. Projectional fibers connect the cortex with the thalamus, hypothalamus, basal ganglia, cerebellum, and other subcortical structures. Commissural fibers connect homologous areas in the two hemispheres. Association fibers connect areas within one hemisphere.

The *cerebral cortex* is the relatively thin mantle of gray matter covering the outer surface of the cerebral hemispheres and forming the gyri of the brain. Each cerebral hemisphere is divided into five lobes: frontal, parietal, occipital, temporal, and limbic. The main function of the *frontal lobe* is motor, with primary motor areas in the precentral gyrus, and speech and eye movement control in Brodmann's areas 44 and 8. In addition, anterior frontal areas have intellectual functions, and the base of the frontal lobe is related to visceral function. The *parietal lobe* mainly has sensory functions and contains the primary sensory receiving area in the postcentral gyrus. Parietal association areas integrate sensory input from multiple sources. The *occipital lobe* contains the visual areas, especially in the calcarine cortex. The *temporal lobe* has a receiving area for auditory and vestibular information and plays a major role in language and memory. The *limbic lobe* on the medial surface includes the orbital frontal region, the cingulate gyrus, and medial portions of the temporal lobe. It plays an integral role in visceral and emotional activity.

Two functional systems are found entirely at the supratentorial level: visual and limbic. The *limbic system* contains diencephalic and telencephalic structures, including olfactory areas (rhinencephalon), hypothalamic nuclei (such as the mammillary bodies), thalamic nuclei (such as the anterior nucleus), and cortex in the limbic lobe. The limbic system integrates emotional, visceral,

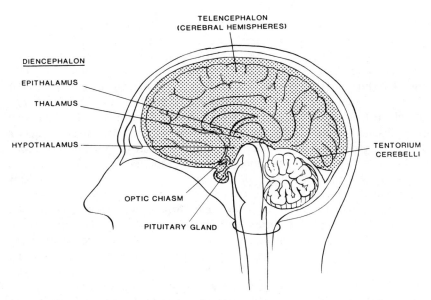

Fig. 15-1. The supratentorial level (stippled area) *includes the diencephalon and telencephalon.*

and behavioral activities and mediates memory and olfaction. The *visual system* includes the eye, retina, visual pathways, and occipital cortex and thus is found at the peripheral level as well as in the diencephalon and the telencephalon.

Disorders at the supratentorial level may alter contralateral motor and sensory functions. Disorders involving the diencephalon impair the relay of information to and from the cerebral hemispheres or impair visceral, endocrine, or emotional functions. The cerebral hemispheres mediate a number of "higher level" functions that result in specific disorders when diseased. Generalized intellectual deterioration (dementia), amnesia, aphasia, agnosia (inability to perceive the meaning of sensory input), apraxia (inability to perform complex motor activities voluntarily), and seizures all occur only with lesions of the cerebral hemispheres.

Diencephalon

The diencephalon lies rostral to the brain stem and includes the structures surrounding the third ventricle. Superiorly, the diencephalon is bounded by the floor of the lateral ventricles, the corpus callosum, and the fornix; laterally, it is bounded by the internal capsule; anteriorly, it extends to the region of the foramen of Monro; and caudally, it merges with the tegmentum of the midbrain.

The diencephalon is subdivided into four regions: dorsal thalamus, hypothalamus, ventral thalamus, and epithalamus (Fig. 15-2). The dorsal thalamus, or, as it is more commonly known, the thalamus, is the largest structure in the diencephalon and contains a number of thalamic nuclei. The hypothalamus lies inferior and anterior to the thalamus and is separated from the thalamus by the hypothalamic sulcus—a groove in the wall of the third ventricle from the foramen of Monro to the aqueduct of Sylvius. The ventral thalamus lies ventral and posterior to the thalamus and merges with the midbrain. The epithalamus forms part of the roof of the diencephalon and lies superior to the ventral thalamus and posterior to the thalamus.

Thalamus (Dorsal Thalamus)

The thalamus is composed of a group of nuclei in the wall of the third ventricle. The thalami sometimes fuse in the midline of the third ventricle, forming the interthalamic adhesion (or massa intermedia). The anterior end of the thalamus, containing the anterior nucleus, is narrow; whereas the posterior end, containing the pulvinar and geniculate bodies, is broad. The Y-shaped internal medullary lamina divides the thalamus into anterior, medial, and lateral areas (Fig. 15-3 and Table 15-1).

The anterior nuclear group is in the anterior area; the dorsomedial and midline nuclei are in the medial area; and the lateral nuclei are ar-

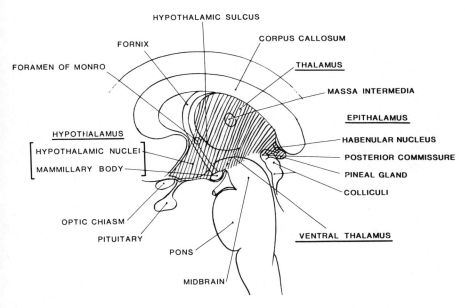

HYPOTHALAMIC SULCUS

FORNIX

CORPUS CALLOSUM

FORAMEN OF MONRO

THALAMUS

MASSA INTERMEDIA

EPITHALAMUS

HYPOTHALAMUS

HABENULAR NUCLEUS

HYPOTHALAMIC NUCLEI

POSTERIOR COMMISSURE

MAMMILLARY BODY

PINEAL GLAND

COLLICULI

OPTIC CHIASM

PITUITARY

VENTRAL THALAMUS

PONS

MIDBRAIN

Fig. 15-2. Diencephalon (shaded area) and its four subdivisions: thalamus, ventral thalamus, epithalamus, and hypothalamus.

ranged in two tiers, a dorsal tier and a ventral tier, in the lateral area. The nuclei in the dorsal tier, from anterior to posterior, are the dorsolateral nucleus, the lateral posterior nucleus, and the pulvinar. The medial geniculate and lateral geniculate bodies project posteriorly from the ventral surface of the pulvinar. In the ventral tier, from anterior to posterior, are the ventral anterior, the ventral lateral, and the ventral posterior nuclei (Fig. 15-3). Between and surrounding these well-defined nuclear groups are layers of cells forming sheetlike nuclei: the intralaminar nuclei in the Y-shaped border between the major groups, the re-

Table 15-1. Summary of Thalamic Nuclei

Anterior area			Anterior nucleus
Medial area			Midline
			Dorsomedial
Intralaminar area			Intralaminar nuclei
Lateral area	Dorsal tier		Dorsolateral
			Lateral posterior
			Pulvinar
			Medial geniculate
			Lateral geniculate
	Ventral tier		Ventral anterior
			Ventral lateral
			Ventral posterior
			Reticular

ticular nuclei around the outside, and the midline nuclei.

The *thalamic nuclei* integrate and relay information for the sensory, motor, consciousness, limbic, and visual systems. The ventral posterior (posterolateral and posteromedial) nuclei relay somatic sensory system information to the cerebral cortex. The ventral posterolateral nucleus is the site of termination of the second-order axons of the spinothalamic and medial lemniscal pathways from the trunk and limbs. Similarly, axons of the trigeminal thalamic pathways from the head terminate in the ventral posteromedial nucleus. Axons from the ventral posterior nuclei project via the middle thalamic radiation in the posterior limb of the internal capsule to the primary somatosensory cortex in the postcentral gyrus of the parietal lobe. The crude perception of, and response to, the sensations of pain, vibration, and coarse touch occur in these nuclei.

The medial geniculate body receives auditory afferent fibers from the inferior colliculus via the brachium of the inferior colliculus and sends efferent fibers through the auditory radiations in the sublenticular portion of the posterior limb of the internal capsule to the auditory cortex of the temporal lobe. The lateral geniculate body relays visual impulses from the optic tract via the retrolenticular portion of the posterior limb of the internal capsule to the calcarine cortex of the occipital lobe and is part of the visual system. Some of these visual projection fibers loop

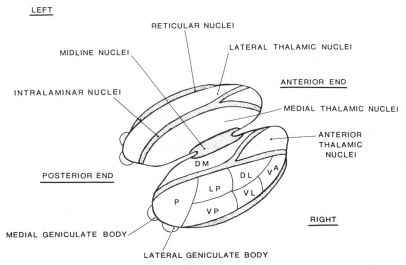

LEFT

RETICULAR NUCLEI

LATERAL THALAMIC NUCLEI

MIDLINE NUCLEI

ANTERIOR END

INTRALAMINAR NUCLEI

MEDIAL THALAMIC NUCLEI

ANTERIOR
THALAMIC
NUCLEI

DM

POSTERIOR END

DL

V A

L P

V L

P

V P

RIGHT

MEDIAL GENICULATE BODY

LATERAL GENICULATE BODY

Fig. 15-3. Four major groups of thalamic nuclei: anterior, medial, lateral, and intralaminar. The medial group includes the midline and dorsomedial (DM) nuclei. The lateral group includes dorsolateral (DL), lateral posterior (LP), pulvinar (P), medial and lateral geniculate bodies, ventral anterior (VA), ventral lateral (VL), and ventral posterior (VP) nuclei. The diffuse includes the intralaminar and reticular nuclei. (Redrawn from F. H. Netter. The Ciba Collection of Medical Illustrations. *Volume I:* The Nervous System. *Summit, N.J.: Ciba Pharmaceutical Products, 1962. P. 48.)*

around the temporal horn of the lateral ventricle (Meyer's loop). The pulvinar also relays visual information to the cerebral cortex.

The ventral anterior and ventral lateral nuclei are specific motor nuclei that integrate and transmit information from the motor control pathways in the motor system to the motor areas of the cerebral cortex. The ventral anterior nucleus receives input from the globus pallidus of the basal ganglia, and the ventral lateral nucleus receives input from the red nucleus and the dentate nucleus of the cerebellum. Both send efferent fibers to widespread areas in the frontal lobe.

Three groups of nuclei—the midline, intralaminar, and reticular—relay information for the consciousness system and are arranged as shells around the specific thalamic nuclei. They receive input from the reticular formation, the hypothalamus, and cortical areas and send efferent fibers diffusely to all areas of the cerebral cortex. They mediate consciousness. The remaining nuclei are part of the limbic system. They have reciprocal connections with other areas of the thalamus and

with associated areas in the frontal and parietal lobes. The anterior and the dorsomedial nuclei are the limbic relay nuclei to the cingulate and orbital frontal cortex.

The blood supply to the posterior thalamus is via branches of the vertebrobasilar circulation. Discrete lesions that destroy the ventral posterior nucleus of the thalamus produce a contralateral hemianesthesia with loss of all sensory modalities in the trunk, limbs, and face. This is often the result of an infarction due to hypertensive vascular disease or thrombosis of one of the branches of the posterior cerebral artery. The initial stage of a contralateral hemianesthesia following a thalamic infarct may in turn be followed by a partial return of sensation associated with a very unpleasant burning sensation referred to as the *thalamic syndrome*. Motor function can be altered by lesions of the motor relay nuclei of the thalamus. Discrete neurosurgical lesions in the ventral anterior thalamic nucleus disrupt connections between the basal ganglia and the cerebral cortex and thereby decrease the tremor and rigidity in some patients with Parkinson's disease.

Ventral Thalamus

The ventral thalamus lies between the thalamus and the midbrain and contains nuclei and pathways related to the control circuits of the basal ganglia. The subthalamic nucleus is the major structure in this region and lies cephalad to the substantia nigra and immediately ventral to the thalamus posteriorly. The ansa lenticularis is the major fiber pathway through the ventral thalamus and carries fibers from the globus pallidus to the ventral anterior nucleus of the thalamus. A lesion of the subthalamic nucleus causes *hemiballismus,* a movement disorder in which there are rapid, flailing movements of one extremity or one side of the body.

Hypothalamus
The hypothalamus is the main control area of the

visceral system. It integrates activity for the limbic, consciousness, visceral, and endocrine systems. The hypothalamus includes those structures in the diencephalon anterior and inferior to the thalamus which are separated from it by the hypothalamic sulcus. The hypothalamus consists of the hypothalamic nuclei in the walls of the third ventricle and the tuber cinereum and mammillary bodies in the floor of the third ventricle (Fig. 15-4).

Fig. 15-4. The hypothalamus. A. Midline section of the hypothalamic nuclei (shaded area), *the pituitary gland in the sella turcica, and the mammillary bodies.*

B. Base of the brain with the optic chiasm, the median eminence of the hypothalamus, the pituitary stalk, and the mammillary bodies.

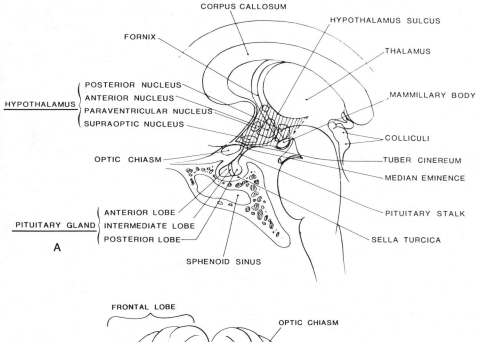

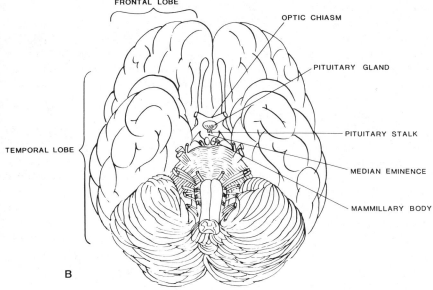

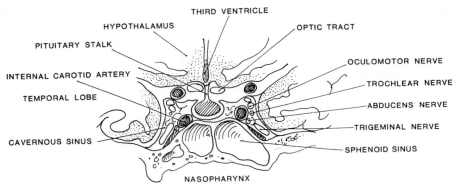

Fig. 15-5. Coronal section of the base of the brain. The structures adjacent to the pituitary gland are in the cavernous sinus located on either side of the pituitary gland: cranial nerves III, IV, V, and VI and the internal carotid arteries. The optic tracts are located adjacent to the pituitary stalk.

The hypophysis, or pituitary gland, is functionally related to the hypothalamus and is attached to it at the tuber cinereum by the infundibulum, or pituitary stalk. Other closely related structures not part of the hypothalamus are the optic chiasm, located immediately below the anterior hypothalamus; the internal carotid arteries in the cavernous sinus, located just lateral to the pituitary gland; and cranial nerves III, IV, V, and VI which lie adjacent to the pituitary gland in the cavernous sinus (Fig. 15-5). The hypothalamus has fiber connections with all areas of the brain stem and cerebral hemispheres, but particularly with the basal frontal and mesial cortical areas and with the reticular formation. The most prominent fiber tracts are the fornix, which ends in the mammillary bodies, and the mammillothalamic tract, which terminates in the anterior nucleus of the thalamus. These tracts and the hypothalamic nuclei are part of the limbic system.

HYPOTHALAMIC NUCLEI. The hypothalamic nuclei are loosely organized groups of cells in the walls of the third ventricle, which can be subdivided into anterior (parasympathetic) and posterior (sympathetic) groups. The anterior group subserves restorative functions, and the posterior group subserves preparative functions, but specific functions have been associated only with the supraoptic and paraventricular nuclei (see Fig. 15-4A). These nuclei give rise to axons that terminate in the posterior pituitary and control water metabolism and uterine contraction by secretion

of vasopressin and oxytocin. The other nuclei (preoptic, anterior, dorsomedial, ventral medial, and posterior) either have fiber connections with other neural structures or secrete hormones that control anterior pituitary secretion. These hormones are called *releasing factors* because they control the release of other hormones from the anterior pituitary gland. There are eight known releasing factors, three of which have been isolated and characterized. These three, all peptides, are somatostatin, thyrotropin-releasing factor, and luteotropin-releasing factor.

The hypothalamic nuclei control the following functions:

1. Visceral. Anterior hypothalamic nuclei mediate parasympathetic activity; posterior nuclei mediate sympathetic activity.
2. Endocrine. Releasing factors act on the anterior pituitary gland to control the release of specific hormones.
3. Water metabolism. The antidiuretic hormone, vasopressin, released from the posterior pituitary gland, regulates the reabsorption of water by the kidneys. Failure of secretion of antidiuretic hormone results in *diabetes insipidus,* in which there is excretion of excessive quantities of urine.
4. Food intake. Satiety and feeding centers in the medial and lateral regions of the posterior hypothalamus, respectively, control the amount of food eaten. Destruction of the satiety center leads to hyperphagia (overeating), whereas destruction of the feeding center results in anorexia (failure to eat).
5. Temperature. A center in the anterior hypothalamus regulates loss of heat, while another in the posterior hypothalamus regulates conservation of heat. Thermoreceptors in these

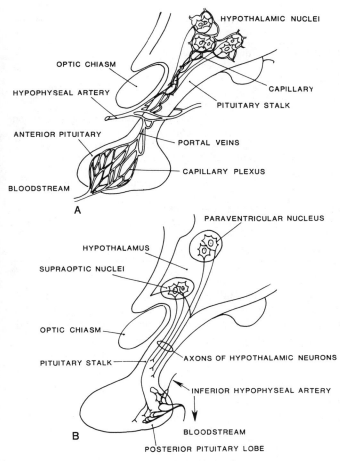

OPTIC CHIASM

HYPOPHYSEAL ARTERY

HYPOTHALAMIC NUCLEI

CAPILLARY

PITUITARY STALK

ANTERIOR PITUITARY

PORTAL VEINS

CAPILLARY PLEXUS

BLOODSTREAM

A

PARAVENTRICULAR NUCLEUS

HYPOTHALAMUS

SUPRAOPTIC NUCLEI

OPTIC CHIASM

AXONS OF HYPOTHALAMIC NEURONS

PITUITARY STALK

INFERIOR HYPOPHYSEAL ARTERY

BLOODSTREAM

B

POSTERIOR PITUITARY LOBE

Fig. 15-6. A. Portal circulation carries releasing factors from hypothalamus to anterior pituitary lobe. B. Axons carry hormones from hypothalamic nuclei to posterior pituitary lobe.

centers respond to the temperature of the blood and initiate heat loss or heat conservation by vasodilation, vasoconstriction, sweating, shivering, or piloerection. Destruction of these regions results in loss of temperature control.

6. Sleep. The consciousness system has connections with the posterior hypothalamus, which has a role in regulating sleep. A lesion in this region can result in hypersomnia, or excessive sleeping.

7. Cardiovascular. Hypothalamic visceral connections affect cardiac rate and output, blood pressure, and respiration.

8. Emotion. As part of the limbic system, the hypothalamus has a role in the neural complex that determines emotions. In experimental ani-

mals, stimulation of the anterior pituitary induces responses resembling fear or rage.

PITUITARY GLAND. The pituitary gland (hypophysis) lies within a bony-walled cavity, the *sella turcica* ("Turk's saddle") in the sphenoid bone at the base of the brain (see Fig. 15-4A). It is connected to the hypothalamus by the *pituitary stalk,* which arises from the median eminence—a midline, ventral projection from the tuber cinereum. The pituitary stalk is located between the optic chiasm and the mammillary bodies.

The pituitary gland consists of three divisions: the anterior lobe, or adenohypophysis; the posterior lobe, or neurohypophysis; and the intermediate lobe. While each lobe is part of a single gland, each has a different embryologic origin. The anterior lobe arises from a neuroectodermal ridge in the oral region, and the posterior lobe arises from a downward evagination of the embryonic diencephalon (see Fig. 2-9). The poste-

Table 15-2. Anterior Pituitary Hormones

Cell type	Hormone	Function
Acidophil	Growth hormone (GH) (somatotropic hormone—STH)	Stimulates body growth
	Prolactin	Stimulates breast growth and induces milk production
Basophil	Thyrotropin (TSH)	Stimulates growth of thyroid gland and secretion of thyroid hormone
	Adrenocorticotropic hormone (ACTH)	Regulates size of adrenal cortex and secretion of cortisol and other adrenal steroids
	Follicle-stimulating hormone (FSH)	Stimulates maturation of ovarian follicle, development of testicular tubules, and spermatogenesis
	Luteinizing hormone (LH)	Induces ovulation and stimulates development of Leydig cells of testes and their secretion of testosterone
Chromophobes	None known	Unknown

rior lobe and the pituitary stalk are formed from this evaginated neural process, which serves as the neural connection with the diencephalon in the adult. The anterior lobe, which fuses with the posterior lobe, has no known neural connections with the brain and receives its hypothalamic control through a system of portal vessels. The release of hormones from the pituitary gland is regulated by a vascular mechanism from the anterior lobe (Fig. 15-6A) and by a neural mechanism from the posterior lobe (Fig. 15-6B).

The anterior pituitary lobe is connected with the hypothalamus by means of a portal circulation (Fig. 15-6A). This consists of hypophyseal arteries located in the median eminence which give rise to capillaries that drain into a series of parallel veins coursing down the pituitary stalk. On reaching the anterior lobe, the veins form a capillary plexus that supplies blood to the anterior lobe. The release of the anterior pituitary hormones is under the control of neurohumoral substances secreted by the hypothalamus. These substances, the releasing factors, are released from nerve endings in the median eminence. They enter the capillaries of the portal circulation, are carried down the pituitary stalk by means of the portal veins, and then empty into the capillary plexus of the anterior pituitary gland where they stimulate the cells of the anterior pituitary gland to release specific hormones.

The posterior pituitary hormones, vasopressin and oxytocin, are synthesized in the cells in the hypothalamus and are transported by axons in the pituitary stalk to the nerve terminals in the posterior lobe for storage or release (Fig. 15-6B). Vasopressin regulates water metabolism and blood osmolality, whereas oxytocin produces uterine musculature contraction after delivery.

The anterior lobe of the pituitary gland contains three types of cells defined by their staining characteristics: the acidophils (red granules), the basophils (blue granules), and the chromophobes (no granules). These cells secrete different hormones (Table 15-2).

CLINICAL CORRELATIONS. Lesions affecting the hypothalamus and surrounding structures can be seen in any type of medical practice because they cause derangements of visceral, endocrine, visual, or homeostatic functions. Lesions of the hypothalamic nuclei result in a disturbance of visceral and homeostatic functions, such as sleep, appetite, temperature regulation, and water metabolism; whereas lesions of the pituitary gland cause endocrine disorders owing to increased or decreased secretion of pituitary hormones. Examples of endocrine disorders include the following:

1. Growth hormone. Increased secretion causes gigantism in children and acromegaly (enlargement of the face, hands, and feet) in adults. Decreased secretion during childhood results in dwarfism.
2. Thyroid-stimulating hormone. Decreased secretion results in hypothyroidism with loss of hair, dry skin, slow pulse, loss of energy,

mental apathy, decreased cold tolerance, and slow deep tendon reflexes.

3. Adrenocorticotropic hormone. Increased secretion results in signs of hyperadrenalism with hirsutism, vascular striae, obesity, and hypertension. Decreased secretion results in hypoadrenalism with generalized weakness, hypotension, and decreased tolerance to stress.
4. Gonadotropic hormone. Decreased secretion results in amenorrhea and decreased libido.

The visual deficits resulting from involvement of structures adjacent to the hypothalamus serve as additional localizing signs of a lesion in this region. A mass lesion in the region of the sella turcica can press on the optic chiasm and cause a characteristic visual field defect, a bitemporal hemianopia. A lesion involving the carotid artery or cranial nerves in the cavernous sinus can cause diplopia and loss of sensation over the forehead and cheek. A mass lesion in or near the sella can cause enlargement of the sella or erosion of the bony margins of the sella which can be seen on a roentgenogram of the skull.

The three most common mass lesions encountered in this region are pituitary adenoma, craniopharyngioma, and aneurysm of the internal carotid artery. A *pituitary adenoma* is a tumor arising from the cells of the anterior pituitary gland. As the tumor expands, it produces enlargement of the sella and compression of the optic chiasm.

Pituitary adenomas were previously classified according to their staining characteristics with acid and basic dyes (acidophilic, basophilic, and chromophobe adenomas). However, with this scheme, correlation with the hormonal activity of the tumor is imprecise. The demonstration of specific secretory granules by electron microscopy and of hormone content by immunostaining (immunoperoxidase, immunofluorescence) permits a more meaningful classification of these biologically active tumors.

Tumors that are acidophilic on routine stains are most often associated with either somatotropin secretion (which causes acromegaly in adults or giantism in children) or prolactin secretion (which causes amenorrhea and galactorrhea in women). Tumors that produce corticotropin (ACTH) are usually basophilic and are associated with Cushing's syndrome.

While all the tumors mentioned contain densely granulated cells, similar hormonal activity may occur in much less densely granulated tumors, classed as chromophobe adenomas on routine staining. Many other chromophobe adenomas, while containing identifiable hormone granules, do not result in clinical evidence of trophic hormone excess. These tumors may grow to enormous size and produce clinical effects by compression of the normal pituitary gland (*panhypopituitarism*) and suprasellar and parasellar structures. Pituitary tumors with no identifiable hormone production, called *oncocytomas*, are rare.

A *craniopharyngioma* is a tumor that arises from an embryonic remnant of Rathke's pouch. Therefore, it is usually located in the region of the pituitary stalk or sella, near the hypothalamus and pituitary gland. It can cause endocrine disturbances, visual symptoms, and erosion of the sella. An *aneurysm* of the internal carotid artery in the region of the sella frequently causes disturbances in extraocular muscle function but rarely disturbs pituitary function.

Epithalamus

The epithalamus lies in the dorsal wall of the posterior part of the third ventricle beneath the overlying splenium of the corpus callosum.

The main structure of the epithalamus is the *pineal gland,* which is formed from an evagination of the roof of the diencephalon. The cavity of the evagination is the pineal recess of the third ventricle. Other structures located in the region of the epithalamus include the habenular nuclei, which lie in the walls of the epithalamus, and the posterior commissure, which crosses the midline ventral to the pineal gland (see Fig. 15-2).

In lower animals, the pineal gland has photoreceptors and nerve cells. The output of a hormone, melatonin, from the pineal gland is regulated by changes in the level of environmental illumination. Melatonin causes clumping of the skin pigment melanin in the granules of melanocytes in the skin. By this means, the animal adaptively darkens in dim illumination and lightens in bright light.

In humans, the pineal gland secretes melatonin, which regulates secretion of gonadotropins. It also secretes melanocyte-stimulating hormones. The latter are lipotropic hormones containing endorphin molecules important in pain control.

In humans after the age of 20 years, the pineal gland also accumulates granules of calcium salts, which are dense enough to be seen on a skull roentgenogram. Because the pineal gland is located in the midline of the skull, the presence of a calcified pineal gland on a roentgenogram of the skull serves as a useful marker of midline structures. A shift of the pineal gland to one side suggests a shift of the brain structures, either from a mass lesion on the opposite side or from an atrophic lesion on the same side.

Telencephalon

The lateral evaginations of the most rostral portion of the embryologic neural tube form the telencephalon, from which the cerebral hemispheres arise. The two cerebral hemispheres fill the entire cranial cavity above the tentorium cerebelli and are separated by the falx cerebri. Each cerebral hemisphere contains three layers of tissue surrounding the ventricular cavities deep within the hemispheres (Fig. 15-7). Immediately adjacent to the ventricles, near the thalamus, are the basal ganglia. Surrounding these deep gray nuclei is the *white matter,* a dense intermingling of axons that connect areas within the cerebral hemispheres with each other and with other areas of the nervous system. The outermost layer, the cerebral cortex, contains neurons that have migrated to this location during fetal development.

Fig. 15-7. Coronal section through cerebral hemispheres. The basal ganglia (caudate nucleus, putamen, globus pallidus) are deep nuclei in the cerebral hemispheres.

This outer layer of gray matter is referred to as *cortical,* whereas the white matter and deep gray matter are referred to as *subcortical.*

Basal Ganglia

Basal ganglia is a term now used to refer to three large subcortical areas of gray matter: the caudate nucleus, the putamen, and the globus pallidus (Fig. 15-7). This term was originally used to designate all the gray matter areas in the diencephalon and telencephalon and is still used by some anatomists to include the amygdala. However, for clinical purposes it refers only to the caudate, putamen, and globus pallidus. Older textbooks used the term *corpus striatum* to refer to the caudate and putamen, because of their striated appearance, and the term *lentiform nucleus* to refer to the putamen and globus pallidus, because of their shape. The individual names are preferred over these older usages. The basal ganglia control circuit includes the caudate nucleus, putamen, globus pallidus, ventral anterior thalamic nucleus, substantia nigra, subthalamic nucleus, and their connections.

The details of the anatomic loops formed by the connections in the basal ganglia control circuit have been detailed in Chapter 9. These areas have connections with many areas of the cerebral hemispheres and the diencephalon and have a major influence on motor behavior, but the precise mechanisms of their action are unknown. Most knowledge of their function has been deduced from clinical findings in patients with lesions in these areas, supported by experimental studies in animals. For instance, the activity in some cells in the globus pallidus is closely related to tonic muscle activity, and reversible lesions in

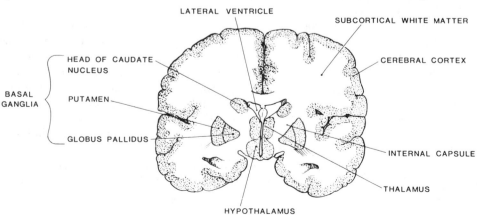

these areas can impair associated or postural movements.

Subcortical White Matter

A large proportion of the cerebral hemispheres between the ventricles and the cortex is composed of myelinated axons that connect multiple areas in the cerebral hemispheres. These fibers carry action potentials from one area to another without synapse or modification. These fibers are named on the basis of the areas that they connect. *Projectional fibers* travel between the cerebral cortex and the subcortical nuclear structures; *commissural fibers* connect homologous areas in the two hemispheres; and *association fibers* connect cortical areas within one hemisphere with one another.

PROJECTIONAL FIBERS. As the axons between subcortical and cortical areas pass between the subcortical nuclei, they are collected into a compact structure, the *internal capsule*. The internal capsule is a broad band flanked medially by the thalamus and laterally by the globus pallidus and putamen (Fig. 15-8). In horizontal section, it is a V-shaped structure pointed medially with an anterior limb, a posterior limb, and a junction called

Fig. 15-8. Internal capsule. The anterior limb carries fibers to the frontal lobe, the genu to the motor areas, and the posterior limb to the sensory areas. The retrolenticular portion of the internal capsule contains the optic radiations; the sublenticular portion contains the auditory radiations.

the genu. The caudate is medial to the anterior limb; the thalamus is medial to the posterior limb; and the globus pallidus and putamen are lateral to the genu. The axons of the projectional fibers carry action potentials either toward the cerebral cortex (afferent) or away from the cerebral cortex (efferent). As the axons of the internal capsule spread out from the internal capsule to reach all areas of cortex, they are known as the *corona radiata*.

The afferent projectional fibers arise in large part from the thalamus and are called *thalamic radiations*. Fibers traveling to the frontal lobe from the anterior and medial thalamic nuclei, carrying visceral and other information, are located in the anterior limb of the internal capsule. Fibers from the ventral anterior and ventral lateral nuclei of the thalamus, projecting to the motor and premotor areas of the frontal lobe, are found in the genu and posterior limb of the internal capsule. Fibers from the ventral posterolateral and medial thalamic nuclei, carrying sensory information to the parietal cortex, travel in the posterior limb of the capsule. Optic radiations, carrying visual information from the lateral geniculate and pulvinar to the occipital and parietal cortex, are in the posterior limb behind the globus pallidus and putamen (retrolenticular portion of the internal capsule). Auditory information is carried from the medial geniculate nucleus to the temporal lobe via the fibers in the posterior limb beneath the globus pallidus and the putamen (sublenticular portion of the internal capsule).

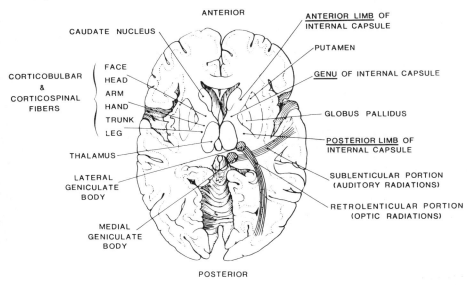

ANTERIOR

CAUDATE NUCLEUS

ANTERIOR LIMB OF INTERNAL CAPSULE

PUTAMEN

CORTICOBULBAR & CORTICOSPINAL FIBERS

FACE
HEAD
ARM
HAND
TRUNK
LEG

GENU OF INTERNAL CAPSULE

GLOBUS PALLIDUS

THALAMUS

POSTERIOR LIMB OF INTERNAL CAPSULE

LATERAL GENICULATE BODY

SUBLENTICULAR PORTION (AUDITORY RADIATIONS)

RETROLENTICULAR PORTION (OPTIC RADIATIONS)

MEDIAL GENICULATE BODY

POSTERIOR

The efferent projectional fibers have several destinations, including the basal ganglia, the hypothalamus, red nucleus, and the brain-stem reticular formation. The largest groups of fibers, however, are in the direct activation pathway from the precentral gyrus via the posterior limb of the internal capsule to the motor nuclei in the brain stem (corticobulbar) and the spinal cord (corticospinal). A second large efferent projection contains fibers primarily from the frontal lobe traveling via the internal capsule and cerebral peduncles to the pontine nuclei of the brain stem, which relay information to the cerebellum. All these fibers are involved in the initiation of voluntary movements, integration of motor function,

modification of reflex activity, modulation of sensory input, regulation of visceral function, and regulation of states of consciousness and attention.

COMMISSURAL FIBERS.   Commissural fibers connect homologous areas in the two hemispheres to integrate the activity on the two sides (Fig. 15-9A). Most of the connections pass through the corpus callosum, which is a large flat bundle of fibers forming the roof of the lateral ventricles. Two smaller bundles connect areas in the temporal lobes. The *anterior commissure* anterior to the third ventricle interconnects anterior temporal areas, whereas the *hippocampal commissure* interconnects the hippocampal formation on the two sides.

ASSOCIATION FIBERS.   A number of fiber tracts known as association pathways run longitudinally within a single hemisphere to correlate activities in different lobes (Fig. 15-9B). Two of the long

Fig. 15-9. A. Coronal section of the cerebral hemispheres. Commissural fibers (corpus callosum and anterior commissure) connect the two hemispheres. The arcuate fibers (short association fibers) connect gyri. B. Medial view of cerebral hemisphere. The long association fibers are the cingulum and the uncinate fasciculus.

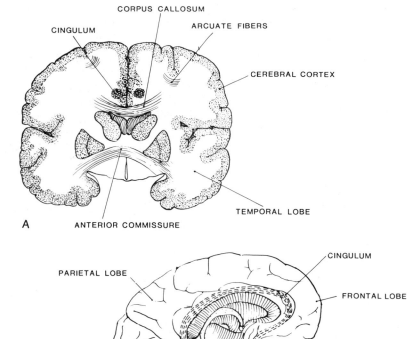

association tracts are the uncinate fasciculus, which joins the temporal and frontal lobes, and the cingulum, which interconnects the medial surfaces of the frontal, parietal, and temporal lobes. Short association fibers connecting adjacent gyri are known as *arcuate fibers* (Fig. 15-9A).

Cerebral Cortex

The cerebral cortex, the outer gray matter of the cerebral hemispheres, contains large numbers of cells intermingled with axons, dendrites, neuroglia, and blood vessels. There are two main types of cortical neurons: the pyramidal cell and the stellate or granule cell. The cells in the cerebral cortex are organized into horizontal layers and vertical columns. Over the surface of the hemispheres, the arrangement of these layers and columns varies with the function of each area, so that differences in function in the lobes of the brain can be correlated with histologic and topographic differences.

HISTOLOGY.   The *pyramidal cell* is triangular in shape, with its upper end giving off an apical

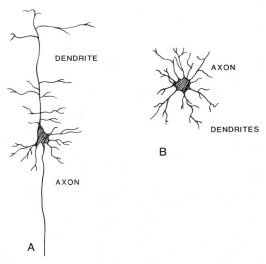

Fig. 15-10. Cells of the cerebral cortex. A. Pyramidal cell. B. Stellate (granule) cell.

dendrite that extends to the surface of the cortex (Fig. 15-10A). The base of the cell gives rise to a long axon that descends to subcortical areas. These cells are found primarily in the motor areas, with the largest, the giant pyramidal cells of Betz, being in the precentral gyrus. The *stellate cell* (granule cell) is a smaller multipolar cell with a dark-staining nucleus, scanty cytoplasm, and a number of dendrites and axons passing in all directions to synapse with other neurons in the cortex (Fig. 15-10B). These cells predominate in sensory areas of the brain, such as the postcentral gyrus.

Fig. 15-11. The six layers of the cerebral cortex: molecular layer (1), external granular layer (2), external pyramidal layer (3), internal granular layer (4), internal pyramidal layer (5), and multiform cell layer (6). A. Cells stained by Nissl stain. B. Selected cells stained by Golgi stain. C. Vertical and horizontal connections of cortical neurons. (AA = afferent association fiber, EA = efferent association fiber, P = efferent projection fiber, R = afferent radiation fiber, CE = commissural efferent fiber.)

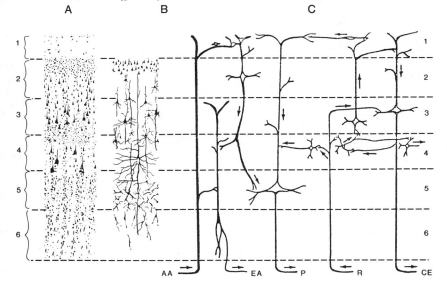

These and other cell types are arranged in layers, which give the cortex a laminated appearance under the microscope. In phylogenetically older areas of the cortex, such as the hippocampus and the piriform areas, there are three layers: a superficial layer of fibers, an intermediate layer of granule cells, and a deep layer of pyramidal cells. Most cortical areas, however, contain six layers (Fig. 15-11):

1. The molecular (plexiform) layer is the outermost superficial layer and contains the apical dendrites of pyramidal cells.
2. The external (outer) granular layer contains many granule cells whose axons synapse in deeper cortical layers or form association fibers.
3. The external (outer) pyramidal layer contains the pyramidal cells whose axons form commissural or association fibers.
4. The internal (inner) granular layer has closely packed granule cells receiving terminal ramifications of the afferent fibers from the thalamus.

Fig. 15-12. The five lobes of the brain. A. Lateral view. B. Medial view of the limbic lobe structures.

5. The internal (inner) pyramidal layer contains the larger pyramidal cells which give rise to association or projectional fibers.
6. The multiform cell layer contains various cell types with axons forming an association of projectional fibers.

Nerve fibers in the cortex run vertically and horizontally, mediating both projectional and associational activity (Fig. 15-11). These fibers separate the cells into columns in some areas of the cortex and into bands in others. The functional correlates of these vertical columns are best demonstrated in the visual cortex.

PHYSIOLOGY.   Bundles of afferent fibers from the thalamus carry action potentials to groups of small cells in layer 4. These cells send axons vertically to the upper cortical layers to end on apical dendrites of pyramidal cells in layers 3 and 5. The ascending fibers organize the cells in the vertical columns of neurons with similar functions (Fig. 15-11).

This circuit constitutes a *vertical cortical unit,* the physiologic basis of cortical activity. Each vertical unit is actually more complex, with collateral branches that relay impulses back and

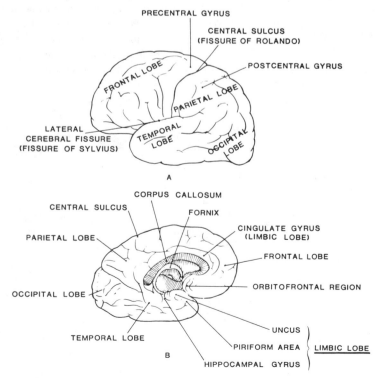

PRECENTRAL GYRUS

CENTRAL SULCUS
(FISSURE OF ROLANDO)

POSTCENTRAL GYRUS

FRONTAL LOBE

PARIETAL LOBE

LATERAL
CEREBRAL FISSURE
(FISSURE OF SYLVIUS)

TEMPORAL
LOBE

OCCIPITAL
LOBE

A

CORPUS CALLOSUM

CENTRAL SULCUS

FORNIX

PARIETAL LOBE

CINGULATE GYRUS
(LIMBIC LOBE)

FRONTAL LOBE

ORBITOFRONTAL REGION

OCCIPITAL LOBE

TEMPORAL LOBE

UNCUS

PIRIFORM AREA   LIMBIC LOBE

HIPPOCAMPAL GYRUS

B

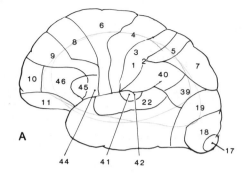

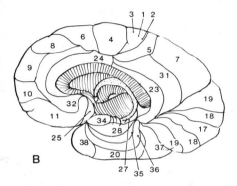

A

B

Fig. 15-13. Brodmann's areas of the cerebral cortex. A. Lateral view. B. Medial view. (44, Broca's motor speech; 11, orbitofrontal; 6, premotor; 4, primary motor; 1, 2, and 3, primary sensory; 5 and 7, sensory association; 18 and 19, visual association; 17, primary visual; 41 and 42, auditory; 22, Wernicke's speech; 23 and 24, cingulate.)

forth between superficial and deep layers. By this means, both excitatory and inhibitory reverberating (feedback) circuits are created that serve either to suppress excitation or to maintain and amplify excitation within the cortex.

The vertical neuronal columns also are interconnected by short axons of granule cells arborizing laterally within a single layer and by lateral processes from other cell types. Activity may spread horizontally in the cortex through these short links. Thus, one vertical column may activate and synchronize the activity of adjacent columns. These horizontal connections can integrate different cortical functions, such as motor and sensory activity.

These general principles of histology and physiology are true for all areas of the cortex, but variations are found in different lobes in relation to differences in function. The cerebral hemi-

spheres are subdivided into frontal, parietal, occipital, temporal, and limbic lobes (Fig. 15-12). Each of these has been subdivided into histologically and functionally distinct areas by the German anatomist Brodmann (Fig. 15-13).

FRONTAL LOBE. The frontal lobe makes up one-third of the hemisphere, extending from the frontal pole to the central sulcus. It has seven major functional areas:

1. The *primary motor area (area 4)* is located on the anterior wall of the precentral sulcus, extending onto the mesial surface of the hemisphere (Fig. 15-13). It has giant pyramidal cells of Betz in the fifth layer, whose axons form part of the corticobulbar and corticospinal tracts. There is a somatotopic arrangement of the contralateral half of the body along the gyrus, with the degree of representation proportional to the discreteness of movement required of that part of the body (see Fig. 7-2). Destructive lesions limited to this area are rare, but when they occur, they cause a flaccid, hyporeflexic paralysis.

2. The *premotor area (area 6)* is located immediately in front of area 4 and gives rise to fibers in the indirect activation pathways to the red nucleus, caudate nucleus, and reticular formation, which coordinate movements and control gross or postural movements. Lesions involving this area as well as area 4 result in a spastic, hyperreflexic paralysis. Isolated destruction of this area produces a motor apraxia.

3. The *supplementary motor area (area 6 medially)* is located immediately in front of the motor area on the mesial surface of the hemisphere (Fig. 15-13B) and is a secondary representation of motor function. Seizures in this area produce a characteristic posturing with elevation of the arm and deviation of the head and eyes toward the elevated arm.

4. The *frontal eye field (area 8)* is located anterior to the premotor area and is concerned with voluntary eye movements. Seizures in this area produce conjugate deviation of the eyes to the opposite side, whereas destructive lesions produce deviation of the eyes toward the side of the lesion.

5. The *motor speech areas (areas 44 and 45)* are

located in the inferior frontal gyrus of the dominant (usually left) cerebral hemisphere, and they control the programming of speech. Lesions in this area (Broca's area) produce a motor speech apraxia.

6. The *prefrontal areas (areas 9, 10, and 46)* are located in the most anterior part of the frontal lobe and are active not only in programming motor function but also in some aspects of memory, emotion, and intellectual functions.

7. The *orbitofrontal area (area 11)* is located at the base of the frontal lobe and is concerned with visceral and emotional activities.

PARIETAL LOBE.   The parietal lobe is bounded anteriorly by the central sulcus, and its posterior margin merges indistinctly with the occipital lobe behind and the temporal lobe below. The parietal lobe has two major areas, the primary and the association cortex.

The *primary sensory cortex (areas 1, 2, and 3)* is in the postcentral gyrus (Fig. 15-13) and receives afferent fibers from the thalamus, particularly from the spinothalamic, trigeminal thalamic, and medial lemniscal pathways. It has a topographic homuncular organization similar to that seen in the motor cortex (see Fig. 7-2).

The *sensory association cortex (areas 5 and 7)* receives input from the primary sensory cortex and coordinates, integrates, and refines the perception of the external sensory input. Cortical analysis here deals primarily with such discriminative aspects of tactile sensation as localization and recognition of spatial relations, texture, shape, size, and recognition of differences. Lesions in this region produce impairment of the ability to recognize a number written on the hand (graphesthesia), of two-point discrimination, of touch localization, of the ability to recognize objects by palpation (stereognosis), and of weight discrimination (barognosis).

OCCIPITAL LOBE.   The occipital lobe forms the posterior pole of the cerebral hemisphere and contains the primary visual cortex (area 17) (Fig. 15-13). The primary visual areas in the banks of the calcarine fissure on the medial aspect of the occipital lobes receive the optic radiations from the lateral geniculate body. Adjacent to the primary visual area are the visual association areas (areas 18 and 19), which organize and integrate

visual stimuli. These areas are an integral part of the visual system.

TEMPORAL LOBE.   The temporal lobe is located on the lateral aspect of the cerebral hemispheres inferior to the lateral (sylvian) fissure. It is continuous posteriorly with the parietal and occipital lobes. The superior temporal gyrus (Heschl's gyrus) contains the primary auditory cortex (areas 41 and 42) (Fig. 15-13), which receives auditory fibers from the medial geniculate body. Sounds coming into either ear reach the auditory cortex bilaterally. Therefore, unilateral lesions of the auditory cortex cause some difficulty in sound localization, but there is no significant hearing deficit. Bilateral ablation of the auditory cortex does not prevent reaction to sounds but does reduce greatly or abolish the ability to discriminate different patterns of sound. The dominant temporal lobe also has a primary role in language functions.

LIMBIC LOBE.   The limbic lobe is on the medial surface of the brain and includes the mesial frontal cortex and some portions of the orbital frontal cortex (area 32), the cingulate gyrus (areas 23 and 24), and the hippocampal gyrus on the medial surface of the temporal lobe (Fig. 15-13B). These areas are an integral part of the limbic system.

Clinical Correlates of the Cerebral Hemispheres

Clinical correlates of some of the areas in the cerebral hemispheres have already been described in this chapter. However, others involve broad areas of cortex and cannot be considered in relation to a single discrete area. The cerebral processes underlying intelligence, sensory-motor integration, language, and certain diseases are in this category and will be discussed in this section. Each of these is unique to the supratentorial level, and a disturbance of any one of them can localize a disease process to this level.

Intelligence

Intelligence is a familiar but difficult term to define precisely. It is best defined as the capacity for the development of cognitive functions. Cognition refers to the operation of the mind in thinking, understanding, and reasoning. Intelligence depends on many cortical areas in the cerebral hemispheres. While specific areas mediating sensory and motor functions have been mapped out in detail and are involved in some aspects of cognition, the more general cognitive functions involve the entire cerebrum and deteriorate in proportion to the loss of total brain substance rather than to damage in specific areas.

Within the limits set by intelligence, the maturation of the cognitive faculties progresses from a reliance on specific information, as seen in the young child, to the use of sophisticated abstractions, as seen in the adult. This progression represents a development in the capacity to solve problems, from the manipulation of objects in physical space to the mental manipulation of symbols. The mind becomes capable of thinking in terms of classes of objects in order to utilize numbers, perform mathematical operations, formulate hypotheses, and test hypotheses in a rigorous, logical manner. Thus, cognition becomes the basis of complex, flexible, adaptive behavior. To the degree that intelligence is limited, regardless of the cause, the ability to develop these cognitive faculties is limited. The failure to develop normal intelligence is referred to as *mental retardation*. Once developed, the cognitive processes may be lost as a result of a wide variety of progressive pathologic conditions, and this results in *dementia*. The processes that cause either mental retardation or dementia affect the cerebral hemispheres in a diffuse manner.

MENTAL RETARDATION. Mental retardation is not a single disease but a group of disorders in which the development of normal intellectual functioning is arrested. Retardation may result from a congenital nonprogressive process, an acquired nonprogressive process, or a progressive disease with onset in infancy or childhood. There are many exogenous causes of mental retardation, such as trauma, anoxia, drugs, toxins, and infections. Three specific examples of endogenous causes are the genetic biochemical defects of Tay-Sachs disease, phenylketonuria, and the chromosomal abnormality of Down's syndrome.

Tay-Sachs disease is an inherited autosomal recessive disorder characterized by an excessive accumulation of the lipid ganglioside in the neurons of the central nervous system (Fig. 15-14). In-

Fig. 15-14. Tay-Sachs disease. Histologic section of cerebral cortex showing massive "ballooning" of neurons due to lipid accumulation. (Bodian stain; ×400.)

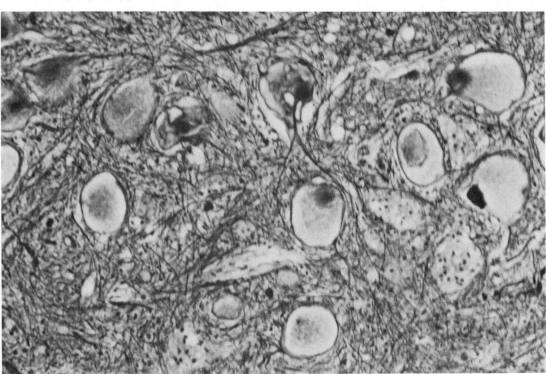

fants with this disorder have normal development during the first few months but then begin to lose previously acquired abilities. The child becomes listless and dull, with weakness, spasticity, and hyperactive reflexes. In the terminal months, there is decerebrate posturing. Death usually occurs as a result of infection. There is also retinal involvement, which produces blindness with a characteristic cherry red spot on funduscopic examination of the retina. There is lipid accumulation in the retinal ganglion cells, which results in a diffuse gray appearance in all areas except the fovea, which is free of ganglion cells and appears as a localized red area surrounded by the gray areas (cherry red spot).

Phenylketonuria is an inherited autosomal recessive disorder in which an enzymatic defect is associated with inability to convert phenylalanine to tyrosine; the increased levels of phenylalanine produce demyelination in the white matter and ultimately neuronal loss, resulting in retardation and seizures. Fortunately, in contrast to Tay-Sachs disease, the biochemical abnormality of phenylketonuria can be detected in the blood or urine and treated with a diet low in phenylalanine to prevent mental retardation. If untreated, severe mental retardation occurs.

Down's syndrome (mongolism), a chromosomal defect with triplication of chromosome 21, is characterized by mental retardation, heart and bladder defects, and a typical physical appearance of a round face, epicanthal folds, a short neck, and a simian crease on the palms of the hands. Children with this syndrome may survive into adulthood and continue to show moderate to severe retardation.

DEMENTIA. The progressive loss of cognitive abilities and memory is dementia. It may range in severity from very mild to severe. As dementia develops, the patient uses simpler, less flexible, more concrete thought mechanisms. The patient finds it difficult to keep two or more things in mind simultaneously or to follow directions. Irrelevant factors become distracting, judgment becomes faulty, and interest in goals is lost. With severe impairment, gross temporal, spatial, and personal confusion become apparent. The fund of knowledge becomes limited to a few highly overlearned memories, such as the patient's name and date of birth and the alphabet. While dementia may occur with a number of disorders, the dementia of Alzheimer's disease and senile dementia are the most common.

Alzheimer's disease is a diffuse degenerative process of unknown cause that affects the cerebral hemispheres. In the past, great emphasis was placed on the distinction between dementia occurring before the age of 65 years (presenile dementia), which was usually diagnosed as Alzheimer's disease, and the same clinical syndrome occurring after the age of 65 years, usually labeled senile dementia. It is now generally agreed that the clinical and pathologic features of these syndromes are identical and that the separation into two different entities based on age is not warranted. Most demented persons older than 65 years have Alzheimer's disease. Clinically, there is progressive loss of memory and other cognitive functions, usually followed later by loss of language and motor functions. Pathologic studies show diffuse atrophy of the cortex, especially the frontal and temporal lobes, due to diffuse neuronal loss (Figs. 15-15A, B). Characteristic histologic features of this disorder are neurofibrillary degeneration and senile plaques (Fig. 15-15C).

Although dementia is usually due to a chronic, diffuse degenerative disease, there are other, potentially treatable causes, which always must be sought in evaluating a patient with the possible diagnosis of an untreatable degenerative brain disease. Generalized processes such as disorders due to drugs and toxins and endocrine or metabolic disorders may begin as dementia. In addition, the widespread hydrodynamic effects of hydrocephalus and some focal lesions (subdural hematoma, neoplasm) may result in apparent dementia and must be excluded in all such patients.

The term *dementia* is usually reserved for the chronic, progressive form of loss of cognitive function without impairment of consciousness, which is sometimes referred to as *chronic organic brain syndrome.* In contrast, acute organic brain syndromes have an impairment of consciousness ranging from confusion to delirium (see Chap. 8). These are usually due to diffuse, toxic, metabolic, or inflammatory disorders and must be distinguished from the psychiatric disorders of schizophrenia, paranoia, depression, and mania.

Sensory and Motor Integration
The central sulcus divides the brain into the fron-

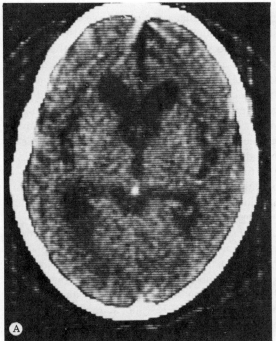
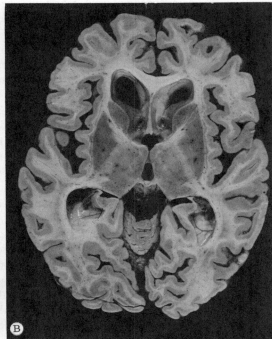
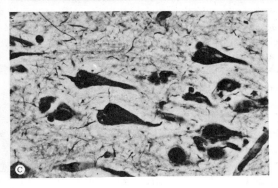

Fig. 15-15. Alzheimer's disease. A. Computed tomogram (CT scan) showing atrophy of brain with widening of cerebral sulci and ventricular dilatation. B. Corresponding horizontal section of brain. C. Histologic section of cortex showing dense neurofibrillary tangles in neurons. (Bodian stain; ×400.)

tal lobe with its motor functions and the parietal lobe with its sensory functions. The motor cortex and the sensory cortex on the precentral and postcentral gyri are the primary sending and receiving stations, but they occupy only a small portion of these lobes. Adjacent to these gyri are large areas of cortex, *association areas,* which integrate information from multiple areas of the body and from other areas of the cortex. The association areas in the parietal lobe integrate the primary sensory input with memories of the past, other sensory input, and cognitive thought processes to enable the person to understand the significance of the sensory input. The association areas of the frontal lobe integrate sensory input, visceral input, and the cognitive thought processes to develop the programs of somatic and visceral motor activity. Disorders in the association areas produce defects that are specific to the supratentorial level, known as agnosias and apraxias.

AGNOSIAS.   The inability to perceive the significance of sensory input that is received in the cerebral hemispheres is known as agnosia and may involve one or more sensory modalities. With a tactile agnosia, known as *astereognosis,* a patient has intact touch, pain, position, and vibration senses but is unable to tell what an object is by touching it. Astereognosis is seen with parietal lobe lesions and is often associated with loss of other cortical sensory functions, such as spatial localization, graphesthesia (recognition of figures written on the skin), and two-point discrimination. Agnosias can also involve visual or auditory input, so that a patient may be able to describe the input but not recognize or comprehend the meaning of objects or sounds, such as running water, music, or jingling coins. These agnosias occur with lesions in the association cortex surrounding the primary visual and auditory receptive areas. Parietal lobe lesions also may be associated with a loss of the body image, *somatagnosia*, in which the patient has right-left disorientation, may be unable to recognize parts of the body, or may neglect body parts. In Gerstmann's syndrome, there is finger agnosia, dysgraphia, and acalculia, with lesions in areas 39 and 40 of the parietal lobe.

APRAXIAS.   A patient with an inability to perform learned complex acts, in the absence of paralysis, sensory loss, or disturbance of coordination, has apraxia. Automatic or unconscious movements may still be normally performed. Apraxias occur as a result of diffuse processes, but in the typical disorder of motor programming—for example, with lesions in the frontal lobe—the patient is able to automatically pull out a handkerchief to cover his nose in sneezing but is unable to perform the same task when asked to do so voluntarily.

Language

Although the cerebral hemispheres usually function in a similar manner in controlling the opposite sides of the body, some functions, such as language, require the simultaneous action of both sides and are controlled entirely by one hemisphere. The hemisphere in which language is mediated is called the *dominant hemisphere.* Other functions, such as spatial orientation, are mediated by the nondominant hemisphere. Ninety-five percent of all patients with disturbance of language function in the cerebral hemispheres have disease in the left cerebral hemisphere. Ninety-nine percent of those who are right-handed and who have a language disorder have left cerebral

hemisphere disease, and 70 percent of left-handed patients with language disorders have left cerebral disease. This dominance of one hemisphere for language function does not occur until after 1 or 2 years of age. Damage to one hemisphere at an earlier age does not impair language. A unilateral lesion occurring in a patient between 4 and 12 years old usually causes only a transient language disorder, presumably because of the ability of the other hemisphere to assume these functions. Cerebral dominance is also manifest in handedness. More than 90 percent of adults are more dexterous with the right hand than with the left. Such handedness is commonly associated with ipsilateral footedness and eye sighting.

Humans communicate with each other by the use of a variety of gestures, expressions, behavioral patterns, and symbols. Communication by the use of symbols such as words or numbers is called language and involves mechanisms both in the cerebral hemispheres and at lower levels of the nervous system. For instance, reading involves peripheral vision and transmission of images to the cerebral hemispheres, as well as the processes of decoding these visual symbols in the cerebral hemispheres. Similarly, writing requires not only the organization of the symbols in the cerebral hemisphere but also the execution of the writing using the descending motor pathways. The central processes will be referred to as *central language processing*, in which the symbols represent meaningful concepts. The conversion of these symbols to sounds or utterances will be referred to as *speech,* which depends on brainstem and peripheral mechanisms.

Central language function involves the reception of spoken, written, or touch (braille) symbols, translation of these symbols into meaningful concepts, and translation of other concepts into appropriate symbols in listening, reading, speaking, and writing. The central language processes include storage of vocabulary, formation and comprehension of word sequences, auditory retention, and selection of appropriate symbols, sequences, and concepts in formulating a communication. Disturbances of language are of two types: (1) disorder of central language processing to produce aphasia and (2) disorder of the mechanisms of speech production to produce dysarthria. Aphasias can be localized in the supratentorial level, whereas dysarthrias may occur with disease at other levels as well.

APHASIA.   A disturbance in the dominant hemisphere may produce a defect in the expression or comprehension of any of the forms of language and is called aphasia. If aphasia involves primarily the understanding of the spoken and written word, it is called *receptive aphasia.* A patient with receptive aphasia may speak fluently but may be unable to recognize what he or she hears or reads. Receptive aphasia is the result of a lesion in the posterior temporal or lower parietal lobe (area 22 or 39) (see Fig. 15-13). In some patients, receptive aphasia is predominantly an impairment of speech recognition (Wernicke's aphasia), while others may have predominantly an impairment of reading.

In contrast, a patient with normal reception of language but who cannot convert thoughts into meaningful speech has an *expressive aphasia.* Most patients have both types of language disturbance. The patient who knows what he or she wants to say but cannot get the words out correctly, at times substituting incorrect words or syllables, has an abnormality of programming the motor functions for language, which is a *motor speech apraxia.* This pattern of language disturbance is seen with lesions in Broca's area in the dominant frontal lobe (areas 44 and 45) (see Fig. 15-13).

DYSARTHRIAS.   Disorders in the motor pathways with weakness, slowness, or incoordination produce characteristic speech disturbances through alteration of respiration, phonation, resonance, articulation, or speech rhythm. *Flaccid dysarthria* occurs with lesions of the final common pathway of cranial nerves IX, X, and XII and is characterized by nasal speech and a breathy voice. *Spastic dysarthria* occurs with upper motor neuron lesions of the direct and indirect pathways and is characterized by a hoarse, strained speech. *Ataxic dysarthria* occurs with lesions of the cerebellum and shows irregular speech patterns with incorrect emphasis or rhythm. *Hypokinetic* and *hyperkinetic dysarthrias* occur with lesions of the basal ganglia. The former is characterized by a low, soft, monotonous speech as seen in parkinsonism. The latter

is characterized by variations in loudness, poor articulation, and inappropriate utterances or silences interrupting the normal flow of speech and occurs in cases of choreas or dystonias.

Seizures

Many of the disorders affecting the cerebral hemisphere result in abnormal excessive discharge of the neurons in the cerebral cortex to produce seizures, which are signs of disease at the supratentorial level. Seizures are transient, physiologic disturbances that may be manifest in different ways with involvement of different cortical areas. They may be focal or generalized in distribution. Focal seizures occur with focal lesions such as vascular disorders, neoplasms, abscess, and trauma. Generalized seizures usually occur with metabolic, toxic, degenerative, and traumatic disorders but may also develop from focal seizures.

GENERALIZED SEIZURES.   Both cerebral hemispheres are involved with abnormal feedback between the cortex and the thalamus to produce widespread discharges in generalized seizures. These seizures involve the consciousness system and are therefore associated with an alteration of consciousness. They may be brief in *absence seizures* or prolonged in *tonic-clonic seizures.* In a *generalized tonic-clonic* (grand mal) *seizure,* the patient abruptly loses consciousness and falls, as the body stiffens in a tonic contraction. This is followed by symmetric, clonic jerking of the extremities and head, urinary incontinence, tongue biting, and apnea. After the seizure, the patient is flaccid and unresponsive, with slow return of consciousness through periods of confusion, drowsiness, and headache. The seizure usually lasts 1 to 2 minutes, with unconsciousness for 10 to 30 minutes. During the seizure an electroencephalogram shows generalized, repetitive spike discharges in the tonic phase, spike and wave discharges during the clonic phase, and depression of activity followed by slow waves after the seizure (Fig. 15-16). Repeated seizures are called *status epilepticus.*

Brief generalized seizures lasting 5 to 30 seconds with impaired consciousness but minimal movement are called *absence* (petit mal) seizures. Usually, the patient abruptly ceases activity, is unresponsive, and stares, sometimes with mild

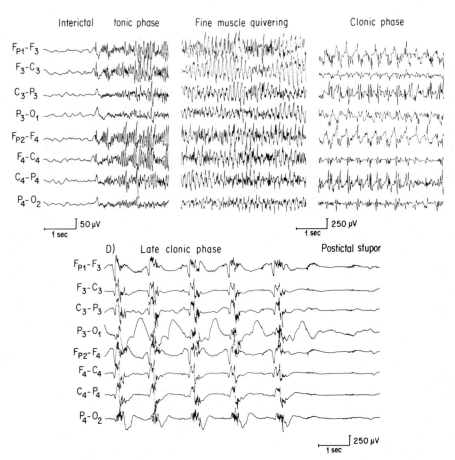

Fig. 15-16. EEG accompaniment to generalized tonic-clonic seizure. Segments of the recording during different phases of the seizure are shown. Interictal is before seizure; tonic phase (body stiff) shows repetitive spikes; clonic phase (body jerking) shows spike and wave discharges; postictal (after seizure) shows suppression of activity.

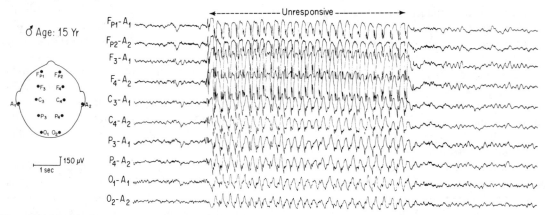

Fig. 15-17. EEG accompaniment during absence seizure consisting of 3-Hz spike and wave pattern during which the patient was unresponsive.

clonic movements of the face or extremities. These seizures usually occur in children and can be induced by hyperventilation. They are associated with a characteristic bilateral, synchronous, generalized 3-Hz spike and wave pattern on the electroencephalogram (Fig. 15-17).

FOCAL SEIZURES.   Seizures arising from a localized area of the cortex are called *partial* or *focal* seizures. They are often due to a focal pathologic process. The symptoms of focal seizures depend on the site of the discharge. Observation of symptoms can localize the pathologic process. Seizures in the precentral gyrus are associated with clonic movements of the contralateral side of the face or the contralateral arm or leg. Postcentral gyrus seizures are accompanied by paresthesias or dysesthesias of the contralateral side of the face or of the contralateral extremities. Occipital lobe seizures produce unformed visual images or impaired vision. Seizures in the temporal lobe are the most common focal seizure. Symptoms are varied and may include strange odors or tastes, formed auditory or visual hallucinations, fear, unusual sensations, mouthing movements, or automatic behavior.

The focal seizure may remain localized in a single area or may spread to other areas. It may spread sequentially along a gyrus via arcuate fibers and thereby spread sequentially through the body in a so-called jacksonian march. It may spread from one lobe to another or from one hemisphere to another via association or commissural fibers. Or it may spread via projectional fibers to the thalamus and thereby become generalized. If focal symptoms precede a generalized seizure, the focal symptoms are called an *aura* and provide evidence of the site of seizure origin.

Diseases of the Cerebral Hemispheres

Just as at other levels, disease at the supratentorial level may be diffuse or focal. Diffuse disorders produce bilateral dysfunction, with alteration in mentation and level of consciousness as well as bilateral motor or sensory abnormalities. Diffuse supratentorial disorders include encephalitis, toxic or metabolic encephalopathies, degenerations, and vascular disorders such as subarachnoid hemorrhage or anoxia. A focal cerebral lesion produces a motor or sensory (or both) deficit in the opposite side of the face and the opposite arm and leg, a contralateral homonymous field defect, language dysfunction, or focal seizures. The most frequent focal lesion is a nonmass lesion, an infarct. The presence of a mass lesion, however, must always be considered and is suggested by a focal, progressive course, with evidence of increased intracranial pressure or distortion of surrounding tissue or both. Abscess, intracerebral hemorrhage, subdural hematoma, and neoplasms are examples of supratentorial mass lesions.

Neoplasms in the cerebral hemispheres seldom metastasize to other body tissues and can be categorized into benign or malignant on the basis of their pathologic characteristics and invasiveness. However, whether they are benign or malignant, intracranial neoplasms are a major threat to life because they enlarge within the confined space of the closed cranial cavity and increase intracranial pressure as well as produce local tissue compression. Although any cell type found within the nervous system may undergo neoplastic change, three major groups account for most brain tumors.

METASTATIC NEOPLASMS.   Focal accumulations of anaplastic cells within the brain parenchyma may arise from tumors originating elsewhere (Fig. 15-18). Metastatic tumors invade locally

Fig. 15-18. Metastatic melanoma. Horizontal section of cerebrum showing multiple pigmented metastatic tumors.

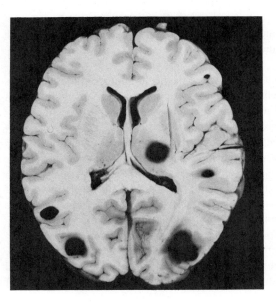

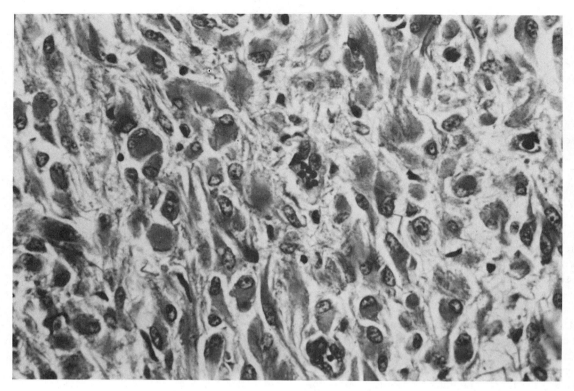

Fig. 15-19. Astrocytoma. Histologic section of an astrocytoma. Note resemblance of cells to reactive astrocytes but with much more irregularity of size, shape, and nuclear morphology. (H & E; ×200.)

and exert a mass effect on the surrounding tissue. The histologic features resemble those of the primary neoplasm, the most common being lung and breast lesions. Frequently surrounding the tumor cells is a large area of cerebral edema, which increases the mass effect of the lesion.

GLIOMAS.   Neoplasms arising from the glial cells constitute the most common primary neoplasm of the brain. These neoplasms are most often derived from astrocytes and are called *astrocytomas*. Astrocytomas vary in malignancy and may arise anywhere in the nervous system. Low-grade astrocytomas are accumulations of astrocytes with some anaplastic features (Fig. 15-19). Invasion of surrounding tissue by an astrocytoma damages adjacent axons or neurons to produce focal neurologic deficit. As size increases, pressure increases. Compared with low-grade astrocytomas, high-grade astrocytomas evolve more rapidly and show more invasiveness, anaplasia, and areas of

hemorrhage (Fig. 15-20). Vascularity and surrounding edema in high-grade lesions further increase the size of the tumor. The clinical course of astrocytomas covers months to many years, depending on the location and degree of malignancy.

MENINGIOMAS.   The neoplastic proliferation of meningothelial cells, the lining cells of the leptomeninges, results in meningiomas. These tumors are almost always histologically benign, slow growing, and produce their clinical effects by compression of the brain and neighboring structures (Fig. 15-21A). Although they have many different histologic appearances, they typically have whorls of cells, which may degenerate and calcify to form psammoma bodies (Fig. 15-21B).

Limbic System
Each of the systems discussed in earlier sections was found at multiple levels, and each mediated a single function or group of closely related functions. In contrast, the limbic system is located at the supratentorial level, has short connections with the periphery, and has functions that at first seem to be more diverse. The limbic system me-

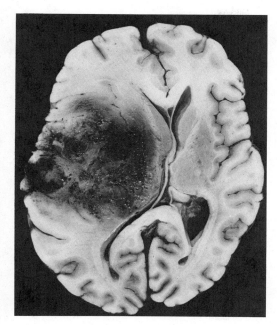

Fig. 15-20. High-grade astrocytoma. Horizontal section of cerebrum showing massive hemorrhagic-necrotic tumor of left hemisphere.

diates the special visceral sensation of olfaction and is the center of emotional or affective behavior and its visceral manifestations. The close anatomic relationship of such apparently disparate functions attests to their common phylogenetic origins.

Anatomy

The structures in the limbic system are arranged in a ring or loop situated deep on the medial surface of the brain and include the cingulate gyrus, hippocampal gyrus, fornix, mammillary bodies, and anterior nucleus of the thalamus. The system has multiple inputs, but a major one is from the specific olfactory structures which, with some of the nuclei and cortex in the ring, have been classified under the term *rhinencephalon* to designate their relationship to olfaction. They are, however, more readily understood under the concept of a single functional system mediating more than just olfaction. The olfactory structures in the limbic system include the short olfactory nerves in the periphery, which go directly to the supratentorial level at the base of the brain, and the connections of this input with nuclei and cortex in the diencephalic and telencephalic regions.

OLFACTORY STRUCTURES. The receptors for cranial nerve I lie in the superior nasal mucosa and respond to the chemical structures of many agents that are perceived as smells. The *olfactory nerve* is composed of multiple small fibers from cell bodies in the olfactory bulb that penetrate the skull through the cribriform plate to innervate the olfactory receptors (Fig. 15-22A). The primary neuron is thus at the supratentorial level. The *olfactory bulb* is a small ovoid structure that lies in the anterior end of the olfactory sulcus on the orbital surface of the frontal lobe. Fibers from the olfactory bulb form the olfactory tract, which passes posteriorly and divides into medial and lateral olfactory striae at the end of the olfactory sulcus. The lateral olfactory striae pass into the medial part of the temporal lobe known as the piriform area and end in the uncus and amygdala (Fig. 15-22B). The medial olfactory striae terminate in the anterior perforated substance and terminal gyri of the medial basal frontal lobe. Most olfactory fibers end in the anterior uncus, the chief cortical olfactory area. These and the connections with the amygdala and adjacent hippocampal gyrus link the olfactory structures with the ring of structures forming the remainder of the limbic system.

TELENCEPHALIC STRUCTURES. Cortical areas and underlying nuclear groups on the medial temporal lobe, the medial parietal lobe, and the orbital and frontal regions of the frontal lobe are part of the limbic system (see Fig. 15-12B). The orbital frontal cortex may have some input from the olfactory structures directly, as well as indirectly from the thalamus and hypothalamus. The *cingulate gyrus* immediately above the corpus callosum is connected with the orbital frontal cortex and hippocampal cortex by the long association pathway, the *cingulum,* which also carries projection fibers from the thalamus. Axons in the cingulum pass posteriorly and inferiorly to the *hippocampal gyrus* in the medial temporal lobe and the underlying hippocampus. One of the major efferent pathways of the telencephalic limbic structures, the *fornix,* arises from the hippocampus and loops anteriorly and inferiorly to the mammillary bodies in the diencephalon. These limbic cortical areas thus form a ring of interconnected areas around the corpus callosum and receive input from olfactory and other cortical ar-

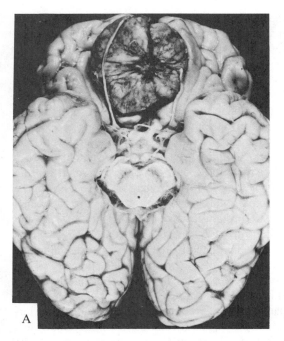

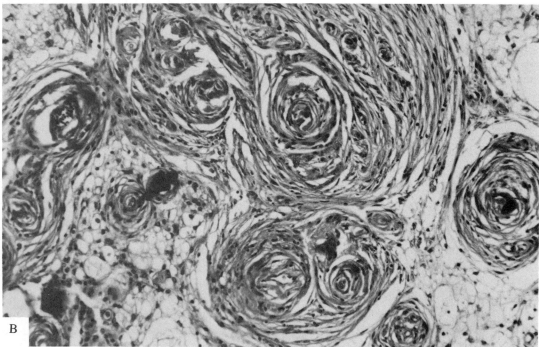

Fig. 15-21. Meningioma. A. Ventral view of brain
showing large meningioma between the frontal lobes.
B. Histologic section showing typical whorl formation
of elongated tumor cells. (H & E; ×250.)

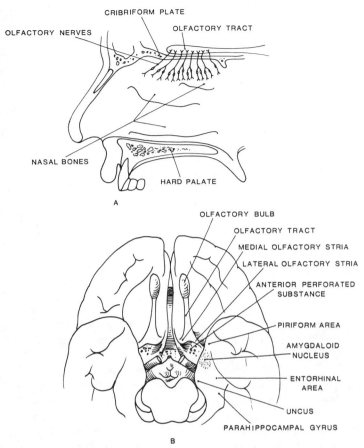

CRIBRIFORM PLATE

OLFACTORY NERVES

OLFACTORY TRACT

NASAL BONES

HARD PALATE

A

OLFACTORY BULB

OLFACTORY TRACT

MEDIAL OLFACTORY STRIA

LATERAL OLFACTORY STRIA

ANTERIOR PERFORATED
SUBSTANCE

PIRIFORM AREA

AMYGDALOID
NUCLEUS

ENTORHINAL
AREA

UNCUS

PARAHIPPOCAMPAL GYRUS

B

Fig. 15-22. Olfactory structures. A. Lateral view of olfactory nerves penetrating skull through cribriform plate. B. Basal view of brain showing termination of lateral olfactory fibers in piriform area of temporal lobe and medial olfactory fibers in the anterior perforated substance.

eas and have their outflow through the hippocampus in the floor of the temporal horn of the lateral ventricle.

DIENCEPHALIC STRUCTURES (FIG. 15-23). The terminations of the fornix in the mammillary bodies and septal area are one of the major connections of the telencephalic to the diencephalic parts of the limbic system. The mammillary bodies are directly connected with the hypothalamus, which also receives other input directly from the orbital frontal cortex. Efferent pathways from this part of the limbic system are the descending neural visceral pathways to the reticular formation and the endocrine pathways to the pituitary. However, the limbic system also has a recurrent loop back

to the telencephalic areas from the mammillary bodies. The *mammillothalamic tract* travels to the anterior nucleus of the thalamus, which in turn projects to the orbital frontal cortex and the cingulate cortex to complete the loop.

Physiology

Because of the system's complexity, the physiologic mechanisms underlying the functions of the limbic system have not been defined. The olfactory receptors in the nasal mucosa can respond uniquely to a wide range of chemical agents in patterns of action potentials whose origins are unclear. Similarly, the manner in which the limbic system structures interact in controlling visceral activities, emotions and affective behavior, the affective quality of sensations (pleasant or unpleasant), and memory is unknown. Stimulation or destruction of limbic structures produces profound alterations in mood, affect, and behavior, associated with such feelings as pleasure, rage, and withdrawal. For example, experimental ani-

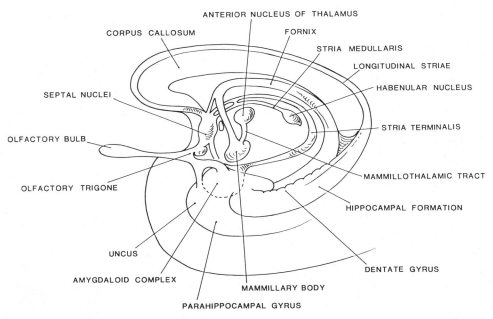

ANTERIOR NUCLEUS OF THALAMUS

CORPUS CALLOSUM

FORNIX

STRIA MEDULLARIS

LONGITUDINAL STRIAE

HABENULAR NUCLEUS

SEPTAL NUCLEI

STRIA TERMINALIS

OLFACTORY BULB

MAMMILLOTHALAMIC TRACT

OLFACTORY TRIGONE

HIPPOCAMPAL FORMATION

UNCUS

DENTATE GYRUS

AMYGDALOID COMPLEX

MAMMILLARY BODY

PARAHIPPOCAMPAL GYRUS

Fig. 15-23. Medial aspect of temporal lobe and interconnections with limbic lobe and diencephalic structures in the limbic system. The cortex of the temporal lobe has been removed to expose the deep fiber pathways. (Modified from R. C. Truex and M. B. Carpenter. Strong and Elwyn's Human Neuroanatomy [5th ed.]. Baltimore: Williams & Wilkins, 1964. P. 446.)

mals voluntarily stimulate electrodes implanted in some areas of their limbic system in preference to any other activity including eating, sleeping, and sex. Such areas have been called pleasure centers. The limbic system is also of major clinical importance because of the key role it has in the process of memory.

MEMORY. This function of the limbic system is difficult to define, but it includes a complex set of neurophysiologic and neurochemical processes involved in the encoding, sorting, storage, retrieval, and transfer of acquired verbal and nonverbal sensory experiences, concepts (products of mental manipulation of symbolic and nonsymbolic material), and sensorimotor behavioral patterns. By this definition, memory is the substrate for all higher mental functions and the prerequisite for learning and adaptive behavior. The anatomic basis of memory is only broadly identified. No localized memory depots have been identified. Since memories can be stored separately in each cerebral hemisphere and normally are readily transferred from one hemisphere to the other,

the loss of memory is roughly proportional to the total amount of cortex removed experimentally in both hemispheres.

However, some structures have a major role in certain phases of the mnemonic process. One of the most important of these is the *hippocampus* in the temporal lobe, a curved eminence 5 cm in length lying in the floor of the temporal horn of the lateral ventricle (Fig. 15-23). Direct stimulation of these areas in humans at surgery with the patient awake produces recall of vivid, complex memories. Seizures arising in this area produce stereotyped recall of past events. Loss of the hippocampus of both temporal lobes is associated with a profound loss of recent memory.

Moreover, there is evidence that different areas of the brain take over memory function at different stages of the storage and retrieval of engrams. Areas in the prefrontal cortex and dorsal medial thalamus are important in short-term memory, and destruction in these areas eliminates retention of sensory information for even 5 seconds. The hippocampus is also needed for recent memory. Later stages of memory involve widespread areas of the cortex.

Memory functions also must be considered at the cellular level in order to gain a full understanding of the complexity of the processes. Experimental data are only now becoming available to explain what physicochemical changes underlying memory occur at the cellular level. In addition to the well-known synaptic alterations lasting milliseconds, there are transient changes at synapses which may alter electrical activity for seconds to hours. These occur with calcium concentration changes and altered ionic conductances caused by the action of serotonin, dopamine, and peptides like oxytocin, which last for minutes to hours—time courses similar to those of some of the memory processes. Many of these changes are mediated by alterations in cyclic AMP. More permanent memory stores, however, imply a greater degree of stability; these stores could be explained on the basis of continuously reverberating local circuits, but they are more likely to be explained by changes in molecular configuration. Such changes could be in either the membrane of established synaptic connections or through the formation of new synaptic connections. It also has been suggested that ribonucleic acid (RNA), whose turnover increases in neural tissue after electrical stimulation, is related to learning. Interference with RNA synthesis impedes learning. Puromycin, an inhibitor of protein synthesis, can erase established memories, suggesting that the role of RNA is secondary to its control of protein synthesis. Recent studies have demonstrated a synaptic process with properties required for an intermediate step in memory storage. Calcium rapidly and irreversibly increases the number of receptors for glutamate in telencephalic synaptic membranes by activating a proteinase that exposes occluded receptors. This process provides a means through which physiologic activity could produce long-lasting changes in synaptic chemistry and ultrastructure.

Clinical Correlations

There are three clinical manifestations of limbic system disease: olfactory, memory, and behavior. The important clinical features of disorders of the limbic system pertain primarily to memory, because of the readily identifiable alterations in memory occurring in neurologic disease. Perhaps of greater overall significance in human behavior than memory disturbances are its effects on emotions and behavior. These latter effects are not yet well enough understood to make them of specific clinical value in understanding disease. In contrast to both memory and behavior, testing olfaction has limited but very specific clinical applications.

OLFACTORY ALTERATIONS.   Olfaction is of limited clinical importance in humans but can be helpful in certain situations. Two types of dysfunction occur: loss of the sense of smell and olfactory hallucinations. Olfactory nerves are the site of disease in some viral infections, traumatic lesions, or toxic poisonings that produce bilateral anosmia. They may also be damaged by lesions in adjacent structures. A tumor in the basal frontal region, for instance a meningioma of the sphenoid ridge, can compress the olfactory bulb or tract and produce a unilateral loss of the sense of smell. Irritative lesions in the region of the uncus of the temporal lobe cause *olfactory hallucinations*. Focal seizures in this region produce sensations of unusual or disagreeable odors. These are called *uncinate seizures* and are evidence of a temporal lobe lesion.

MEMORY ALTERATIONS.   Disorders of memory are classified clinically on the basis of the type of memory loss involved, since this can be correlated with anatomic structures. Memory loss may involve short-term memory, recent memory, or long-term memory. The *short-term memory mode* has limited storage capacity, with data being held for only seconds. After this time, the engrams either are dropped (forgotten) as new material is registered in short-term memory or are transferred to a more stable memory mode. These memories can be retrieved rapidly for conscious awareness and then recycled into short-term memory. Short-term memory is tested clinically by asking a patient to recall series of numbers of increasing length.

Information successfully processed through short-term memory for longer retention is then transferred to the *recent memory mode*. The engrams are stored here by categories rather than by temporal sequence of arrival and may be held in this mode for periods of minutes to years. Recycling through short-term memory by conscious review enhances the probability of storage in recent memory. Retrieval of memories from this storage area is slower than from short-term memory, probably reflecting the time needed for searching in the larger storage system. Engrams are lost from recent memory by decay through disuse at an exponential rate, regardless of the ease with which they were acquired. They also can be lost by interference with previously stored material. Recent memory is tested by asking the patient to recall recent events of the past day or two, or by asking the patient to recall specific items after 5 minutes or more have elapsed. Recent memory depends on an intact hippocampus; therefore, if both temporal lobes are damaged, recent memory is lost.

Some memories become nearly permanent for a person; for example, his name, birth date, family, the alphabet, the days of the week, and the months of the year. This information is stored in *long-term memory,* which has a vast capacity and which may be retained despite the major loss of other functions. Transfer of information into this mode takes months or years of repeated learning. Recall of engrams in this area is very fast. This mode of memory is diffusely distributed in both cerebral hemispheres and perhaps elsewhere, whereas recent memory is mainly localized in the hippocampus and short-term memory is localized in the prefrontal cortex and the dorsomedial nuclei of the thalamus. Disorders of the cerebral hemispheres affect one or more of these modes of memory, depending on location and severity of the damage.

Memory disturbances also have been classified on the basis of whether they affect memories that already have been established (as in retrograde amnesia) or memories that would have been established after the damage occurred (as in antegrade amnesia). A patient with *antegrade amnesia* has a defect in the process of registration and storage of recent or long-term memory stores. Typically, this occurs as a result of impaired consciousness or a diffuse disturbance of cerebral function. As the effects of the insult to the brain recede, mnemonic functions gradually improve and the amount of information that can be processed and recalled grows in quality and quantity. *Korsakoff's syndrome,* seen in habitual alcoholics, is a chronic, anterograde amnesia that occurs even though levels of consciousness are normal and other mental faculties are preserved. The patient cannot retain new information and cannot remember what has happened minutes earlier. Rehearsal of material does not aid the registration of memories. In an effort to cover this disturbance in memory, the patient frequently will elaborately fabricate answers to questions (confabulate). Lesions in this disorder are found in particular in the medial dorsal nucleus of the thalamus and in the medial pulvinar as well as the mammillary bodies.

The failure of retention or retrieval of recent and long-term memory traces formed for a variable period before a brain insult has occurred is called *retrograde amnesia.* This amnesia is most common in patients with head trauma and unconsciousness, who have difficulty in recalling events that occurred minutes to days before the injury. The extent of retrograde amnesia correlates roughly with the severity of the head injury. With recovery from the injury, there is gradual reduction in the extent of the retrograde amnesia, but there is often some permanent inability to remember events that took place just prior to the injury.

The Visual System

The second of the two systems that are limited to the supratentorial level and are associated with cranial nerve function is the visual system. This system has the single function of transforming visual representations of the external world into a pattern of neural activity which the person can use. As a system devoted entirely to the reception of one sensation, it has peripheral receptive structures in the eye and has central pathways in the diencephalon and telencephalon. The eye is a peripheral receptor organ specialized to respond to the complexity of visual stimuli. It has nonneural components whose function is the transmission of the light stimuli to the neural receptors, and it has neural structures that respond to the light. The supratentorial level contains the central neural pathways through the diencephalon and telencephalon, which analyze and synthesize the visual information.

Nonneural Peripheral Structures

Most of the nonneural structures of the eyeball are derivatives of embryonic ectoderm, although the muscles that control the eye are mesodermal in origin. These structures include the cornea, sclera, anterior chamber, iris, lens, and vitreous humor (Fig. 15-24).

The eyeball is located in a bony orbit that supports and protects the eye. There are six muscles responsible for eye movement: the lateral, medial, superior, and inferior recti and the superior and inferior oblique muscles. The actions of these muscles have already been described in Chapter

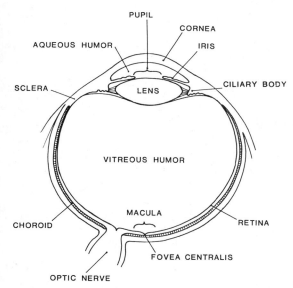

Fig. 15-24. Nonneural structures of the eye form the anterior portion and the outer coats. The retina and optic nerve are the neural components.

14. There are also muscles of the eyelids: the orbicularis oculi, which acts to close the eyelids, and the levator palpebrae and Müller's muscle, which elevate the eyelids. Impaired functioning of the levator palpebrae causes a ptosis or drooping of the eyelid.

The *cornea* is a transparent membrane that covers the anterior part of the eye and joins the opaque white sclera at the limbus. The *sclera* is a supporting tissue that covers the rest of the eyeball, to which the extraocular muscles are attached. The *iris* is a circular diaphragm with a central aperture, the *pupil,* through which the light projects to the posterior part of the eye. The ciliary body supports the *lens,* a biconvex, transparent, elastic structure that accommodates for vision at varying distances. The *vitreous humor* is a transparent gelatinous material separating the lens and retina and serving to hold both in place. The *choroid* lies between the sclera and the retina and functions to decrease the scatter of light inside the eye.

These nonneural structures transmit and focus the light rays to the neural structures in the back of the eye. The iris opens or closes in response to varying intensity of light, to control the illumination of the retina. The lens inverts the image and changes its configuration to focus the light rays from near or distant objects on the retina.

Peripheral Neural Structures

Two components of the eyeball are derived embryologically from the evagination of the embryonic diencephalon (see Figs. 2-2C, D). As this evaginating pouch extends, the optic vesicle grows; it invaginates into itself to form a two-layered optic cup. The inner layer forms the retina with its sensory receptors, and the outer layer forms the pigmented choroid. The retina contains the light receptors, the rods and cones.

The *cones* are responsible for daylight (photopic) vision, color vision, and discriminative vision. The *rods* are responsible for nighttime (scotopic) vision. The rods and cones communicate with *bipolar cells,* the first-order neurons occupying an intermediate layer in the retina. Bipolar cells, in turn, synapse with the *ganglion cells,* which are the second-order neurons in the visual pathway. The axons of the ganglion cells make up the nerve fiber layer of the retina. This is the innermost layer of the retina, lying adjacent to the vitreous humor. Light rays must pass through all the layers of the retina (0.5 mm thick) to reach the photoreceptors (rods and cones) (Fig. 15-25). The ganglion cells give rise to unmyelinated axons that converge from all parts of the retina on the *optic disk.* The disk lies to the nasal side of the posterior pole of the globe. Here, the ganglion cell axons become myelinated, imparting a yellow color to the cuplike optic disk (see Fig. 6-8A). They leave the eye via the lamina cribrosa, perforating the sclera to form the *optic nerve.*

The retina is modified at the posterior pole of the eye. Those layers near the vitreous humor are pushed apart to form a pit, the *macula lutea.* The apex of the macula lutea consists of the *fovea centralis* (see Fig. 15-24). Here, visual acuity and color discrimination are most acute. Although cones are found throughout the retina, their density increases abruptly at the macula. They are the only photoreceptors found in the fovea. However, rods are in greater abundance in the more peripheral portions of the retina and respond to low-intensity illumination (i.e., they have a low threshold to excitation). Rods are responsible for twilight and night (scotopic) vision, when visual acuity is low.

The rods and cones are the receptors in the visual sensory system. They are most readily activated by a narrow band of electromagnetic

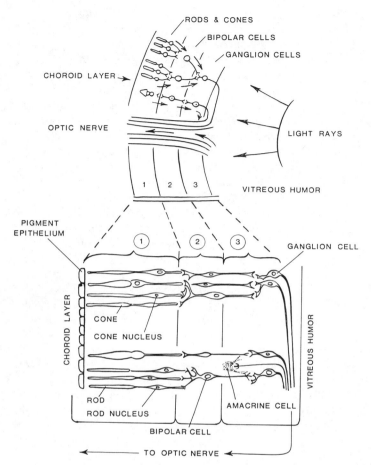

Fig. 15-25. The retina has three cell layers from outside to inside: rods and cones, the receptor cells (1); the bipolar cells (2); and the ganglion cells (3). Note that the light rays have to pass through the inner layers to reach the receptor cells in the outer layer.

wavelengths lying between the longer infrared and the shorter ultraviolet spectra. Within this energy range, the photoreceptors are generally more sensitive to the middle energies. At any particular wavelength, "light" is detected as a color (hue).

There are about 100 million rods in each eye. They are abundant in the more peripheral portions of the retina, but are not found in the fovea. The rods contain *rhodopsin* (visual purple), a high molecular weight (270,000) red compound consisting of a protein moiety *(opsin)* to which is bound a prosthetic group called *retinene*. Retinene is formed from vitamin A. When exposed to as little as one quantum of light, rhodopsin breaks down into retinene and opsin. The process

is reversed in darkness over a period of 5 to 30 minutes. The breakdown of rhodopsin on exposure to dim light somehow produces the receptor potential. Light having a wavelength of 500 nm is most effective in producing the breakdown of rhodopsin. This is predominantly in the blue end of the visual spectrum. Light in the red region has very little effect on rhodopsin.

Scotopic vision is night vision. Because of their low threshold, rods are responsible for vision in dim light. Therefore, night vision relies on the more peripheral portions of the retina. The discriminative capacity of the rod system is low compared with that of the cones; therefore, visual acuity is low in dim light. Because bright light blocks the regeneration of rhodopsin, vision is reduced for 10 to 15 minutes after entering a dark room. As rhodopsin in the rods regenerates, the eyes become adapted to the dark. Rods also have an important role in detection of movement. A deficiency of vitamin A causes a deficiency of retinene and rhodopsin, which results in a condition known as *night blindness,* with inability to see in the dark.

Most cones are concentrated in the macular area, particularly at the fovea. Cones have a relatively high threshold for excitation, requiring a minimum of 6 or 7 quanta of light. Cones are more sensitive than rods to light frequencies lying toward the red end of the visual spectrum. Reflecting their role in color vision, individual cones differ in their sensitivity to narrow spectral bands. Cones are densely concentrated and thereby provide discriminatory (detailed) vision. Such vision lies within a 10-degree angle of the center of the visual field.

The precise chemical bases for color vision have not been definitely established. Three basic types of cones have been identified electrophysiologically; each is sensitive to one fundamental color—red, green, or blue-violet. Equal stimulation of all groups of cones produces the sensation of white. All other colors represent combinations of stimulations of different intensity of these three types of receptors. There are probably three distinct retinal pigments, corresponding to the three types of cones. Each pigment may be composed of an opsin and a prosthetic group similar to retinene. Color selectivity is due to the unique structure of the opsin.

Thus, rods and cones code the location and color of objects in the visual fields. These receptors also undergo adaptation in response to a constant stimulus. Because of adaptation, images experimentally stabilized (immobilized) on the retina rapidly fade away. Normally, the eyes make continuous, small, rapid, irregular oscillations (microsaccades) when gaze is fixed on an object. Therefore, no retinal image remains immobile. The retina reports on what is changing in the visual field, thereby avoiding the effects of adaptation. The mechanism of the transduction process, whereby the breakdown of the visual pigments produces the receptor potentials and the activation of generator potentials in the dendrites of bipolar cells, is obscure.

Central Neural Structures

The visual structures within the cranial cavity at the supratentorial level include the optic nerve and optic chiasm, the optic tracts and lateral geniculate bodies in the diencephalon, and the optic radiations and occipital cortex in the telencephalon.

DIENCEPHALIC STRUCTURES. The optic nerve consists of axons arising from ganglion cells in the retina. These axons converge at the optic disk, become myelinated, and then leave the back of the eye via the lamina cribrosa. The optic nerve leaves the orbit and enters the cranial cavity via the optic foramen. Although the optic nerve is considered one of the cranial nerves (cranial nerve II), it is actually a nerve tract similar to the nerve tracts within the central nervous system and consists of axons of second-order neurons with myelin sheaths formed by oligodendroglia cells rather than by Schwann cells. Thus, disease processes such as multiple sclerosis, which affect myelin of the central nervous system, produce similar lesions in the optic nerve.

After passing through the optic foramen, the optic nerves unite to form the *optic chiasm,* beyond which the axons continue as the *optic tracts.* Within the chiasm, a partial decussation occurs; the fibers from the nasal half of each retina cross to the opposite side, whereas those from the temporal halves of the retina remain uncrossed. In binocular vision, each visual field, right and left, is projected upon one-half of both right and left retinas. Thus, the images of objects in the right field of vision are projected on the right nasal and the left temporal halves of the two retinas. In the chiasm, the fibers from these two retinal segments are combined to form the left optic tract, which then represents the complete right field of vision. By this arrangement, the whole right visual field is projected upon the left hemisphere, and the left visual field is projected upon the right hemisphere (Fig. 15-26).

After the partial decussation in the optic chiasm, the visual pathways, which are now known as the optic tracts, course laterally and posteriorly to terminate in the lateral geniculate bodies. A few fibers leave the optic tract before it reaches the lateral geniculate body to go to the pretectal area. These fibers constitute the afferent limb of the light reflex. The *lateral geniculate body* receives the fibers from the optic tract and gives rise to the *geniculocalcarine tract,* which forms the last relay of the visual pathway.

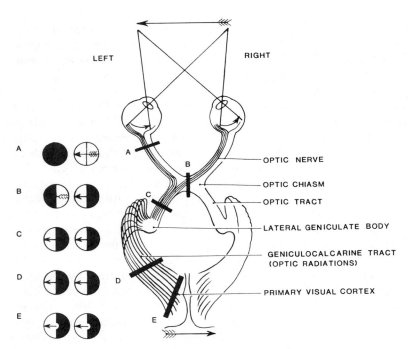

Fig. 15-26. Visual pathways as seen from the base of the brain. The visual impulses from the right half of the visual field project to the left half of each retina and to the left occipital lobe. On the left are the visual field defects (black areas) *produced by lesions affecting:* A, *optic nerve;* B, *optic chiasm;* C, *optic tract;* D, *optic radiation; and* E, *occipital cortex.*

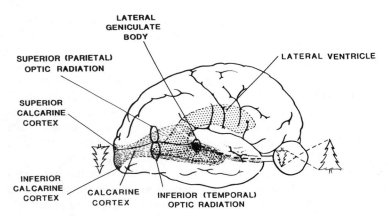

Fig. 15-27. Course of superior and inferior optic radiations. Fibers from the upper part of the retina (which receive impulses from the inferior visual field) form the superior optic radiations (located in the parietal lobe) and terminate in the superior calcarine cortex. Fibers from the inferior half of the retina (which receive impulses from the superior visual field) form the inferior optic radiations (located in the temporal lobe) and terminate in the inferior calcarine cortex.

TELENCEPHALIC STRUCTURES. The geniculo-calcarine tract arises from the lateral geniculate body, passes through the retrolenticular portion of the internal capsule, and forms the *optic radiations*. The upper or dorsal fibers of the optic radiations run posteriorly in the parietal lobe and terminate in the superior part of the calcarine cortex of the occipital lobe. The lower or ventral fibers loop anteriorly and laterally around the temporal horn in the temporal lobe (Meyer's loop) before turning posteriorly to end in the inferior calcarine cortex (Fig. 15-27).

The primary visual (calcarine) cortex is organized into columns of cells running from the surface to the white matter. These columns function as units that respond to specific patterns of visual stimuli, such as moving lines or bars. Each column is activated by a particular pattern or array of cells in the lateral geniculate body, which, in turn, are activated by retinal ganglion cells.

The visual images impinging on the retina are inverted so that the superior part of the visual field projects to the inferior part of the retina and the inferior visual field projects to the superior part of the retina. Fibers from the upper part of the retina form the superior part of the optic radiations, which run in the parietal lobe and terminate in the superior calcarine cortex. Fibers from the lower part of the retina form the inferior optic radiations, which run in the temporal lobe to terminate in the inferior calcarine cortex (Fig. 15-27).

The calcarine cortex thus has a topographic organization such that the superior part of the

visual field terminates in the inferior calcarine cortex and the inferior visual field terminates in the superior calcarine cortex (Figs. 15-27, 28). In addition, the posterior portion of the occipital pole is primarily concerned with macular (central) vision, and the more anterior parts of the visual cortex are concerned with peripheral vision. The primary visual cortex (Brodmann's area 17), located in the walls of the calcarine fissure, receives the primary visual stimuli. The visual association areas (Brodmann's areas 18 and 19) lie lateral to the primary visual area (see Fig. 15-13B). The visual association areas synthesize visual impressions, integrate visual impressions with other sensory modalities, and help form visual memory traces.

The visual association areas also are responsible for eye movements induced by visual stimuli. The analysis of visual information by the visual cortex is performed by columns of cells with specific functions. Some columns respond to input from one eye, while adjacent ones respond to that from the opposite eye. Some columns respond to images with one orientation, while others respond to images with a particular direction of motion. The complexity of this analysis increases in the surrounding visual association areas. The visual association areas have connections with the pulvinar.

The ability to perceive visual signals correctly is highly dependent on the coordinated control of the eyes, especially in looking at moving objects. Visual cortical areas control the brain-stem centers that mediate eye movements (see Chap. 14). The major function of the extraocular muscles is to move the eyes in such a way that the images of objects in the binocular visual fields always fall on corresponding points in the retinas and to direct the eyes to such images. This requires the

Fig. 15-28. Medial aspect of occipital lobe showing superior and inferior calcarine cortices separated by the calcarine fissure, the location of the primary visual area (17), and the visual association areas (18 and 19).

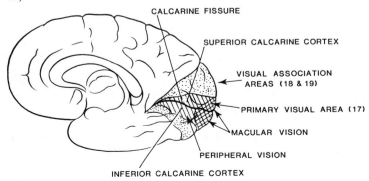

CALCARINE FISSURE

SUPERIOR CALCARINE CORTEX

VISUAL ASSOCIATION AREAS (18 & 19)

PRIMARY VISUAL AREA (17)

MACULAR VISION

PERIPHERAL VISION

INFERIOR CALCARINE CORTEX

simultaneous coordinated contraction of yoke muscles of the eyes (along with relaxation of their antagonists) to produce voluntary and reflex conjugate ocular movements. While such movements are under the control of several different regions of the brain, a few of these control centers are of particular significance: those in the cerebral cortex, the frontal and occipital eye fields, and those in the brain stem.

The *frontal eye fields* are responsible for voluntary control of conjugate gaze. One such center is located in the posterior portion of the middle frontal gyrus (Brodmann's area 8, see Fig. 15-13) of each frontal lobe immediately rostral to the precentral gyrus. Stimulation of this center causes the eyes to move conjugately to the opposite side; that is, if the right frontal field is stimulated, the eyes turn to the left. If one center is acutely destroyed, the unbalanced activity of the other center will cause the eyes to deviate to the side of the lesion; that is, if the right side is destroyed, the eyes will deviate to the right.

The *occipitoparietal centers* are responsible for involuntary visual pursuit. These centers are located in each hemisphere in the visual association area (Brodmann's area 19, see Fig. 15-13) at the parietooccipital junction. Stimulation of this area causes contralateral deviation of the eyes in a similar fashion to that outlined for the frontal fields. The involuntary visual pursuit center is responsible for fixing the eyes on an object in the visual field and maintaining that visual fixation as the object moves through the visual field. Because of the action of this center, the eyes of a person casually looking out the window of a moving car will automatically fix on some point in the environment and follow the object involuntarily until it approaches the limits of the person's visual fields. Then visual fixation is broken, and the eyes make a quick conjugate movement in the opposite direction to fix on a new point of interest. Such involuntary visual pursuit of a moving target is the basis for the optokinetic nystagmus produced by a rotating drum containing dark bands alternating with white bands (optokinetic nystagmus is the nystagmus produced by looking at a moving object).

Voluntary movement of the eyes to a point of interest in the visual fields occurs via the frontal eye centers. The occipitoparietal centers help keep the eyes fixed on an object once it has been located.

The term *visual acuity* denotes the smallest distance by which two parallel lines may be separated visually. Visual acuity depends on the ability of the retina to perceive a separation between the images that fall on it (resolving power). Resolving power, in turn, depends on the adequacy of illumination, the fidelity with which the light rays are transmitted by the optical system, and the diffraction pattern of the image on the retina. In addition, the density of packing of the retinal receptors (retinal grain) is a determining factor in the resolution of images. If separation of images on the retina is to be perceived, a receptor must be present in the intervening space between the images. Since diffraction patterns tend to diffuse the edges of an image, such separation may not be clear-cut. There may be, in fact, a "gray" zone between two images, which the retina codes as a separation. Thus, the resolving power of the eye is determined primarily by retinal receptor density and the diffraction of rays. Clinically, both far and near visual acuity are tested.

Clinical Correlations

Disorders of the visual system produce specific, readily identifiable visual defects that depend on the part of the visual system damaged. Knowledge of these defects permits precise localization of many lesions involving the visual system. Damage may occur at any site along the visual pathways and will be considered in terms of the observed differences between lesions at each site.

EYE DISEASE.   Most visual system disorders are due to abnormalities in the nonneural structures of the eye and are seen as abnormalities in visual acuity due to inability to focus visual images properly. Common examples are nearsightedness or farsightedness, distortion of light rays by diseases of the cornea or lens such as a cataract, and glaucoma, in which there is increased pressure within the eye. Each of these causes monocular visual loss (unless both eyes are involved) and can be identified by tests of visual acuity and direct inspection of the eye.

RETINAL DISEASE.   Disorders of the retina also cause monocular visual loss, often with reduced visual acuity. Retinal detachment and retinal degenerations are associated with progressive loss of vision. Some retinal degenerations produce changes seen on funduscopic examination, such as the cherry red spot of Tay-Sachs disease. Vascular diseases involving the retina also are reflected in visible changes in the retinal arteries with arteriosclerosis, small emboli, or hemorrhages. *Amaurosis fugax* is a transient loss of vision in one eye due to reduced blood supply (see Chap. 11). In elderly persons, it is most often the result of atherosclerotic disease in the ipsilateral internal carotid artery.

OPTIC NERVE. Focal lesions may involve a single optic nerve to produce a focal defect in the field of vision known as a *scotoma*, which also may be seen in some retinal diseases. Some disorders of the optic nerve head may be seen with the ophthalmoscope. *Optic atrophy* is seen as a pale disk and occurs with degenerative diseases of the retina or nerve. *Optic neuritis* is an inflammation of the optic nerve and may be associated with blurring of the disk margin and decreased visual acuity. *Papilledema,* a sign of increased intracranial pressure, is seen as swelling and elevation of the disk, with blurring of the disk margin (see Chap. 6).

OPTIC CHIASM. Lesions of the chiasm cause several kinds of defects. Most commonly, the crossing fibers from the nasal portions of the retina are involved, with consequent loss of the two temporal fields of vision (bitemporal hemianopia) (see Fig. 15-26B). Rarely, both lateral angles of the chiasm are compressed; in such cases, the nondecussating fibers from the temporal retinas are affected, and the result is loss of the nasal visual fields (binasal hemianopia).

OPTIC TRACT AND OPTIC RADIATIONS. Lesions affecting the optic tract, the lateral geniculate body, or optic radiations on one side produce homonymous defects in the opposite visual field (see Figs. 15-26C, D). For example, a lesion affecting the optic tract or radiations on the right side results in a homonymous field defect in the left visual field of both eyes. Complete destruction of the optic tract or radiation on one side

produces a *homonymous hemianopia,* that is, a loss of vision in the opposite half of the visual field of both eyes. A partial lesion produces a *homonymous quadrantanopia,* a loss of vision in one quadrant of the vision fields. A lesion in the temporal lobe on one side destroys the fibers running in the lower portion of the optic radiation and thus results in a *superior quadrantic field defect,* that is, a loss of vision in the superior portion of the visual fields of the opposite side. A lesion in the parietal lobe destroys the superior optic radiations and thus results in an *inferior quadrantic field defect,* that is, a loss of vision in the inferior visual fields of the opposite side.

Axons mediating the pupillary light reflexes and other visual reflexes leave the optic tract at or before the lateral geniculate to terminate in the pretectal area. Optic radiation lesions, therefore, differ from optic tract lesions in that the pupillary light reflex is preserved in the former. Secondary visual fibers can reach the visual association cortex via the pulvinar, but there are no known clinical syndromes associated with this thalamic nucleus.

OCCIPITAL LOBE. Lesions affecting the visual cortex in the occipital lobe on one side also cause a homonymous loss of vision in the contralateral visual fields; however, with occipital lesions, there is often macular sparing (see Fig. 15-26E). *Macular sparing,* or the persistence of central vision with involvement of one occipital lobe, occurs because of widespread representation of the macular fibers in the occipital cortex, incomplete destruction of the visual cortex by the lesion, overlapping of blood supply, and the constant physiologic shift of fixation of central gaze. Bilateral destruction of the occipital lobes results in a form of blindness in which there is often a denial of the visual loss. Cortical disorders in the occipital lobe can be associated with subjective transient anomalies of vision, such as scintillating scotomas and visual hallucinations.

Scintillating scotomas consist of the hallucination of flashing lights in a field of vision. This condition usually occurs secondary to a disturbance of functioning in the occipital lobes and is seen most commonly with migraine headaches but may also occur with retinal disease. *Visual hallucinations* are perceptions of visual images for which there is no external stimulus. The scintillating scotoma previously described is one characteristic type of visual hallucination. These may be unformed in nature and consist of flashing or twinkling lights, or they may be formed visual hallucinations in which an actual scene or picture is visualized. Such hallucinations may occur as part of a seizure involving the posterior temporal lobes or as an imagined phenomenon in psychotic states.

Neurologic Examination

Assessment of functions specific to the supratentorial level includes tests of cranial nerves I and II; evaluation of intellectual function, including in particular memory and language; and tests of cortical motor and sensory functions. In addition, the distribution of findings with involvement of longitudinal systems can aid in the localization of supratentorial damage. For example, the presence of weakness in the face, arm, and leg on one side is evidence of a unilateral cerebral lesion.

Cranial Nerve I (Olfactory)

Olfaction is tested by having the patient sniff a substance that has an odor (camphor, coffee, wintergreen) with each nostril separately while the other nostril is held closed. Since it is not possible to quantitate this sensation, the appreciation of the odor is sufficient to exclude anosmia. Intranasal disease is a common cause of impaired olfactory sensation and must be excluded before a diagnosis of neurogenic anosmia is made.

Cranial Nerve II (Optic)

Visual system testing requires attention to four aspects of visual function: the appearance of the nonneural components of the eye, visual acuity, visual field, and ophthalmoscopic examination of the optic fundus. The nonneural structures are examined by direct inspection of the external appearance and by visualization of internal features, such as the lens, with the ophthalmoscope. Tests of the extraocular muscles are described in Chapter 14.

VISUAL ACUITY.   The resolving power of vision depends on the ability of the retina to distinguish a separation between two images, and it is measured as acuity. Visual acuity is tested separately for each eye, for near and distant vision. A pa-

tient who wears glasses should be tested with and without the glasses. Available are eye charts (Snellen's chart) that are read at fixed distances (20 feet for distant vision, 14 inches for near vision). The smallest size of print the patient can read is compared with what a person with normal vision can read at the same distance, and acuity is reported as a comparison of these numbers. For example, visual acuity of 20/200 means that the patient can read at 20 feet what a person with normal vision can read at 200 feet. With major visual loss, acuity can be tested with large objects such as fingers or hands.

VISUAL FIELD.   Localized loss of vision in one area of the field of vision is tested by confrontation in which the examiner faces the patient and compares his or her visual field with the patient's. Each eye is tested separately by having the patient look straight ahead at the examiner's nose while an object is moved in the field of vision. This is usually a finger but may be smaller for more precise testing. Two methods of testing can be used. In one, a finger is wiggled and gradually brought in from the periphery in all four quadrants of the visual field to determine where it is first seen. In the second, one to four fingers are briefly extended in each of the four quadrants, and the patient is asked to identify the number of fingers that are shown. With uncooperative patients or those who cannot respond directly, the field can be tested grossly by swiftly moving the hand toward the eye from one direction and looking for defensive blinking. Very precise plots of the visual field can be obtained with a perimeter or tangent screen.

VISUAL EVOKED POTENTIALS.   A low-amplitude, surface-positive electrical potential can be recorded over the occipital areas in response to a visual stimulus. Highly contrasting linear profiles are the most effective visual stimuli for generating reliable and reproducible cortical responses. A black and white checkerboard pattern is ideal for this purpose. As each new stimulus is presented to the eye, by rapidly reversing the black and white checks, a volley of action potentials is relayed to the visual cortex. With appropriate amplification and computer averaging of a hundred or more successive responses, the evoked response is clearly distinguished from random

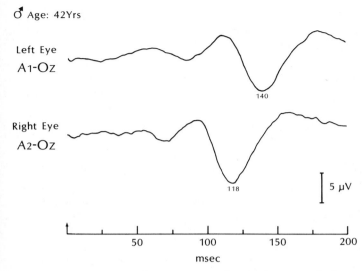

♂ Age: 42Yrs

Left Eye
A₁-Oz

140

Right Eye
A₂-Oz

118

5 μV

50   100   150   200

msec

Fig. 15-29. Visual evoked responses to television pattern reversal stimuli in a 42-year-old man with multiple sclerosis. Stimulation of the left eye (top segment) shows an abnormal peak-positive response of 140 msec secondary to demyelination of the left optic nerve. Stimulation of the right eye (bottom segment) shows a normal response of 118 msec. Responses represent an average of 128 responses. Recording electrodes: A2 = right ear, A1 = left ear, Oz = midline occipital.

background electroencephalographic activity (Fig. 15-29). The major, surface-positive potential occurs approximately 100 msec after the stimulus. A latency of the response prolonged beyond the upper limit of normal is suggestive of delayed conduction in the visual pathway of that eye.

FUNDUSCOPIC EXAMINATION. Both of the optic fundi should routinely be examined with an ophthalmoscope as part of a neurologic examination. The optic disk, the blood vessels, and the retina should be examined. The disk should be examined for variation from its usual yellow color and for flat appearance with distinct margins. In papilledema, the margins are blurred and elevated; in optic atrophy, the disk is pale. The arteriolar caliber and appearance and the venous pulsation should be examined. Areas of exudates, hemorrhage, and abnormal pigmentation may be seen in the retina.

Cortical Functions
The specific functions mediated by the cerebral cortex are tested as a group in the *mental status examination*. The mental status examination includes assessment of the level of consciousness, cognitive functions, cortical motor and sensory functions, and language.

LEVEL OF CONSCIOUSNESS. Evaluation of the level of consciousness is performed by testing the patient's awareness of (or response to) his external environment, by stimulating him with verbal, visual, tactile, and painful stimuli. His responses allow him to be characterized as alert, confused, somnolent, stuporous, or comatose (as described in Chap. 8). As part of the assessment of the level of consciousness, the patient's orientation and affect also should be noted. Does the patient know who he is, where he is, and what the date is? Is his emotional state one of anger, hostility, fear, suspicion, or depression?

COGNITIVE FUNCTIONS. The patient's intellectual functions are tested with a series of specific tests, most of which depend on diffuse cortical processes. The tests can be helpful in determining the extent of dementia or retardation or in distinguishing organic intellectual impairment from psychiatric diseases. The evaluation should include memory, fund of knowledge, calculation, ability to think abstractly, and judgment. *Memory function* should be tested in the three memory modes of short-term, recent, and long-term memory. Short-term memory is tested by having the patient repeat a sequence of digits of increasing length and recall the names of items after 5 minutes. Normal subjects can readily repeat up to six digits immediately and can recall the names of three cities or objects after 5 minutes. Recent memory is tested by having the patient recall events of the past few days, such as where he has been, whom he has seen, or what he has eaten. Long-term memory is tested by asking about events, such as date of birth and marriage, or overlearned material, such as the alphabet or names of the months.

The *general fund of information* should be tested in the light of the patient's intellectual level, cultural background, and geographic origin. Inquiry can be made into knowledge of the presidents, other public figures, dates of major events such as world wars, or knowledge of geographic features such as rivers, lakes, and distances. Ability to *calculate* is usually tested by serial 7s, in which the patient is asked to subtract 7 sequentially from 100 and then from each subsequent answer. For some patients, simpler tasks such as simple addition or serial 3s may be more appropriate for their level of education. The *ability to abstract* is tested by determining the patient's ability to detect similarities such as those between gold and silver or a book and a newspaper. It also may be tested by asking for an interpretation of a well-known proverb such as "People who live in glass houses shouldn't throw stones." A patient's *judgment* is tested by asking such questions as "Why are laws needed?" or "What would you do if there were a fire in a theater?"

CORTICAL SENSORY FUNCTION. The general tests for agnosias have been described in detail in Chapter 7 and include assessment of stereognosis, graphesthesia, two-point discrimination, and tactile localization. Additional tests for visual or auditory agnosia or somatagnosia may be needed in some patients. These tests might include tests of ability to recognize visual objects, to identify sounds, to recognize parts of the body, or to know right from left. The last may be tested with commands such as "Show me your thumb" or "Touch your left ear with your right thumb."

CORTICAL MOTOR FUNCTION. The general tests of motor function have been described in Chapter 9, but additional special tests may be needed for a patient suspected of having disease in the frontal association areas and a resultant apraxia—particularly if the results of standard tests of strength and coordination are normal. The patient's motor activities during the entire examination should be observed, and comparisons should be made between facility in performing automatic acts and facility in performing voluntary acts. In addition, asking the patient to demonstrate how to drink a cup of water or light a match may reveal apraxia that is not apparent on routine testing.

LANGUAGE. The four modalities of central language processing are listening, speaking, reading, and writing. Each should be tested in a patient with a suspected language disorder. Listening is evaluated by judging a patient's ability to recognize and appropriately respond to verbal input. The patient may be asked to perform acts, point to objects, move part of the body, and so forth. If there is a defect of speaking, the patient should be asked to respond in ways other than with language. Speaking is evaluated through conducting an ordinary conversation, but it also may be specifically tested by having the patient repeat certain phrases, or name objects. Reading may be tested directly if the patient can speak, but if not, it should be evaluated by having the patient point to specific words or letters or to objects that are symbolized by the words. Writing can be tested by having the patient write something from dictation or copy a written message.

Objectives
Diencephalon
1. Name the four main subdivisions of the diencephalon, list the component parts of each of these subdivisions, and localize the structures on a diagram or brain model.
2. List the four main functional subgroups of the thalamic nuclei and their connections and projections to other parts of the central nervous system.
3. List the regulatory functions of the hypothalamic nuclei.
4. Describe the clinical significance of the pituitary gland, and list the neurohormones secreted by the adenohypophysis and the neurohypophysis and their functions.
5. Describe how a mass lesion in the region of the hypothalamus may affect vision and endocrine function.

6. Describe the clinical significance of the pineal gland.

Telencephalon
1. List the component nuclei of the corpus striatum, and identify them on a brain model or diagram.
2. Define projectional fibers, commissural fibers, and association fibers.
3. Localize the internal capsule on a gross specimen, and describe what occurs with a lesion involving the internal capsule.
4. Localize on a diagram and describe the functions of the primary motor and premotor areas, frontal eye fields, motor speech area, primary somesthetic area, primary visual cortex, primary auditory cortex, Broca's area, and Wernicke's area.
5. Define agnosia, and describe the various types of agnosia.
6. Define apraxia.
7. Define aphasia and the two main types of aphasia, and be able to localize the lesion that produces these two types of aphasia. Define motor speech apraxia.
8. List the types of lesions that may produce dysarthria.
9. List the various types of cortical sensory deficit, and describe how the type of deficit is useful as a localizing sign.
10. Describe short-term memory, recent memory, long-term memory, amnesia, dementia, and mental retardation.
11. Differentiate focal from generalized seizures.
12. Describe absence and generalized tonic-clonic seizure.
13. Given the clinical manifestations of a focal seizure, localize the site of origin of the seizure; given the site of origin of a focal seizure, describe the clinical manifestations of the seizure.

Limbic System
1. List the structures of the limbic system.
2. List the functions of the limbic system.
3. Describe what happens with bilateral lesions involving the limbic system.
4. List the structures involved with olfaction.

5. Discuss the clinical significance of smell as a localizing sign.

Visual System
1. Describe the anatomy of the optic pathways.
2. Describe what effect a lesion has on the visual fields at the level of the optic nerve, optic chiasm, optic tract, optic radiations, and occipital cortex.
3. Given a visual field defect, localize the lesion.
4. Define and describe the significance of papilledema.
5. Describe the function of the rods and cones.
6. Localize on a diagram: cornea, sclera, iris, ciliary body, lens, vitreous humor, retina, and choroid.
7. Define hemianopia, quadrantanopia, homonymous, heteronymous, macular sparing, scotoma, and visual hallucination.

Clinical Problems
1. A 30-year-old woman noted the onset of amenorrhea 1 year ago. In the past 6 months, she noted that she tired very easily, could not tolerate stress or cold weather, and had lost weight. Physical examination revealed a dull, apathetic, thin woman with low blood pressure, a slow pulse, a bitemporal hemianopia, and deep tendon reflexes with a slow relaxation phase.
   a. Where is the primary lesion?
   b. What structures are affected by the lesion?
   c. What are the two component parts of the pituitary gland?
   d. Which lobe of the pituitary gland is involved?
   e. What hormones are secreted by this lobe? What regulates the release of these hormones?
   f. Which hormones are affected in this patient?
   g. How do you explain the visual symptoms?
   h. What might you expect a roentgenogram to show?
   i. What structures are near the pituitary gland?
   j. What is the lesion?
2. A 10-year-old boy had become fat and listless during the past year. He also drank water and urinated excessively. For the past several months, he had complained of headaches and

had experienced nausea and vomiting on arising in the morning. Neurologic examination revealed an obese boy with papilledema and bitemporal hemianopia.

a. Where is the primary lesion?
b. What regulates the release of the hormones?
c. Which hormone is affected in this patient?
d. What are the functions of the hypothalamic nuclei?
e. What is the lesion?

3. A 65-year-old man had the sudden onset of numbness of the right side of his face and body, and he noted difficulty in seeing in his right visual field. Neurologic examination performed 2 hours later revealed that he could not identify objects or written numbers in his right hand; nor could he localize sensory stimuli on the right side, or distinguish right from left. Further testing revealed that he had difficulty with arithmetic calculations and writing his name.

a. Where is the lesion?
b. What is the lesion?
c. What kinds of agnosia are manifested by this patient?
d. What are the other types of agnosia, and where would the lesion be located to produce these?
e. What type of visual field defect might be expected in this patient?

4. A 50-year-old woman had the gradual onset of memory loss 3 years ago. This loss has become progressively worse, so that now she cannot remember from one minute to the next what she has been doing. She also has had difficulty in carrying out various household activities such as sewing, cooking, and washing dishes, even though she denies being weak or having trouble with coordination. Neurologic examination revealed that she could not recall numbers just presented to her, what she had had for breakfast, or even where she was born. She was unable to perform activities such as pretending to light a cigarette or showing how a key would work.

a. Where is the lesion?
b. What is the disease process?
c. What types of memory functioning were affected in this patient?

d. What is the difference between dementia and mental retardation?
e. What is the name given to the inability to perform learned complex motor activities, in the absence of weakness?
f. Name three other types of neurologic dysfunction that signify a lesion or disease process affecting cortical structures.

5. Three years ago, a 28-year-old man had the onset of transient spells lasting 1 to 2 minutes in which he experienced an unpleasant odor. Immediately following the odor, he felt as if he were in a dream state in which he saw and heard things that he had experienced before. He also was aware that he was unable to understand what other people were saying to him during these episodes. In the past year, the spells have changed somewhat, in that now he hears the sound of a bell and at the same time experiences a mental picture of a country scene from his childhood. In the past 3 months, he has been bothered by increasingly severe headaches, nausea, and vomiting; and he has difficulty understanding what people are saying to him even when he is not having his spells. Neurologic examination showed bilateral blurring of the disk margins, a visual field defect, aphasia, and Babinski's reflex on the right.

a. Where is the lesion?
b. What is the lesion?
c. What visual field defect would you expect this patient to show?
d. What do the transient spells represent?
e. What was the initial site of origin for the spells?
f. What clues are present that show progression of the underlying process?
g. What tests would be most helpful for this patient?
h. What might these tests show?
i. What type of language problem did the patient have?
j. The olfactory structures are part of what system? Name the other structures that are associated with this system. What are the functions of this system?

6. What type of visual field defect might be expected in each of the following clinical situations?

a. A 47-year-old woman with a large tumor protruding from the pituitary fossa and pushing the optic chiasm forward.

b. An 81-year-old man who sustained an occlusive vascular event involving the right posterior cerebral artery.

c. A 44-year-old woman with a right parietal lobe tumor.

d. A 14-year-old boy with an abscess of the left temporal lobe after a chronic infection of the left middle ear.

Suggested Reading

Ajmone Marsan, C., and Matthies, H. *Neuronal Plasticity and Memory Formation*. New York: Raven, 1982.

Allen, M. B., Jr., and Mahesh, V. B. (eds.). *The Pituitary: A Current Review*. New York: Academic, 1977.

Ashworth, B., Isherwood, I., and Rosen, E. S. *Clinical Neuro-ophthalmology* (2nd ed.). Boston: Blackwell, 1981.

Benson, D. F. *Aphasia, Alexia, and Agraphia*. New York: Churchill Livingstone, 1979.

Browne, T. R., and Feldman, R. G. *Epilepsy: Diagnosis and Management*. Boston: Little, Brown, 1983.

Cummings, J. L., and Benson, D. F. *Dementia: A Clinical Approach*. Boston: Butterworth, 1983.

Darley, F. L. *Aphasia*. Philadelphia: Saunders, 1982.

Darley, F. L., Aronson, A. E., and Brown, J. R. *Motor Speech Disorders*. Philadelphia: Saunders, 1975.

Gazzaniga, M. S., and LeDoux, J. E. *The Integrated Mind*. New York: Plenum, 1978.

Hubel, D. H., and Wiesel, T. N. Brain Mechanisms of Vision. *Sci. Am.* 241:150, September 1979.

Answers to Clinical
Problems

Chapter 2
Organization of the Nervous System:
Neuroembryology
1. a. Fusion of neural tube, posterior neuropore.
   b. Neural tube at 4 weeks of development.
   c. Motor, sensory, and visceral.
   d. Neural tube and somites (myotome, sclerotome, dermatome).
   e. Ependymal, mantle, and marginal.
   f. Myelomeningocele.
2. a. Tumor formation in ectodermal derivatives: skin, eye, brain.
   b. Ectoderm and diencephalon.
   c. Neuroblast and spongioblast.
   d. Special somatic afferent.
   e. Tuberous sclerosis.

Chapter 3
Diagnosis of Neurologic Disorders:
Anatomic Localization
1. Supratentorial, focal-left.
2. Supratentorial, focal-left.
3. Posterior fossa, focal-left.
4. Posterior fossa, focal-right.
5. Spinal, focal-midline.
6. Peripheral, focal-right.
7. Spinal, focal-left.

Chapter 4
Diagnosis of Neurologic Disorders:
Neurocytology and the Pathologic
Reactions of the Nervous System
1. Supratentorial, focal-right, nonmass, vascular.
2. Supratentorial, focal-right, mass, inflammatory.
3. Supratentorial, focal-left, mass, neoplastic.
4. Multiple levels, nonfocal-diffuse, nonmass, vascular.
5. Multiple levels, nonfocal-diffuse, nonmass, inflammatory.
6. Supratentorial, nonfocal-diffuse, nonmass, degenerative.
7. Posterior fossa, focal-left, nonmass, vascular.
8. Multiple levels, nonfocal-diffuse, nonmass, degenerative.
9. Spinal, focal-right, nonmass, vascular.
10. Peripheral, focal-right, mass, neoplastic.

Chapter 5
Diagnosis of Neurologic Disorders:
Transient Disorders and
Neurophysiology
1. Anoxia produces block of sodium pump, with accumulation of extracellular potassium. Reduction in ionic concentration gradient reduces resting potential and makes cells inexcitable. Recovery occurs with opening of collateral vessels or restoration of blood flow.
2. a. Both reduced with possible block of action potential conduction.
   b. Reduced
3. Slow or block conduction in axons with reduction in visual acuity.
4. a. The resting membrane potential moves closer to threshold.
   c. Increased extracellular potassium concentration.
5. a. Decreased.
   b. None.
   c. Decreased.
   d. None.
6. a. Equilibrium.
   b. Steady state.
   c. Active transport.

Chapter 6
The Cerebrospinal Fluid System
1. a. By comparison with standardized tables of normal head circumference, 50 cm at 10 months is more than 2 standard deviations above the norm.
   b. An increase in the volume of any of the constituents of the skull. At this age, subdural hematomas and hydrocephalus due to several causes are common.
   c. Computed tomography and magnetic resonance imaging are safe, noninvasive procedures. This patient was found to have aqueductal stenosis.
   d. Noncommunicating hydrocephalus.
   e. (1) Enlargement of lateral and third ventricles with obstruction at the aqueduct. The fourth ventricle would not be visualized.
      (2) Uniform dilatation of the ventricular system proximal to the blockage (of the lateral and third ventricles, aqueduct,

and fourth ventricle), with no extraventricular air present.
(3) Uniform dilatation of the entire ventricular system, with some air escaping into the basal extraventricular cisterns.
(4) Usually no changes (but the cerebrospinal fluid would probably be bloody).
2. In the infant, intracranial volume can be increased by modest expansion of the sutures, which increases the head size and results in a less significant rise in intracranial pressure. In the adult, such compensation is impossible, and intracranial pressure increases.
3. a. Spinal, focal-midline, mass, neoplastic.
  b. Assuming that the lesion is at the midthoracic level, producing near complete blockage of cerebrospinal fluid pathways, then the opening pressure in the lumbar sac would be low normal; some respiratory pulsations transmitted via the abdomen would be seen but cardiac pulsations would not; compression of abdominal contents would result in an increase in pressure transmitted to the lumbar sac below the blockage, while jugular compression, which increases intracranial pressure, would not result in a pronounced pressure increase because compression-induced pressure would not be fully transmitted beyond the blockage to the lumbar sac.
  c. Skin, subcutaneous tissues, intraspinous ligaments, epidural space, dura mater, subdural space, and arachnoid and subarachnoid spaces.
  d. Myelography.
4. a. Multiple levels, diffuse, nonmass, an unidentified inflammation.
  b. An inflammatory process and a traumatic tap.
  c. Possibly bacteria; growth of the offending organism.
  d. In the presence of bacterial meningitis, the cerebrospinal fluid glucose level is often significantly lowered.
  e. No. It is indicated only in cases of suspected intraspinal lesions.

Chapter 7
The Sensory System
1. a. Peripheral, focal-right, nonmass, traumatic or vascular.

  b. The lateral femoral cutaneous nerve (refer to Fig. 7-12).
  c. Refer to Figure 7-12.
2. a. Spinal, focal-midline and bilateral, mass, neoplastic.
  b. Dorsal roots or spinal nerves of the C-2 segment.
  c. Structures listed in 2b and dorsal columns (fasciculus cuneatus and fasciculus gracilis) bilaterally.
  d. The segmental loss at C-2 suggests that this is the level of the lesion.
  e. Meningioma, neurofibroma.
  f. The segmental sensory loss would be at the level of the nipples, and the dorsal-column deficit would spare the upper extremities and be present mainly in the lower extremities.
3. a. Spinal, focal-midline, mass, neoplastic.
  b. The second-order axons transmitting pain and temperature impulses (bound for the lateral spinothalamic tracts bilaterally), as they decussate in the ventral white commissure at the involved levels.
  c. Syringomyelia; but the same clinical pattern could be produced by an intramedullary neoplasm at that level.
4. a. Spinal, focal-left, nonmass, traumatic.
  b. T-10 (refer to Fig. 7-13).
  c. Brown-Séquard's syndrome.
  d. The lesion involves only the left side of the spinal cord; the sensation of touch ascends bilaterally.
  e. Wallerian degeneration occurs in the distal axon when it is severed from its cell body of origin. Above the level of the lesion, the left lateral spinothalamic tract would show degeneration up to the level of the thalamus. The left fasciculus gracilis would show degeneration only to the level of its second-order neuron—the nucleus gracilis. The left corticospinal tract would show degeneration below the lesion.
5. a. Supratentorial, focal-right, nonmass, vascular.
  b. Thalamus (ventral posterolateral nucleus).
  c. In the right thalamocortical radiations.
6. a. Supratentorial, focal-right, mass, neoplastic.
  b. Focal sensory seizures.

c. The lesion is suprathalamic, producing a cortical sensory loss. Crude perceptions of touch, pain, temperature, and vibration occur at the thalamic level, while discriminative sensations require intact thalamocortical pathways for perception.

Chapter 8
The Consciousness System

1. a. Multiple levels (supratentorial and posterior fossa), nonfocal and diffuse, nonmass, metabolic.
   b. Widespread areas of cerebral cortex and portions of the ascending reticular activating system in the cerebrum, thalamus, and brain stem.
   c. Hypoglycemia.
   d. Diffuse slow-wave abnormality.
2. a. Supratentorial, focal-right, mass, vascular.
   b. Intracerebral hemorrhage.
   c. Although unilateral cerebral lesions do not ordinarily cause a loss of consciousness, a mass lesion (such as is present in this case) may compress diencephalic structures bilaterally or produce herniation of the supratentorial structures (or do both) with secondary involvement of diencephalic and brain-stem structures bilaterally.
   d. In addition to the focal slow-wave abnormality present over the right cerebral hemisphere, a more diffuse (projected) slow-wave disturbance may be seen.
3. a. Supratentorial, nonfocal-diffuse, indeterminate. The only abnormalities present were transient symptoms. As noted in Chapter 5, transient symptoms alone may be associated with various disorders and do not allow a pathologic diagnosis to be established.
   b. Epileptiform abnormalities generalized in distribution, occurring in repetitive and rhythmic fashion (see Fig. 8-16).
   c. Inflammatory (encephalitis), vascular, neoplastic, degenerative, toxic-metabolic, traumatic.
   d. The presence of focal seizures would increase the likelihood of an underlying structural lesion involving one cerebral hemisphere. In a patient of this age, a neoplasm should be suspected.

Chapter 9
The Motor System

1. a. Supratentorial, focal-right, mass, neoplastic.
   b. Corticospinal.
   c. It is higher than normal.
   d. Focal clonic seizures secondary to local ionic changes in the area of the tumor.
   e. No. It would be dangerous and perhaps fatal to the patient.
2. a. Multiple levels, diffuse, nonmass, degenerative.
   b. Basal ganglia control, cerebellar control.
   c. It is degenerative according to temporal profile, so toxic and metabolic causes must be considered. This is a case of hepatolenticular degeneration, or Wilson's disease, a genetic error in copper metabolism.
   d. Basal ganglia—caudate nucleus, putamen, globus pallidus, thalamus, and cortex; cerebellum—dentate nucleus, red nucleus, thalamus, cortex, and pons.
   e. Hypokinesia, hyperkinesia, athetosis, dystonia, tremor, and rigidity.
3. a. Multiple levels, diffuse, nonmass, vascular.
   b. Traumatic and toxic. This is an example of carbon monoxide poisoning.
   c. Indirect and direct activation pathways.
   d. By damage at midbrain level with release of vestibulospinal and excitatory reticulospinal activation of lower motor neurons.
   e. Type II (secondary) muscle spindle endings.
4. a. Multiple levels, diffuse, nonmass, inflammatory.
   b. Yes, typical of viral infection—in this case, poliomyelitis.
   c. Final common pathway.
   d. Weakness, atrophy, hypotonia, hyporeflexia, and fasciculations.
   e. Sensory from peripheral afferents, corticospinal, vestibulospinal, reticulospinal, rubrospinal, tectospinal, and input from other cord levels.
5. a. Supratentorial, left, nonmass, vascular.
   b. Direct activation, precentral gyrus inferiorly on the left, including Broca's area.
   c. Babinski's sign present, abdominal reflexes absent.
   d. Speech apraxia or aphasia.

e. Lower motor neurons to upper facial muscles receive bilateral cortical innervation.

6. a. Posterior fossa, right, mass, inflammatory.
   b. Cerebrospinal fluid pressure might be increased, and cerebellar tonsil herniation might occur.
   c. Cerebellar control.
   d. Superior cerebellar peduncle in the midbrain, pontocerebellar fibers entering the middle cerebellar peduncle, olivocerebellar fibers entering the inferior cerebellar peduncle.
   e. Equilibration in the flocculonodular lobe, posture and gait in the anterior lobe, skilled extremity movements in the posterior lobes, speech in the vermis.

Chapter 10
The Visceral System

1. a. Multiple levels, diffuse.
   b. Nonmass, degenerative.
   c. Blackouts, impotence, lack of sweating.
   d. It would produce sweating.
   e. All four.
2. a. Spinal, focal-midline.
   b. Mass, neoplastic.
   c. Nonreflex, autonomous neurogenic bladder dysfunction.
   d. Impotence.
3. a. Peripheral, focal-left.
   b. Mass, neoplastic.
   c. Superior cervical ganglion or sympathetic trunk.
   d. Sympathetic.
   e. Midbrain, pons, medulla, cervical cord, T-1 spinal nerve, sympathetic trunk, carotid plexus.
   f. Postganglionic or ganglionic lesion.
   g. Preganglionic lesion.
4. a. Peripheral, diffuse.
   b. Nonmass, vascular (toxic).
   c. Parasympathetic.
   d. Mushroom poisoning (muscarine).
   e. It would enlarge the pupils.
   f. (1), (2), (3), (4) altered by fear; (4) by blushing; (5) by crying.
5. a. Supratentorial, focal-midline.
   b. Mass, neoplastic.
   c. Hypothalamus and optic chiasm.
   d. Fornix, cortex, reticular formation—afferents; mammillothalamic, pituitary, reticular formation—efferents.
   e. Osmoreceptors, temperature receptors.
   f. Blocking of releasing factors that control the pituitary gland, and optic chiasm compression, producing visual loss.

Chapter 11
The Vascular System

1. a. Supratentorial, focal-right, nonmass, vascular.
   b. Vertebrobasilar system. The complete loss of vision suggests involvement of both posterior cerebral arteries; with resolution, only the distribution of the right posterior cerebral artery was involved.
   c. Infarction (right occipital lobe).
   d. Embolization from the heart.
   e. Decrease in PaO_2, increase in $PaCO_2$, increase in lactic acid, decrease in pH.
2. a. Supratentorial, focal-right, nonmass, vascular.
   b. Right carotid system—middle cerebral artery distribution.
   c. Infarction.
   d. May be related to extracranial carotid artery disease: thrombosis or embolization.
   e. True.
3. a. Supratentorial, focal-left, mass, vascular initially. (The loss of consciousness and bilateral Babinski's signs suggest secondary bilateral involvement at supratentorial or posterior fossa levels.)
   b. Intracerebral hemorrhage (with secondary early herniation).
   c. Hypertension, rupture of a vascular anomaly (arteriovenous malformation, aneurysm), trauma.
   d. Focal signs, headache, alteration in consciousness.
   e. Computed tomography.
4. a. Posterior fossa, focal-left, nonmass, vascular.
   b. Vertebrobasilar system, left posterior inferior cerebellar artery distribution.
   c. Infarction (in the left lateral medulla).
   d. Mechanism indeterminate; many patients have thrombotic occlusion of the vertebral artery.
   e. Vertigo—vestibular nucleus involvement;

dysarthria, dysphagia, and left palatal weakness—left cranial nerves IX and X; loss of pain sensibility over left face—left descending tract and nucleus of cranial nerve V; loss of pain sensibility of the right limbs and trunk—left spinothalamic tract; left Horner's syndrome—left descending sympathetic fibers.

5. a. Multiple levels, diffuse, nonmass, vascular. There are no focal abnormalities. The loss of consciousness suggests diffuse involvement of supratentorial and posterior fossa levels. Full recovery suggests no pathologic change in the central nervous system.
   b. Diffuse ischemia (syncope)—secondary to decreased cardiac output.
   c. The ability of an organ to maintain a constant blood supply in spite of variations in blood pressure. This regulation applies for all but the widest extremes in pressure.
   d. Only inhalation of carbon dioxide.
   e. Transient ischemic attacks are episodes of focal neurologic dysfunction; syncope is diffuse ischemia.

6. a. Multiple levels (supratentorial, posterior fossa, and spinal), diffuse, nonmass, vascular. The diffuse involvement, meningeal signs, and bloody cerebrospinal fluid suggest subarachnoid hemorrhage.
   b. At this age, rupture of an intracranial aneurysm is suspected.
   c. Immediate centrifugation of the specimen. The presence of a xanthochromic supernatant would suggest that it was not a traumatic puncture.

Chapter 12
The Peripheral Level

1. a. Peripheral (motor, sensory, and visceral), diffuse, nonmass, degenerative (metabolic).
   b. Peripheral neuropathy.
   c. They indicate loss of nerve or muscle fibers.
   d. It indicates loss of innervation of muscle fibers.
   e. Fibrillation is repetitive, rhythmic discharge of single muscle fiber. Fasciculation is single, spontaneous discharge of a motor unit.

2. a. Size of quanta and number of quanta.
   b. Number of quanta released.
   c. 11.
   d. EPP below action potential threshold; no muscle fiber contraction.
   e. Myasthenic syndrome associated with carcinoma.

3. a. Myositis.
   b. Peripheral, diffuse, nonmass, inflammatory.
   c. Muscle and nerve.
   d. Increased rate of firing, recruitment of more motor units.
   e. By making them of lower amplitude and shorter duration.
   f. Inflammatory cells, fiber degeneration, central nuclei.
   g. No.
   h. Neurogenic atrophy.
   i. As a result of collateral sprouting of intact axons.
   j. They all mediate excitation-contraction coupling.
   k. Because of leakage of enzyme from damaged muscle fibers.

Chapter 13
The Spinal Level

1. a. Spinal, midline, nonmass, vascular.
   b. L-1 to L-3, all of spinal cord except posterior columns.
   c. No.
   d. Reflex (automatic) bladder, nonreflex (autonomous bladder).
   e. Anterior spinal artery occlusion.

2. a. Spinal, midline, mass, neoplastic.
   b. Motor: final common pathway, direct and indirect activation pathways. Sensory: spinothalamic.
   c. C-4 to T-1; central gray matter affecting commissural fibers, anterior horn cells, and corticospinal tracts.
   d. Spinal cord mass—tumor or syrinx (possibly syringomyelia).

3. a. Multiple levels, diffuse, nonmass, degenerative.
   b. Posterior columns.
   c. Peripheral and spinal cord involvement.
   d. Biochemical (vitamin B_{12} deficiency in this patient).

4. a. Spinal, right mass, traumatic.
   b. Right L-5 spinal nerve.
   c. Peroneal nerve, sciatic nerve, sacral plexus, L-5 spinal nerve, L-5 ventral roots, and lumbar spinal cord.
   d. Traction on sacral spinal nerves.

Chapter 14
The Posterior Fossa Level

1. a. Posterior fossa, left, nonmass, vascular.
   b. Left lateral medulla.
   c. Left posterior inferior cerebellar artery—a branch of the left vertebral artery (which is often the site of occlusion in this syndrome).
   d. The left descending tract of cranial nerve V, the left spinothalamic tract.
   e. Involvement of the descending sympathetic pathways en route to the spinal cord (producing Horner's syndrome).
2. a. Posterior fossa, right, mass, neoplastic.
   b. Cranial nerves IX, X, and XI on the right.
   c. Jugular foramen.
   d. Jugular vein.
   e. Chemodectoma.
3. a. Posterior fossa, left, nonmass, vascular.
   b. Left medullary pyramid (weakness), left medial lemniscus (decreased proprioception), left hypoglossal nerve (tongue weakness).
   c. Infarction of left medial medulla in the paramedian zone.
4. a. Posterior fossa, left, nonmass, vascular.
   b. Special visceral afferent fibers of the facial nerve supply taste to the anterior two-thirds of the tongue.
   c. General visceral efferent fibers of the facial nerve supply the lacrimal gland.
   d. Bell's palsy.
5. a. Posterior fossa, right, mass, neoplastic.
   b. Auditory division of cranial nerve VIII (decreased hearing, tinnitus), vestibular division of cranial nerve VIII (absent caloric response, disequilibrium), facial nerve (weakness of muscles of facial expression), cerebellar control circuit (decreased coordination).
   c. Cerebellopontine angle.
   d. Acoustic neuroma.

   e. Skull roentgenogram and petrous tomograms (enlargement of the internal auditory meatus), computed tomography, rhombencephalography.
6. a. Posterior fossa, left, nonmass, vascular.
   b. Cranial nerve VI (lateral rectus weakness), cranial nerve VII (facial weakness), medial lemniscus (loss of joint position and vibratory sense), descending (direct and indirect activation) motor pathways (hemiparesis).
   c. Infarction, left paramedian region of the pons.
7. a. Posterior fossa, right, nonmass, vascular.
   b. Cranial nerve III on right (diplopia, ptosis, mydriasis), right cerebral peduncle (left hemiparesis).
   c. Right medial and superior rectus muscles.
   d. The efferent limb of the pupillary light reflex travels via general visceral efferent fibers contained in cranial nerve III.
   e. Infarction, right paramedian region of the mesencephalon.
8. a. Posterior fossa, left, mass, neoplasm.
   b. The left cerebellar hemisphere (ataxia).
   c. Headache, nausea, vomiting, papilledema.
   d. Cerebellar astrocytoma. (These tumors are often cystic and have an excellent prognosis.)
9. a. Multiple levels, diffuse, nonmass, degenerative.
   b. Motor system only, at the posterior fossa and spinal levels.
   c. Final common pathway (weakness, fasciculations), direct activation pathways (bilateral Babinski's signs).
   d. Motor neuron disease (amyotrophic lateral sclerosis).
10. a. Supratentorial, left, mass, inflammatory (abscess).
    b. Secondary involvement of the consciousness system by the expanding mass lesion causing herniation.
    c. Compression of cranial nerve III on the left by an expanding temporal lobe mass.
    d. With increasing herniation, there is also secondary compression of the cerebral peduncle.
    e. Uncal herniation.
    f. Mesencephalon.

g. Decerebrate rigidity.

h. Transtentorial or central herniation.

Chapter 15
The Supratentorial Level

1. a. Supratentorial, midline (region of pituitary gland).

   b. Pituitary gland and optic chiasm.

   c. Anterior lobe and posterior lobe.

   d. Anterior lobe.

   e. TSH, STH, ACTH, gonadotropins (FSH, LH), and prolactin; releasing factors from the hypothalamus, which descend to the anterior lobe via a portal circulation.

   f. TSH, ACTH, and gonadotropin.

   g. Compression of the optic chiasm by the lesion.

   h. Enlarged sella.

   i. Optic chiasm; internal carotid artery; cavernous sinus with cranial nerves III, IV, V, and VI.

   j. Mass, neoplastic (chromophobe adenoma).

2. a. Supratentorial, midline (in the region of the hypothalamus).

   b. Hypothalamus via nerve fibers.

   c. Vasopressin.

   d. Regulate visceral functions, regulate releasing factors for the anterior pituitary lobe, regulate water metabolism, regulate food intake, regulate body temperature, regulate sleep, regulate the cardiovascular system, regulate emotion.

   e. Mass, neoplastic (craniopharyngioma).

3. a. Supratentorial, left (left parietal cortex).

   b. Nonmass, vascular (infarct).

   c. Astereognosia, graphesthesia, somatagnosia.

   d. Visual agnosia, occipital lobe. Auditory agnosia, temporal lobe.

   e. A right inferior homonymous quadrantanopia.

4. a. Supratentorial, diffuse (cerebral cortex).

   b. Nonmass, degenerative (Alzheimer's disease).

   c. Short-term, recent, and long-term memory.

   d. Mental retardation is the failure to develop normal intelligence; dementia is the loss of cognitive processes after these have developed.

   e. Apraxia.

   f. Seizures, aphasia, agnosia.

5. a. Supratentorial, left (left temporal lobe).

   b. Mass, neoplastic (glioma).

   c. Right superior homonymous quadrantanopia.

   d. Temporal lobe seizures.

   e. Uncus.

   f. Change in the seizures with involvement of more posterior portions of the temporal lobe, the development of aphasia, increasingly severe headaches, and nausea and vomiting.

   g. EEG, computed tomographic scan, skull roentgenogram, and arteriogram.

   h. EEG: focal slowing and spike discharges over the left temporal region. Computed tomographic scan: decreased density, left temporal lobe. Skull roentgenogram: shift in pineal gland from left to right. Arteriogram: mass lesion.

   i. Receptive aphasia.

   j. Limbic system. Anatomic structures: telencephalic structures—orbitofrontal cortex, cingulate gyrus, hippocampus, fornix; diencephalic structures—mammillary bodies, septal area, anterior nucleus of the thalamus. Functions: olfaction, memory, emotion, affective behavior, and visceral manifestations of olfaction.

6. a. Bitemporal hemianopia.

   b. Left homonymous hemianopia with macular sparing.

   c. Left inferior homonymous quadrantanopia.

   d. Right superior homonymous quadrantanopia.

Index

Index